FOUNDATIONS
OF MEDICAL IMAGING

FOUNDATIONS OF MEDICAL IMAGING

Z. H. Cho

University of California
Irvine, CA
Korea Advanced Institute of Science
Seoul, Korea

Joie P. Jones

University of California
Irvine, CA

Manbir Singh

University of Southern California
Los Angeles, CA

A WILEY-INTERSCIENCE PUBLICATION

JOHN WILEY & SONS, INC.

New York / Chichester / Brisbane / Toronto / Singapore

Library of Congress Cataloging in Publication Data:
Cho, Z.-H. (Zang-Hee), 1936–
    Foundations of medical imaging / Z. H. Cho, Joie P. Jones,
      Manbir Singh.

        p.   cm
      "A Wiley-Interscience publication."
      Includes index.
      ISBN 0-471-54573-2 (cloth)
      1. Diagnostic imaging.   I. Jones, Joie P.   II. Singh, Manbir.
    III. Title.
    RC78.7.D53C48   1993
    616.07'54–dc20   92-26906

PREFACE

This book is, in large part, the result of interactions over the last several years with the graduate program in Radiological Sciences at the University of California, Irvine, and with various courses in medical imaging at the University of Southern California, Los Angeles.

Since the introduction of computerized tomography (CT) over 20 years ago, medical imaging and the general disciplines of imaging science and imaging technology have grown at a remarkable pace. In fact, the introduction of CT created the contemporary field of medical imaging, transforming classical two-dimensional *qualitative* imaging into a *quantitative* three-dimensional format. Although the CT concept was first applied to X-rays, it has since been utilized with a host of interaction parameters leading to a variety of imaging modalities, some of which are still in an early stage of development. Today there are more than 15,000 X-ray CT units and over 5000 magnetic resonance imaging (MRI) units in place worldwide. For some time medical imaging has represented the fastest growing area of diagnostic medicine. Consequently large numbers of scientists and engineers continue to be involved in developing various techniques and methods associated with this emerging technology.

Because of the complexity and sophistication of modern medical imaging, it is imperative to understand the underlying principles of the entire discipline. Our goal with this book is to provide the reader with just such an understanding. The foundations upon which medical imaging is based include the basic physics and mathematics associated with each modality and interaction parameter as well as the mathematics and computational tools associated with image reconstruction.

Historically medical imaging has been a set of distinct and separate disciplines, each defined by a particular imaging modality. Here we have tried to provide the student as well as the independent researcher with a coherent and unified view of medical imaging as a whole. Our hope is that this book will help medical imaging coalesce into a single discipline.

The book is divided into five sections, each of which, with the exception of Part I, includes the basic principles as well as the imaging details associated with a common set of interaction parameters or imaging modalities. First,

Part I provides the basic mathematical formalism necessary for the understanding of imaging in several different disciplines. Here also is included an introduction to image processing in which the Wiener and inverse filtering, for example, play important roles, as well as two- and three-dimensional projection reconstruction algorithms of various forms developed for computerized tomography.

In Part II we describe imaging based on various forms of ionizing radiation. After a review of radiation physics and radiation detection, we detail three radiation-related tomographic imaging techniques: X-ray CT, SPECT (single photon emission computed tomography), and PET (positron emission tomography). The formalism developed here provides the basis for describing newly emerging radiation-related imaging techniques such as particle transmission tomography using high-energy particles.

In Part III we describe a variety of MRI (magnetic resonance imaging) techniques, all of which are based on various aspects of NMR (nuclear magnetic resonance) physics. This modality is currently developing so rapidly that it is difficult to cover the entire field in a timely manner. We therefore have attempted to describe those areas that presently seem important, together with some basic NMR physics, related imaging fundamentals, and some discussion of spectroscopy and spectroscopic imaging.

Ultrasound, unlike the other imaging modalities covered in Parts II and III, has yet to utilize, at least on a clinical basis, contemporary reconstruction methods. However, ongoing research suggests that quantitative ultrasound imaging has considerable potential and may well open new horizons for medical imaging. In Part IV we provide sufficient background in ultrasound physics so the reader can appreciate the potentials as well as understand the challenges of contemporary ultrasound imaging. Here we review the various imaging methods that have been proposed and develop a formalism for evaluating them on a unified basis.

Finally, in Part V we introduce biomagnetic imaging. This new modality uses a very sensitive magnetic field measurement device known as SQUID (*s*uperconducting *qu*antum *i*nterference *d*evice), together with 3-D image reconstruction techniques to produce mappings of neuronal current.

The authors have regularly used the material in this book for graduate level courses in medical imaging. We believe this book is suitable for a two-quarter or possibly a one-semester course for first- or second-year graduate students. With supplementary materials, the text could serve as the basis for a full year's course in medical imaging for graduates and upper division undergraduates. We believe this book will also be of interest to graduate students in physics and engineering and to practitioners in these fields who are interested in medical imaging.

The authors would like to thank the many students who worked with them to develop this material. Particular thanks must go to the graduate students in Radiological Sciences at the University of California, Irvine. One of us (ZHC) acknowledges with pleasure the many students at the Korea Advanced Institute of Science who have participated in editing and correcting a large part of the volume, particularly the sections on MRI and PET. Finally, the authors would like to thank Andrew Naglestad, who prepared most of the manuscript, patiently assisted with the many revisions, and systematically organized everything.

ZANG-HEE CHO
JOIE PIERCE JONES
MANBIR SINGH

Irvine, CA
April 1993

CONTENTS

BASICS
FOR MEDICAL IMAGING

1

INTRODUCTION

The study of medical imaging is concerned with the interaction of all forms of radiation with tissue and the development of appropriate technology to extract clinically useful information from observations of this interaction. Such information is usually displayed in an image format. Medical images can be as simple as a projection or shadow image—as first produced by Röntgen nearly 100 years ago and utilized today as a simple chest X-ray—or as complicated as a computer reconstructed image—as produced by computerized tomography (CT) using X-rays or by magnetic resonance imaging (MRI) using intense magnetic fields.

Although, strictly speaking, medical imaging began in 1895 with Röntgen's discoveries of X-rays and of the ability of X-rays to visualize bones and other structures within the living body [1], contemporary medical imaging began in the 1970s with the advent of computerized tomography [2, 3]. Early, or what we call *classical*, medical imaging utilizes images that are a direct manifestation of the interaction of some form of radiation with tissue. Three examples will illustrate what we mean by classical imaging. First is the conventional X-ray procedure in which a beam of X-rays is directed through the patient onto a film. The developed film provides a shadow image of the patient which is a direct representation of the passage of X-rays through the body. Although such images are not quantitative, they do provide some measure of the attenuation of X-rays in tissue. Thus a section of soft tissue will appear darker than an equally thick section of bone, which attenuates more of the X-rays. It should be noted that even with current technological developments

3

conventional X-ray imaging still represents the major imaging procedure at most medical facilities.

As a second example of classical imaging, consider a conventional nuclear medicine procedure. Here a radioactive material is injected into the patient and its course followed by a detector which is moved over the patient in a specified manner. Although the image recorded by the detector generally has poor spatial resolution, its real advantage is that it provides a measure of physiological function from the time course of the radioisotope uptake. Clearly the conventional nuclear medicine image is a direct measure of the location and concentration of the radioactive isotope used.

As a final example of classical imaging, consider conventional medical ultrasound. Here, a pulse of ultrasonic energy is propagated into the patient and the backscattered echo signal is recorded by the same transducer. By angulating or moving the transducer (or by using a transducer array) positionally sequential echo signals are recorded, and a cross-sectional image of the subject is displayed directly on a video monitor. Ultrasound images are really a mapping of echo intensities and are a direct result of the interaction of the ultrasound pulse with tissue.

In this text we will define modern or contemporary medical imaging operationally as a two-part process: (1) the collection of data concerning the interaction of some form of radiation with tissue, and (2) the transformation of these data into an image (or a set of images) using specific mathematical methods and computational tools. Note that our definitions for both classical and modern imaging are consistent with our general definition of medical imaging, given in the first paragraph of this chapter. Note also that modern imaging can be represented as a generalization of classical imaging and that classical imaging is simply a special case of modern imaging in which the image forms directly from the interaction process. Whereas classical imaging is direct and intuitive, modern imaging is indirect and, in many cases, counter intuitive. Since modern images are formed by processing, reformulating, or reconstructing an image from the tissue/radiation interaction data base, the process is often referred to as "reconstruction" and the image as a "reconstructed image."

The first device capable of producing true reconstructed images was developed by G. N. Hounsfield [2] in 1972 at EMI in England. Hounsfield's X-ray computerized tomograph device was based in part on mathematical methods developed by A. M. Cormack [4] a decade earlier. For their efforts Hounsfield and Cormack were awarded the Nobel Prize in medicine in 1979. Put quite simply, CT imaging is based on the mathematical formalism that states that if an object is viewed from a number of different angles, then a cross-sectional image of it can be computed (or "reconstructed"). Thus X-ray CT yields an image that is essentially a mapping of X-ray attenuation or tissue density.

The introduction of X-ray CT in 1972 represents the real beginning of modern imaging and has altered forever our concept of imaging as merely

Table 1-1   3-D image reconstruction algorithms

2-D and 3-D Projection Reconstruction	2-D Projection Reconstruction	Parallel-Beam Mode
		Fan-Beam Mode
	3-D Projection Reconstruction	Parallel-Beam Mode
		Cone-Beam Mode
Iterative Method	Algebraic Reconstruction Technique (ART)	
	Maximum Likelihood Reconstruction (MLR) or Expectation Maximization (EM) Reconstruction	
Fourier Reconstruction	Direct Fourier Reconstruction (DFR)	
	Direct Fourier Imaging (DFI) in NMR	

taking a picture. It has also led to the development of 3-D imaging and is making quantitative imaging a reality. The application of reconstructive tomography to conventional nuclear medicine imaging has led to the development of two new imaging modalities: single photon emission computed tomography (SPECT) and positron emission tomography (PET). Similar applications to the laboratory technique of nuclear magnetic resonance (NMR) has led to magnetic resonance imaging (MRI). The CT concept is currently being extended to 3-D magnetoencephalography, electrical impedance tomography, and photon migration tomography, to name a few. Inherent to the development of these new imaging modalities has been the development of new reconstruction techniques, which are detailed in Table 1-1.

In this chapter we seek to provide a brief historical perspective for the various medical imaging modalities that are currently important. The various techniques are shown in Figs. 1-1 and 1-2 where they are characterized by the interrogation wavelengths. A parallel sequence will be followed in the succeeding chapters which provide more detailed discussions of the various imaging modalities. Although the various imaging techniques will, of necessity, be treated separately, our goal is to provide a unified approach to the field of medical imaging.

1-1   THE BEGINNING WITH X-RAYS

The history of medical imaging really began on November 8, 1895, when Wilhelm Konrad Röntgen reported the discovery of what he called "a new

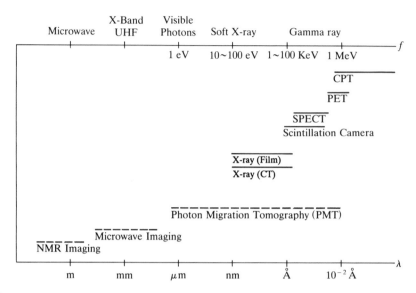

Figure 1-1 Ionizing radiation for imaging. CPT, charged particle tomography; PET, positron emission tomography; SPECT, single photon emission computed tomography. ---- represents the nonionizing radiation imaging given for comparison.

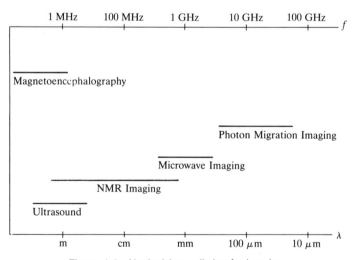

Figure 1-2 Nonionizing radiation for imaging.

kind of rays," a form of energy that was more penetrating than anything previously described [1]. He had serendipitously discovered the phenomenon some months earlier and applied the term "X-rays" to indicate its mysterious nature. By the time his initial report was published, he had spent nearly a full year in characterizing the new phenomenon, which became the focus of the remainder of his career. One of his earliest observations was that in using photographic dry plates sensitive to X-rays, it was possible to exhibit a shadow of the bones of the hand. Röntgen's first (now famous) radiograph happened to be of the hand of his wife Bera.

The earliest English translation of Röntgen's 1895 paper appeared in the journal *Nature* on January 23, 1896; this journal subsequently began running a special section entitled, "The Röntgen Rays" as a designated forum to publish the vast amount of experimental results on the phenomenon being submitted from scientists throughout the world. In an apparent frenzy of scientific enthusiasm, within 12 months of Röntgen's initial paper, there appeared over 1000 publications related to the "Röntgen rays." Perhaps the most significant of these were subsequent papers by Röntgen himself, who has been described by scientific historians as one of the greatest experimentalists of his time.

The impact of his discovery on medicine was obvious to Röntgen when he noted that the new ray could not only penetrate the human body, but that different tissues were penetrated to different degrees, thus forming complex images on photographic glass plates or phosphor luminescent screens. Thus penetrability, as demonstrated on the X-ray photograph (which became known as the "Röntgenogram"), was a direct extension of Röntgen's own observations. The reasons for the differences in tissue absorption in what has now become known as the "diagnostic range" of X-ray energies, specifically the photoelectric and Compton effects, were not understood until many years later. Despite this lack of fundamental understanding of the mechanism underlying the interactions of X-rays with body tissues, the utility of the discovery and its far-reaching potential for medicine was clear to Röntgen's contemporaries. The significance to the science of physics was appreciated as well. Röntgen received the first Nobel Prize in physics in 1901.

Application to medicine quickly followed, and clinical use of X-rays for diagnosis soon became routine. The first clinical use of X-rays in the United States was on February 3, 1896. The patient was a young boy named Eddie McCarthy of Hanover, New Hampshire, who had fallen while ice skating two weeks earlier, injuring his wrist. His physician, Dr. Gilman Frost of Hanover, contacted his brother Edwin Frost who was a professor of astronomy at Dartmouth. Eddie was brought to the physics laboratory at Reed Hall, Dartmouth College, where Professor Edwin Frost used a battery-powered Crookes' vacuum tube apparatus and a photographic glass plate to produce the first American Röntgenogram, revealing a colles' fracture. The exposure required 20 minutes.

The first report of an experiment designed to demonstrate the ability of the X-ray photograph to characterize tissue appeared in *Nature* within three months of Röntgen's original paper. Cormack and Ingle, using two essentially identical human finger bones, demonstrated that the X-ray opacity of bone was due to the concentration of calcium [5]. From this a series of experiments designed to demonstrate the underlying nature of particular "shadows" (i.e., densities") and "blackenings" (i.e., "lucencles") on the images was developed.

The new technologies of radiography and fluoroscopy were of great interest to the American inventor Thomas Alva Edison. Edison accepted a challenge from Randolph Hearst in 1896 to produce a radiograph of the living human brain. He was not successful of course, due to the limitations of the technique in discriminating the subtle differences in electron densities of the different tissues. This limitation was partially ameliorated in subsequent years by the development of pneumoencephalography by W. Dandy in 1918, a technique in which intracranially injected air provides contrast to delineate the normally fluid-filled compartments of the brain [6]. However, X-ray imaging of the actual brain was not accomplished until 1972 with the introduction of the CT scanner by its inventor Sir Godfrey Hounsfield of EMI, who was, in a very real sense, a successor of Edison.

Significant advances in radiography occurred prior to World War I with the first application of gastrointestinal contrast materials, such as ingested bismuth, to examine the stomach. There of course were technical improvements. Perhaps the most important of these was the development of equipment that could allow faster imaging times (on the order of seconds rather than minutes), that enabled better evaluation of complex moving tissues such as the lungs. Cerebral angiography was serendipitously invented by the French physician Egaz Moniz in 1927 while attempting to opacify the brain in a similar fashion to the gallbladder by arterial injection of opaque contrast media.

From the standpoint of physics and instrumentation, the first 75 years of research in radiology brought very few advances. There of course was a tremendous improvement in the technical quality of the images. The underlying physics of X-ray production and absorption was clarified, providing both a theoretical framework and a practical basis for engineering improvement. Within medicine, a considerable body of empirical knowledge on medical image interpretation was also accumulated during this period. This knowledge was primarily derived from rigorous integration of the most fundamental principles of differential X-ray absorption (e.g., the fact that air-containing structures appear less dense on Röntgenograms than do fat-containing structures or fluid-containing structures) with classical anatomy and expanding knowledge on the anatomic pathology of the diseases detected and characterized on the images.

The vast body of empirical knowledge led to the inception of a new medical specialty, which became known as Röntgenology, or radiology. Specialty societies and academic departments became established, and research in radiology received increasing governmental financial support. As a result a new scientific discipline, radiological sciences, found a permanent home in universities throughout the world. Still imaging remained limited to two areas: (1) the "plain" radiograph, and (2) new applications of opaque contrast materials that served to outline the structure and physiologic function of what would otherwise be radiographically indistinct tissue elements. It was not until the early 1950's, however, with the simultaneous development of nuclear and ultrasonic imaging, that any truly new physical methods were developed.

1-2 NUCLEAR MEDICINE WITH RADIOACTIVE ISOTOPES

In contrast to the science of radiography, the birthdate of nuclear isotope imaging (now known as nuclear medicine or nuclear radiology) is less well defined. The very beginning can of course be traced to the discovery of natural radioactivity by Antoine Henri Becqurel in 1896. The discovery of polonium by Pierre Curie and Marja Sklodowska-Curie in 1898 soon followed. The significance of these contributions to physics was such that these three scientists shared the third Nobel Prize in physics in 1903. The concept of producing diagnostic images using radioactive materials is much more recent, as is the use of the term "nuclear medicine," which dates from the 1950s and can be traced to the contributions of the nuclear chemist Paul Kohman who proposed the concept of the radionuclide as an atom, with a composition of its nucleus such that it had a measurable life span (longer than 10^{-10} sec). It may come as a surprise that the term "atomic medicine" was still in common use in many clinical departments and in the literature of the field as recently as 1969.

The initial primary application of radionuclides in medicine was not in diagnosis but in radiotherapeutic applications, including treatment of metastatic thyroid cancer by radioactive iodine and the use of radium and radioactive isotopes of cobalt and cesium (used primarily, but not exclusively) for the treatment of malignant tumors. In fact the first reported medical use of a radioactive substance was by Eugene Bloch and the French physicians Henri Danlos when they placed radium in contact with a tuberculous skin lesion.

Although the concept of using radioactive tracers in physiologic research had been introduced by George de Hevesy in 1923, the first report of the clinical use of the technique for imaging comes from G. E. Moore, reporting in the journal *Science* in 1947. Moore administered I-131 to patients in order to detect the presence of brain tumors. This was not an imaging technique in the strict sense but rather a means of external, relatively noninvasive detection. Similarly in 1949 Benedict Cassen at the University of California, Los

Angeles, administered I-131 to compare the function of thyroid nodules in patients to normal thyroid tissue in volunteers, using crude instrumentation which he later refined in the early 1950s to produce the first rectilinear scanner [7]. These experiments by Cassen were arguably the true beginning of modern nuclear medicine.

Technetium was discovered in 1937 by Perrier and Emilio Segrè, and the metastable isotope 99m-Tc was first applied to clinical use in 1961. The history of this development has been well reviewed by Lindeman [8]. Technetium compounds soon became generally available for clinical diagnostic use for a variety of applications (e.g., the localization and characterization of tissues using technetium tracers) both in the form of pertechnitate salt and as a radio label for a diverse group of pharmaceutical agents. A wide variety of such Tc-labeled biologically active molecules known as "radiopharmaceuticals" are now in everyday clinical use. Nuclear medicine techniques, deriving from the physiologic localization of just such isotopically labeled, biologically active molecules to particular tissues, are intrinsically tissue-characterizing imaging techniques.

One of the most significant developments in imaging instrumentation was the scintillation camera developed by Hal Anger in 1952. [9]. This scintillation camera, known as an Anger camera, is still a workhorse for nuclear medicine, and constitutes a major component of nuclear medicine facilities even when expanded into computerized or computed tomography methods such as single photon emission tomography (SPECT). Today SPECT systems using two or more Anger scintillation cameras are common tools for nuclear medicine imaging. Obviously, nuclear medicine visualizes physiological functions or functional metabolisms in comparison to X-ray imaging in which visualization of the structure is the main function.

As will be discussed in the computerized or computed tomography section, the introduction of CT not only stimulated the development of single photon tomography (SPECT), but also positron emission tomography (PET). The first SPECT of the pre-CT period was developed by Kuhl and Edward in the early 1960s [10]. Their system had four banks of detectors with linear and rotational scanning capability and provided the basic essential framework for the modern SPECT. It was a great success despite its inability to quantitatively visualize the radionuclide distribution, apparently due to the lack of modern 3-D image reconstruction algorithms. During or even preceding Kuhl's effort to visualize the radionuclide distribution using the scanning concept, Brownell and colleagues had long attempted to do the same, using positron-emitting radionuclides such as C^{11} and N^{13} [11]. Parallel to Brownell's effort, Rankowitz et al. [12] had attempted to visualize the positron-emitting radionuclide distribution using a multidetector array in the form of a ring much the same way as today's PET scanners. Although close to today's SPECTs and PETs, all of those attempts from the so-called pre-CT period were disappointing in the real usage of the methods and techniques.

Nevertheless, through those efforts much of the groundwork was established. When the CT concept was introduced in 1972, it became clear that both SPECT and PET could be made fully quantitative devices using the newly introduced 3-D image reconstruction algorithm [13].

The first wave of post-CT PETs were the PETT, a hexaganal type detector array, developed by Ter-Pogossian, Phelps, and Hofmann [14] at Washington University, and the circular ring type by Cho et al. [15] at UCLA and Budinger et al. [16] at UC Berkeley. Those early PET systems, however, not only suffered poor resolution (resolution of the early systems was on the order of 2 cm fwhm [full width at half maximum]) but also suffered from a lack of sensitivity. They captured only a fraction of the radiation emitted in 4π with relatively poor detection sensitivity using existing detectors, namely NaI(T1). Great advances with the PET scanner were realized with the introduction of high Z detectors such as BGO (bismuth germanate, $Bi_4Ge_3O_{12}$) in 1977 [17]. BGO not only improved resolution through use of small-size detectors, it improved sensitivity, especially the coincident detection sensitivity which in effect improved more than an order of magnitude in comparison to NaI(T1) of the same size. It soon became apparent that the detection geometry could be improved by using more rings or by extending the geometry to the cylindrical or even spherical multiple ring systems. Today's PET boasts resolution down to 3 ~ 6 mm fwhm by utilizing small and narrow detectors of 8- to 16-layer rings. In the 1980s many more detection schemes were developed, such as the positology developed by Tanaka et al. [18].

There have also been great advances in SPECT through better construction of detector schemes and arrangements, such as three-head camera systems rather than the conventional two-head camera systems [19]. Resolution of SPECT has been improved dramatically and is approaching 6 to 7 mm fwhm. The ultimate performance of SPECT, however, still remains inferior to PET in resolution by almost a factor of two and sensitivity by as much as an order of magnitude, since the electronic collimation used in the PET is vastly superior to the physical collimation employed in SPECT.

The integration of CT methods into classical nuclear medicine imaging has dramatically expanded the range of diagnostic applications by introducing a greater degree of anatomic specificity and by providing far greater contrast resolution than was previously available. Another noteworthy point is the radiopharmaceutical development. Classical, as well as contemporary nuclear medicine imaging, has benefited considerably from the development of numerous new radiopharmaceuticals. These chemicals have greatly expanded the range of organ systems that can be studied.

In concluding this section, we should note that whereas the goal of X-ray imaging is to visualize structure, the objective of nuclear medicine imaging is to visualize physiological function or functional metabolism. Clearly such goals are complementary and not mutually exclusive.

1-3 X-RAY COMPUTED TOMOGRAPHY WITH THREE-DIMENSIONAL IMAGE RECONSTRUCTION

The introduction of X-ray computed tomography (or CT) in 1972 was perhaps the most revolutionary development in the field of medical imaging since the time of Röntgen. For the first time the computer played a central role in the creation of the images. The digital acquisition of data was in itself a revolutionary idea and brought with it a new concept, that of quantitative imaging. Perhaps even more important was the new concept of image processing, the ability to alter and enhance the image after it was created, potentially extracting even more diagnostically relevant information. Another advantage of CT was that the method was tomographic and potentially three-dimensional, allowing the viewer to analyze isolated cross-sectional visual slices of the body. Technical advances with improved detectors, computers, mathematics, and software, plus changes in mechanical components and system geometry, have produced images of much higher spatial and density resolution.

Computed tomography allows much finer discrimination of the intrinsic X-ray attenuation of the body tissues than was possible with plain radiography. Typical equipment allows discrimination of a range of tissue densities 1000-fold wider than was possible with even the best film-screen techniques. This new ability led investigators to make use of the quantitative CT data in attempts to characterize tissue and make relatively noninvasive discriminations between normal and pathologic tissues. The CT density data was standardized by the introduction of the "EMI unit," which later became known as the "Hounsfield number," a calculated standardized index based on the mathematical estimate of the linear attenuation coefficient of the subject, standardized with reference to the measured attenuation coefficient of pure water. The Hounsfield scale was thus a fairly reproducible measure of the tissue's ability to attenuate X-rays.

The introduction of computed tomography engendered an enthusiastic response of basic and clinical investigators to apply the new technique for the purpose of tissue characterization based primarily on the Hounsfield number. In addition there were numerous published articles describing the characterization of tissues by measuring the Hounsfield number of the tissue(s) in question following injection of intravenous iodinated contrast materials. Within three years of Hounsfield's original report, over 1000 publications appeared in the English language imaging literature. The number of books and articles had more than quadrupled by 1980, in a burst of enthusiastic research reminiscent of that which followed Röntgen's original report. Despite high hopes and expectations for the new technology, reliable discrimination between normal and pathologic tissues by virtue of their Hounsfield numbers was largely unsuccessful, except for a few and limited examples.

Interestingly, this very observation prompted a new line of experimentation in which the energy of the X-ray beam was changed during the course of the study and a new image, derived from the mathematical subtraction or other manipulation of the two component images (obtained at different X-ray energies), was constructed. This method became known as dual-energy CT imaging; it has generated considerable interest with regard to CT-based tissue characterization, primarily with regard to quantification of high atomic number tissue elements, such as calcium in trabecular bone and pathologic tissue iron stores [20, 21].

Much of the physics of contrast by the different energies of X-ray and tissue atomic composition has been studied by Cho et al. [22] and also by McCullough [23]. Their studies have introduced in addition to the mean value of attenuation, a new index, the "effective atomic number" Z_{eff} or $\tilde{Z}$. As mentioned earlier, another important area of research spurred by the development of X-ray CT was the image reconstruction algorithm, now known as 2-D and 3-D image reconstruction (see [13, 24, 25]; and Table 1-1) which will be discussed in detail in later chapters. For the past two decades 3-D image reconstruction mathematics has been the backbone of modern medical imaging and will likely remain so.

1-4 MAGNETIC RESONANCE IMAGING AND TOMOGRAPHY

It is rather a coincidence that in 1972, the birthday of X-ray CT, a crude mode of NMR (nuclear magnetic resonance) imaging began to appear, or at least some preliminary form of NMR imaging commonly known now as MRI (magnetic resonance imaging) had been suggested in the medical imaging community. At the time, however, it was premature and was greatly over-shadowed by the overwhelming X-ray CT "fever." First, two papers appeared at nearly the same time: one by Paul C. Lauterbur in 1973 [26] and the other by Raymond Damadian in 1971 [27]. At that time the phenomenon of nuclear magnetic resonance was not new. It had been discovered independently by Felix Bloch and Edward Purcell (for which the pair shared the 1952 Nobel Prize for physics) and extended by Richard R. Ernst whose work, using the Fourier transform of the raw NMR signal, was introduced in 1966 for production of NMR spectra. Subsequently, largely inspired by P. C. Lauterbur's work, a two-dimensional Fourier transform method using field gradient pulses and phase encoding was introduced by Kumar, Welti, and Ernst in 1975 [28], forming the basis of modern MRI. For this contribution Richard Ernst received the Nobel Prize in chemistry in 1991. Soon after, MR imaging from point mapping to the projection reconstruction type has emerged from many different research groups all over the world [29, 30, 31, 32].

The inherent advantages of MRI as an imaging tool are many. Chief among these are unprecedented contrasts between the various organs and tumors essential for image quality and the three-dimensional nature of the method. Although there are a large number of different modalities within MR imaging—for example, flow imaging, T_1 and T_2 weighted imaging, and spectroscopic imaging—the single most important advantage of MR imaging is the contrast provided by the T_1 and T_2 relaxation mechanisms. As we will elaborate later, MR imaging has now expanded into many different imaging modes—namely simple T_1 and T_2 weighted imaging, chemical shift imaging for tissue discrimination such as normal tissue to fatty tissue, flow-related imaging including angiography or bulk flow, and susceptibility enhanced dynamic functional imaging. Spectroscopic NMR and imaging have also been developed extensively, especially in the fields of proton and phosphorus spectroscopies with both localization and imaging. A great future for MRI also lies in the field of spectroscopic imaging, where it might eventually provide tissue characterization with chemical specificity. Today, although not in common clinical use, many high-field MRI scanners above 1.5 tesla are capable of providing a limited usage of the systems for in-vivo spectroscopic investigation of the human body for medical diagnosis.

In the beginning a somewhat cumbersome feature of MR imaging was its slow speed. Today the speed of imaging has been greatly improved. The fastest imaging times, which had been in the range of tens of minutes, are now reduced to as short as 50 msec. Since MRI is capable of imaging magnetic susceptibility in relation to microvascularity, MR imaging is now moving from static imaging to dynamic imaging such as microvascular diffusion and perfusion imaging. When this development is achieved, MRI will join in the competition with PET and SPECT in the race among dynamic physiological functional studies.

1-5 ULTRASOUND AND ACOUSTIC IMAGING

The history of imaging and tissue characterization by ultrasound has been adequately reviewed elsewhere ([33, 34]). Here we only outline some of the modalities' important features. Modern clinical ultrasound, including all systems currently in commercial use, is based on construction of an image from the backscattered echo strength. These systems have their origin in World War II navy sonar technology, from which the field ultimately derives. Such methods are limited in that they utilize only a fraction of the acoustical information available in the echo wave form. In particular they exclude signal features which standard ultrasonic transducers are capable of detecting. Most technical advances in the field have served merely to improve upon the spatial and intensity discriminations of the equipment by producing improved transducers and improvements in post-acquisition image-enhancement circuitry. The additional signal data available has unfortunately been of only academic interest up to the present time. These "unused features" of the ultrasound signal, however, contain potentially useful information that is currently being discarded in routine clinical application.

The interaction of sound with tissue structures is complex and is not fully understood; the science of ultrasound tissue characterization is derived from the belief that it may be possible to identify and utilize particular features of the interaction of ultrasound energy that are characteristic of certain tissues. These features could then be utilized to make specific tissue diagnoses noninvasively. Yet, despite years of disciplined experimentation and considerable advances in basic knowledge of the underlying physics of the propagation of ultrasound in tissue, as well as in the interactions of high frequency sound waves with different types of tissues, no technique has evolved that will allow the desired end point of determination of specific "ultrasonic signatures" by which specific tissues can be characterized.

Scattering of the ultrasound beam by inhomogeneities in the tissue has received attention as a potential tissue-discriminating property. Recently a number of investigators have demonstrated that scatter can be correlated with structural periodicity in the tissue sample, and they have found differences in benign and malignant diseases of the liver in tissue samples that correlated with structural features evident in microscopy [35, 36, 37]. Other investigators have used backscattered echoes to distinguish between normal and diseased myocardium [38, 39].

The frequency dependence of attenuation (due to changes in the scattering process) was also studied, and a difference in myocardial infarction was found. Ultrasound attenuation in normal and infarcted myocadium has been studied for several years, and many differences between normal and ischemic/infarcted tissues have been found. For example, if there is an initial decrease in the attenuation in the early stages of the infarct, it was felt to be related to tissue edema. As scar tissue forms, attenuation increases, probably as a reflection of the increased collagen matrix of the necrotic tissues.

While data on ultrasound attenuation remain primarily empirical, without a comprehensive unifying theory, a large number of observations have revealed significant trends: (1) Attenuation increases with increasing collagen content and decreases with increasing water content, and (2) with the current diagnostic range of ultrasound frequencies, the frequency dependence of sound attenuation in tissue is approximately linear in soft tissues. Consequently, tissues can be characterized, at least to some extent, by application of sound wave velocity and attenuation measurements. Measurements of this sort are still being reported.

The role of density and elasticity fluctuations in acoustical scattering was first described by Lord John Rayleigh over 100 years ago with reference to the propagation of sound in air. This "classical" approach has value with regard to the propagation of sound in tissue as well, and to some degree it can be described by classical acoustics. Assuming classical acoustical behavior, it is possible to calculate the effective impedance of sound of various tissues. This concept was first introduced to describe tissue ultrasound scattering in quantitative terms [40, 41] and recently it has provided a theoretical framework for the approach to ultrasonic tissue characterization by acoustical measurement [42].

Within the last few years there have been increased efforts to measure the "backscattering coefficient" of various tissue samples and to relate this parameter to the pathological state of the tissues. One method [43] utilizes the angle of diffraction—the Bragg scattering method, which measures the variations of a particular frequency component of the backscattering coefficient of a small region of interest (interrogated from different directions). In theory this index should reflect components of the tissue structure; despite its inherent merits and a great deal of interest in the technique, its clinical application has been limited to date.

The application of particular signal-processing approaches to extract tissue-specific information has been pursued by several investigators, all of whom have proposed using a post-acquisition homomorphic filtering algorithm to provide a measure of the frequency-dependent attenuation by estimation of changes in the shape of the ultrasound pulse. The method is complex and computationally intensive, presenting a practical limitation in implementation [44]. However, it would allow accurate measurements of tissue sound impedance and attenuation in a single measurement with a single index that could be compared between tissue types. A similar method involving an "adaptive filtering technique" has been proposed and used [45].

Ferrari and Jones et al. in 1982 proposed an "FM" ultrasound system [46]. This system incorporated phase information (the "FM" signal) along with reflected echo amplitude (the "AM" signal) in the generation of a single image that combined information on both the echo amplitude and its inherent phase information. By incorporating this phase information into the acoustical image, more specific tissue characterization might be possible. This technique was unfortunately fraught with technical difficulties and has had poor clinical acceptance.

Very recently prototype equipment has been produced that employs very high frequency ultrasound to produce high-resolution images on a microscopic scale, thereby creating a new science called "ultrasound microscopy." The new technique requires extensive instrumentation, but it has shown promise in "noninvasive" microscopy (i.e., unfixed and largely unprepared tissue samples can be studied) as well as serving to extend the knowledge of how very high frequency ultrasound (in the gigahertz range) interacts with tissue [47, 48]. In limited clinical applications the images have been favorable compared to conventional fixed and stained tissue specimens in a variety of skin lesions, and their microscopic information content has proved to be of diagnostic quality similar to conventional hematoxalin/eosin stained tissue specimens [49].

1-6 NEUROMAGNETIC IMAGING — AN EMERGING IMAGING MODALITY

The recent development of SQUID (*s*uperconducting *qu*antum *i*nterference *de*vice), with which one can measure magnetic field variations as small as 10^{-15} tesla, will enable neuroscience researchers to observe accurately the site of neuronal activity in the brain and eventually to reconstruct the activity in three-dimensional form. SQUID's fast temporal resolution and better localization capability, compared with methods such as EEG, makes it a unique method for measuring neuronal activity. Thus magnetoencephalography (MEG) is a potentially powerful tool for studying the spatiotemporal distribution of neuronal activity.

More recent developments in neuromagnetic imaging include the tomographic imaging of the neuronal activity using 3-D reconstruction algorithms. Singh and Doria, in 1984 [50], were the first to develop and demonstrate the feasibility of imaging neuronal activity using CT–like image reconstruction algorithms. Subsequently neuromagnetic localization has been performed in conjunction with MRI. Although neuromagnetic research is a relatively new area, it has unprecedented potential for examining and observing the various neuronal activities in the brain, thereby enabling one to study brain functions with a time response much faster than any other imaging modalities. Currently, with the advent of a 37-channel SQUID neuromagnetometer which is commercially available and suitable processing techniques, it has become possible to locate or image the center of the 3-D distribution of the neuronal activity evoked by external stimulation such as vision and hearing [51].

REFERENCES

1. W. K. Röentgen (transl. by A. Stanton). On a new kind of rays. *Nature* 53:274–276 (23 January 1896).

2. G. N. Hounsfield. A method of and apparatus for examination of a body by radiation such as X-ray or gamma radiation. British Patent No. 1283915. London (1972).

3. G. N. Hounsfield. Potential uses of more accurate CT absorption values by filtering. *AJR* 131:103 (1978).

4. A. M. Cormack. Representation of a function by its line integrals, with some radiological applications. *J. Appl. Physics* 34:2722–2727 (1963).

5. J. D. Cormack and H. Ingle. The Roentgen rays. *Nature* 53:437 (12 March 1896).

6. W. E. Dandy. Ventriculography following the injection of air into the cerebral ventricles. *Am. J. Surgery* 68:5 (1918).

7. B. Cassen, L. Curtis, C. Reed, and R. Libby. Instrumentation for ^{131}I used in medical studies. *Nucleonics* 9:46 (1951).

8. J. F. Lindeman. The recent history of nuclear medicine intrumentation. In *Diagnostic Nuclear Medicine*, A. Gottschalk and E. I. Potchen, ed. Baltimore: Waverly Press, 1976, pp. 5–12.

9. H. O. Anger. Use of a gamma-ray pinhole camera for in-vivo studies. *Nature* 170:200 (1952).

10. E. Kuhl and R. Q. Edwards. Reorganizing data from transverse section scans using digital processing. *Radiology* 91:975–983 (1968).

11. G. Brownell and W. H. Sweet. Localization of brain tumors. *Nucleonics* 11:40–45 (1953).

12. S. Rankowitz, J. S. Robertson, and W. A. Higginbotham. Positron scanner for locating brain tumors. *IRE Intern. Conv. Record*, Part 9:49–56 (1962).

13. Z. H. Cho (ed). Special issue on physical and computational aspects of 3-dimensional image reconstruction. *IEEE Trans. Nucl. Sci.* NS-21 (1974).

14. M. Ter-pogossian, M. E. Phelps, E. J. Hoffman, et al. A positron emission transaxial tomograph for nuclear imaging (PETT). *Radiology* 114:89–98 (1975).

15. Z. H. Cho, J. K. Chan, and L. Eriksson. Circular ring transverse axial positron camera for 3-D reconstruction of radionuclide distribution. *IEEE Trans. Nucl. Sci.* NS-23:613–622 (1976).

16. T. F. Budinger, S. E. Derenzo, G. T. Gullberg, W. L. Greenberg, and R. H. Huesman. Emission computed tomography with single photon and positron annihilation photon emitters. *J. Comput. Assist. Tomogr.* 1:131–145 (1977).

17. Z. H. Cho and M. R. Farukhi. Bismuth germinate (BGO) as a potential scintillation detector in positron camera. *J. Nucl. Med.* 18:840–844 (1977).

18. E. Tanaka, N. Nohara, T. Tomitani, M. Yamaoto, and M. Murayama. Stationary positron emission tomography and its image reconstruction. *IEEE Trans. Med. Imag.* MI-5:199–206 (1986).

19. R. Jaszczak, L. Chang, N. Stein, and F. Moore. Whole body SPECT using dual, large-field of-view scintillation cameras. *Phys. Med. Biol.* 24:1123–1143 (1979).

20. R. E. Alvarez and A. Macovski. Energy selective reconstruction in X-ray computerized tomography. *Phys. Med. Biol.* 21:733–744 (1976).

21. G. Di Chiro, R. A. Brooks, R. M. Kessler, et al. Tissue signatures with dual-energy CT. *Radiology* 131:521 (1979).

22. Z. H. Cho, C. M. Tsai, and G. Wilson. Study of contrast and modulation mechanisms in X-ray/photon transverse axial transmission tomography. *Phys. Med. Biol.* 20:879–889 (1975).

23. E. C. McCullough. Factors affecting the use of quantitative information from a CT scanner. *Radiology* 124:99 (1977).

24. Z. H. Cho, I. Ahn, C. Bohm, and G. Huth. Computerized image reconstruction methods with multiple photon/X-ray transmission scanning. *Phys. Med. Biol.* 19:511–522 (1974).

25. L. Shepp and B. Logan. The Fourier reconstruction of a head section. *IEEE Trans. Nucl. Sci.* NS-21:21 (1974).

26. P. Lauterbur. Image formation by induced local interactions: Example employing nuclear magnetic resonance. *Nature* 242:190 (1973).

27. R. Damadian. Tumor detection by NMR *Science* 171:1151 (1971).
28. A. Kumar, D. Welti, and R. Ernst. NMR Fourier zeugmatography. *J. Magn. Reson.* 18:69 (1975).
29. W. Hinshaw, P. Bottomley, and G. Holland. *Nature* 270:722 (1977).
30. P. Mansfield and A. Maudsley. Fast scan proton density imaging by NMR. *J. Phys. E: Sci. Instrum.* 9:271 (1976).
31. Z. H. Cho, H. S. Kim, H. B. Song, and J. Cummings. Fourier transform nuclear magnetic resonance tomographic imaging. *Proc. IEEE* 70:1152–1173 (1982).
32. W. Hinshaw and A. Lent. An introduction to NMR imaging: From the Bloch equation to the image equation. *Proc. IEEE* 71:338 (1983).
33. K. R. Erikson, F. J. Fry, and J. P. Jones. Ultrasound in medicine—A review. *IEEE Trans. Sonics Ultrasonics* SU-21:144–170 (1974).
34. J. P. Jones and S. Leeman. Ultrasonic tissue characterization: A review. *Acta Electronica* 26(1–2):3–31 (1984).
35. J. P. Jones and R. Kovack. A computerized data analysis system for ultrasonic tissue characterization. *Acoustical Imaging* 9:503–512 (1980).
36. F. G. Sommer, L. Joynt, B. Carroll, and A. Macovski. Ultrasonic characterization of abdominal tissues via digital analysis of backscattered waveforms. *Radiology* 141:811–817 (1981).
37. J. M. C. Gallet and J. P. Jones. The envelope correlation spectrum as a means for characterizing tissue structure. *Ultrasound in Medicine and Biology* (in press).
38. M. R. Milunski, G. A. Mohr, J. E. Perez, Z. Vered, K. A. Wear, C. J. Gessler, B. E. Sobel, J. G. Miller, and S. A. Wickline. Ultrasonic tissue characterization with integrated backscatter. *Circulation* 80:491–503 (1989).
39. L. J. Thomas, B. Barzilai, J. E. Perez, B. E. Sobel, S. A. Wickline, and J. G. Miller. Quantitative real-time imaging of myocardium based on ultrasonic integrated backscatter. *IEEE Trans. Ultrasonic, Ferroelectrics and Frequency Control* 36:466–470 (1989).
40. J. P. Jones. Ultrasonic impediography and its application to tissue characterization. In *Recent Advances in Ultrasound in Biomedicine*, D. N. White, ed. Research Studies Press, 1977, pp. 131–156.
41. S. Leeman. Impediography equations. *Acoustical Imaging* 8:517–525 (1980).
42. S. Leeman. Impediography revisited. *Acoustical Imaging* 9:513–520 (1980).
43. D. Nicholas and A. M. Nicholas. Two-dimensional diffraction scanning of normal and cancerous human hepatic tissue in vitro. *Ultrasound Med. and Biol.* 9:283–296 (1983).
44. J. P. Jones. Current problems in Ultrasonic impediography. In *Ultrasonic Tissue Characterization*, M. Linzer, ed. NBS Spec. Publ. 453:253–258 (1976).
45. L. Hutchins and S. Leeman. Pulse and impulse response in human tissues. *Acoustical Imaging* 12:459–467 (1982).
46. L. Ferrari, J. P. Jones, V. Gonzalez, et al. Acoustical imaging using the phase of the echo waveforms. Presented at the 12th International Symposium on Acoustical Imaging, London, 1982. Also in *Acoustical Imaging*, vol. 12, E. A. Ash and C. R. Hill, eds. New York: Plenum, 1982, pp. 635–642.

47. R. J. Barr, L. B. Shaw, P. A. Ross, and J. P. Jones. Evaluation of skin biopsy samples using acoustical microscopy and comparison with conventional pathological studies and light microscopy. *Acoustical Imaging* 18:205–219 (1991).

48. L. K. Ryan, G. R. Lockwood, B. G. Starkoski, D. S. Holdsworth, D. W. Rickey, M. Drangova, A. Fenster, and F. S. Foster. A high frequency intravascular ultrasound imaging system for investigation of vessel wall properties. *Proceedings of the 1992 IEEE Ultrasonics Symposium* (in press).

49. R. J. Barr, G. M. White, J. P. Jones, L. B. Shaw, and P. A. Ross, Scanning acoustic microscopy of neoplastic and inflammatory cutaneous tissue specimens. *J. Investigative Dermatology* 96:38–42 (1991).

50. M. Singh, D. Doria, V. Henderson, et al. Reconstruction of images from neuromagnetic fields. *IEEE Trans. Nucl. Sci.* NS-31:585–589 (1984).

51. M. Singh, R. Brechner, and V. W. Henderson. Neuromagnetic localization using magnetic resonance images. *IEEE Trans. Med. Imag.* 11(1):129–134 (1992).

2

MATHEMATICAL PRELIMINARIES FOR IMAGE PROCESSING

Since its introduction in the early 1960s, digital image processing has grown remarkably. There has been a rise in the utilization of various aspects of image processing in many fields, often coupled with recent developments in digital computers and related signal processing techniques. Image processing now plays an important role in medicine; it can be used by physicians, medical engineers, and physicists to educe maximal information from detected images and to diagnose diseases.

This chapter describes the mathematical preliminaries for image processing. The first two sections discuss 2-D and 3-D Fourier transforms [1] and other transform techniques and methods that are the basis of image processing [2–6]. The third section explores other related image processing techniques such as sampling, interpolation, and image reformation [5, 6]. The fourth section presents the mathematical tools necessary for image enhancement and restoration for viewing the image [7]. The last section gives brief descriptions of the image quantizations that are necessary for the image data archive and transmission [3, 6].

2-1 FOURIER TRANSFORMS OF TWO- AND THREE-DIMENSIONAL IMAGES

2-1-1 Two- and Three-dimensional Fourier Transforms

The 2-D Fourier transform of the image function $f(x, y)$ is defined as

$$F(\omega_x, \omega_y) = \iint_{-\infty}^{\infty} f(x, y) \exp\{-i(\omega_x x + \omega_y y)\} \, dx \, dy \qquad (2-1)$$

21

where $\omega_x = 2\pi f_x$ and $\omega_y = 2\pi f_y$ with f_x and f_y being the spatial frequencies corresponding to the spatial coordinates x and y, respectively, and $i = \sqrt{-1}$. The 3-D extension of Eq. (2-1) is given by

$$F(\omega_x, \omega_y, \omega_z) = \iiint_{-\infty}^{\infty} f(x, y, z) \exp\{-i(\omega_x x + \omega_y y + \omega_z z)\} \, dx \, dy \, dz$$

$$(2\text{-}2)$$

Notationally the 2-D and 3-D Fourier transforms and their inverse Fourier transform operators are noted as

$$\mathscr{F}_2[f(x, y)] = F(\omega_x, \omega_y), \qquad \mathscr{F}_2^{-1}[F(\omega_x, \omega_y)] = f(x, y)$$

$$\mathscr{F}_3[f(x, y, z)] = F(\omega_x, \omega_y, \omega_z), \quad \mathscr{F}_3^{-1}[F(\omega_x, \omega_y, \omega_z)] = f(x, y, z)$$

$$(2\text{-}3)$$

where $\mathscr{F}_2, \mathscr{F}_3$, and $\mathscr{F}_2^{-1}, \mathscr{F}_3^{-1}$ are the 2-D and 3-D Fourier transforms and their corresponding inverse Fourier transform operators, respectively. In general, the Fourier coefficients $F(\omega_x, \omega_y)$ is a complex number that may be represented in real and imaginary form as

$$F(\omega_x, \omega_y) = R(\omega_x, \omega_y) + iI(\omega_x, \omega_y) \qquad (2\text{-}4a)$$

or in complex phasor form as

$$F(\omega_x, \omega_y) = M(\omega_x, \omega_y) \exp\{i\phi(\omega_x, \omega_y)\} \qquad (2\text{-}4b)$$

where

$$M(\omega_x, \omega_y) = \left[R^2(\omega_x, \omega_y) + I^2(\omega_x, \omega_y)\right]^{1/2} \qquad (2\text{-}5)$$

$$\phi(\omega_x, \omega_y) = \tan^{-1}\left\{\frac{I(\omega_x, \omega_y)}{R(\omega_x, \omega_y)}\right\} \qquad (2\text{-}6)$$

A sufficient condition for the existence of the Fourier transform of $f(x, y)$ is that the function be absolutely integrable and finite. This applies in both the spatial domain as well as the spatial frequency domain (Fourier domain). That is, a Fourier transform pair exists such that

$$F(\omega_x, \omega_y) \underset{\mathscr{F}_2^{-1}}{\overset{\mathscr{F}_2}{\rightleftharpoons}} f(x, y) \qquad (2\text{-}7)$$

The input function $f(x, y)$ then can be recovered from its Fourier transform by the inversion formula, which is given by

$$f(x, y) = \frac{1}{4\pi^2} \iint_{-\infty}^{\infty} F(\omega_x, \omega_y) \exp\{i(\omega_x x + \omega_y y)\} \, d\omega_x \, d\omega_y \quad (2\text{-}8)$$

or in operator form [see Eq. (2-3)] as

$$f(x, y) = \mathcal{F}_2^{-1}\{F(\omega_x, \omega_y)\} \quad (2\text{-}9)$$

The functions $f(x, y)$ and $F(\omega_x, \omega_y)$ are called a *Fourier transform pair*. As is clear from Eqs. (2-1) and (2-8), a 1-D Fourier transform pair can easily be deduced:

$$F(\omega_x, 0) = F(\omega_x) = \int_{-\infty}^{\infty} f(x, 0) \exp(-i\omega_x x) \, dx \quad (2\text{-}10)$$

$$f(x, 0) = f(x) = \frac{1}{2\pi} \int_{-\infty}^{\infty} F(\omega_x, 0) \exp(i\omega_x x) \, d\omega_x \quad (2\text{-}11)$$

or

$$F(0, \omega_y) = F(\omega_y) = \int_{-\infty}^{\infty} f(0, y) \exp(-i\omega_y y) \, dy \quad (2\text{-}12)$$

$$f(0, y) = f(y) = \frac{1}{2\pi} \int_{-\infty}^{\infty} F(0, \omega_y) \exp(i\omega_y y) \, d\omega_y \quad (2\text{-}13)$$

Similarly the 2-D Fourier transform can be computed in two steps using the property of separability of the kernel:

$$F(\omega_x, y) = \int_{-\infty}^{\infty} f(x, y) \exp(-i\omega_x x) \, dx \quad (2\text{-}14)$$

From Eq. (2-14) the final 2-D Fourier transform can be derived as

$$F(\omega_x, \omega_y) = \int_{-\infty}^{\infty} F(\omega_x, y) \exp(-i\omega_y y) \, dy \quad (2\text{-}15)$$

The above two-step Fourier transform is an important procedure universally used in most digital Fourier transforms in image processing.

2-1-2 Some Useful Properties of Fourier Transforms

Separability

The spatially separable function $f(x, y)$ can be written as

$$f(x, y) = f_x(x) f_y(y) \quad (2\text{-}16)$$

Similarly, in the Fourier domain, a separable function can be written as

$$F(\omega_x, \omega_y) = F(\omega_x)F(\omega_y)$$

where $F(\omega_x)$ and $F(\omega_y)$ are 1-D Fourier transforms of $f_x(x)$ and $f_y(y)$, respectively.

Two-Dimensional Complex Conjugate and Symmetry

If $f(x, y)$ and $F(\omega_x, \omega_y)$ are a 2-D Fourier transform pair, the Fourier transform of $f^*(x, y)$, the complex conjugate of $f(x, y)$, is given by

$$\mathscr{F}_2[f^*(x, y)] = F^*(-\omega_x, -\omega_y) \qquad (2\text{-}17)$$

where $f^*(\cdot)$ and $F^*(\cdot)$ represent complex conjugates of $f(\cdot)$ and $F(\cdot)$, respectively. If $f(x, y)$ is symmetric, that is, if $f(x, y) = f(-x, -y)$, then the Fourier domain function $F(\omega_x, \omega_y)$ is also symmetric:

$$F(\omega_x, \omega_y) = F(-\omega_x, -\omega_y) \qquad (2\text{-}18)$$

In general when $f(x, y)$ is a real function, the Fourier transform of $f(x, y)$ results in a complex Fourier domain function that has symmetry in the real part but antisymmetry in the imaginary part. This is sometimes called the *Hermitian property*, and it is one of the most often encountered and useful properties in digital image processing.

Linearity

The Fourier transform is a linear operator; thus the Fourier transform of two additive functions is also additive in the Fourier domain:

$$\mathscr{F}_2\{af_1(x, y) + bf_2(x, y)\} = aF_1(\omega_x, \omega_y) + bF_2(\omega_x, \omega_y) \qquad (2\text{-}19)$$

where a and b are constants. An example of linearity illustrated in one dimension is shown in Fig. 2-1.

Scaling

A linear scaling of the spatial variables results in an inverse scaling in the Fourier domain as given by

$$\mathscr{F}_2\{f(ax, by)\} = \frac{1}{|ab|} F\left(\frac{\omega_x}{a}, \frac{\omega_y}{b}\right) \qquad (2\text{-}20)$$

Equation (2-20) indicates that an increase along an axis in the spatial domain means a decrease along the corresponding axis in the Fourier domain together with an increase in the amplitude. A well-known example of this property is the Fourier transform of a Gaussian function which often relates

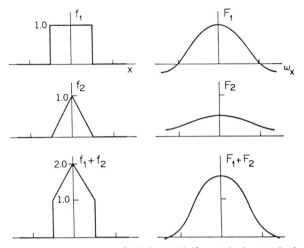

Figure 2-1   Linearity: $\mathscr{F}[af_1(x) + bf_2(x)] = aF_1(\omega_x) + bF_2(\omega_x)$.

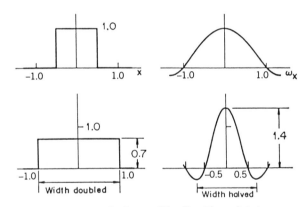

Figure 2-2   Scaling: $\mathscr{F}[f(ax)] = F(\omega_x/a)/|a|$.

to the uncertainty principle. An example of scaling illustrated in 1-D is shown in Fig. 2-2.

Shifting
A spatial domain positional shift in the input plane results in a phase shift in the spatial frequency or Fourier (transform) domain:*

$$\mathscr{F}_2\{f(x - a, y - b)\} = F(\omega_x, \omega_y)\exp\{-i(a\omega_x + b\omega_y)\} \quad (2\text{-}21)$$

*Note here that we have freely interchanged the terminology "spatial frequency domain," "Fourier domain," and "Fourier transform domain."

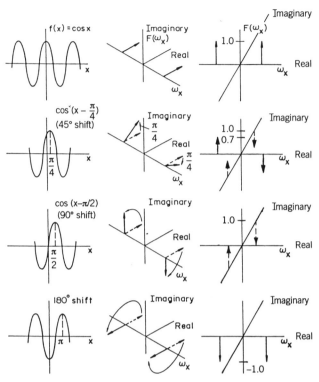

Figure 2-3 Shifting: $\mathscr{F}[f(x-a)] = F(\omega_x)\exp(-ia\omega_x)$ with $a = 0, \pi/4, \pi/2$, and π.

Inversely, a frequency shift in the Fourier domain results in a phase shift in the spatial domain as

$$\mathscr{F}_2^{-1}\{F(\omega_x - a_x, \omega_y - b_y)\} = f(x, y)\exp\{i(a_x x + b_y y)\}. \quad (2\text{-}22)$$

Here, both $\exp\{-i(a\omega_x + b\omega_y)\}$ and $\exp\{i(a_x x + b_y y)\}$ are phase factors. An example of shifting illustrated in one dimension is shown in Fig. 2-3.

Convolution Theorem (Fourier-Convolution Theorem)

The 2-D Fourier transform of two spatial-domain-convolved functions is equal to the product of the transforms of the two functions in the Fourier domain. Thus

$$\mathscr{F}_2\{f(x, y) * h(x, y)\} = F(\omega_x, \omega_y)H(\omega_x, \omega_y) \quad (2\text{-}23)$$

The inverse theorem states that

$$\mathscr{F}_2\{f(x, y)h(x, y)\} = \frac{1}{4\pi^2}\{F(\omega_x, \omega_y) * H(\omega_x, \omega_y)\} \quad (2\text{-}24)$$

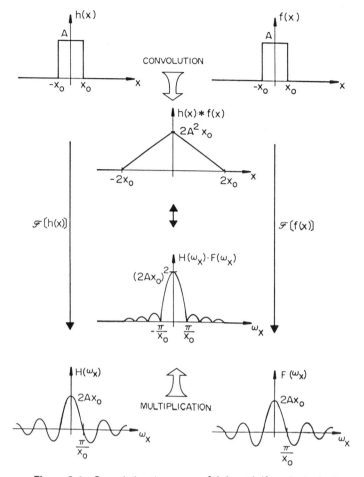

Figure 2-4   Convolution theorem: $\mathscr{F}[f(x) * h(x)] = F(\omega_x)H(\omega_x)$.

where $*$ denotes the convolution operation. This Fourier convolution theorem is one of the most often used and important theorems both in 1-D and 2-D signal processing. An example of the convolution theorem illustrated in one dimension is shown in Fig. 2-4.

Parseval's Theorem
The energies in the spatial and the spatial frequency or Fourier domains are related by

$$\iint_{-\infty}^{\infty} |f(x,y)|^2 \, dx \, dy = \frac{1}{4\pi^2} \iint_{-\infty}^{\infty} |F(\omega_x, \omega_y)|^2 \, d\omega_x \, d\omega_y \qquad (2\text{-}25a)$$

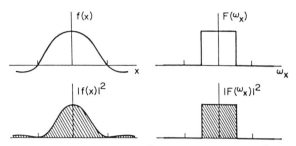

Figure 2-5 Parseval's theorem: $\int_{-\infty}^{\infty}|f(x)|^2\,dx = 1/2\pi[\int_{-\infty}^{\infty}|F(\omega_x)|^2\,d\omega_x]$ (the shaded areas are equal).

or

$$\iint_{-\infty}^{\infty} f(x,y)f^*(x,y)\,dx\,dy = \frac{1}{4\pi^2}\iint_{-\infty}^{\infty} F(\omega_x,\omega_y)F^*(\omega_x,\omega_y)\,d\omega_x\,d\omega_y$$

(2-25b)

where $f^*(\cdot)$ and $F^*(\cdot)$ are the complex conjugates of $f(\cdot)$ and $F(\cdot)$, respectively.

Equations (2-25a) and (2-25b) state that the total energy in the spatial domain function is the same as the total energy in the Fourier domain function. An example of Parseval's theorem illustrated in one dimension is shown in Fig. 2-5.

Autocorrelation Theorem

In some cases, such as random signals, it is difficult to obtain the Fourier transforms, and therefore the power spectra. The autocorrelation of a random signal and its Fourier transform often conveniently leads to the power spectrum of the random signal, since the Fourier transform of the autocorrelation of a function in the spatial domain is equal to the square of the absolute value of its Fourier transform which is known as the power spectrum:

$$\mathscr{F}_2\left\{\iint_{-\infty}^{\infty} f(\alpha,\beta)f^*(\alpha - x, \beta - y)\,d\alpha\,d\beta\right\} = \left|F(\omega_x,\omega_y)\right|^2 \quad (2\text{-}26)$$

Symbolically Eq. (2-26) can also be written as

$$\mathscr{F}_2\{f(\alpha,\beta) \otimes f^*(\alpha,\beta)\} = \left|F(\omega_x,\omega_y)\right|^2 \quad (2\text{-}27)$$

where $\otimes$ denotes the correlation operation. An example of the autocorrelation theorem illustrated in one dimension is shown in Fig. 2-6.

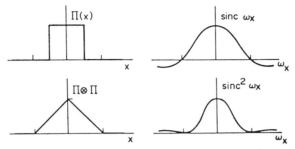

Figure 2-6 Autocorrelation theorem: $\mathscr{F}[f(x) \otimes f^*(x)] = |F(\omega_x)|^2$. (Reproduced from ref. [1]). Here Π denotes a rectangular function.

Stochastic Random Signals and Their Power Spectra

As was discussed in the autocorrelation theorem, stochastic random signals and their power spectra are an efficient measure of the power of a signal. There are actually two avenues to estimate the power spectrum: the square of the amplitude of the Fourier transform of the signal itself and the Fourier transform of the autocorrelation of the signal. Both of these can be useful for deterministic signals; however, for a stochastic random signal, the power spectrum can only be derived by the Fourier transform of the autocorrelation of the signal. For a deterministic signal the power spectrum is therefore simply obtained by

$$S(\omega_x, \omega_y) = |F(\omega_x, \omega_y)|^2 \tag{2-28a}$$

where $F(\omega_x, \omega_y) = \mathscr{F}_2[d(x, y)]$. Here, $d(\cdot)$ denotes a deterministic image field. For a stochastic random image field, however, the power spectrum can only be derived through its autocorrelation operation:

$$S(\omega_x, \omega_y) = \mathscr{F}_2[r(\alpha, \beta) \otimes r^*(\alpha, \beta)]$$
$$= \mathscr{F}_2\left[\int_{-\alpha}^{\alpha} \int_{-\beta}^{\beta} r(\alpha, \beta) r^*(\alpha - x, \beta - y)\, d\alpha\, d\beta\right] \tag{2-28b}$$

where $r(\alpha, \beta)$ and $r^*(\alpha, \beta)$ are the random image field and its complex

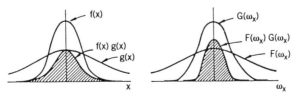

Figure 2-7 Power spectrum theorem: $\int_{-\infty}^{\infty} f(x) g^*(x)\, dx = \int_{-\infty}^{\infty} F(\omega_x) G^*(\omega_x)\, d\omega_x$ or $fg = FG$. Note the equal size of the shaded areas. (Reproduced from ref. [1]).

conjugate, respectively. An example of the power spectrum theorem illustrated in 1-D is shown in Fig. 2-.7

Fourier Transforms of Derivatives

The Fourier transforms of the directional derivatives of an image function are given by

$$\mathscr{F}_2\left\{\frac{\partial f(x,y)}{\partial x} + \frac{\partial f(x,y)}{\partial y}\right\} = i(\omega_x + \omega_y)F(\omega_x, \omega_y) \quad (2\text{-}29a)$$

The Fourier transforms of the second-order derivatives or Laplacians of an image function are given by

$$\mathscr{F}_2\left\{\frac{\partial^2 f(x,y)}{\partial x^2} + \frac{\partial^2 f(x,y)}{\partial y^2}\right\} = -\left(\omega_x^2 + \omega_y^2\right)F(\omega_x, \omega_y) \quad (2\text{-}29b)$$

An example of the Fourier transform of a derivative illustrated in one dimension is shown in Fig. 2-8.

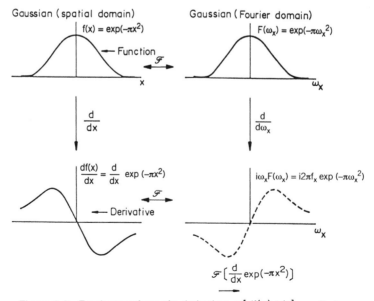

Figure 2-8 Fourier transform of a derivative: $\mathscr{F}[df(x)/dx] = \omega_x F(\omega_x)$.

Example 2-1   Shifting and Convolution Theorems

Let us consider an output image function when an image function $f(x, y)$ is convolved with an impulse response or point spread function $h(x, y)$:

$$g(x, y) = \iint_{-\infty}^{\infty} f(\alpha, \beta) h(x - \alpha, y - \beta)\, d\alpha\, d\beta \qquad (2\text{-}30)$$

Equation (2-30) is a well-known 2-D convolution operation. The Fourier transform of the above equation, after reversing the order of integration on the right-hand side, results in

$$G(\omega_x, \omega_y) = \mathscr{F}_2\{g(x, y)\}$$

$$= \iint_{-\infty}^{\infty} f(\alpha, \beta) \left[\iint_{-\infty}^{\infty} h(x - \alpha, y - \beta) \right.$$

$$\left. \times \exp\{-i(x\omega_x + y\omega_y)\}\, dx\, dy \right] d\alpha\, d\beta$$

$$(2\text{-}31)$$

Using the shifting theorem, Eq. (2-31) can be written as

$$G(\omega_x, \omega_y) = \iint_{-\infty}^{\infty} f(\alpha, \beta) H(\omega_x, \omega_y) \exp\{-i(\alpha\omega_x + \beta\omega_y)\}\, d\alpha\, d\beta$$

$$= F(\omega_x, \omega_y) H(\omega_x, \omega_y) \qquad (2\text{-}32)$$

This is an interesting example of how the shifting theorem leads to the Fourier convolution theorem by converting the shifts in the spatial domain to phase factors in the Fourier domain. Equation (2-32) also proves that the convolution operation in the spatial domain is equivalent to multiplication in the Fourier domain. Since the convolution operation is often more complicated than the simple multiplicative operation, convolution operation is performed in Fourier domain where Fourier transform of the input data are simply multiplied and then inverse transformed to obtain the final results (i.e., the convolution theorem is used). These seemingly twice repetitive Fourier transform operations could, sometimes, still be more advantageous than the one direct convolution operation due to the recent development of the FFT (fast Fourier transform) algorithm.

2-1-3   Fourier Transform of Circularly Symmetric Functions

Hankel Transform

Two-dimensional systems, such as optical systems, often show circular symmetry. If a system is symmetrical, simplifications can be made; for example, two cartesian variables (x, y) can be replaced by one radial variable. The Hankel transform is an example of a 1-D transform which is often used for such purposes.

When circular symmetry exists, a two-dimensional function $f(x, y)$ can be written as

$$f(x, y) = f(r) \tag{2-33a}$$

where r is a spatial domain radial variable. In polar coordinates, r is related to x and y by

$$r^2 = x^2 + y^2 \quad \text{or} \quad re^{i\theta} = x + iy \tag{2-33b}$$

where $x = r \cos \theta$, $y = r \sin \theta$, and $\theta = \tan^{-1}(y/x)$. Then the Fourier transform equivalent becomes

$$F(\omega_x, \omega_y) = F(\rho) \tag{2-34a}$$

where ρ is the spatial frequency or Fourier domain radial variable. Note that ρ is related to ω_x and ω_y as

$$\rho^2 = \omega_x^2 + \omega_y^2 \quad \text{or} \quad \rho e^{i\phi} = \omega_x + i\omega_y \tag{2-34b}$$

where $\omega_x = \rho \cos \phi$, $\omega_y = \rho \sin \phi$, and $\phi = \tan^{-1}(\omega_y/\omega_x)$. Then the two 1-D radial functions $f(r)$ and $F(\rho)$ are related as

$$F(\rho) = 2\pi \int_0^\infty f(r) J_0(2\pi\rho r) r \, dr \tag{2-35a}$$

$$f(r) = 2\pi \int_0^\infty F(\rho) J_0(2\pi\rho r) \rho \, d\rho \tag{2-35b}$$

where $J_0(\cdot)$ is the Bessel function of zero order. We refer to $F(\rho)$ as the Hankel transform (of zero order) of $f(r)$. Note that we deliberately used ρ instead of ω which is $2\pi f_r$, where f_r is the radial spatial frequency. We may consider the kernel J_0 as a Fourier kernel in the broad sense of a kernel associated with a reciprocal transform. Eq. (2-35a) can be derived from cartesian coordinate to polar coordinate transformation using the relation given in Eq. (2-34b),

$$F(\rho) = \int_0^\infty \int_0^{2\pi} f(r) \exp\{-i\rho r \cos(\theta - \phi)\} |J| \, d\theta \, dr$$

$$= \int_0^\infty f(r) \left[\int_0^{2\pi} \exp\{-i\rho r \cos \theta\} \, d\theta \right] r \, dr$$

$$= 2\pi \int_0^\infty f(r) J_0(2\pi\rho r) r \, dr \tag{2-35c}$$

where $J_0(2\pi\rho r) = 1/2\pi \int_0^{2\pi} \exp\{-i\rho r \cos \theta\} \, d\theta$. It should be noted that r in

Eq. (2-35c) is the Jacobian $|J|$ which can be derived from the coordinate transformation of the cartesian to the polar coordinates (r, θ) and is given by

$$|J| = \begin{vmatrix} \dfrac{\partial x}{\partial r} & \dfrac{\partial x}{\partial \theta} \\[2mm] \dfrac{\partial y}{\partial r} & \dfrac{\partial y}{\partial \theta} \end{vmatrix} = r \qquad (2\text{-}35d)$$

where (x, y) are related to (r, θ) as

$$x = r \cos \theta \quad \text{and} \quad y = r \sin \theta \qquad (2\text{-}35e)$$

As will be shown later in the section on 3-D image reconstruction from projections, the spatial domain rotated coordinates (x', y') in reference to the spatial domain coordinates (x, y) are also related as

$$\begin{bmatrix} x' \\ y' \end{bmatrix} = \begin{bmatrix} \cos \theta & \sin \theta \\ -\sin \theta & \cos \theta \end{bmatrix} \begin{bmatrix} x \\ y \end{bmatrix} \qquad (2\text{-}35f)$$

where x' and y' are the rotated coordinates in relation to the spatial domain polar coordinates (r, θ) and are given by

$$x' = x \cos \theta + y \sin \theta$$
$$y' = -x \sin \theta + y \cos \theta \qquad (2\text{-}35g)$$

The same is true for the spatial frequency domain coordinates,

$$\omega_{x'} = \omega_x \cos \phi + \omega_y \sin \phi \quad \text{and} \quad \omega_{y'} = -\omega_x \sin \phi + \omega_y \cos \phi \quad (2\text{-}35h)$$

In summary,

$$F(\rho) = F(\omega_x, \omega_y) = \iint_{-\infty}^{\infty} f(x, y) \exp\{-i(\omega_x x + \omega_y y)\} \, dx \, dy$$

$$= \int_0^{\infty} \int_0^{2\pi} f(r) \exp\{-i\rho r \cos(\theta - \phi)\} |J| \, d\theta \, dr \qquad (2\text{-}35i)$$

For above notations, note that $\omega_x = \rho \cos \phi$ and $\omega_y = \rho \sin \phi$.

Some useful zero order Hankel transforms are shown in Fig. 2-9.

Abel Transform

In optical image formation, television raster display, mapping by radar or passive detection, and so forth, the Abel transform can be used with great convenience. The Abel transform is particularly useful when circularly symmetrical distributions in 2-D are projected in one dimension. The Abel

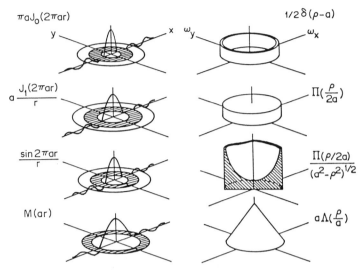

Figure 2-9 Some useful zero-order Hankel transforms. $\Pi(\cdot)$ and $\Lambda(\cdot)$ represent circularly symmetric rectangular and triangular functions, respectively. (Reproduced from ref. [1]).

transform $f_A(x)$ of the function $f(r)$ is commonly defined as

$$f_A(x) = 2 \int_x^\infty \frac{f(r) r \, dr}{(r^2 - x^2)^{1/2}} \tag{2-36}$$

$$f(r) = -\frac{1}{\pi} \frac{d}{dx} \left(\int_r^\infty \frac{f_A(x) r \, dx}{(x^2 - r^2)^{1/2}} \right) \tag{2-37}$$

As the symbols suggest, x and r represent an abscissa and a radius, respectively, in the same plane.

The Abel transform can be used to calculate the line spread function from the point spread function. If the point spread function is rotationally symmetric, it will be completely specified by a section of $f(r)$ or by the one-dimensional line spread function $f_A(x)$. In practice, the line spread function is often more useful, and may also be easier to measure experimentally. The line spread function of an imaging system is defined as the response of the system to a line input. An ideal line input may be represented by a single delta function, $\delta(x)$, which lies along the y_1-axis. The line spread function depends only on the x-variable, and using the convolution relationship between the input and the output, it is defined as

$$f_A(x) = \iint_{-\infty}^\infty \delta(x - x_1) f(x_1, y_1) \, dx_1 \, dy_1 \tag{2-38}$$

Table 2-1 Some useful two-dimensional Fourier transform pairs

$f(x, y)$ or $f(r)$	$F(\omega_x, \omega_y)$ or $F(\rho)$
$\delta(x, y)$	1
$\delta(x + x_0, y + y_0)$	$\exp(+i2\pi x_0 \omega_x)\exp(+i2\pi y_0 \omega_y)$
$\exp\{+i2\pi(\eta_1 x + \eta_2 y)\}$	$\delta(\omega_x - \eta_1, \omega_y - \eta_2)$
$\Pi(x, y)$ or $\text{rect}(x, y)$	$\text{sinc}(\omega_x, \omega_y)$
$\Lambda(x, y)$ or $\text{tri}(x, y)$	$\text{sinc}^2(\omega_x, \omega_y)$
$\text{comb}(x, y)$	$\text{comb}(\omega_x, \omega_y)$
$\exp\{+i2\pi(\eta_1 x + \eta_2 y)\}f(x, y)$	$F(\omega_x - \eta_1, \omega_y - \eta_2)$
$c(x, y) = f(x, y)*h(x, y)$	$C(\omega_x, \omega_y) = F(\omega_x, \omega_y)H(-\omega_x, -\omega_y)$
$I = \iint_{-\infty}^{\infty} f(x, y)h^*(x, y)\, dx\, dy$	$I = 1/4\pi^2 \iint_{-\infty}^{\infty} F(\omega_x, \omega_y)H^*(\omega_x, \omega_y)\, d\omega_x\, d\omega_y$
$1/r$	$1/\rho$
$\exp\{-\pi r^2\}$	$\exp\{-\pi\rho^2\}$

By the shifting property of the delta function, Eq. (2-38) can be written as

$$f_A(x) = \int_{-\infty}^{\infty} f(x, y_1)\, dy_1 \qquad (2\text{-}39)$$

Thus the line spread function is obtained from the point spread function by integrating over one variable provided that the point spread functions are rotationally symmetric; that is, $f(r) \equiv f(x, y)$, where $r^2 = x^2 + y^2$. The point spread function and the line spread function are therefore related as an Abel transform pair as shown in Eqs. (2-36) and (2-37). Table 2-1 contains a list of some useful 2-D Fourier transform pairs.

2-2 TRANSFORM TECHNIQUES AND METHODS

2-2-1 Fourier Transform as a Series

The Fourier transform for 1-D sequence $u(m)$, real or complex, is defined as the series [1, 2, 6, 10]

$$U(\omega) = \sum_{m=-\infty}^{\infty} u(m)\exp(-im\omega), \qquad -\pi \leq \omega < \pi \qquad (2\text{-}40)$$

Note that $U(\omega)$ is periodic with period 2π; hence it is sufficient to specify it over one period. The natural extension of the Fourier transform of 1-D sequence $u(m)$ to 2-D sequence $u(m, n)$ is defined as

$$U(\omega_x, \omega_y) = \sum_{n=-\infty}^{\infty} \sum_{m=-\infty}^{\infty} u(m, n)\exp\{-i(m\omega_x + n\omega_y)\},$$

$$-\pi \leq \omega_x, \omega_y < \pi \quad (2\text{-}41)$$

In Eq. (2-41) we have assumed that (m, n) has a Fourier domain correspondence of (ω_x, ω_y). Since $U(\omega_x, \omega_y)$ is periodic in each argument with period 2π, it can also be written as

$$U(\omega_x + 2\pi, \omega_y + 2\pi) = U(\omega_x, \omega_y) \quad (2\text{-}42)$$

2-2-2   Discrete Fourier Transform

The discrete Fourier transform (DFT) of a sequence $\{u(n), n = 0, \ldots, N - 1\}$ is defined as

$$v(k) = \sum_{n=0}^{N-1} u(n)\exp\left\{\frac{-i2\pi}{N}kn\right\}, \qquad k = 0, 1, \ldots, N - 1 \quad (2\text{-}43a)$$

or

$$v(k) = \sum_{n=0}^{N-1} u(n)W_N^{kn}, \qquad k = 0, 1, \ldots, N - 1 \quad (2\text{-}43b)$$

where

$$W_N = \exp\left\{\frac{-i2\pi}{N}\right\} \quad (2\text{-}43c)$$

The inverse transform is given by

$$u(n) = \frac{1}{N} \sum_{k=0}^{N-1} v(k)W_N^{-kn}, \qquad n = 0, 1, \ldots, N - 1 \quad (2\text{-}44)$$

Equations (2-43) and (2-44) are not properly scaled and therefore are not considered to be unitary transformations. In image processing it is more convenient to consider the unitary DFT, which is defined as

$$v(k) = \frac{1}{\sqrt{N}} \sum_{n=0}^{N-1} u(n)W_N^{kn}, \qquad k = 0, 1, \ldots, N - 1 \quad (2\text{-}45)$$

$$u(n) = \frac{1}{\sqrt{N}} \sum_{k=0}^{N-1} v(k)W_N^{-kn}, \qquad n = 0, 1, \ldots, N - 1 \quad (2\text{-}46)$$

The DFT is one of the most important transforms in digital image processing. It has a number of distinctive properties that make it useful for many image processing applications.

2-2-3 Discrete Cosine Transform

The 1-D discrete cosine transform (DCT) of a sequence $u(n)$ is defined as

$$v(k) = \alpha(k) \sum_{n=0}^{N-1} u(n)\cos\left[\frac{\pi(2n+1)k}{2N}\right], \qquad 0 \le k \le N-1 \quad (2\text{-}47)$$

where

$$\alpha(0) = \sqrt{\frac{1}{N}}, \qquad k = 0$$

$$\alpha(k) = \sqrt{\frac{2}{N}}, \qquad 1 \le k \le N-1 \qquad (2\text{-}48)$$

The inverse transformation is given by

$$u(n) = \sum_{k=0}^{N-1} \alpha(k)v(k)\cos\left[\frac{\pi(2n+1)k}{2N}\right], \qquad 0 \le n \le N-1 \quad (2\text{-}49)$$

Some important observation about the cosine transform are (1) the cosine transform is not the real part of a unitary DFT, and (2) the cosine transform is a fast transform and similar to the FFT in that the cosine transform of a vector of N elements can be calculated by $N \log_2 N$ operations via an N-point FFT. By reordering the even and odd elements of $u(n)$, we set up a new sequence $\tilde{u}(n)$ and Eq. (2-47) rearrange as

$$v(k) = \text{Re}\left[\alpha(k)\exp\left(\frac{-i\pi k}{2N}\right) \sum_{n=0}^{N-1} \tilde{u}(n)\exp\left(\frac{-i2\pi kn}{N}\right)\right]$$

$$= \text{Re}\left[\alpha(k)W_{2N}^{k/2}\,\text{DFT}\{\tilde{u}(n)\}\right], \qquad (2\text{-}50)$$

where we have assumed that $\tilde{u}(n)$ and $\tilde{u}(N-n-1)$ represent even and odd terms; that is, $\tilde{u}(n) = u(2n)$ and $\tilde{u}(N-n-1) = u(2n+1)$. To obtain the inverse cosine transform, we write Eq. (2-49) for even data points as

$$u(2n) = \tilde{u}(2n) = \text{Re}\left[\sum_{k=0}^{N-1} \left\{\alpha(k)v(k)\exp\left(\frac{i\pi k}{2N}\right)\right\}\exp\left(\frac{i2\pi nk}{N}\right)\right],$$

$$0 \le n \le \left(\frac{N}{2}\right) - 1 \quad (2\text{-}51)$$

The odd data points are obtained by noting that

$$u(2n + 1) = \bar{u}\{2(N - 1 - n)\}, \qquad 0 \le n \le \left(\frac{N}{2}\right) - 1 \qquad (2\text{-}52)$$

As seen from Eq. (2-50), $v(k)$ is now written in a DFT format that allows us to perform a fast transform. Finally, the cosine transform has excellent energy compaction for highly correlated data.

2-2-4   Discrete Sine Transform

The 1-D forward and inverse discrete sine transforms (DSTs) are given by

$$v(k) = \sqrt{\frac{2}{N + 1}} \sum_{n=0}^{N-1} u(n)\sin\left[\frac{\pi(k + 1)(n + 1)}{N + 1}\right], \qquad 0 \le k \le N - 1$$
$$(2\text{-}53)$$

$$u(n) = \sqrt{\frac{2}{N + 1}} \sum_{k=0}^{N-1} v(k)\sin\left[\frac{\pi(k + 1)(n + 1)}{N + 1}\right], \qquad 0 \le n \le N - 1$$
$$(2\text{-}54)$$

Note that the forward and inverse transforms are identical. Some important observations about the sine transform are as follows: First, the sine transform is real, symmetric, and orthogonal. Second, it is not the imaginary part of the unitary DFT. Finally, the sine transform is also a fast transform, and the sine transform (or its inverse) of a vector of N elements can be calculated by $N \log_2 N$ operations via a $2(N + 1)$ point FFT. Typically this requires $N + 1 = 2n\pi$; that is, the fast sine transform is usually defined for $N = 3, 7, 15, 31, 63, 255, \ldots$.

2-3   SAMPLING, INTERPOLATION, AND RECONSTRUCTION

In digital image processing, arrays of data are obtained by sampling from a physical image. After processing, another array of data is produced, and these data are interpolated. The interpolated data are then used to construct a new array which will be used for viewing or displaying the final image. Interpolation is therefore one step before the construction of the final image data array. In this section we will examine sampling, interpolation, and reconstruction in some detail and study the correlation between these operations.

2-3-1 Sampling

Let $f_I(x, y)$ denote an ideal image field representing such characteristics as the density, the activity distribution, and the brightness. To obtain a sampled data, the spatial domain image function is multiplied by a two-dimensional spatial sampling function that consists of a series of delta functions similar to "the bed of nails":

$$s(x, y) = \sum_{j_1 = -\infty}^{\infty} \sum_{j_2 = -\infty}^{\infty} \delta(x - j_1 \Delta x, y - j_2 \Delta y) \qquad (2\text{-}55)$$

where Δx and Δy are the spacings and $\delta(\cdot)$ is the Dirac delta function. The sampled image function is then given by

$$f_S(x, y) = f_I(x, y)s(x, y) = \sum_{j_1 = -\infty}^{\infty} \sum_{j_2 = -\infty}^{\infty} f_I(j_1 \Delta x, j_2 \Delta y)\delta(x - j_1 \Delta x, y - j_2 \Delta y)$$

$$(2\text{-}56)$$

Let us now consider the spatial frequency domain representations $F_S(\omega_x, \omega_y)$ which is the Fourier transform of the sampled image $f_S(x, y)$:

$$F_S(\omega_x, \omega_y) = \iint_{-\infty}^{\infty} f_S(x, y)\exp\{-i(\omega_x x + \omega_y y)\} \, dx \, dy \qquad (2\text{-}57)$$

Using Eq. (2-56) and the convolution theorem, the Fourier transform of $f_S(x,y)$ (i.e., the Fourier transform of the sampled image) can be expressed as the convolution of the Fourier transforms of two functions, namely the image function $F_I(\omega_x, \omega_y)$ and the sampling function $S(\omega_x, \omega_y)$ and can be given by

$$F_S(\omega_x, \omega_y) = \frac{1}{4\pi^2} F_I(\omega_x, \omega_y) * S(\omega_x, \omega_y) \qquad (2\text{-}58)$$

Since the 2-D Fourier transform of an infinite array of delta functions is also an infinite array of delta functions in the spatial frequency domain, it is natural to write the Fourier transform of the sampling function $S(\omega_x, \omega_y)$ as

$$S(\omega_x, \omega_y) = \frac{4\pi^2}{\Delta x \, \Delta y} \sum_{j_1 = -\infty}^{\infty} \sum_{j_2 = -\infty}^{\infty} \delta(\omega_x - j_1 \omega_{xs}, \omega_y - j_2 \omega_{ys}) \qquad (2\text{-}59)$$

where $\omega_{xs} = 2\pi/\Delta x$ and $\omega_{ys} = 2\pi/\Delta y$ represent the Fourier domain sampling frequencies corresponding to ω_x and ω_y, respectively. Since the convolution of a function with a delta function is the function itself, Eq. (2-58) can

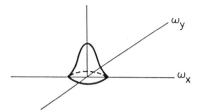

(a) Original image spectrum $F_I(\omega_x, \omega_y)$ in Fourier domain.

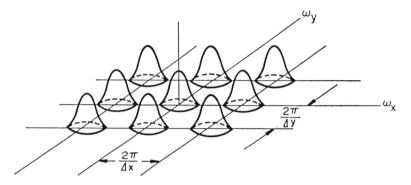

(b) 2-Dimensional display of the sampled image spectra $F_S(\omega_x, \omega_y)$ in Fourier domain.

Figure 2-10   Repetitiveness is a characteristic of the sampled data.

be rewritten as

$$F_S(\omega_x, \omega_y) = \frac{1}{\Delta x\, \Delta y} \sum_{j_1 = -\infty}^{\infty} \sum_{j_2 = -\infty}^{\infty} F_I(\omega_x - j_1\omega_{xs}, \omega_y - j_2\omega_{ys}) \quad (2\text{-}60)$$

Equation (2-60) represents the replica of the Fourier transform $F_I(\cdot)$ of the original image function $f_I(\cdot)$ in the spatial frequency or Fourier domain with separations of $2\pi/\Delta x$ and $2\pi/\Delta y$. An example of a bandlimited spectrum $F_I(\omega_x, \omega_y)$ and its repeated replica in the spatial frequency domain is illustrated in Figs. 2-10 (a) and (b).

2-3-2   Interpolation or Reconstruction

After the sampled data are processed by computer or by other physical image processors, they must be reconstructed by interpolation for final display or viewing. Interpolation is usually performed by convolution of the discrete data array with some interpolation function to form a continuous function.

For example, the discrete array $f_S(x, y)$ convolved with an interpolation function $r(x, y)$ can be expressed as

$$f_R = f_S(x, y) * r(x, y)$$

or

$$f_R = \sum_{j_1 = -\infty}^{\infty} \sum_{j_2 = -\infty}^{\infty} f_S(j_1 \Delta x, j_2 \Delta y) r(x - j_1 \Delta x, y - j_2 \Delta y) \quad (2\text{-}61)$$

where Δx and Δy are the sampling intervals in the x- and y-coordinates. The Fourier domain representation of Eq. (2-61), as is obvious from the Fourier convolution theorem, becomes

$$F_R(\omega_x, \omega_y) = F_S(\omega_x, \omega_y) R(\omega_x, \omega_y) \quad (2\text{-}62)$$

where $R(\cdot)$ is the Fourier transform of the interpolation function $r(\cdot)$ in the spatial domain and is known as the reconstruction filter function in the Fourier domain. Even if there is no spectral overlap in $F_S(\cdot)$ (see Fig. 2-10(b) series of 2-dimensional spectra, exact replicas of the original image spectrum $F_I(\cdot)$ that are distributed repeatedly over all the Fourier domain), it is necessary to single out the $F_I(\cdot)$ from the $F_S(\cdot)$. This requires, ideally, that the reconstruction filter function be a rectangular bandlimited filter of the form

$$R(\omega_x, \omega_y) = \begin{cases} K, & \text{for } |\omega_x| \le \omega_{xc} \text{ and } |\omega_y| \le \omega_{yc} \\ 0, & \text{otherwise} \end{cases} \quad (2\text{-}63)$$

where K is a scaling constant and ω_{xc} and ω_{yc} are the cutoff frequencies in the ω_x and the ω_y directions in the Fourier domain that satisfy the condition of exact reconstruction if $\omega_{xc} \le \omega_{xs}/2$ and $\omega_{yc} \le \omega_{ys}/2$. Since the reconstruction filter in the Fourier domain is equivalent to the interpolation function in the spatial domain, the Fourier transform of Eq. (2-63) is the desired interpolation function and is given by

$$r(x, y) = \frac{K \omega_{xc} \omega_{yc}}{\pi^2} \frac{\sin(\omega_{xc} x)}{(\omega_{xc} x)} \frac{\sin(\omega_{yc} y)}{(\omega_{yc} y)} \quad (2\text{-}64)$$

Another type of reconstruction filter that could be employed is the circular filter of the form

$$R(\omega_x, \omega_y) = \begin{cases} K, & \text{if } \sqrt{\omega_x^2 + \omega_y^2} \le \omega_0 \\ 0, & \text{otherwise} \end{cases} \quad (2\text{-}65)$$

provided that $\omega_{xc}^2 + \omega_{yc}^2 \le \omega_0^2$ where ω_0 is the diameter of the circle. The corresponding interpolation function would be

$$r(x, y) = 2\pi\omega_0 \frac{J_1\left\{\omega_0\sqrt{x^2 + y^2}\right\}}{\sqrt{x^2 + y^2}} \qquad (2\text{-}66)$$

where $J_1(\cdot)$ is a Bessel function of the first order. As we will see shortly, there are a number of reconstruction filters or equivalent interpolation wave forms that can be employed to provide good image reconstruction.

Aliasing and Imperfect Sampling

To achieve perfect image reconstruction in a sampled imaging system, it is necessary to band-limit the image to be sampled or spatially sample the image at the Nyquist rate or higher and, at the end, to properly interpolate the processed image samples. Let us first consider the effect of undersampling an image. A spectral overlap resulting from undersampling is shown in Fig. 2-11 and indicated by the shaded regions. This is called *aliasing*, and an

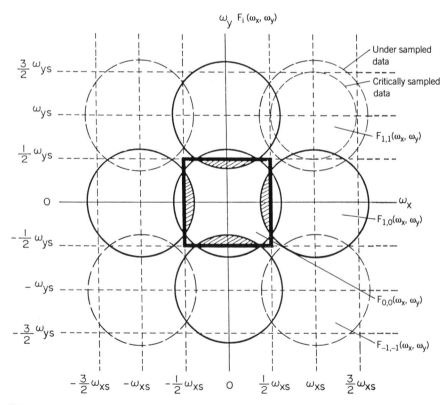

Figure 2-11 Two-dimensional illustration of the spectral overlaps in the case of undersampling. Shaded areas shown within the rectangular region are the aliasing components. (Reproduced from ref. [6]).

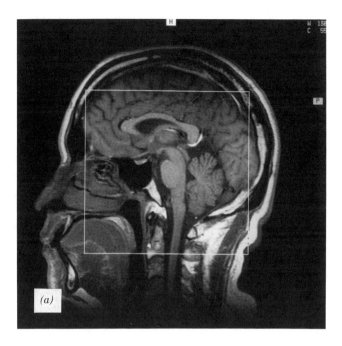

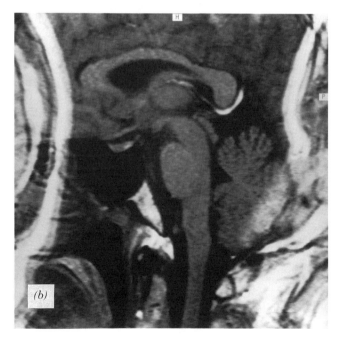

Figure 2-12 An example of aliasing in an image due to undersampling. (*a*) Original, (*b*) undersampled image distorted by aliasing.

example of the effects of aliasing in an actual MRI (magnetic resonance imaging) image is shown in Fig. 2-12. The unaliased image in Fig. 2-12(a) shows a perfect reconstruction of the image, while the undersampled and aliased image in Fig. 2-12(b) shows image field overlap. To further illustrate this aliasing effect, let us assume a spectrum of a sampled image using a zonal filter of the form (see the square box in Fig. 2-11):

$$F_S(\omega_x, \omega_y) = \frac{1}{\Delta x \, \Delta y} \left[F_I(\omega_x, \omega_y) + F_A(\omega_x, \omega_y) \right] \qquad (2\text{-}67)$$

where $F_I(\omega_x, \omega_y)$ and $F_A(\omega_x, \omega_y)$ represent the spectra of the original image and the aliasing component sampled at period $(\Delta\omega_x, \Delta\omega_y)$, respectively. The term $F_A(\cdot)$ here represents the aliasing component and is quantitatively given as

$$F_A(\omega_x, \omega_y) = \sum_{j_1=-\infty}^{\infty} \sum_{j_2=-\infty}^{\infty} F_I(\omega_x - j_1\omega_{xs}, \omega_y - j_2\omega_{ys}),$$

$$j_1 \neq 0 \text{ and } j_2 \neq 0 \quad (2\text{-}68)$$

$F_A(\cdot)$ now represents the spectral components other than $F_I(\omega_x, \omega_y)$, that is, spectral components belonging to high-order replicas other than $j_1, j_2 = 0$ which are smeared into the bandwidth of the rectangular or zonal filter $R(\omega_x, \omega_y)$. From Eqs. (2-62) and (2-67) and by Fourier transform, the final image can be obtained,

$$f_R(x, y) = f_I(x, y) + f_A(x, y) \qquad (2\text{-}69)$$

where the aliasing component $f_A(\cdot)$ is

$$f_A(x, y) = \frac{1}{4\pi^2} \int_{-\omega_{xs}/2}^{\omega_{xs}/2} \int_{-\omega_{ys}/2}^{\omega_{ys}/2} F_A(\omega_x, \omega_y) \exp\{i(\omega_x x + \omega_y y)\} \, d\omega_y \, d\omega_x$$

$$(2\text{-}70)$$

Equation (2-70) is the aliasing component resulting from a 2-D interpolation when an ideal zonal reconstruction filter is used or an ideal sinc function interpolation is performed. Figure 2-13 illustrates several often-used, one-dimensional interpolation functions. The sinc function, as stated previously, provides an exact reconstruction but is usually difficult to realize in practical

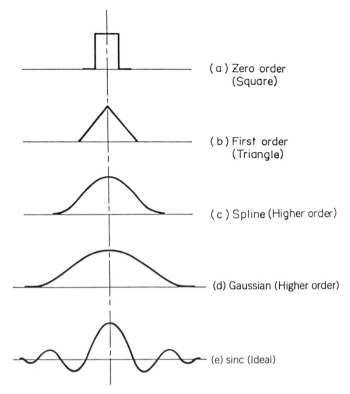

(a) Zero order
(Square)

(b) First order
(Triangle)

(c) Spline (Higher order)

(d) Gaussian (Higher order)

(e) sinc (Ideal)

Figure 2-13   Various spatial domain interpolation functions.

image processing. The simplest interpolation waveform is the rectangular pulse function that results in a zero-order interpolation of the samples. A triangle function provides first-order linear interpolation. The triangle function may be considered to be the result of convolving two rectangular pulse functions. Repeated convolution of the rectangular pulse function yields various bell-shaped interpolation waveforms and eventually converges to the Gaussian-shaped waveform (see Fig. 2-13). Polynomials of order two or greater can also be employed as interpolation waveforms. Thecubic B-spline is a particularly attractive candidate for the interpolation because of its properties of continuity and smoothness at its extremities. Another useful property of the cubic B-spline is the fact that the function is nonzero only over a short span of the sample period and can be obtained by a convolution of four square pulses. Figure 2-14 illustrates typical one-dimensional interpolations using the square, the triangle, spline, Gaussian, and the sinc functions. As mentioned earlier, the sinc function interpolation will result in an ideal reconstruction provided that the Nyquist sampling criterion is satisfied.

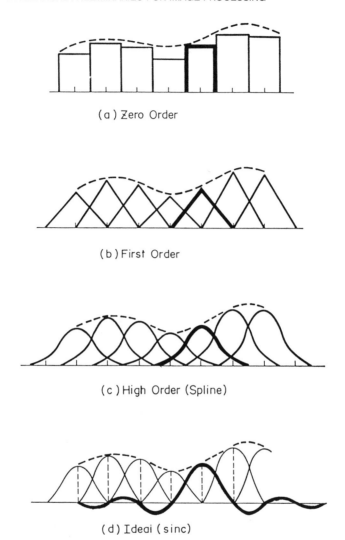

(a) Zero Order

(b) First Order

(c) High Order (Spline)

(d) Ideal (sinc)

Figure 2-14 Interpolation procedures of three interpolation functions of different orders (a – c). Ideal sinc interpolation would reconstruct the image in perfect shape (d).

2-3-3 Errors in Interpolation or Reconstruction

For the analysis of the performance of reconstruction processes, it is assumed that the input to the reconstruction system is composed of samples of an ideal image obtained by sampling at the Nyquist rate. Figure 2-15 provides a graphic example of the effects of an interpolation function or reconstruction filter. A typical cross section of the spectral distribution of a sampled image is shown at the top of Fig. 2-15(a). An ideal reconstruction filter employing a

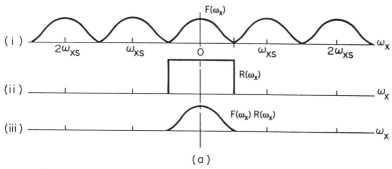

(a)

Ideal sinc function interpolation or rectangular zonal filtering

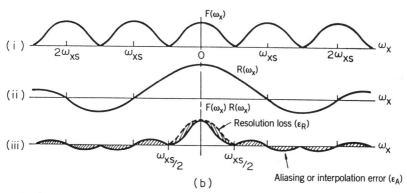

(b)

Nonideal rectangular function interpolation or zero order interpolation

Figure 2-15 Example of two interpolation processes: (a) an interpolation with the sinc function [the sinc function in the spatial domain is equivalent to the rectangular function in the Fourier domain as shown in (ii)]; (b) a nonideal interpolation with a zero-order rectangular function [the rectangular function in the spatial domain is equivalent to the sinc function in the Fourier domain as shown in (ii)]. Note the spectral loss and other spatial frequency domain spectral leakages. (Reproduced from ref. [6]).

sinc function for interpolation can perfectly extract only the central image spectrum as shown at the bottom of Fig. 2-15(a). On the other hand a nonideal reconstruction using e.g. zero-order or rectangular function interpolation results in both aliasing and resolution loss. The resulting spectrum due to this zero-order reconstruction filter can be easily seen by simple multiplication of the original spectra with a sinc function [see Fig. 2-15(b)]. It shows both spectral loss at the central spectrum (resolution loss) and leakages of the higher-order spectral components (aliasing or interpolation error) due to the imperfect zonal filtering.

The resolution loss resulting from the use of a nonideal interpolation function $r(x, y)$ or reconstruction filter function $R(\omega_x, \omega_y)$ may be quantitatively evaluated as

$$\varepsilon_R = \frac{E_{RM} - E_R}{E_{RM}} \qquad (2\text{-}71)$$

where E_{RM} and E_R are the energy of the ideal reconstruction obtained by a sinc function interpolation or an ideal rectangular zonal filter and the energy of the nonideal reconstruction filter, respectively, and are given by

$$E_{RM} = \int_{-\omega_{xs}/2}^{\omega_{xs}/2} \int_{-\omega_{ys}/2}^{\omega_{ys}/2} W_{F_I}(\omega_x, \omega_y) \, d\omega_x \, d\omega_y \qquad (2\text{-}72)$$

$$E_R = \int_{-\omega_{xs}/2}^{\omega_{xs}/2} \int_{-\omega_{ys}/2}^{\omega_{ys}/2} W_{F_S}(\omega_x, \omega_y) \left| R(\omega_x, \omega_y) \right|^2 \, d\omega_x \, d\omega_y \qquad (2\text{-}73)$$

where $W_{F_I}(\omega_x, \omega_y)$ is the power spectrum of the ideal image and $R(\cdot)$ is the nonideal reconstruction filter function. These represent the actual interpolated image energies in the Nyquist sampling band limits. As seen from Eq. (2-72), in the ideal case, $R(\omega_x, \omega_y)$ will simply become unity.

On the other hand, the aliasing or interpolation error may be defined as the artifact resulting from the high spatial frequency components outside the zonal bandwidth ($|\omega| = \omega_{xs}/2$ for the one-dimensional case) as schematically illustrated in Fig. 2-15 (b):

$$\varepsilon_A = \frac{E_T - E_R}{E_T} \qquad (2\text{-}74)$$

where E_T and E_R represent the total energy over the entire frequency band and the energy of the ideal image field filtered with a zonal filter, respectively. The total energy E_T is given by

$$E_T = \iint_{-\infty}^{\infty} W_{F_S}(\omega_x, \omega_y) \left| R(\omega_x, \omega_y) \right|^2 \, d\omega_x \, d\omega_y \qquad (2\text{-}75)$$

where W_{F_S} is the sampled image data power spectrum which is given by

$$W_{F_S} = \left| F_S(\omega_x, \omega_y) \right|^2 \qquad (2\text{-}76)$$

Table 2-2 contains a list of the resolution and interpolation or aliasing errors obtained with several separable two-dimensional interpolation functions.

Table 2-2 **Approximate resolution and interpolation errors for various separable interpolation functions**

Interpolation Function	Percent Resolution Error, $\varepsilon_R(\%)$	Percent Interpolation or Aliasing Error, $\varepsilon_A(\%)$
Sinc	0%	0%
Square	~ 30%	~ 20%
Triangle	~ 45%	~ 5%
B-spline	~ 65%	~ 0.5%

2-4   IMAGE ENHANCEMENT AND RESTORATION

Two types of image manipulation processes are applied for image enhancement and improvement. One is image enhancement, and the other is image restoration [3, 6, 11]. Image enhancement includes operations that improve the appearance of an image to a human viewer or on a display. Image restoration includes such operations as the reconstruction or correction of an image which is degraded, for instance, by noise or local shifts.

2-4-1   Image Enhancement

For visualization or machine processing of an image, it is often necessary to improve the image. For this purpose a number of image enhancement techniques have been developed and are in use today. Image enhancement commonly refers to accentuation or sharpening of the image features. Image enhancement includes gray level and contrast manipulation, noise reduction,* edge sharpening, smoothing,* filtering,* interpolation, and magnification or zooming, and pseudocoloring. Image enhancement is often subjective and requires human judgment; it is, nevertheless, an important class of image processing.

Histogram Modeling and Manipulations
The histogram of an image represents the relative frequency of occurrence of the various gray levels in the image. A histogram of the gray level content provides the characteristics of an image. Histogram manipulation techniques therefore can be used to provide a desired histogram that would be better for the viewers or the machines. With histogram modification the original histogram of an image is rescaled or redistributed so that the histogram of the enhanced image follows some desired characteristics. Histogram manipulation is found to be a useful technique for many classes of image enhancement, such as the equalization of X-ray CT images where bones and soft tissues are distributed in a well-separated bimodal form with relatively narrow distributions.

---

*These features are also available in image filtering and restoration.

Histogram Equalization   One of the most often used histogram manipulations is the histogram equalization. The goal of equalization involves a
histogram modification that makes the output histogram uniform. Let us
consider a histogram having a distribution function or a probability function
$p(f)$ as an input and a desired output distribution function $p(g)$. Two
distribution functions with different configurations, such as different numbers
of gray levels, will be equal if

$$\int_0^J p(f)\, df = \int_0^K p(g)\, dg \qquad (2\text{-}77)$$

where J and K represent the number of gray levels in each distribution that
satisfy the relation

$$\sum_{j=0}^J p(f_j) = \sum_{k=0}^K p(g_k) = 1 \qquad (2\text{-}78)$$

To make Eq. (2-78) more general, we can define minimum bounds for the
input and the output histograms, and Eq. (2-78) can be rewritten as

$$\int_{f_{min}}^f p(f)\, df = \int_{g_{min}}^g p(g)\, dg \qquad (2\text{-}79)$$

or

$$P_f(f) = \int_{g_{min}}^g p(g)\, dg \qquad (2\text{-}80)$$

where $P_f(f)$ now represents the cumulative input histogram or distribution
function.

A simple example of a uniform output distribution function $p(g)$ would be

$$p(g) = \frac{1}{g_{max} - g_{min}} \qquad (2\text{-}81)$$

when the output distribution function is defined as [see Eq. (2-80)]

$$\int_{g_{min}}^g p(g)\, dg \bigg|_{g=g_{max}} = 1$$

$$= P_f(f) \qquad (2\text{-}82)$$

From Eqs. (2-81) and (2-82), for a uniform output distribution, the output

Table 2-3   Some useful histogram transfer functions

Output Probability or Distribution Function	Transform or Transfer Function
Uniform	
$p(g) = \dfrac{1}{g_{max} - g_{min}}, \; g_{min} \leq g \leq g_{max}$	$g = [g_{max} - g_{min}]P_f(f) + g_{min}$
Exponential	
$p(g) = \alpha \exp\{-\alpha(g - g_{min})\}, \; g_{min} \leq g$	$g = g_{min} - \dfrac{1}{\alpha}\ln[1 - P_f(f)]$
Hyperbolic	
$p(g) = \dfrac{1}{g[\ln(g_{max}) - \ln(g_{min})]}$	$g = g_{min}\left[\dfrac{g_{max}}{g_{min}}\right]^{P_f(f)}$

Note: $P_f(f)$ is the cumulative probability distribution of the input image histogram [see Eq. (2-80)].

value g can be written as

$$g = (g_{max} - g_{min})P_f(f) + g_{min} \qquad (2\text{-}83)$$

Equation (2-83) is an example of a histogram transfer function (for a uniform output distribution) from among the many transfer functions available (see Table 2-3). Figure 2-16 provides a reference example of the transform process of histogram equalization. Note that the number of input gray levels

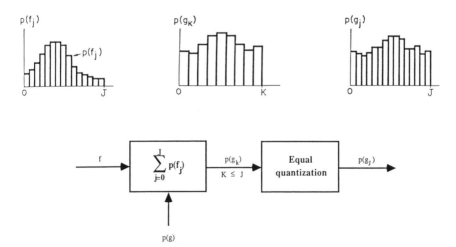

Figure 2-16   Transform process of histogram equalization. Note $K < J$.

is always larger than the number of transformed gray levels (i.e., $K \leq J$). Since the available gray levels are J, the K levels of the transform image can again be scaled back to J for finer display or viewing.

Histogram Modification Histograms can be modified to provide a more comprehensive image for the human eye or for machine interpretation. An example of histogram modification is illustrated in Fig. 2-17 where both histogram equalization and additional manipulations, such as the hyperbolization, are employed. Figure 2-18 shows an example of histogram hyperbolization to optimally match the human eye response.

Table 2-3 presents several forms of the desired distribution function and their corresponding transform functions. For example, the uniform distribution function is nothing but the histogram equalization function discussed above.

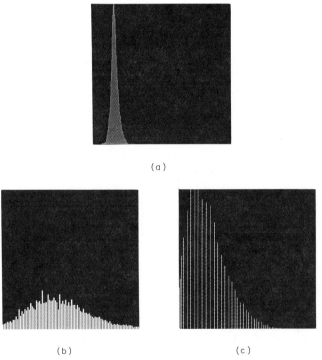

(a)

(b)   (c)

Figure 2-17 Example of histogram modification: (a) In the original histogram most of the information is concentrated in a narrow band with most of the gray levels unoccupied; (b) the histogram is segmented and expanded; (c) the equalized histogram is further modified for a specific purpose, such as to make it suitable for viewing (hyperbolization). (Reproduced from ref. [6]).

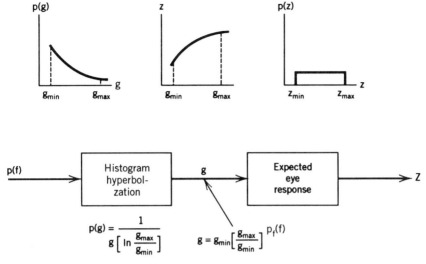

Figure 2-18 Example of histogram hyperbolization that optimally matches the response of the human eye.

Generalized Histogram Modification   The preceding consideration of histogram modification gave examples of uniform distribution or histogram hyperbolization that fit some specific applications involving human eye response. The more general unknown cases, however, are treated mathematically as an inverse problem. A cumulative input histogram can be defined as

$$\int_0^f p(f)\, df = P_f(f) = s \qquad (2\text{-}84)$$

Similarly an output cumulative histogram can be defined as

$$\int_0^g p(g)\, dg = P_g(g) = v \qquad (2\text{-}85)$$

Since Eqs. (2-84) and (2-85) are identical [i.e., $P_f(f) = P_g(g)$], the desired output variable g can be given as

$$g = P_g^{-1}\big[P_f(f)\big] \qquad (2\text{-}86)$$

Example 2-2   Generalized Histogram Modification

Consider a 128×128, eight-level image that has the gray level distribution shown in Table 2-4a. To be useful for digital image processing, Eq. (2-84)

Table 2-4a.

f_k	$f_0 = 0$	$f_1 = \dfrac{1}{7}$	$f_2 = \dfrac{2}{7}$	$f_3 = \dfrac{3}{7}$	$f_4 = \dfrac{4}{7}$	$f_5 = \dfrac{5}{7}$	$f_6 = \dfrac{6}{7}$	$f_7 = 1$
n_k	2458	4096	4259	2458	1475	819	655	164
$p(f_k) = n_k/n$	0.15	0.25	0.26	0.15	0.09	0.05	0.04	0.01

Table 2-4b.

s_k	s_0	s_1	s_2	s_3	s_4	s_5	s_6	s_7
$\displaystyle\sum_{j=0}^{k} p(f_j)$	0.15	0.40	0.66	0.81	0.90	0.95	0.99	1
Closest valid level	1/7	3/7	5/7	6/7	6/7	1	1	1
Redefining level	1/7	3/7	5/7	6/7	1			

Table 2-4c.

$f_j \to s_k$	n_k	$p_s(s_k)$
$f_0 \to s_0 = \dfrac{1}{7}$	2458	0.15
$f_1 \to s_1 = \dfrac{3}{7}$	4096	0.25
$f_2 \to s_2 = \dfrac{5}{7}$	4259	0.26
$f_3, f_4 \to s_3 = \dfrac{6}{7}$	3933	0.24
$f_5, f_6, f_7 \to s_4 = 1$	1638	0.10

Table 2-4d.

g_k	g_0	g_1	g_2	g_3	g_4	g_5	g_6	g_7
$p(g_k)$	0.00	0.00	0.00	0.15	0.25	0.30	0.20	0.10

Table 2-4e.

v_k	v_0	v_1	v_2	v_3	v_4	v_5	v_6	v_7
$\displaystyle\sum_{j=0}^{k} p(g_j)$	0.00	0.00	0.00	0.15	0.40	0.70	0.90	1.00

Table 2-4f.

g_k	$g_0 = 0$	$g_1 = \dfrac{1}{7}$	$g_2 = \dfrac{2}{7}$	$g_3 = \dfrac{3}{7}$	$g_4 = \dfrac{4}{7}$	$g_5 = \dfrac{5}{7}$	$g_6 = \dfrac{6}{7}$	$g_7 = 1$
$p(g_k)$	0.00	0.00	0.00	0.15	0.25	0.26	0.24	0.10

must be formulated in discrete form. For gray levels that assume discrete values, we deal with a probability given by the relation

$$s_k = P_f(f_k) = \sum_{j=0}^{k} p(f_j) \qquad (2\text{-}87a)$$

where

$$p(f_k) = \frac{n_k}{n}, \qquad 0 \le f_k \le 1, \; k = 0, 1, 2, \ldots, L-1 \qquad (2\text{-}87b)$$

In Eq. (2-87), L is the number of levels, $p(f_k)$ is the probability of the kth gray level, n_k is the number of times this level appears in the image, and n is the total number of pixels in the image. To transform from the original probability density [see Fig. 2-19(a)] to the desired probability density [see Fig. 2-19(d)], the following algorithm might be applied:

1. Equalize the histogram of the original image according to Eq. (2-84).
2. Specify the desired density function, and obtain the equaling transformation $P_g(g)$ in Eq. (2-85).
3. Apply the inverse transformation as shown in Eq. (2-86) to the previously equalized image $P_f(f)$.

According to the first step the transformation function is obtained by using Eq. (2-87) for digital image processing as shown in Table 2-4b [also see Fig. 2-19(b)]. Since only eight equally spaced levels are allowed in this case, each of the transformed values must be assigned to its closest valid level (see Table 2-4b). It is noted that there are only five distinct histogram equalized levels. Redefining the notation to take this into account yields five new levels (see Table 2-4b), and the histogram equalization mappings can be obtained as shown in Table 2-4c [also see Fig. 2-19(c)]. Since a histogram is an approximation of a probability density function, the result is seldom obtained when working with discrete levels.

The second step is to obtain the transformation function of the desired histogram using a discrete form of Eq. (2-85) similar to Eq. (2-87). The desired transformed function shown in Fig. 2-19(e) (see also Table 2-4e)

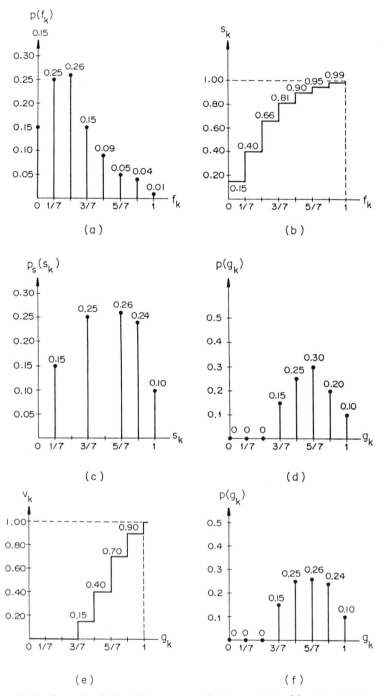

Figure 2-19 Example of the histogram specification method: (a) original histogram, (b) transformation function for histogram equalization of the original histogram, (c) equalized histogram from the original histogram, (d) specified histogram, (e) transformation function for histogram equalization of the specified histogram, and (f) resulting histogram.

can be obtained from the desired probability density shown Fig. 2-19(d) (see also Table 2-4d).

For the final step the inverse mapping is obtained from the histogram equalized s_k levels to the g_k levels. The g_k levels can be obtained by referring to Table 2-4b and Table 2-4e as follows:

$$s_0 = \frac{1}{7} \to g_3 = \frac{3}{7}$$

$$s_1 = \frac{3}{7} \to g_4 = \frac{4}{7}$$

$$s_2 = \frac{5}{7} \to g_5 = \frac{5}{7}$$

$$s_3 = \frac{6}{7} \to g_6 = \frac{6}{7}$$

$$s_4 = \frac{7}{7} \to g_7 = \frac{7}{7}$$

These results can be combined with those of histogram equalization to yield the following direct mappings:

$$f_0 \to s_0 \to g_3, \quad f_1 \to s_1 \to g_4, \quad f_2 \to s_2 \to g_5$$
$$f_3, f_4 \to s_3 \to g_6, \quad f_5, f_6, f_7 \to s_4 \to g_7$$

Redistributing the pixels according to these mappings results in the histogram shown in Fig. 2-19(f). The values are listed in Table 2-4f.

Edge Enhancement

Unsharp Masking   Human eyes perceive an image as more subjectively pleasing with accentuated edges than without. This accentuation of edges and boundaries can be accomplished with a variety of filtering and other image-enhancement techniques such as "unsharp masking." In this process the image is scanned by two apertures, one with normal resolution and the other with a lower resolution, and then an unsharp mask is produced using the normal and low resolution images $F_N(j, k)$ and $F_L(j, k)$. Using the "unsharp mask," a masked or sharpened image is produced and is

$$F_M(j, k) = F_N(j, k) + \lambda[F_N(j, k) - F_L(j, k)]$$
$$= F_N(j, k) + \lambda[Fu(j, k)] \tag{2-88}$$

where λ is a proportionality constant smaller than 1 and $Fu(j, k) = F_N(j, k) - F_L(j, k)$. Figure 2-20 illustrates a typical sharpening process using an "unsharp mask." The masked or sharpened signal has both overshoot as

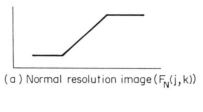

(a) Normal resolution image $(F_N(j,k))$

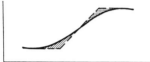

(b) Smoothed low resolusion image $(F_L(j,k))$

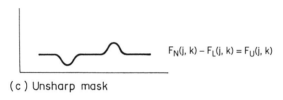

$F_N(j, k) - F_L(j, k) = F_U(j, k)$

(c) Unsharp mask

$F_N(j, k) + \lambda[F_U(j, k)]$

(d) Sharpened image

Figure 2-20 Sharpening process using an image-sharpening mask. The sharpening mask is produced by addition and subtraction of the processed images.

Table 2-5   Several high-pass masks

Mask 1 $H = \begin{bmatrix} 0 & -1 & 0 \\ -1 & 5 & -1 \\ 0 & -1 & 0 \end{bmatrix}$

Mask 2 $H = \begin{bmatrix} -1 & -1 & -1 \\ -1 & 9 & -1 \\ -1 & -1 & -1 \end{bmatrix}$

Mask 3 $H = \begin{bmatrix} 1 & -2 & 1 \\ -2 & 5 & -2 \\ 1 & -2 & 1 \end{bmatrix}$

well as undershoot which accentuate the edges. Subjectively the apparent sharpness of the image is improved.

High-Pass Masking   Edge crispening can also be accomplished by discrete convolutional filtering with convolution kernels that have high-pass filtering characteristics. Several typical high-pass masks are listed in Table 2-5. Note that these masks possess the property that the sum of their elements is unity.

Statistical Differencing   Another interesting edge-enhancement technique is the statistical differencing technique. It uses the statistical standard deviation $\sigma(j, k)$ of the image; for example, an enhanced image $G(\cdot)$ is obtained by dividing the original image $F(\cdot)$ with its standard deviation $\sigma(\cdot)$:

$$G(j, k) = \frac{F(j, k)}{\sigma(j, k)} \tag{2-89}$$

The result tends to improve low contrast in the image or low contrast portions of the image. The standard deviation is calculated in this case as

$$\sigma^2(j, k) = \sum_j \sum_k \left[F(j, k) - \bar{F}(j, k) \right]^2 \tag{2-90}$$

where σ is usually computed over some neighborhood of the pixel and the function $\bar{F}(j, k)$ is the mean value of the original image at the point (j, k) and is approximated by blurring or smoothing the original image by some form of low-pass filter. In the enhanced image the $G(j, k)$ amplitude will be increased with respect to the original image $F(j, k)$ in the regions such as edge points where the $\sigma(\cdot)$ values are lower and will be decreased in regions where $\sigma(\cdot)$ values are relatively high.

2-4-2   Image Filtering and Restoration [11, 12]

Spatial Image Filtering Techniques

In a linear system spatial degradation of an image can be modeled by a linear space invariant point spread function (PSF) or by the impulse response and the noise, which is additive. Restoration of the image then can be performed by linear filtering techniques, some of which are described in this section.

Inverse Filter   The simplest form of restoration filter is the inverse filter in which the degrading transfer function is inverted and used to restore the image. Figure 2-21 presents a block diagram for the analysis of inverse filtering of a continuous image field. An ideal image $f_I(x, y)$ passes through a linear degrading system with an impulse response $h_D(x, y)$ and is combined

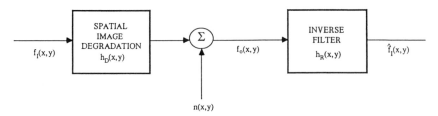

Figure 2-21   Image restoration using inverse filtering.

with uncorrelated noise $n(x, y)$. The observed image $f_O(\cdot)$ is then the ideal image two-dimensionally convolved with the point spread function $h_D(\cdot)$ plus noise:

$$f_O(x, y) = \iint_{-\infty}^{\infty} f_I(\alpha, \beta) h_D(x - \alpha, y - \beta) \, d\alpha \, d\beta + n(x, y) \quad (2\text{-}91)$$

Image restoration then can be described by convolution of the impulse response $h_R(x, y)$ which would be the inverse filter designed on the basis of the image degrading impulse response $h_D(\cdot)$:

$$\hat{f}_I(x, y) = [f_I(x, y) * h_D(x, y) + n(x, y)] * h_R(x, y) \quad (2\text{-}92)$$

Using the Fourier transform and the Fourier convolution theorem, the Fourier domain image corresponding to Eq. (2-92) becomes

$$\hat{F}_I(\omega_x, \omega_y) = [F_I(\omega_x, \omega_y) H_D(\omega_x, \omega_y) + N(\omega_x, \omega_y)] H_R(\omega_x, \omega_y) \quad (2\text{-}93)$$

where $\hat{F}_I(\omega_x, \omega_y)$, $F_I(\omega_x, \omega_y)$, $H_D(\omega_x, \omega_y)$, $N(\omega_x, \omega_y)$, and $H_R(\omega_x, \omega_y)$ are the two-dimensional Fourier transforms of $\hat{f}_I(x, y)$, $f_I(x, y)$, $h_D(x, y)$, $n(x, y)$, and $h_R(x, y)$, respectively. Now, if the restoration filter transfer function $H_R(\omega_x, \omega_y)$, the Fourier transform of the inverse function of the impulse response $h_R(x, y)$, is chosen such that

$$H_R(\omega_x, \omega_y) = \frac{1}{H_D(\omega_x, \omega_y)} \quad (2\text{-}94)$$

then the spectrum of the reconstructed image becomes

$$\hat{F}_I(\omega_x, \omega_y) = F_I(\omega_x, \omega_y) + \frac{N(\omega_x, \omega_y)}{H_D(\omega_x, \omega_y)} \quad (2\text{-}95)$$

Upon inverse Fourier transformation, the restored image function $\hat{f}_I(\cdot)$ can

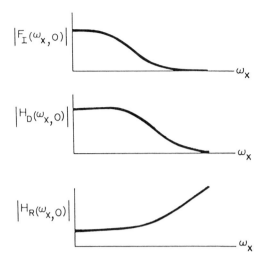

Figure 2-22   One-dimensional version of the inverse filtering process and related spectra. The upper, middle, and lower spectra are the image function, the point spread or degrading function, and the corresponding inverse filter function, respectively. Note the diverging tendency of the restoration filter power spectrum, which will amplify the noise at high frequency. (Reproduced from ref. [6]).

be written as

$$\hat{f}_I(x, y) = f_I(x, y) + \frac{1}{4\pi^2} \iint_{-\infty}^{\infty} \left[\frac{N(\omega_x, \omega_y)}{H_D(\omega_x, \omega_y)} \right] \exp\{i(\omega_x x + \omega_y y)\} \, d\omega_x \, d\omega_y$$

$$(2\text{-}96)$$

In the absence of noise, a perfect restoration will result, but if noise is present, there will be an additive restoration error whose value can become quite large at some spatial frequencies for which $H_D(\omega_x, \omega_y)$ is small. Typically both $H_D(\omega_x, \omega_y)$ and $F_I(\omega_x, \omega_y)$ are small at high spatial frequencies; therefore the fine structure of the image becomes severely degraded. Figure 2-22 illustrates sketches of typical frequency spectra involved in simple inverse filtering.

Wiener Filter with Additive Noise   One of the basic problems of inverse filtering is the extreme sensitivity of the filter to noise since the filter design ignores the noise process. This can be remedied with the Wiener filtering technique, since it incorporates a priori statistical knowledge of the noise in the image. It is assumed that the noise is a zero-mean Gaussian and is independent of the image. It is also assumed that the noise power spectral density $W_N(\omega_x, \omega_y)$ is known. In Wiener filtering the impulse response of the

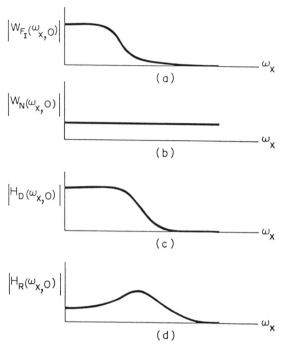

Figure 2-23 One-dimensional version of the derivation process for the Wiener filter and the related spectra. Shown, from the top, are the power spectra of the image function, the noise, the point spread or image degrading function, and the derived Wiener filter function. (Reproduced from ref. [6]).

restoration filter is designed to minimize the mean square error:

$$\varepsilon = E\left\{\left[f_I(x, y) - \hat{f}_I(x, y)\right]^2\right\} \qquad (2\text{-}97)$$

The transfer function of the resultant restoration filter has been found to be

$$H_R(\omega_x, \omega_y) = \frac{H_D^*(\omega_x, \omega_y)}{\left|H_D(\omega_x, \omega_y)\right|^2 + W_N(\omega_x, \omega_y)} \qquad (2\text{-}98)$$

where $H_D(\omega_x, \omega_y)$ and $H_D^*(\omega_x, \omega_y)$ are the transfer function of the spatial degradation and its complex conjugate. As can be seen from Eq. (2-98), in the case of negligible noise [i.e., $W_N(\omega_x, \omega_y) = 0$] the Wiener filter is reduced to the inverse filter. Figure 2-23 illustrates the typical image and noise spectra, image-degrading transfer function, and the resultant Wiener filter transfer function. The basic difference between the inverse filter and the Wiener filter is the noise power spectral density term in the Wiener filter transfer function. The noise power spectral density term makes the filter function smooth and nonsingular with respect to noise even at the high-frequency region in the image.

Wiener Filter—Dynamic Stochastic Blur   In many imaging systems the impulse response of the blur is not fixed or constant; rather, it changes shape in a random manner. A practical example is the blur caused by imaging through a turbulent atmosphere. Obviously the Wiener filter would perform better if it could dynamically adapt to the changing blur impulse response. If this is not possible, a design improvement in the Wiener filter can be obtained by considering the impulse response to be a sample of a 2-D stochastic process with a known mean shape and with a random perturbation about the mean described by a known power spectral density. Transfer functions for this type of restoration filter have been developed by Slepian [7] for several error measures.

Image Power Spectrum Filter   Wiener filters of different forms have also been developed for image restoration for a variety of specific applications. A variation of the Wiener filter known as the *image power spectrum filter* is proposed by Stockham [8] and is given by

$$H_R(\omega_x, \omega_y) = \left[W_{F_I}(\omega_x, \omega_y) \right]^{1/2} \left\{ |H_D(\omega_x, \omega_y)|^2 W_{F_I}(\omega_x, \omega_y) + W_N(\omega_x, \omega_y) \right\}^{-1/2}$$

(2-99)

The power spectrum of the estimated output image from the above filter is given by

$$W_{\hat{F}_I}(\omega_x, \omega_y) = |H_R(\omega_x, \omega_y)|^2 W_{F_O}(\omega_x, \omega_y)$$ (2-100)

where $W_{F_O}(\omega_x, \omega_y)$ represents the power spectrum of the input image data (observed data), which is given by

$$W_{F_O}(\omega_x, \omega_y) = |H_D(\omega_x, \omega_y)|^2 W_{F_I}(\omega_x, \omega_y) + W_N(\omega_x, \omega_y)$$ (2-101)

By assuming that $W_{\hat{F}_I}(\cdot) = W_{F_I}(\cdot)$ and using Eqs. (2-100) and (2-101), it can be shown that the right-hand side of Eq. (2-99) also leads to $H_R(\cdot)$, thus proving the validity of Eq. (2-100). From Eq. (2-100), the restoration filter function can be derived as

$$H_R(\omega_x, \omega_y) = \left\{ \frac{W_{F_I}(\omega_x, \omega_y)}{W_{F_O}(\omega_x, \omega_y)} \right\}^{1/2}$$ (2-102)

Because of the form of Eq. (2-102), this restoration filter is often called the *image power spectrum filter*.

The power spectrum of the restored image as obtained by the Wiener filter with the image spectral density $W_{F_I}(\omega_x, \omega_y)$ thus is given by

$$W_{\hat{F}_I}(\omega_x, \omega_y) = \left\{ W_{F_I}(\omega_x, \omega_y) | H_D(\omega_x, \omega_y) |^2 + W_N(\omega_x, \omega_y) \right\} | H_R(\omega_x, \omega_y) |^2$$

or from Eq. 2-100,

$$W_{\hat{F}_I}(\omega_x, \omega_y) = W_{F_I}(\omega_x, \omega_y) | H_D(\omega_x, \omega_y) |^2 W_{F_I}(\omega_x, \omega_y) / W_{F_O}(\omega_x, \omega_y)$$

$$= | H_D(\omega_x, \omega_y) |^2 W_{F_I}(\omega_x, \omega_y)^2$$

$$\Big/ \left\{ | H_D(\omega_x, \omega_y) |^2 W_{F_I}(\omega_x, \omega_y) + W_N(\omega_x, \omega_y) \right\} \quad (2\text{-}103)$$

Equation (2-103) implies that the power spectra of the restored and the ideal images become identical if they are free of noise.

Geometrical Mean Filter   Stockham and Cole [8, 13] have also proposed a geometrical mean filter, which is defined as

$$H_R(\omega_x, \omega_y) = \left[H_D(\omega_x, \omega_y) \right]^{-S} \left[H_D^*(\omega_x, \omega_y) W_{F_I}(\omega_x, \omega_y) \right]^{1-S}$$

$$\times \left\{ | H_D(\omega_x, \omega_y) |^2 W_{F_I}(\omega_x, \omega_y) + W_N(\omega_x, \omega_y) \right\}^{S-1} \quad (2\text{-}104)$$

where $0 \leq S \leq 1$ is a design parameter. If $S = 1/2$ and $H_D = H_D^*$, the geometrical mean filter reduces to the image power spectrum filter as given in Eq. (2-99).

Constrained Least Squares Filter   Hunt [9] has developed another parametric restoration filter known as the constrained least squares filter, which is given by

$$H_R(\omega_x, \omega_y) = H_D^*(\omega_x, \omega_y) \left\{ | H_D(\omega_x, \omega_y) |^2 + \gamma | \varepsilon(\omega_x, \omega_y) |^2 \right\}^{-1} \quad (2\text{-}105)$$

where γ is a design constant and $\varepsilon(\omega_x, \omega_y)$ is a design spectral variable. The spectral variable can be used to minimize higher-order derivatives of the estimate.

Some Useful Nonlinear Filters

Median Filter   There are several simple nonlinear filters useful in medical imaging, such as the median filter. The median filter is a nonlinear filter particularly useful in reducing impulsive noise, yet preserving the edges in an image while reducing random noise. In a median filter a window slides along

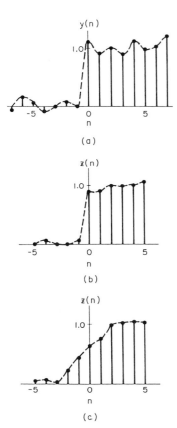

Figure 2-24 Examples of filtering a noisy image: (a) a noisy image with a notable step, (b) results of median filtering, and (c) results of conventional low pass filtering. Note the superior performance of median filtering for certain applications.

the image in one or two dimensions, and the median intensity value of the pixels within the window replaces the intensity of the pixel being processed. For example, if the pixel values within a window are 4, 6, 30, 8, and 16, then the center pixel value 30 is replaced by one of the median values, in this case 8. Figure 2-24 illustrates an example of median filtering and a corresponding conventional low-pass filtering operation for comparison. In Fig. 2-25 additional examples of median filter performance for several different image shapes—such as a discrete step function, a ramp function, and a spike function, operated with a window of five pixels—are given for reference. It is seen from these examples that the median filter has the unusual property of preserving the step and pulse functions without degrading the overall image resolution. An important characteristic of the median filter is that it also smooths the image, the same as a low-pass filter; therefore the median filter is useful in reducing noise. Unlike low-pass filtering, median filtering can preserve the sharpness of the step function and yet smooth a few pixels whose values differ from their surroundings without affecting the other pixels.

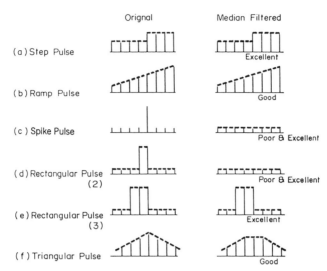

Figure 2-25 Results of median filtering for several image shapes. Note the excellent performance for the steplike and the rectangular images. The median filter is also an ideal filter for the elimination of spike noise [see (c)]. Elimination of the spikes and narrow rectangular pulses, however, can also be considered as loss of information, and therefore, can be categorized as poor performance.

Statistical Scaling Filter   The ability of our visual system to detect an object in a uniform background depends on its size (resolution) and the contrast ratio c, which is defined as

$$c = \frac{\sigma(m, n)}{\mu(m, n)} \tag{2-106}$$

where $\mu(\cdot)$ is the average luminance of the object and $\sigma(\cdot)$ is the standard deviation of the luminance of the object plus its surrounding. $\mu(m, n)$ and $\sigma(m, n)$ are the local mean and the standard deviation of $u(m, n)$ measured over a window W and are given by

$$\mu(m, n) = \frac{1}{N} \sum\sum_{(k, l) \in W} u(m - k, n - l)$$

$$\sigma(m, n) = \left\{ \frac{1}{N} \sum\sum_{(k, l) \in W} [u(m - k, n - l) - u(m, n)]^2 \right\}^{1/2} \tag{2-107}$$

Statistical scaling is then performed by transformation of an image where the weak (i.e., low-contrast) edges are enhanced while the high-contrast edges are surpressed. A special case of this transformation can be performed by assuming that the mean can be written as

$$\nu(m,n) = \frac{\mu(m,n)}{\sigma(m,n)} \qquad (2\text{-}108)$$

Eq. (2-108) now represents that each pixel is scaled by its standard deviation to generate an image whose pixels have unity variance.

2-5 IMAGE QUANTIZATION

Quantization, like other applications, is the first step necessary for the interface to the computer and other digital processors, and requires the speed and the accuracy. In this section some often used quantization methods are discussed in conjunction with image processing.

2-5-1 Scalar Quantization

Quantization usually means discretization of a continuous analog signal and is achieved by processing the amplitude of an analog signal sample by comparing it with a set of decision levels. If the sample amplitude falls between two decision levels, it is quantized to a fixed reconstruction level lying in the quantization band. In a digital system each quantized sample is assigned to a binary code.

Let f and $\hat{f}$ represent the amplitude of a real analog signal and its quantized value, respectively. It is assumed that f is a random process with known probability density $p(f)$ and that f is bound to

$$a_{\min} \leq f \leq a_{\max} \qquad (2\text{-}109)$$

where $a_{\min}$ and $a_{\max}$ represent upper and lower limits of the sample values. The quantization problem includes the specification of a set of decision levels d_j and reconstruction levels r_j. If decision levels are set as

$$d_j \leq f < d_{j+1} \qquad (2\text{-}110)$$

then, the reconstruction levels r_j will also fall between those decision levels:

$$d_j < r_j < d_{j+1} \qquad (2\text{-}111)$$

Figure 2-26 illustrates the manner in which the decision levels d_j and reconstruction levels r_j are placed along a line and along the staircase format for J quantization levels.

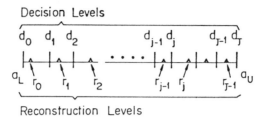

Decision Levels

Reconstruction Levels

Figure 2-26   Decision and reconstruction levels in the quantization process. (Reproduced from ref. [6]).

Decision and reconstruction levels are chosen to minimize some desired quantization error between f and $\hat{f}$. The quantization error measure usually used is the mean square error defined for J quantization levels which is given by

$$\varepsilon = E\left[(f - \hat{f})^2\right] = \int_{a_{\min}}^{a_{\max}} (f - \hat{f})^2 p(f)\, df = \sum_{j=0}^{J-1} \int_{d_j}^{d_{j+1}} (f - r_j)^2 p(f)\, df$$

(2-112)

For a large number of quantization levels J, the probability density $p(f)$ might be represented as a constant value k over each quantization band. Hence

$$\varepsilon = \sum_{j=0}^{J-1} k \int_{d_j}^{d_{j+1}} (f - r_j)^2 \, df$$

(2-113)

which leads to

$$\varepsilon = \frac{1}{3} \sum_{j=0}^{J-1} k\left[(d_{j+1} - r_j)^3 - (d_j - r_j)^3\right]$$

(2-114)

When the range d_{j-1} to d_j is large, an optimum reconstruction level r_j can be determined by minimization of ε with respect to r_j (i.e., $d\varepsilon/dr_j = 0$). The optimum r_j value is found to be a geometrical mean value, which is given by

$$r_j = \frac{d_{j+1} + d_j}{2}$$

(2-115)

Using the result of Eq. (2-115) and after some algebra, the quantization error given in Eq. (2-114) can be written as

$$\varepsilon = \frac{1}{12} \sum_{j=0}^{J-1} k(d_{j+1} - d_j)^3$$

(2-116)

2-5-2 Companding Techniques for Nonlinear Quantization

Finally, let us briefly review nonlinear quantization, which often requires some signal manipulations. It is possible to perform nonlinear quantization with a companding operation; that is, the sample is transformed nonlinearly, and then linear quantization is performed followed by an inverse nonlinear transformation. In the companding system of quantization, the probability density of the transformed samples is forced to be uniform. General notation of transformation from a nonlinear value to a linear value can be written as

$$g = T\{f\} \tag{2-117}$$

where the nonlinear transformation $T(\cdot)$ is chosen such that the probability density of g becomes uniform and is given as

$$p\{g\} = 1 \tag{2-118}$$

The nonlinear transformation function given in Eq. (2-117) is equivalent to the cumulative probability distribution of f. An example of a Gaussian function, its companding transformations, and inverse are given by

$$p(f) = (2\pi\sigma^2)^{-1/2} \exp\left\{-\frac{f^2}{2\sigma^2}\right\} \qquad \text{(source function)} \quad (2\text{-}119)$$

$$g = \frac{1}{2}\operatorname{erf}\left\{\frac{f}{\sqrt{2}\,\sigma}\right\} \qquad \text{(companding transformation)} \quad (2\text{-}120)$$

$$\hat{g} = g \qquad \text{(uniform quantization)} \tag{2-121}$$

$$\hat{f} = \sqrt{2}\,\sigma\,\operatorname{erf}^{-1}\{2\hat{g}\} \qquad \text{(inverse transformation)} \tag{2-122}$$

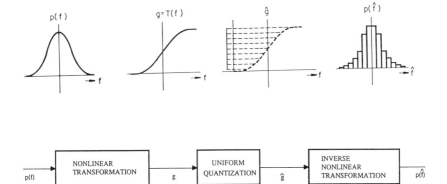

Figure 2-27   Companding and quantization used for uniformity improvement.

where $\operatorname{erf}(x) = 2/\sqrt{\pi} \int_0^x \exp(-y^2)\, dy$ and g is a uniform quantizer. In Fig. 2-27 a corresponding companding quantizer and its operating procedures are illustrated.

REFERENCES

1. R. Bracewell. *The Fourier Transform and Its Application*. New York: McGraw-Hill, 1965.

2. E. O. Brigham. *The Fast Fourier Transform*. Englewood Cliffs, NJ: Prentice Hall, 1974.

3. A. K. Jain. *Fundamentals of Digital Image Processing*. Englewood Cliffs, NJ: Prentice Hall, 1980.

4. N. Ahmed, T. Natarajan, and K. R. Rao. Discrete cosine transform. *IEEE Trans. Comput*. C-23:90–93 (1974).

5. P. Yip and K. R. Rao. A fast computational algorithm for the discrete sine transform. *IEEE Trans. Comm*. COM-28:304–307 (1980).

6. W. K. Pratt. Digital image processing. New York: Wiley, 1978.

7. D. Slepian. Restoration of photographs blurred by image motion. *Bell Sys. Tech. J*. 46:2253–2362 (1967).

8. T. G. Stockham Jr. Image processing in the context of a visual model. *Proc. IEEE*, Vol. 60, No. 7, 828–842 (1972).

9. B. R. Hunt. The application of constrained least squares estimation to image restoration by digital computer. *IEEE Trans. Comput*. C-23:805–812 (1973).

10. J. W. Tukey. *Exploratory Data Analysis*. Reading, MA: Addison-Wesley, 1971.

11. H. C. Andrews and B. R. Hunt. *Digital Image Restoration*. Englewood Cliffs, NJ: Prentice Hall, 1977.

12. J. S. Lim. *Two-dimensional Signal and Image Processing*. Englewood Cliffs, NJ: Prentice Hall, 1990.

13. E. R. Cole. The removal of unknown image blurs by homomorphic filtering. Ph.D. dissertation. Department of Electrical Engineering, University of Utah, Salt Lake City, June 1973.

IMAGE RECONSTRUCTION FROM PROJECTIONS IN TWO DIMENSIONS

Image reconstruction, which is sometimes known as "image reconstruction from projection," is now a well-known mathematical image processing technique. It was mainly developed for X-ray computerized tomography. Besides its original application in X-ray CT, the projection reconstruction technique is now widely used in many scientific and medical disciplines such as X-ray crystallography, nuclear emission tomography, and nuclear magnetic resonance imaging. As will be seen in this chapter, 2-D and 3-D images can be reconstructed with remarkable accuracy, with the extent of accuracy limited only by statistics [1–4].

The reconstruction algorithms to be discussed are the two main schemes, namely 2-D planar imaging and 3-D volume image reconstructions. In terms of the available data configurations, parallel-beam and divergent- (fan- or cone-) beam data sets are the two generally available data forms; they are therefore treated separately. In addition we will briefly consider an alternative image reconstruction algorithm based on the statistical properties of the data, namely the "expectation maximization" algorithm. Image reconstruction algorithms are categorically arranged as a reference in Table 3-1. In this chapter, mainly 2-D planar imaging is treated and 3-D volume imaging or true three dimensional reconstruction will be treated separately in Chapter 4.

3-1 MATHEMATICAL PRELIMINARIES FOR TWO- AND THREE-DIMENSIONAL IMAGE RECONSTRUCTIONS

The basic data to be used in the reconstruction are the projection data, and the simplest form of the projection data is illustrated in Fig. 3-1. In this figure

Table 3-1 Image reconstruction algorithms

Projection Reconstruction (PR)	2-D PR	Filtered Backprojection (FB)	Parallel-Beam Mode
			Fan-Beam Mode
		Backprojection Filtering (BF)	Parallel-Beam or Fan-Beam Mode
	3-D PR	True Three-Dimensional Reconstruction (TTR)	Parallel-Beam Mode
			Cone-Beam Mode
		Generalized TTR (GTTR)	
		Planar-Integral Projection Reconstruction (PPR)	
Iterative Method	Algebraic Reconstruction Technique (ART)		
	Maximum Likelihood Reconstruction (MLR) or Expectation Maximization (EM) Reconstruction		
Fourier Reconstruction (FR)	Direct Fourier Reconstruction (DFR)		
	Direct Fourier Imaging in NMR		

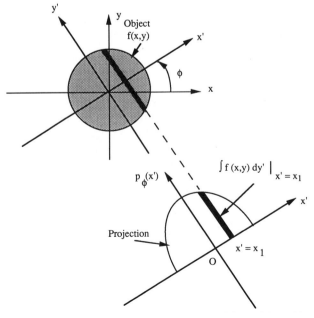

Figure 3-1 Radon transform or line-integral projection in relation to an image function $f(x,y)$. Radon transform or projection data at a given view angle ϕ are shown at the bottom.

the line integrals of a physical object are estimated along straight lines. Each line integral, in practice, represents a physical property of a strip with a finite width which is determined mainly by the detector width. At each view ϕ a set of line-integral data is obtained. Complete projection data sets can be obtained by repeated assessment of the data round 180° or 360° with a specified angular interval $\Delta\phi$. All the measured line-integral sets around 180° or 360° are referred to as *line-integral projection data* or simply *projections*.

3-1-1   Radon Transform

The Radon transform of a function $f(x, y)$, represented as $p_\phi(x')$, is defined as its line integral along a line that is parallel with the y'-axis at a distance x' from the origin. Here (x', y') are the rotated coordinates of (x, y) with the rotation angle ϕ (see Fig. 3-1).*

We denote the Radon transform operator for a given function f as $\mathscr{R}[f]$. Mathematically it is given by

$$p_\phi(x') \equiv \mathscr{R}[f(x, y)]$$

$$= \iint_{-\infty}^{\infty} f(x, y)\delta(x \cos \phi + y \sin \phi - x') \, dx \, dy$$

$$= \int_{-\infty}^{\infty} f(x' \cos \phi - y' \sin \phi, x' \sin \phi + y' \cos \phi) \, dy' \quad (3\text{-}1)$$

where

$$\begin{bmatrix} x' \\ y' \end{bmatrix} = \begin{bmatrix} \cos \phi & \sin \phi \\ -\sin \phi & \cos \phi \end{bmatrix} \begin{bmatrix} x \\ y \end{bmatrix}$$

or

$$\begin{bmatrix} x \\ y \end{bmatrix} = \begin{bmatrix} \cos \phi & -\sin \phi \\ \sin \phi & \cos \phi \end{bmatrix} \begin{bmatrix} x' \\ y' \end{bmatrix} \quad (3\text{-}2)$$

Since the function $p_\phi(x')$ is the 1-D projection of $f(x, y)$ at an angle ϕ, the Radon transform operator performs the line integral of the 2-D image data along y'. As is known, these projection data will be the base data for the image to be reconstructed, and this is the most important theme of 2-D and 3-D image reconstruction.

---

*Note that the role of the angle θ in Eqs. (2-33) to (2-35) is now changed to ϕ in this chapter for simple notational convenience.

The Radon transform or projection operation has the following properties:

1. The projections are periodic in ϕ with a period of 2π and symmetric; therefore, $p_\phi(x') = p_{\phi \pm \pi}(-x')$.
2. The Radon transform leads to the projection or central slice theorem through a 1-D or 2-D Fourier transform.
3. The Radon transform domain data provide a sinogram (see subsection 3-1-3).

3-1-2   Projection Theorem or Central Slice Theorem

Let us now consider the basic relationship between the 2-D Fourier transform of the object function $f(x, y)$ and the 1-D Fourier transform of its Radon transform or the projection data $p_\phi(x')$. This relationship provides the fundamental basis of projection-based image reconstruction. One-dimensional Fourier transform of the projection data $p_\phi(x')$ will result in

$$P_\phi(\omega) \equiv \mathscr{F}_1\left[p_\phi(x')\right]$$

$$= \int_{-\infty}^{\infty} p_\phi(x')\exp(-i\omega x')\, dx'$$

$$= \iint_{-\infty}^{\infty} f(x' \cos \phi - y' \sin \phi, x' \sin \phi + y' \cos \phi)\exp(-i\omega x')\, dx'dy'$$

$$(3\text{-}3)$$

By transforming the coordinates from (x', y') to (x, y) using Eq. (3-2), Eq. (3-3) can be rewritten as

$$P_\phi(\omega) = \iint_{-\infty}^{\infty} f(x, y)\exp\left[-i\omega(x \cos \phi + y \sin \phi)\right] dx\, dy \quad (3\text{-}4\mathrm{a})$$

Knowing that the Fourier domain coordinates $\omega_{x'}$ and $\omega_{y'}$ correspond to $\omega_{x'} = \omega \cos \phi$ and $\omega_{y'} = \omega \sin \phi$, Eq. (3-4a) can also be written as

$$P_\phi(\omega) = F(\omega \cos \phi, \omega \sin \phi)$$

$$= F(\omega_{x'}, \omega_{y'})\big|_\phi \quad \text{or} \quad F(\omega_x, \omega_y)\big|_\phi$$

$$= F(\omega, \phi) \quad (3\text{-}4\mathrm{b})$$

where $F(\omega_x, \omega_y)$ is the 2-D Fourier transform of $f(x, y)$, and $(\omega_{x'}, \omega_{y'})$ or (ω_x, ω_y) and (ω, ϕ) represent the cartesian and polar coordinates in the Fourier domain, respectively.

Equation (3-4b) states that a 1-D Fourier transform of the projection data $p_\phi(x')$ at a given view angle ϕ is the same as the radial data passing through the origin at a given angle ϕ in the 2-D Fourier transform domain data. This is the *projection theorem* (also known as the *central slice theorem*) which plays a key role in 2-D and 3-D image reconstruction from projections.

3-1-3 Sinogram

It is interesting to see how the Radon transform maps data from the object space domain (x, y) to the projection data space domain (x', ϕ). Let us consider an arbitrary point q at (x, y) or (r, θ) in the object space, as shown in Fig. 3-2. Since all the points on the line L (same as the ray direction) in the object domain are mapped onto a single point corresponding to (x', ϕ) in the projection domain through the Radon transform, the point q at (r, θ) is also mapped onto a point in the (x', ϕ) domain according to the relation $x' = r \cos(\phi - \theta)$. This sinusoidal equation implies that a point q at (r, θ)

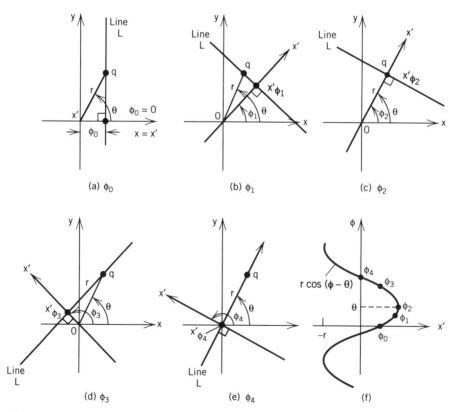

Figure 3-2 Sinogram of a point q at a various angles ϕ_i for a given θ: (a) $\phi_0 = 0$, (b) $\phi_1 = 45°$, (c) $\phi_2 = 60°$, (d) $\phi_3 = 135°$, and (e) $\phi_4 = 150°$. At $i = 0$ or $\phi_i = 0$, the rotated coordinates x' coincide with the reference x-axis and give $x' = r \cos(\phi - \theta) = r \cos \theta$.

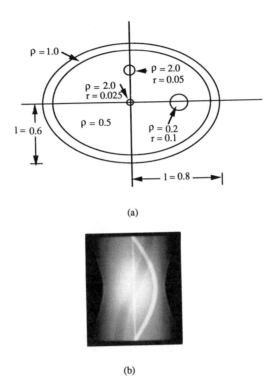

(a)

(b)

Figure 3-3 (a) Phantom with several distinct objects at various positions; (b) corresponding sinogram.

will follow a locus or *sinogram* in the projection space (x', ϕ), as shown in Fig. 3-2. In the figure the sinogram translates the rotational behavior of each pixel in the spatial domain onto the Radon transform domain. For example, a point at the center represents the straight line at the center in the sinogram, while a point at the utmost periphery represents a sinusoidal trace with the largest amplitude. Any point in the image represented by polar coordinates (r, θ) therefore will simply follow the equation $x' = r \cos(\phi - \theta)$. The sinusoidal trajectory of a point q is illustrated for various view angles ϕ_i. An example of a simple object phantom and its projection data in a sinogram format are shown in Figs. 3-3(a) and (b), respectively.

3-1-4 Inverse Radon Transform

As will be shown, image reconstruction from the projection can be thought of as the inverse Radon transform of the projection data $p_\phi(x')$. Before we invoke the inverse Radon transform directly from projection data $p_\phi(x')$, let us consider the 2-D inverse Fourier transform operation of $F(\omega_x, \omega_y)$. As we have learned, once the 2-D Fourier domain data are available, the estimated image function $\hat{f}(x, y)$ can be obtained simply by the inverse Fourier transform:

$$
\begin{aligned}
\hat{f}(x, y) &= \mathscr{F}_2^{-1}\big[F(\omega_x, \omega_y)\big] \\
&= \iint_{-\infty}^{\infty} F(\omega_x, \omega_y)\exp\big[i(x\omega_x + y\omega_y)\big]\, d\omega_x\, d\omega_y \\
&= \hat{f}(r, \theta)
\end{aligned}
\tag{3-5}
$$

If we write (ω_x, ω_y) in Eq. (3-5) in polar coordinates (ω, ϕ), it can easily be shown that

$$
\hat{f}(r, \theta) = \int_0^{\pi}\int_0^{\infty} F(\omega, \phi)\exp\big[i\omega(x\cos\phi + y\sin\phi)\big]|J|\, d\omega\, d\phi
\tag{3-6}
$$

where $x\cos\phi + y\sin\phi = x'$, $\omega = \sqrt{\omega_x^2 + \omega_y^2}$, $\phi = \tan^{-1}[\omega_y/\omega_x]$, $\omega_x = \omega\cos\phi$, $\omega_y = \omega\sin\phi$, and $|J|$ is the Jacobian. The Jacobian $|J|$ again is given as

$$
\begin{aligned}
|J| &= \begin{vmatrix} \dfrac{\partial\omega_x}{\partial\omega} & \dfrac{\partial\omega_y}{\partial\omega} \\[2ex] \dfrac{\partial\omega_x}{\partial\phi} & \dfrac{\partial\omega_y}{\partial\phi} \end{vmatrix} \\[2ex]
&= \begin{vmatrix} \cos\phi & \sin\phi \\ -\omega\sin\phi & \omega\cos\phi \end{vmatrix} \\[1ex]
&= \omega\cos^2\phi + \omega\sin^2\phi \\
&= |\omega|
\end{aligned}
\tag{3-7}
$$

By changing the limits of integration in Eq. (3-6) to $0 \le \phi < \pi$ and $-\infty < \omega < \infty$, and replacing $F(\omega, \phi)$ with $P_\phi(\omega)$, Eq. (3-6) can be rewritten as

$$
\begin{aligned}
\hat{f}(r, \theta) &= \int_0^{\pi}\int_{-\infty}^{\infty} |\omega|P_\phi(\omega)\exp\big[i\omega(x\cos\phi + y\sin\phi)\big]\, d\omega\, d\phi \\
&= \int_0^{\pi} p_\phi^*(x')\, d\phi
\end{aligned}
\tag{3-8}
$$

where

$$
\begin{aligned}
p_\phi^*(x') &= \int_{-\infty}^{\infty} |\omega|P_\phi(\omega)\exp(i\omega x')\, d\omega \\
&= \mathscr{F}_1^{-1}\big[|\omega|P_\phi(\omega)\big] \\
&= \mathscr{F}_1^{-1}\big[|\omega|\big] * p_\phi(x')
\end{aligned}
\tag{3-9}
$$

In Eq. (3-9) the asterisk ($*$) denotes the 1-D convolution operator. Note that $p_\phi^*(x')$ represents the filtered projection data (note this operation does not include noise filtering).

We may also consider the above reconstruction process as an inverse Radon transform. An inverse Radon transform therefore involves both filtering and backprojection; that is, the estimated image function $\hat{f}(x, y)$ or $\hat{f} = (r, \theta)$ is notationally given as

$$\hat{f}(x, y) = \beta \mathcal{H}\{\mathcal{R}[f(x, y)]\}$$
$$= \mathcal{R}^{-1}\{\mathcal{R}[f(x, y)]\} \tag{3-10}$$

where β and $\mathcal{H}$ denote the backprojection and the spatial domain filtering operators, respectively, and $\mathcal{R}^{-1}$ represents the inverse Radon transform operator. The inverse Radon transform therefore can be represented as a filtering followed by a backprojection operation:

$$\mathcal{R}^{-1} = \beta \mathcal{H} \tag{3-11}$$

Alternatively, the filtered Radon transform or the filtered projection $p_\phi^*(x')$ can also be derived as [6]

$$p_\phi^*(x') = \mathcal{F}_1^{-1}[\omega P_\phi(\omega)] * \mathcal{F}_1^{-1}[\text{sgn}(\omega)]$$
$$= \frac{1}{i2\pi}\left(\frac{\partial p_\phi(x')}{\partial x'}\right) * \left(\frac{-1}{i\pi x'}\right)$$
$$= \frac{1}{2\pi^2}\int_{-\infty}^{\infty}\frac{\partial p_\phi(t)}{\partial t}\left(\frac{1}{x' - t}\right)dt \tag{3-12}^*$$

where t is a variable of x'. Equation (3-12) can be derived simply by using the following relationships and integral notation of the convolution operation:

$$\mathcal{F}_1^{-1}[\omega P_\phi(\omega)] = \frac{1}{i2\pi}\frac{\partial p_\phi(x')}{\partial x'}$$
$$\mathcal{F}_1^{-1}[\text{sgn}(\omega)] = \frac{-1}{i\pi x'} \tag{3-13}$$

Equation (3-8) can therefore be written as

$$\hat{f}(r, \theta) = \frac{1}{2\pi^2}\int_0^\pi\int_{-\infty}^{\infty}\frac{\partial p_\phi(t)}{\partial t}\frac{1}{x' - t}\,dt\,d\phi \tag{3-14}$$

Considering the fact that the operation $\{\int_{-\infty}^{\infty}(\partial p_\phi(t)/\partial t)[1/(x' - t)]\,dt\}/2\pi^2$ is a filtering process while the operation $\int_0^\pi d\phi\, 1/\pi$ is a backprojection

---

*Sign sgn($\cdot$) is a function which is negative unity in minus x and positive unity in plus x.

process, Eq. (3-14) can be written again as

$$\hat{f}(r,\theta) = \beta\mathcal{H}\{p_\phi(x')\}$$

$$= \beta\mathcal{H}\{\mathcal{R}[f(x,y)]\}$$

$$= \mathcal{R}^{-1}\{\mathcal{R}[f(x,y)]\} = \hat{f}(x,y) \qquad (3\text{-}15)$$

This result is identical to Eq. (3-10). It is also interesting to note that the operation $\{\int_{-\infty}^{\infty}(\partial p_\phi(t)/\partial t)[1/(x'-t)]\,dt\}/2\pi^2$ is also equivalent to the Hilbert transform of the derivative of $p_\phi(x')$ representing a bidirectional filtering operation in the Fourier domain.

3-2 TWO-DIMENSIONAL PROJECTION RECONSTRUCTION

Although 2-D projection reconstruction is also known as "3-D reconstruction," it is a common practice to refer to it as 2-D slice image reconstruction to distinguish it from 3-D volume image reconstruction, which will be discussed in the next chapter. In this section therefore we will discuss several variations of 2-D slice image reconstruction derived from the basic formulation discussed above.

3-2-1 Filtered Backprojection (FB) Algorithm

The filtered backprojection (FB) or convolution backprojection algorithm is the most popular, and perhaps most frequently used, reconstruction method so far and is used in both transmission and emission CT. It should be noted that although the FB type of projection reconstruction algorithm is not used in NMR imaging as frequently as in X-CT or emission CT, it can be effectively used for NMR imaging depending on the situation. There are two basic approaches to the FB algorithm depending on the system and the detection scheme employed. Generally the FB algorithm is divided into two schemes: namely the parallel-beam and divergent or fan-beam modes.

Parallel-Beam Mode
The parallel-beam mode is perhaps the simplest and the most often used mode. It is also the foundation of the other reconstruction algorithms that are to be derived. From the projection theorem and Eqs. (3-8) and (3-9), it can easily be shown that the estimated object function $\hat{f}(x, y)$ can be recovered from projection data $p_\phi(x')$ as

$$\hat{f}(x,y) = \frac{1}{\pi}\int_0^\pi d\phi \int_{-\infty}^\infty dx'\, p_\phi(x')h(x\cos\phi + y\sin\phi - x') \quad (3\text{-}16)$$

where $h(x)$ is derived from the inverse Fourier transform of the Jacobian $|\omega|$:

$$h(x) = \mathscr{F}_1^{-1}[|\omega|]$$
$$= \mathscr{F}_1^{-1}[H(\omega)] \tag{3-17}$$

Note here that we have noted the convolution kernel $h(x)$ in Eq. (3-17) as an inverse Fourier transform of $|\omega|$ or the filter function $H(\omega)$, for simplicity, as will be discussed further in the following sections. Equation (3-17), however, is not attainable in practice due to its divergent nature. It is worth noting that $h(x)$ and $H(\omega)$ are the one-dimensional operators in the spatial and the Fourier domains, respectively, and are used for the deblurring operation of the $1/r$ blur arising in the backprojection operation. Several modified filter functions that consider the sampled nature of the digital data and the noise behavior have been developed. The choice of the optimum filter function is certainly an important factor in image reconstruction.

Let us consider a basic filter function derived from the ramp function $H(\omega) = |\omega|$ developed by Ramachandran and Lakshiminarayanan [5]. Here we assume that the number of view angles and the data sampling along the x'-axis are sufficiently fine so that effects such as aliasing do not affect the reconstructed image; that is $f(x, y)$ is band-limited in the spatial frequency by B. If we assume that $f(x, y)$ is band-limited in the spatial frequency by B, the filter kernel $H(\omega) = |\omega|$ can be given by a simple windowed filter function, which is the same as the one defined by Ramachandran and Lakshiminarayanan (often called the "Ram–Lak filter"):

$$H_{RL}(\omega) = \begin{cases} |\omega|, & (|\omega| \leq 2\pi B) \\ 0, & (\text{otherwise}) \end{cases} \tag{3-18a}$$

For this case the corresponding spatial domain filter kernel $h_{RL}(x)$ can be obtained by the inverse Fourier transform of $H_{RL}(\omega)$:

$$h_{RL}(x) = \frac{1}{2\pi} \int_{-\infty}^{\infty} H_{RL}(\omega) \exp(ix\omega) \, d\omega$$

$$= \frac{1}{2\pi} \int_{-2\pi B}^{2\pi B} |\omega| \exp(ix\omega) \, d\omega$$

$$= 2B^2 \, \text{sinc}(2\pi Bx) - B^2 \, \text{sinc}^2(\pi Bx) \tag{3-18b}$$

where $\text{sinc}(x) = \sin(x)/x$. The filter function and kernel given in Eq. (3-18(a) and (b)) are sketched in Fig. 3-4(a) and (b).

Since the projection data are discrete, the filter kernel should also be discrete in the spatial domain. By applying the Nyquist sampling criteria with uniformly spaced $\Delta x = 1/(2B)$, the sampled version of the Ram–Lak filter

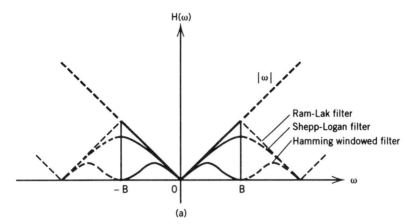

Figure 3-4   (a) Examples of the band-limited filter function of sampled data. Note the cyclic repetitiveness of the digital filter.

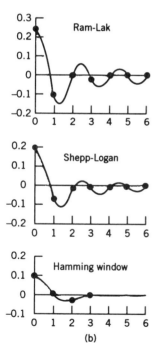

Figure 3-4 (b) Spatial domain filter kernals corresponding to the filter functions shown in the Ram-Lak filter is a high-pass filter with a sharp response but results in some noise enhancement, while the Shepp-Logan and the Hamming window filters are noise-smoothed filters and therefore have better SNR.

kernel can be obtained by discretizing Eq. (3-18b) at discrete positions $x_k = k\,\Delta x$. This filter kernel is given by

$$h_{\mathrm{RL}}(0) = B^2 = \frac{1}{4\,\Delta x^2} \qquad\qquad (\text{if } k = 0)$$

$$h_{\mathrm{RL}}(k) = 0 \qquad\qquad (\text{if } k \text{ even})$$

$$h_{\mathrm{RL}}(k) = \frac{-4B^2}{\pi^2 k^2} = \frac{-1}{\pi^2 k^2\,\Delta x^2} \qquad (\text{if } k \text{ odd}) \qquad (3\text{-}18c)$$

Since the Ram–Lak filter kernel is sampled in the spatial domain, the filter function in the Fourier domain will be a set of periodically repeating band-limited spectra, as shown in Fig. 3-4(a). This periodicity or cyclic nature necessarily requires smooth and continuous functions at the repeated frequency bandwidth; that is, nB where $n = 1, 2 \ldots$. As is known, the sharp boundary of a filter function such as the Ram–Lak filter often makes the spatial domain filter kernel oscillatory and therefore introduces a ringing artifact in the reconstructed image.

Shepp and Logan [6] have suggested an alternative filter function by introducing a sine-weighted function into the $|\omega|$ filter function, effectively removing the ringing artifact. The filter function derived is given by (see also Fig. 3-4(a))

$$H_{SL}(\omega) = \begin{cases} |\omega|\,\sin\!\left(\dfrac{\omega}{4B}\right), & |\omega| < 2\pi B \\ 0, & \text{otherwise} \end{cases} \qquad (3\text{-}19)$$

The corresponding filter kernel in the spatial domain is given by

$$h_{SL}(x) = \frac{B}{\pi^2}\left\{ \frac{1 - \cos 2\pi B[(1/4B) + x]}{(1/4B) + x} + \frac{1 - \cos 2\pi B[(1/4B) - x]}{(1/4B) - x} \right\} \qquad (3\text{-}20)$$

A sampled version of Eq. (3-20) can be easily obtained simply by replacing x with $x_k = k\,\Delta x$ and is given by

$$h_{SL}(k) = \frac{-2}{\pi^2\,\Delta x^2(4k^2 - 1)}$$

$$= \frac{-8B^2}{\pi^2(4k^2 - 1)} \qquad (3\text{-}21)$$

The spatial domain of the Shepp–Logan filter kernel is also shown in Fig. 3-4 (b). Similarly many weighted $|\omega|$ filter functions can also be derived, such as the filter function weighted by the Hamming window, as shown in Fig. 3-4 (a), and its corresponding filter kernel, as shown in Fig. 3-4(b).

Let us now consider the generalized filter function or kernel, applicable to a noisy condition [2, 7]. Consider a noisy projection data $\dot{p}_\phi(x')$ which is given by

$$\dot{p}_\phi(x') = p_\phi(x') + n_\phi(x') \tag{3-22}$$

It is worth noting that most of the previous filterings [e.g., Eq. (3-9)] have been referred for deblurring without consideration of the noise in the projection data; however, the noisy projection data given in Eq. (3-22) requires deblurring as well as noise filtering. By introducing an optimum filter $H_{\text{opt}}(\omega, \phi)$, the noisy projection data $\dot{p}_\phi(x')$ can be both deblurred and noise filtered:

$$\mathscr{F}_1^{-1}\left[H_{\text{opt}}(\omega, \phi)\right] * \dot{p}_\phi(x') = \dot{p}_\phi^*(x'). \tag{3-23}$$

Now $\dot{p}_\phi^*(x')$ represents the noise filtered as well as deblurred version of the noisy projection data $\dot{p}_\phi(x')$ [compare with Eq. (3-9)]. Note here that the optimum filter $H_{\text{opt}}(\omega, \phi)$ now has both noise filtering and deblurring operations in contrast to the previous filter, which has only the deblurring operation; that is, $H_\phi(\omega) = H(\omega)$ was simply the weighted $|\omega|$ function without consideration of the noise in the projection data.

The optimum filter function $H_{\text{opt}}(\omega, \phi)$ can be derived in terms of the minimum mean square error criteria (i.e., from the viewpoint of a Wiener filter) and can be formulated as

$$H_{\text{opt}}(\omega, \phi) = |\omega| H_W(\omega, \phi) \tag{3-24}$$

where $H_W(\omega, \phi)$ denotes the Wiener filter. A Wiener filter with known power spectra for both the image function and noise is given by

$$H_W(\omega, \phi) = \frac{H_D^*(\omega, \phi) W_P(\omega, \phi)}{|H_D(\omega, \phi)|^2 W_P(\omega, \phi) + W_{PN}(\omega, \phi)} \tag{3-25}$$

where $H_D(\omega, \phi)$ and $H_D^*(\omega, \phi)$, $W_P(\omega, \phi)$, and $W_{PN}(\omega, \phi)$ are the image degradation function and its complex conjugate, the signal power spectrum of the projection data at view angle ϕ, and the power spectrum of the noise in the projection data, respectively. Moreover, Eq. (3-25) can also be simplified to

$$H_W(\omega, \phi) = \frac{H_D^*(\omega, \phi)}{|H_D(\omega, \phi)|^2 + (W_{PN}(\omega, \phi)/W_P(\omega, \phi))} \tag{3-26}$$

In Eq. (3-26), $[W_P(\omega, \phi)]/[W_{PN}(\omega, \phi)]$ is approximately equivalent to the SNR (signal-to-noise ratio). Consequently the optimum filter function can be represented as

$$H_{\text{opt}}(\omega, \phi) = |\omega| H_W(\omega, \phi)$$

$$= \frac{|\omega| H_D^*(\omega, \phi)}{|H_D(\omega, \phi)|^2 + 1/\text{SNR}(\omega, \phi)} \qquad (3\text{-}27)$$

where $\text{SNR}(\omega, \phi)$ is the signal to noise ratio of the projection at a given view angle ϕ.

Fan-Beam Mode

Although the parallel-beam reconstruction algorithm has been a basic tool for image reconstruction, the fan-beam reconstruction algorithm is, nevertheless, widely used, for example, in X-CT where X-ray beams are emitted in a diverging fan-beam mode. In addition image reconstruction using the fan-beam algorithm often provides better resolution with the same dimension of sampled data as the parallel case due to improved sampling at the central region [8, 9]. The resolution improvement with fan-beam mode reconstruction is found to be of importance, for example, in positron emission tomography where the intrinsic image resolution is restricted by the detector size.

Among the various approaches to the derivation of the fan-beam reconstruction algorithm, use of a coordinate transformation from the parallel-beam algorithm is found to be useful [10–12]. If the fan-beam projection data set is represented by $p_\alpha(\beta)$ where α and β represent rotation angles of the center ray of the fan-beam and the detector position, respectively (see Fig. 3-5), the relation between the parallel- and fan-beam projection data with coordinates (x', ϕ) and (α, β) is given by

$$x' = R_d \sin \beta$$

$$\phi = \alpha + \beta \qquad (3\text{-}28)$$

where R_d is the distance between the center point and the apex of the fan. Since the reconstruction formula derived for the parallel projection data set given in Eq. (3-16) is equally valid for 0 to 2π, one can start from the basic equation, which is given by

$$\hat{f}(x, y) = \frac{1}{2\pi} \int_0^{2\pi} d\phi \int_{-\infty}^{\infty} dx' \, p_\phi(x') h(x \cos \phi + y \sin \phi - x') \quad (3\text{-}29)$$

where $p_\phi(x')$ is the projection data we have discussed in parallel-beam reconstruction. Using Eqs. (3-28) and (3-29), the fan-beam analogy can be

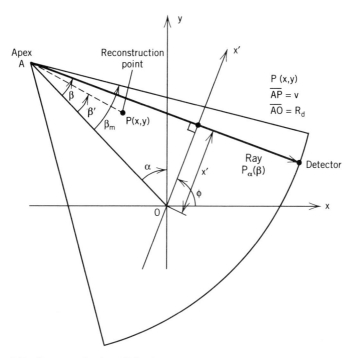

Figure 3-5   Geometry for the 2-D fan beam projection data and reconstruction process.

derived as

$$\hat{f}(x, y) = \frac{1}{2\pi} \int_0^{2\pi} d\alpha \int_{-\beta_m}^{\beta_m} d\beta$$
$$\times p_\alpha(\beta) h\{x \cos(\alpha + \beta) + y \sin(\alpha + \beta) - R_d \sin \beta\} |J| \quad (3\text{-}30)$$

where β_m is the maximum range of β depending on both the object size and the distance between the apex of the fan and the center point of the image, and $|J|$ is the Jacobian of the coordinate transformation from the parallel-beam to the diverging fan-beam which is given by

$$|J| = \left| \frac{\partial(x', \phi)}{\partial(\alpha, \beta)} \right| = R_d \cos \beta \quad (3\text{-}31)$$

After some rearrangement, Eq. (3-30) can be rewritten as

$$\hat{f}(x, y) = \frac{1}{2\pi} \int_0^{2\pi} d\alpha \int_{-\beta_m}^{\beta_m} d\beta \, p_\alpha(\beta) h\{v \sin(\beta' - \beta)\} |J| \quad (3\text{-}32)$$

where

$$v = \sqrt{(x \cos \alpha + y \sin \alpha)^2 + (x \sin \alpha - y \cos \alpha + R_d)^2} \quad (3\text{-}33)$$

$$\beta' = \tan^{-1}\left[\frac{x \cos \alpha + y \sin \alpha}{x \sin \alpha - y \cos \alpha + R_d}\right] \quad (3\text{-}34)$$

Note that β' represents an angle between the central line and the line passing through the reconstruction point at (x, y). Using the relation given in Eq. (3-17), the filter function in Eq. (3-32) can be written as

$$h\{v \sin(\beta' - \beta)\} = \frac{1}{2\pi}\int_{-\infty}^{\infty} d\omega \, |\omega| \, \exp[i\omega v \sin(\beta' - \beta)] \quad (3\text{-}35)$$

If we define a new variable ω', which is given by

$$\omega' = \omega \frac{v \sin(\beta' - \beta)}{\beta' - \beta}$$

or

$$\omega = \omega' \frac{\beta' - \beta}{v \sin(\beta' - \beta)} \quad (3\text{-}36)$$

and substitute it into Eq. (3-35), Eq. (3-35) becomes

$$h\{v \sin(\beta' - \beta)\} = \frac{1}{2\pi}\int_{-\infty}^{\infty} d\omega' \left[\frac{\beta' - \beta}{v \sin(\beta' - \beta)}\right]^2 |\omega'| \exp[i\omega'(\beta' - \beta)]$$

$$= \frac{1}{v^2}\left[\frac{\beta' - \beta}{\sin(\beta' - \beta)}\right]^2 h(\beta' - \beta) \quad (3\text{-}37)$$

Using the new filter kernel given in Eq. (3-37), the fan-beam reconstruction algorithm given in Eq. (3-32) is reduced to

$$\hat{f}(x, y) = \int_0^{2\pi} d\alpha \, W_2 \int_{-\beta_m}^{\beta_m} d\beta [W_1 p_\alpha(\beta)] g(\beta' - \beta) \quad (3\text{-}38)$$

where

$$W_1 = |J| = R_d \cos \beta \quad (3\text{-}39)$$

$$W_2 = \frac{1}{2\pi}\frac{1}{v^2} \quad (3\text{-}40)$$

$$g(\beta) = \left[\frac{\beta}{\sin(\beta)}\right]^2 h(\beta) \quad (3\text{-}41)$$

Note here that W_1 and W_2 are the two functions that perform the β- and v-dependent angular and distance weightings, respectively, while $g(\beta)$ is the space-invariant filter function newly defined for the fan-beam algorithm.

3-2-2 Backprojection Filtering Algorithm

Although the filtered backprojection (FB) algorithm is by far the most popular algorithm in CT and provides a high-quality reconstructed image with computational efficiency, it requires uniformly sampled data both in the linear translational and angular directions. The FB algorithm also often requires rebinning and interpolation which would, in some cases, be difficult and cumbersome.

An alternative approach to image reconstruction starting from simple backprojection and filtering later, is also possible, rather than filtered back-projection, and is known as the *backprojection-filtering (BF) algorithm*. If the data collection method employed has a general transverse axial scanning format without any other specific knowledge of the data collection process itself, one can assume that the simple backprojected image would follow the well-known $1/r$ blur. Therefore the resultant simple backprojected or blurred image $b(x, y)$ will appear as

$$b(x, y) = f(x, y) * * \left(\frac{1}{r}\right) \qquad (3\text{-}42)$$

where $f(x, y)$ is the object function and $**$ represents the 2-D convolution operator. From Eq. (3-42), and using the Hankel transform relation, the estimated image $\hat{f}(x, y)$ can be obtained as

$$\hat{f}(x, y) = \mathscr{F}_2^{-1}\left[\rho B(\omega_x, \omega_y)\right] \qquad (3\text{-}43)$$

where $B(\omega_x, \omega_y) = \mathscr{F}_2[b(x, y)]$ and ρ is the radial spatial frequency.*

Although the BF algorithm appears to be attractive, it is rarely used because the resultant images are usually poor in comparison with the images obtained by the conventional FB algorithm. Assume an $N \times N$ image in the spatial domain and that image reconstruction follows the BF algorithm. Image degradation in this case would occur mainly due to the following two reasons:

1. The backprojection process itself generates an image that extends beyond matrix size $N \times N$ in the spatial domain and thus requires truncation of the 2-D blurred image to match the original matrix size of the $N \times N$. This means loss of information.
2. The 2-D filter function to be used in rectangular cartesian coordinates has a slope discontinuity near the cutoff frequency that results in the ringing artifact.

---

*ρ and ω are used freely depending on the situation.

The above two aspects should be considered to obtain high-quality images through the BF algorithm given in Eq. (3-43). Although this is not a fundamental problem, the following algorithmic precaution have to be taken if BF algorithm is to be used for high quality image reconstruction. First, if backprojection precedes convolution filtering, the extension of the blurred backprojection image should be allowed beyond an $N \times N$, for example, $2N \times 2N$ or larger. Similar to the case of 1-D filtering, optimum selection of the 2-D filter function with an appropriate windowing will also be an important consideration for the BF algorithm, since the slope discontinuity of the 2-D filter at the boundary near the cutoff frequency will result in the ringing artifact. Finally, the step-by-step image reconstruction procedure for the BF algorithm based on Eq. (3-43) is as follows:

1. Obtain the backprojected image at least up to $2N \times 2N$ if the size of the original image matrix is $N \times N$.
2. Obtain the 2-D FFT of the full $2N \times 2N$ data array.
3. Obtain the optimum filtering in 2-D in Fourier domain by multiplication of ρ filter.
4. Obtain the 2-D inverse FFT and select the $N \times N$ image in the central region.
5. Normalize the image.

REFERENCES

1. Z. H. Cho (ed.). *IEEE Trans. Nucl. Sci.* NS-21, Special issue on 3-D Image Reconstruction (June 1974).
2. Z. H. Cho and J. R. Burger. *IEEE Trans. Nucl. Sci.* NS-24 (April 1977).
3. Z. H. Cho. Computerized tomography. *Encyclopedia of Physical Science and Technology*, vol. 3. San Diego: Academic Press, 1987, pp. 507–544.
4. H. J. Scudder, *IEEE Proc.* Vol. 66, pp. 628–637 (June 1978).
5. G. N. Ramachandran and A. V. Lakshiminarayanan, *Proc. Nat. Acad. Sci. U.S.* 68:2236–2240 (1971).
6. L. A. Shepp and B. F. Logan. *IEEE Trans. Nucl. Sci.* NS-21:21–41 (1974).
7. E. T. Tsui and T. F. Budinger. *IEEE Trans. Nucl. Sci.* NS-26:2687–2690 (1979).
8. G. T. Herman. *J. Comp. Assist. Tomog.* 3:361–366 (1979).
9. Z. H. Cho, K. S. Hong, J. B. Ra, and S. Y. Lee. *IEEE Trans. Nucl. Sci.* NS-28:94–98 (1981).
10. G. T. Herman, A. V. Lakshiminarayanan, and A. Naparastek. *Comput. Biol. Med.* 6:259–271 (1976).
11. C. B. Lim, L. T. Chang, and R. J. Jaszczak. *IEEE Trans. Nucl. Sci.* NS-27:559–568 (1980).
12. B. K. P. Horn. *IEEE Proc.* 67:1616–1623 (1979).

4

IMAGE RECONSTRUCTION FROM PROJECTIONS IN THREE-DIMENSIONS AND OTHER RELATED TECHNIQUES

4-1 THREE-DIMENSIONAL PROJECTION RECONSTRUCTION

4-1-1 True Three-dimensional Reconstruction (TTR) Algorithm for the Complete Sphere

In the conventional reconstruction algorithm, the 3-D volume image of an object is formed by stacking 2-D slice images, each of which has been reconstructed by the conventional 2-D reconstruction algorithm using projection data. In emission CT (ECT) such as PET, photons are emitted from the radionuclides in the object in 4π directions. It is therefore necessary to utilize all the emitted photons in 4π directions instead of restricting the data collection to a plane or transaxial direction for a given image plane (in conventional 2-D slice imaging only a small fraction of the emitted photons are utilized and, consequently, produce images of low signal to noise ratio). In ECT all the emitted photons can be collected by use of a complete or a near complete spherical detection geometry and those data collected can then be used for the direct reconstruction of the 3-D volume image.

Let us consider a detection geometry in the form of a complete sphere and assume that all the photons emitted in 4π directions are measured by the detectors on the surface of the sphere and are rearranged into 2-D parallel line projection data sets. In the case of direct 3-D volume image reconstruction by backprojection of the projection data in three dimensions in analogy to the 2-D backprojection algorithm, the PSF would be $1/r^2$, and the simple backprojected image function would be given by*

$$b(x, y, z) = f(x, y, z) * * * \left(\frac{1}{r^2} \right) \tag{4-1}$$

where $* * *$ represents a 3-D convolution operator. Since $\mathscr{F}_3[1/r^2] = 1/\rho$, where ρ is the radial spatial frequency, that is, $\rho = (\omega_x^2 + \omega_y^2 + \omega_z^2)^{1/2}$, and $\mathscr{F}_3[\cdot]$ is a 3-D Fourier transform operator, the object function obtained is given by

$$f(x, y, z) = \mathscr{F}_3^{-1}\left[\rho B(\omega_x, \omega_y, \omega_z) \right] \tag{4-2}$$

where $\mathscr{F}_3^{-1}[\cdot]$ is a 3-D inverse Fourier transform operator and $B(\cdot) = \mathscr{F}_3[b(x, y, z)]$. Equation (4.2) defines a process of 3-D filtering of a simple backprojected (blurred) image by backprojection filtering (BF) which would require long computation time, especially when the backprojected image extends to infinity, as we have discussed in the previous sections.†

As an alternative approach, the filtered backprojection (FB) algorithm based on the 3-D version of the projection theorem is considered (i.e., the Fourier transform of a 2-D projection data in spatial domain corresponds to a 2-D data passing through the coordinate center in the 3-D Fourier transform domain). Let 2-D projection data $p_{\theta, \phi}(s, t)$ has a Fourier transform relation as

$$\mathscr{F}_2\left[p_{\theta, \phi}(s, t) \right] = F(\omega_s, \omega_t; \theta, \phi) \tag{4-3}$$

where (ω_s, ω_t) are the spatial frequency domain coordinates corresponding to the spatial coordinates (s, t). As is known, the 3-D backprojected data in the Fourier domain will result in a $1/\rho$, and it therefore requires compensation by a ρ filter,* where $\rho = (\omega_s^2 + \omega_t^2)^{1/2}$.

Then the 3-D FB algorithm can be written as

$$f(x, y, z) = \frac{1}{4\pi^2} \int_0^\pi d\theta \cos \theta \int_0^{2\pi} d\phi \left[\mathscr{F}_2^{-1}[\rho] * * p_{\theta, \phi}(s, t) \right] \tag{4-4}$$

As mentioned earlier, the 2-D filter kernel or 2-D convolution kernel is $\mathscr{F}_2^{-1}[\rho]$.

4-1-2 True Three-dimensional Reconstruction Algorithm of Generalized Form [1, 2]

The ideal detector configuration for ECT is a complete sphere where the 3-D images can be reconstructed by the FB algorithm using the 2-D line-integral

---

*Note here that $\mathscr{F}_1[1/r] = 1/\rho$, $\mathscr{F}_2[1/r] = 1/\rho$, and $\mathscr{F}_3[1/r^2] = 1/\rho$.
†In three dimensional case, the extent of blur may not be as large as in the two-dimensional case due to the $1/r^2$ blur. BF is, therefore, more suitable for the 3-D case than the 2-D case.

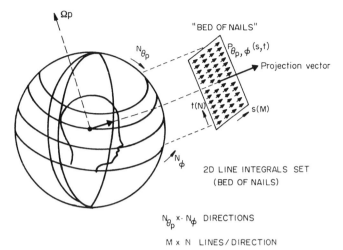

Figure 4-1   2-D bed of nails projection data that can be acquired at a given view angle (ϕ, θ) or orientation vector Ω_p.

data sets. Such an ideal case is illustrated in Fig. 4-1 where the 2-D projection data $p_{\theta_p, \phi}(s, t)$ or the bed of nails forms a basic data set in direct 3-D volume reconstruction. Practical system design, however, prohibits the construction of such an ideal system and requires modifications so that the system can accommodate several different object shapes other than a simple sphere (e.g., an elongated object such as the human body). In a practical situation a truncated spherical geometry (Fig. 4-2) is considered and a generalized true three-dimensional reconstruction (GTTR) algorithm suitable for such a configuration is developed [1]. This algorithm will eventually lead to a generalized algorithm for both 2-D slice reconstruction and 3-D volume image reconstruction of a complete sphere.

Consider the detector geometry of a truncated sphere where parts of the surface have been truncated along the body axis to allow access of the elongated shapes such as the human body (see Fig. 4-2). For a given truncated spherical detection geometry, the 3-D image can be obtained by using the slice-by-slice reconstruction technique at a given slice orientation in which a complete set of 2-D projection data is available. All the 3-D images reconstructed for all the available slice orientations are then summed for statistical improvement of the final image. Essentially this is the basis of the generalized true three-dimensional reconstruction algorithm developed for a truncated spherical geometry. Naturally, this algorithm is a general form from which both a single slice image reconstruction and a full 3-D volume image reconstruction can be derived, with each treated as a special case.

For a generalized detection geometry with a certain degree of truncation, each 2-D parallel line-integral data set corresponding to a given object size has only a fixed number of slice orientations. Conceptually, one set of 2-D

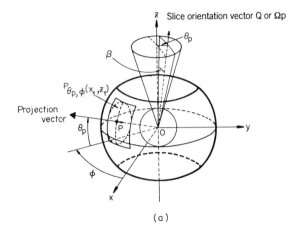

(a)

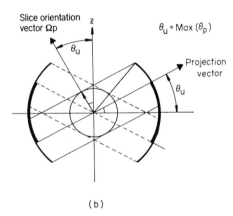

(b)

Figure 4-2 (a) Basic configuration of the truncated spherical geometry for the generalized TTR algorithm. (b) Maximum value of θ_p for a given object size and degree of truncation, for example, $\theta_p \rightarrow \theta_u$.

projection data in the bed of nails can be repeatedly used for the reconstruction of a set of slice images for a number of different slice orientations. For each slice orientation vector therefore a set of slice images perpendicular to the orientation vector exists. The number of slice orientation vectors, which is given for each 2-D projection data set for a given θ_p, allows us to treat a certain projection data set in a unified fashion; that is, a 2-D projection data set at a given θ_p can be processed with one filter function called a composite filter function, as will be discussed in the following.

Let us consider a 2-D projection data set or bed of nails projected on a direction parallel with the line $\overline{OP}$ in Fig. 4-2(a) where O and P are the center of the coordinates and the projection plane, respectively. Considering the truncated geometry, the projection data (the bed of nails) are shared <u>only</u> by the limited slice orientations rotated from $-\beta$ to $+\beta$ around the line $\overline{OQ}$, as shown in Fig. 4-2(a). The angle β depends on the polar angle θ_p of the center line of the 2-D projection data as well as the angle θ_u, which is defined as the maximum limiting angle within which a set of parallel-beam data are assumed and is given by

$$\beta = \cos^{-1}\left[\frac{\cos\theta_u}{\cos\theta_p}\right] \tag{4-5}$$

where $\theta_u = \max[\theta_p]$. This situation is illustrated in Fig. 4-2(b) in relation to the truncation angle and the size of the object. Using a composite filter yet to be defined, a simplified and unambiguous 2-D filtering can be performed instead of the repeated 1-D filtering used in slice-by-slice reconstruction and the superposition of those images to form a true volumetric image.

Let the reconstructed image function $f(\bar{r})$, using a composite filter $h(s, t: \alpha)$ be defined as

$$f(\bar{r}) = \frac{\int_0^\pi d\phi \int_{-\theta_u}^{\theta_u} d\theta_p \cos\theta_p \int_{-\beta}^{\beta} d\alpha \left[p_{\theta_p,\phi}(s,t) * * h(s,t:\alpha) \right]}{\int_0^\pi d\phi \int_{-\theta_u}^{\theta_u} d\theta_p \cos\theta_p \int_{-\beta}^{\beta} d\alpha}$$

$$= \frac{\int_0^\pi d\phi \int_{-\theta_u}^{\theta_u} d\theta_p \cos\theta_p \left[p_{\theta_p,\phi}(s,t) * * \int_{-\beta}^{\beta} d\alpha\, h(s,t:\alpha) \right]}{\int_0^\pi d\phi \int_{-\theta_u}^{\theta_u} d\theta_p \cos\theta_p \int_{-\beta}^{\beta} d\alpha} \tag{4-6}$$

where $\int_{-\beta}^{\beta} d\alpha\, h(s, t: \alpha)$ is the composite filter to be derived for each $p_{\theta_p,\phi}(s, t)$ which is the 2-D parallel projection data at the polar angle θ_p with the azimuthal angle ϕ, α is the rotation angle variable which is proportional to the θ_p, $h(s, t: \alpha)$ is the filter kernel to be convolved with the projection data at each given slice orientation α and $\bar{r}$ is a three dimensional coordinate vector. The denominator of Eq. (4-6) is the normalization factor, which is the sum of all the weighting coefficients of the projection data. Here the t-axis lies in the direction of the line $\overline{OQ}$, and the s-axis is normal to both the line $\overline{OP}$ and the line $\overline{OQ}$ given in Fig. 4.2(a).

Since it is often easier to comprehend a filter concept in the frequency domain, let us define the relation between the filter kernel $h(s, t: \alpha)$ and its Fourier counterpart $H(\omega_s, \omega_t; \alpha)$ as

$$h(s, t; \alpha) = \mathscr{F}_2^{-1}\left[H(\omega_s, \omega_t; \alpha) \right] \tag{4-7a}$$

where $H(\cdot)$ is defined as

$$H(\omega_s, \omega_t: \alpha) = |\omega_{s'_\alpha}|$$
$$= \rho|\cos(\xi - \alpha)| \tag{4-7b}$$

where ξ is the spatial frequency domain angular variable. Note here that $\omega_{s'_\alpha}$ is the rotated version of the axis ω_s with angle α in the frequency domain and (ρ, ξ) represents the polar coordinates of (ω_s, ω_t). One can define the composite filter by integration of the filter function over β given in Eq. (4-7b):

$$H_\beta(\omega_s, \omega_t) = \mathcal{F}_2\left[\int_{-\beta}^{\beta} d\alpha\, h(s, t; \alpha) \right]$$

$$= \int_{-\beta}^{\beta} d\alpha\, \mathcal{F}_2[h(s, t; \alpha)]$$

$$= \int_{-\beta}^{\beta} d\alpha\, \rho |\cos(\xi - \alpha)|$$

$$= H_{\theta_p}(\omega_s, \omega_t) \tag{4-7c}$$

or

$$= H_{\theta_p}(\rho, \xi) \tag{4-7d}$$

This frequency domain composite filter concept is the key element in the GTTR algorithm. Examples of the composite filters derived for several different θ_p, therefore different β, are shown in Fig. 4-3.

In Eq. (4-6) note that the projection data set $p_{\theta_p, \phi}(s, t)$ is practically independent of the rotation angle α, Eq. (4-6) can therefore be replaced by a simple 2-D filtering process, with the composite filter function given in Eq. (4-7c):

$$f(\bar{r}) = \frac{\int_0^\pi d\phi \int_{-\theta_u}^{\theta_u} d\theta_p \cos\theta_p \mathcal{F}_2^{-1}\left[P_{\theta_p}(\omega_s, \omega_t) H_{\theta_p}(\omega_s, \omega_t) \right]}{\int_0^\pi d\phi \int_{-\theta_u}^{\theta_u} d\theta_p \cos\theta_p \int_{-\beta}^{\beta} d\alpha} \tag{4-8}$$

where $\mathcal{F}_2^{-1}[\cdot]$ denotes 2-D inverse Fourier transform.

The $H_{\theta_p}(\omega_s, \omega_t)$ or $H_{\theta_p}(\rho, \xi)$ can be obtained by simply integrating Eq. (4-7c) over β. The results are given as

$$H_{\theta_p}(\rho, \xi) = \begin{cases} 2\rho \cos\xi \sin\beta, & 0 \le \xi \le \dfrac{\pi}{2} - \beta \\[2mm] 2\rho(1 - \sin\xi \cos\beta), & \dfrac{\pi}{2} - \beta < \xi \le \dfrac{\pi}{2} \end{cases} \tag{4-9}$$

$H_{\theta_p}(\omega_s, \omega_t)$ also has interesting behavior; it will lead to a conventional 2-D $|\omega|$ filter as well as a 2-D ρ filter in the case of a complete sphere or ideal spherical case.

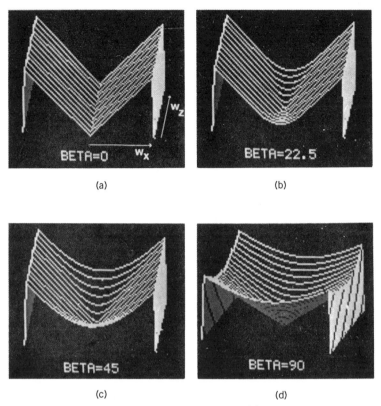

(a)   (b)

(c)   (d)

Figure 4-3 Composite 2-D filter functions for various β: (a) conventional 2-D reconstruction filter, (b) composite filter function for $\beta = 22.5°$, (c) composite filter function for $\beta = 45°$, and (d) composite filter function for $\beta = 90°$.

Let us first consider $\theta_u \rightarrow \pi/2$. This is the case of a complete spherical data collection and naturally $\beta \rightarrow \pi/2$. Therefore, Eq. (4-9) leads to

$$H_{\theta_p}(\rho, \xi) = 2\rho(1 - \sin \xi \cos \beta)|_{\beta \rightarrow \pi/2}$$

$$= 2\rho \qquad (4\text{-}10)$$

Equation (4-10) is the expected result and is consistent with the well-known 2-D ρ filter for 3-D volume image reconstruction. In the second case, where $\theta_u \rightarrow 0$, Eq. (4-9) leads to a conventional 1-D $|\omega|$ filter:

$$H_{\theta_p}(\rho, \xi) = 2\rho \cos \xi \sin \beta$$

$$= 2\omega_s \sin \beta$$

$$= k|\omega_s| \qquad (4\text{-}11)$$

Note that $\sin \beta$ is independent of frequency and can eventually be normalized. Equation (4-11) is also an important result, since it is the conventional 1-D $|\omega|$ filter for 2-D slice image reconstruction. It has therefore been proved that the filter $H_{\theta_p}(\cdot)$ is a generalized filter that can be applied to 2-D slice image reconstruction at one extreme (i.e., $\theta_u = 0$) and 3-D volume image at the other extreme (i.e., the complete spherical object when $\theta_u = \pi/2$). Clearly Eq. (4.8) will lead to any intermediate form of image reconstruction such as the truncated sphere.

4-1-3   Planar-Integral Projection Reconstruction

Fourier NMR imaging techniques suggest the possibility of exciting the entire volume of an object, thereby obtaining planar-integral data sets with which an efficient volume image reconstruction can be performed [3]. Let us consider the 1-D planar-integral projection data of a 3-D object along a given direction T at an angle (θ, ϕ), which is given by

$$p_{\theta, \phi}(t) = \iiint\limits_{-\infty}^{\infty} f(x, y, z)\delta(T - t)\, dx\, dy\, dz \qquad (4\text{-}12)$$

where

$$T = x \cos \phi \sin \theta + y \sin \phi \sin \theta + z \cos \theta \qquad (4\text{-}13)$$

In Eq. (4-13), θ and ϕ represent the polar and azimuthal angle, respectively in spherical coordinates (see Fig. 4-4). By taking the 1-D Fourier transform of $p_{\theta, \phi}(t)$, one obtains

$$P_{\theta, \phi}(\rho) = \int_{-\infty}^{\infty} p_{\theta, \phi}(t)\exp(-i\rho t)\, dt$$

$$= F(\omega_x, \omega_y, \omega_z)\big|_{\theta, \phi} \qquad (4\text{-}14)$$

where $F(\omega_x, \omega_y, \omega_z)$ is the 3-D Fourier transform of the spatial domain object function $f(x, y, z)$ and ρ is the radial frequency. Equation (4-14) is another 3-D projection theorem that states that the 1-D Fourier transform of the planar-integral data at a given polar angle θ and azimuthal angle ϕ gives the 1-D radial frequency data in 3-D Fourier space $F(\omega_x, \omega_y, \omega_z)$. The spatial 1-D planar integral projection data along a direction t and the corresponding 1-D Fourier domain data are shown in Figs. 4-4 (a) and (b).

Conceptually direct volume image reconstruction can be achieved through the 3-D inverse Fourier transform of the complete set of Eq. (4-14). Using the spatial domain planar-integral data given in Eq. (4-12) and the relation of the Fourier transform of a derivative, it can be shown that the resultant

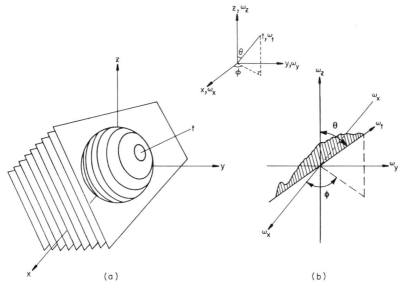

Figure 4-4 Data set for planar-integral projection reconstruction: (a) a planar-integral data set in the spatial domain representing $p_{\theta,\phi}(t)$ and (b) the Fourier domain correspondence to (a).

reconstruction image is obtained by

$$f(x, y, z) = -\frac{1}{8\pi^2} \int_0^{2\pi} d\phi \int_0^{\pi} d\theta \sin \theta p''_{\phi,\theta}(t) \qquad (4\text{-}15)$$

where $p''_{\phi,\theta}(t)$ is the second derivative of $p_{\phi,\theta}(t)$ with respect to t. Some planar-integral-projection-reconstruction-related applications are given in Chapter 10, "Magnetic Resonance Imaging: Mathematics and Algorithms."

4-2 ITERATIVE RECONSTRUCTION TECHNIQUES

4-2-1 Algebraic Reconstruction Technique [4]

Iterative techniques are often used in image reconstruction as an alternative to projection reconstruction, especially in the areas of emission tomography. The algebraic reconstruction technique (ART) was the first of its kind based on the iterative procedures and was first used in the EMI brain scanner developed by Hounsfield. ART is, however, not the major algorithm used in commercial scanners these days mainly due to its computational inefficiency. Another drawback of the ART is that the iteration procedure can start only after all the projection data are measured or collected. Currently the ART algorithm is used only in some specific applications such as the case of limited view angle reconstruction. A brief illustration of the ART algorithm is given in this section.

Let us consider a square grid superimposed on the image $f(x, y)$ with f_n representing the image value of the nth cell in $f(x, y)$ and assumed to be a constant value within the cell. Then a ray can be defined by a strip of a certain width passing through the xy-plane. If a ray integral is called a *ray sum*, the ray sum of the mth ray p_m can be represented as

$$p_m = \sum_{n=1}^{N} W_{nm} f_n, \qquad m = 1, 2, \ldots, M \qquad (4\text{-}16)$$

where N and M are the total number of cells per ray and the number of rays, respectively, and W_{nm} is a weighting factor that represents the contribution of the nth cell to the mth ray sum. W_{nm} is the area of the nth image cell

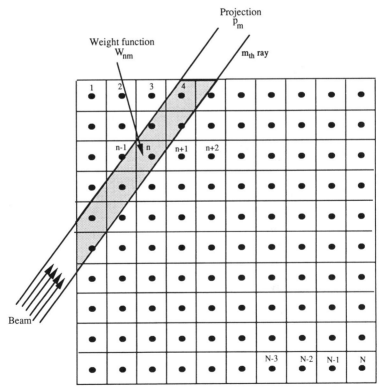

Figure 4-5 Reconstruction process in the iterative technique. Each ray p_m overlaps a pixel element with a different fraction. These overlapping areas are called *weight functions*, and denoted W_{nm}, representing the weight function of the nth pixel and the mth ray.

covered by the mth ray, most of which are zero with the exception of those overlapping the image cells. Note here that the ray is a strip with finite width. The width is usually the size of the square pixel dimension, as shown in Fig. 4-5.

Now the value of the image cell f_n can be obtained by using the measured projection data p_m. It is an inversion problem in the general sense and can be solved by using the conventional matrix inversion. It is found, however, that the computational efficiency of such a method is extremely low, especially for large M and N values.

Instead of a direct solution by matrix inversion, an iteration method can be sought. In this case Eq. (4-16) can be thought of as M linear equations with N unknowns. The solution is sought by checking the consistency of the equations by iteratively searching the f_n values. A suitable initial guess for the solution should be given before the start of the iteration. Although this type of iteration technique works well in many types of image reconstruction problems, iteration techniques of various types based on statistical properties, such as the EM (expectation maximum) or ML (maximum likelihood) iterations algorithms are more useful and are commonly used.

4-2-2 Expectation Maximization Reconstruction [5]

The expectation maximization (EM) algorithm is an iterative method that maximizes the likelihood function or the probability of the reconstructed image for a given set of measured projection data [5].

If each emitted photon in a box or pixel b ($b = 1, 2, \ldots, B$) in the object is detected by a detector unit d with a probability $p(b, d)$, $d = 1, 2, \ldots, D$, then the unknown emission density $f(b)$ can be estimated using the measured projection data $n^*(d)$ in the detector d. Let $\lambda^*(d)$ be the expected counts in detector d due to the emitted photons from every pixel b; that is, $\lambda^*(d)$ is given by

$$\lambda^*(d) = \sum_{b=1}^{B} f(b)p(b, d) \qquad (4\text{-}17)$$

Assuming that the photon emissions follow the Poisson distribution, the likelihood function $\mathscr{L}$ can be defined as follows:

$$\mathscr{L} = \prod_{d=1}^{D} \exp[-\lambda^*(d)] \frac{[\lambda^*(d)]^{n^*(d)}}{n^*(d)!}$$

$$= \prod_{d=1}^{D} P_{n^*(d)}[\lambda^*(d)] \qquad (4\text{-}18)$$

where $p_{n^*(d)}[\lambda^*(d)]$ is the Poisson distribution and $\lambda^*(d)$ is the expectation of $n^*(d)$. The goal of this algorithm is to find an estimate of the unknown image $f(b)$ by maximizing the likelihood function defined in Eq. (4-19).

In implementing the iterative computation, differences between steps k and $k + 1$ are measured until the differences are minimized. The decision rule for stopping the iteration operation can be determined, in reality, by the measurement of the logarithm of the likelihood ratio:

$$\log\left(\frac{\mathscr{L}^{k+1}}{\mathscr{L}^k}\right) = \log(\mathscr{L}^{k+1}) - \log(\mathscr{L}^k) \tag{4-19}$$

By substituting the likelihood function given in Eq. (4-18), Eq. (4-19) can be written as

$$\log\left(\frac{\mathscr{L}^{k+1}}{\mathscr{L}^k}\right) = \sum_{d=1}^{D}\left[\lambda^{(k)*}(d) - \lambda^{(k+1)*}(d) + n^*(d)\log\frac{\lambda^{(k+1)*}(d)}{\lambda^{(k)*}(d)}\right] \tag{4-20}$$

Equation (4-20) is calculated using Eq. (4-17) where the $p(b, d)$'s are known and $f(b)$ is the calculated pixel value. Initially $f(b)$ can be assumed uniform or can be derived from convolution backprojection image data.

The EM algorithm has been found to be an effective reconstruction algorithm for ECT, especially in positron emission tomography where positron emission follows Poisson statistics.

4-3   FOURIER RECONSTRUCTION

4-3-1   Fourier Reconstruction from Projections [6, 7]

From the projection theorem given in the previous section, the radial data set of the 2-D Fourier transform of the object function can be obtained through the 1-D Fourier transform of the projection data. The interpolation of this radial data from polar to cartesian coordinates followed by the 2-D or 3-D inverse Fourier transform provides an alternative way of reconstructing the 2-D and 3-D images. Currently the FB algorithm provides a high-quality reconstructed image and is the most popular, although a considerable amount of computation time is required primarily due to the backprojection operation.

The above algorithm is considered to be a direct Fourier reconstruction (DFR) technique. The DFR algorithm requires, however, a fast and accurate polar to cartesian coordinate interpolation. Since the quality of the reconstructed image is often dependent on the accuracy of the interpolation. If the interpolation to be performed is in the form of a 2-D interpolation, a DFR algorithm will require a long computation time. Although several efficient interpolation schemes have been developed and proposed, 2-D interpolations still take substantially longer times than the 1-D interpolation. One of the promising data acquisition schemes that could lead to 1-D sampling is the concentric square raster scan shown in Fig. 4-6 [5]. The DFR technique with this concentric square raster sampling is attractive in some applications, for example, in NMR imaging where the measured data themselves are in the Fourier domain and the sampling interval is controllable simply by varying the magnitude of the gradient field at each projection data acquisition. In Fig. 4-6(a) a spatial domain sampling density variation which could fit the proposed concentric raster scan is shown. Shown in Fig. 4-6(b) is an example of the concentric square sampling resulting from the Fourier transform of the

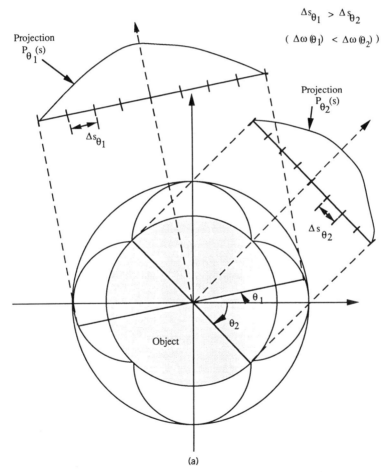

(a)

Figure 4-6 (a) Spatial domain path of concentric square sampling; (b) resulting sampled concentric square raster in the Fourier domain.

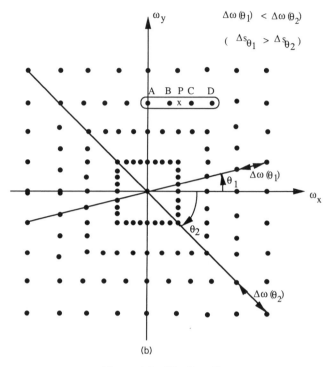

(b)

Figure 4-6   *(Continued)*

sampling pattern shown in Fig. 4-6(a). The advantage of this concentric raster sampling is clear from the example of the 1-D interpolation shown in Fig. 4-6(b), where a point P is one-dimensionally interpolated by using points A, B, C, and D, instead of two-dimensional interpolation which is needed for the data in the conventional polar grids.

4-3-2   Fourier Imaging in NMR

Another interesting image reconstruction method ideally suited for NMR imaging is the simple 2-D Fourier transform [8, 9]. This Fourier imaging method, which was originally suggested by Kumar, Welti, and Ernst, can be explained in conjunction with the inherent characteristics of the detected NMR signal. (Details of NMR imaging and image reconstruction will be discussed in later chapters.)

In NMR imaging the measured signal $s(t_x, t_y)$ is usually known as the "free induction decay" (FID) or "echo signal." It can be represented as

$$s(t_x, t_y) = M_0 \iint_{-\infty}^{\infty} f(x, y) \exp(i\gamma x G_x t_x + i\gamma y G_y t_y)\, dx\, dy \quad (4\text{-}21)$$

where M_0 is the equilibrium magnetization, $f(x, y)$ is the 2-D spin density (e.g., proton density) distribution, γ is the gyromagnetic ratio, and G_x and G_y are the x- and y-directional gradient fields, respectively. If in Eq. (4-21) we let $\omega_x = \gamma x G_x$ and $\omega_y = \gamma y G_y$, it will become

$$s(t_x, t_y) = M_0 \int\!\!\!\int_{-\infty}^{\infty} f(x, y) \exp\left[i(\omega_x t_x + \omega_y t_y)\right] dx\, dy \qquad (4\text{-}22)$$

Note that $dx \simeq d\omega_x$ and $dy \simeq d\omega_y$. As shown, the measured signal $s(t_x, t_y)$ is the 2-D inverse Fourier transform of the spin density $f(x, y)$. The spin density image can therefore be reconstructed simply by taking the 2-D Fourier transform of the measured FID signal $s(t_x, t_y)$.

If we represent the reconstructed image as $\tilde{f}(\omega_x, \omega_y)$, then we have

$$\tilde{f}(\omega_x, \omega_y) = \int\!\!\!\int_{-\infty}^{\infty} s(t_x, t_y) \exp\left[-i(t_x \omega_x + t_y \omega_y)\right] dt_x\, dt_y \qquad (4\text{-}23)$$

The reconstructed image $\tilde{f}(\omega_x, \omega_y)$ is then related to the original density function $f(x, y)$ as

$$\tilde{f}(\omega_x, \omega_y) = kf(\gamma G_x x, \gamma G_y y)$$
$$\cong k'f(x, y) \qquad (4\text{-}24)$$

where k and k' are constants. In conjunction with the previously discussed concentric data sampling, the measured data can easily be obtained in the equi-sampled cartesian domain simply by varying the gradient strength. Then the NMR image reconstruction can proceed without additional interpolation processes. Thus the reconstruction process can be substantially simplified.

REFERENCES

1. Z. H. Cho, J. B. Ra, and S. K. Hilal. *IEEE Trans. Med. Imag.* MI-2:6–8 (1983).
2. J. Colsher. *Phys. Med. Biol.* 25:103–105 (1980).
3. L. A. Shepp. *J. Comput. Assit. Tomogr.* 4:94–107 (1980).
4. R. Gordon, R. Bender, and G. T. Herman. *J. Theor. Biol.* 29:471 (1970).
5. L. A. Shepp and Y. Vardi. *IEEE Trans. Med. Imag.* MI-1:113–122 (1982).
6. R. M. Mersereau and A. V. Oppenheim. *IEEE Proc.* 62:1319–1338 (1974).
7. Z. H. Cho, J. C. Jung, and H. B. Song. Direct Fourier reconstruction techniques in NMR tomography. In *Selected Topics in Imaging Science*, vol. 23. O. Nalcioglu and Z. H. Cho, eds. Berlin: Springer-Verlag, 1984, pp. 40–61.
8. A. Kumar, D. Welti, and R. Ernst. *J. Mag. Res.* 18:69–83 (1975).
9. Z. H. Cho, H. S. Kim, H. B. Song, and J. Cumming. *Proc. IEEE* 70:1152–1173 (1982).

II

IMAGING WITH IONIZING RADIATION

5

RADIATION PHYSICS AND DETECTORS

Electronic methods for the investigation of radiation are based on the interaction between the nuclear particles or quanta with a substance contained in a special device, detector, or transducer in which the energy of the registered particle E is transformed into some electrical quantity such as a current pulse $i(t)$, a charge Q, or a voltage V. The passage of a particle or a quantum through the sensitive volume of the detector is accompanied by the appearance of a short-duration current pulse $i(t)$ in the output circuit. This current pulse charges the output capacitor of the detector in such a way that a voltage pulse $v(t)$ is produced at its output. The amplitude of this pulse is proportional to the charge $Q = \int i(t)\,dt$ which is supplied to the capacitor by the detector current.

If a one-to-one correspondence exists between the energy E of the gamma quanta or particle slowed down in the sensitive volume of the detector and the amplitude of the output electric current or voltage pulse, then it is possible to measure the energy of the particles or the quanta striking the detector. The most interesting cases are those in which the amplitude of the pulse is proportional to the energy E. Such a spectrometer has a linear scale and has some form of linear relationship between the energy and amplitude of the electrical signal.

Detectors that possess a unique connection between E and V do not exist in actuality. Even if the investigated radiation is monoenergetic, the amplitudes of the detector output pulses are always fluctuate with some uncertainty in accordance with the laws of probability. The smaller the fluctuation, the more distinguishable the lines, or as it is customarily stated, the higher its resolution. Detectors that linearly convert the energy E into an amplitude V with sufficient resolution are called *spectrometrometers*, and in this chapter we will study such detectors in detail.

5-1   INTERACTION OF RADIATION WITH MATTER

Charged particles passing through matter gradually lose their energy as a result of multiple collisions with the atomic electrons. The energy lost by the charged particle is consumed in the ionization and excitation of the atoms of the medium. Radiation that bears no charge, such as neutrons and gamma quanta, loses its energy not gradually but in discrete events accompanied by the transfer of a considerable part or all of the energy to the secondary particle. If one of the secondary particles is charged, then its energy is measured by the detector in terms of its ionizing action. Knowing the laws of interaction of uncharged particles and quanta with the substance in the detector, it is possible to establish the connection between the energies of the secondary charged particle and the primary, even through this connection may not always turn out to be unique.

5-1-1   Interaction of Heavy Charged Particles with Matter

Heavy particles are usually considered to be those whose mass M greatly exceeds the mass of the electron m, for example, protons, deutrons, and alpha particles. A heavy particle moving in a medium gradually loses energy by ionization and excitation of the particles and the electrons of the atoms of the medium. If the heavy charged particle has an energy E, then in a single interaction it can transfer to the atomic electron a maximum energy $E_{max} = 4mE/M$.

Fast secondary electrons naturally participate in the ionization and excitation of the atoms of the medium. As a result a large number of ionized and excited atoms are produced along the track of the particle. The ionization energy losses of the heavy particles can be expressed approximately by

$$-\frac{dE}{d\zeta} = 0.072 \frac{q^2}{E/A} \ln\left(\frac{160}{Z} \frac{E}{A}\right) \qquad (5\text{-}1)$$

where $dE/d\zeta$ (MeV/mg-cm^{-2}) is the energy loss per unit path length expressed in mg/cm^2, E is the particle energy in MeV, A is the mass number of the particle, q is the charge of the particle in units of elementary charge, and Z is the atomic number of the medium. Thus, for example, for an alpha particle ($Z = 2$, $A = 4$) with energy $E = 5$ MeV the specific ionization loss in air ($Z = 7$) is equal to $dE/d\zeta = 0.8$ MeV/mg-cm^{-2}.

An important characteristic of the deceleration of particles in matter is the range R, that is, the distance traversed by the particle in the matter until it stops completely. To measure the energy of the particle, it is necessary that its range be smaller than the volume of the detector. In the case of a detector volume that is smaller than the range R, the results of the measurement turn out to be underestimated by the amount of energy lost outside the detector volume.

It is obvious that the range can be determined by analytically integrating the equation for the ionization losses:

$$R = \int_0^E \frac{E/A}{(0.072)q^2 \ln[(160/Z)(E/A)]} \, dE \qquad (5\text{-}2)$$

For alpha particles the most accurate values of the range in air at atmospheric pressure are given by the empirical formula R (cm) $= 0.32 E^{3/2}$ with energy E in MeV. From this formula one obtains a range R of 3.6 cm in air for a particle of energy 5 MeV.

5-1-2   Interaction of Fast Electrons with Matter [3, 4, 5]

The energy lost by electrons when passing through matter are due essentially (at least for energies up to 3 MeV) to inelastic collisions with the atomic electrons. Such collisions, as in the case of heavy particles, lead to the excitation and ionization of atoms. Since the electron velocity is close to the velocity of light even with a kinetic energy of only 1 MeV, the time/space and also probability of interaction between the beta particle and the shell electron of the atom is much smaller than that for heavy particles. The specific ionization losses of the beta particles are therefore also considerably smaller than those of the heavy particles. The ionization losses of electrons with an energy of 5 MeV are approximately 500 times smaller than for alpha particles of the same energy. The dependence of dE/dx on the atomic number of the absorber is, however, rather weak, and the specific losses in lead and aluminum differ by less than a factor of 2.

The deceleration of the electrons in the medium is accompanied by strong scattering. The path therefore is tortuous, since the masses of the incident and scattering particles are the same. The equality of the masses of the interacting particles leads to a more intense exchange in energy between them; that is, the fast particle can transfer all or a part of its energy in a single collision. The strong scattering and the intense exchange of energy make even the distances traversed by monochromatic electrons in the substance differ greatly. Therefore the concept of range for electrons is less well defined than for the heavy particles.

However, for monochromatic electrons, as well as for heavy particles, one frequently uses the concept of extrapolated or practical range determined by extrapolation of the linear part of the experimental absorption curve. Such a range is equivalent to the thickness of matter containing 97% of all the

Table 5-1   Approximate values of μ/ρ for several different energies
of incident particle (electron)

E_β^{max} (MeV)	0.1	0.3	1.0	3.5
$\dfrac{\mu}{\rho} 10^3 \left(\dfrac{cm^2}{g} \right)$	0.21	0.090	0.018	0.0028

particles incident on the absorber. The connection between the extrapolated range and energy of the electrons, for $E > 0.6$ MeV, is satisfactorily described by the empirical relation $R = 0.526E$ minus a 0.004 unit of the range in grams per square centimeter.

If the electrons incident on the absorber are not monochromatic but have an energy distribution characteristic of beta radiation, then the attenuation of the beta-particle flux obeys a near-exponential law $N = N_0 e^{-\mu x/\rho}$, where μ/ρ is the mass attenuation coefficient of absorption in cm^2/g and x is the thickness of the absorber layer in g/cm^2. The value of μ/ρ depends on the maximum energy of the beta spectrum. The approximate values of μ/ρ corresponding to different energies are listed in Table 5-1.

5-1-3   Interaction of Electromagnetic Radiations (X-rays and Gamma rays) with Matter [3]

Gamma radiation interacts with matter through three independent processes: photoelectric absorption, Compton scattering, and pair production. The end result of the interaction is the appearance of secondary ionizing particles (electrons, and also positrons in the case of pair production), which are registered by the detector. Due to the fact that the energy of the gamma quanta are not lost gradually, as in the case of charged particles, but in single interaction events that occur in accordance with a probability law, the attenuation in the intensity of a collimated beam of gamma quanta as the beam passes through matter follows an exponential law $I = I_0 e^{-\mu x}$, where I_0 and I are the intensities before and after passage through an absorber of thickness x, respectively, and μ (cm^{-1}) is the coefficient of linear attenuation of the gamma rays. The quantity μ, known as the linear attenuation coefficient, can be expressed as the ratio of several parameters including the atomic attenuation coefficient μ_a $(cm^2/atom)$, the atomic number Z, and the number of electrons n_e:

$$\mu = \frac{\mu_a}{Z} \frac{N_0 \rho Z}{A}$$

$$= \mu_e n_e \tag{5-3}$$

where $\mu_e = \mu_a/Z$ (cm^2/electron) and $n_e = N_0\rho Z/A$ (electrons/cm^3). From Eq. (5-3), μ can be written as

$$\mu \; (\text{cm}^{-1}) = \frac{\Delta I}{I} \frac{1}{\Delta x} = \mu_a \frac{N_0}{A}\rho$$

where N_0 is Avogadro's number ($= 6.02 \times 10^{23}$ mol^{-1}), A is the atomic mass number, and ρ is the density.

It is often convenient to use the mass independent attenuation coefficient μ_m which is simply the linear attenuation coefficient normalized for the density of the material involved; that is, $\mu_m = \mu/\rho$ (cm^2/g). As mentioned, there are three types of independent interactions, and the result is usually the sum of these cross sections:

$$\mu_a = \tau_a + \sigma_a + \kappa_a \tag{5-4}$$

where τ_a is the cross section of the photoelectric effect per atom, σ_a is the cross section of the Compton scattering per atom, and κ_a is the cross section of pair production per atom.

Photoelectric Absorption of Gamma Photons

The photoelectric effect involving gamma photons is analogous to the ordinary photoelectric effect, that is, the liberation of an orbital electron under the influence of electromagnetic radiation. In this case, however, the electron is removed from one of the internal shells of the atom. The fundamental equation of the photoelectric effect, which expresses the energy balance, is also valid for photoelectric absorption on the K shell, $E = E_e^K + I_K$, where E is the gamma-photon energy, E_e^K is the kinetic energy of the photoelectron knocked out of the K shell, and I_K is the binding energy of the electron in the K shell.

It is difficult to analyze theoretically the photoelectric absorption process in the general form. There are several equations for different energy regions that are in contact with one another in the transition regions. The probability of the photoelectric effect occurring is larger when the gamma-photon energy is close to the binding energy. Then resonance sets in, and the cross section of the photoelectric effect is particularly large. As the energy of the gamma quanta increases relative to the value of I_K, the cross section decreases rapidly. A similar effect is produced by a decrease in the atomic number of the absorber, since here the binding energy of the internal electrons also decreases ($I_K \approx Z$). As a result of the fact that the K electrons, which are the closest to the nucleus, have a maximum binding energy, the photoelectric absorption on the K shell for $E > I_K$ always predominates. Photoelectric absorption in the subsequent shells, despite the large number of electrons they contain, is negligibly small. For example, a theoretical estimate gives the ratio of the total atomic cross section of the photoelectric effect τ_a to the particle cross section on the K shell τ_{aK} as $\tau_{aK}/\tau_a = 0.8$. Theory also gives an equation for the photoelectric absorption cross section on the K shell when $E \gg I_K$ as

$$\tau_{aK} = 10^{-33} \frac{Z^5}{E^{3.5}} \left(\frac{cm^2}{atom} \right) \tag{5-5}$$

where E is in MeV. Although this formula has been obtained under the aforementioned assumptions, it describes well the character of the dependence of the cross section on the atomic number of the absorber ($\sim Z^5$) and the energy of the gamma quanta ($\sim E^{-3.5}$).

Compton Scattering
Gamma quanta, interacting with the weakly bound electrons, lose part of their energy and transfer it to the electron in the form of kinetic energy and momentum through inelastic scattering. Knowing this, it is possible to establish a connection between the energies of the primary gamma quantum E_γ, the scattered quantum $E_{\gamma'}$, and the electron E_e, and also their scattering angles relative to the direction of the primary quantum, namely θ of the scattered quantum and ϕ of the electron as

$$E_{\gamma'} = \frac{E_\gamma}{1 + \alpha(1 - \cos\theta)} \tag{5-6}$$

$$E_e = E_\gamma - E_{\gamma'} \tag{5-7}$$

$$\cot\phi = (1 + \alpha)\tan\frac{\theta}{2} \tag{5-8}$$

where $\alpha = E_\gamma/mc^2$ and $mc^2 = 0.511$ MeV. For the energy distribution of the secondary electrons, there is a characteristic upper limit $E_e^{max} = E_\gamma - E_{\gamma'}|_{\theta=\pi} = E_\gamma 2\alpha/(1 + 2\alpha)$. Thus, for example, given $E_\gamma = 0.511$ MeV, the limiting energy of the distribution of the Compton electrons is $E_e^{max} = 0.34$ MeV.

A polar diagram of the differential cross section σ_e' is shown in Fig. 5-1(a). As can be seen from the diagram, the distribution of scattered photons becomes more and more peaked forward with increasing energy. The values presented are those of the differential cross section per electron per unit solid angle ($cm^2/electron/\Omega$).

The integral of the differential cross section over all possible angles gives the total cross section σ_e of the interaction, which is only a function of the energy. The dependence of the integral cross section σ_e, calculated per electron, on the energy is shown in Fig. 5-1(b). It has the form of a broad distribution, which decreases slowly with increasing energy. Thus Compton interaction is probable for gamma quanta over a wide range of energies.

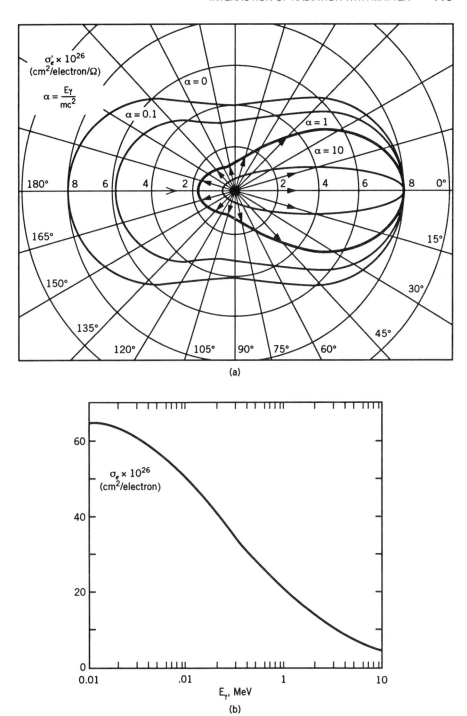

Figure 5-1 Dependence of the cross section of Compton interaction on (a) the scattering angle and (b) energy. σ_e' and σ_e are the differential and total cross section, respectively and Ω is the unit solid angle.

For almost all atomic electrons (with the exception of the K and L electrons in heavy atoms), the weak coupling condition is satisfied ($I_K \ll E_\gamma$). Therefore the atomic cross section for the Compton effect σ_a, calculated per atom, is equal to the product of σ_e and the number of atomic electrons; that is to say, $\sigma_a = \sigma_e Z$.

Pair Production

Suppose that the gamma-photon energy exceeds $2mc^2 = 1.02$ MeV. Then, as a result of the interaction of such a quantum with the field of the nucleus, the creation of an electron-positron pair is possible. The resulting kinetic energy E of the produced charged particles is equal to $E = E_\gamma - 2mc^2$.

Theory yields the following expression for the total effective cross section for pair production per atom κ_a as

$$\kappa_a = 10^{-27} Z^2 F(\alpha) \left(\frac{cm^2}{atom} \right) \tag{5-9}$$

where Z is the atomic number of the absorber and $F(\alpha)$ is a function of the energy ($\alpha = E_\gamma/mc^2$), the values of which are given in Table 5-2. Knowing the partial cross sections of the individual processes τ_a, σ_a, and κ_a, we can determine the total cross section of the substance absorber or detector.

Let us note some general laws governing the absorption of gamma radiation or electromagnetic radiation in the energy range of a few keV to 100 MeV. First, photoelectric absorption plays a noticeable role for an absorber with a large atomic number and decreases rapidly with increasing radiation energy. Second, the Compton-scattering cross section is significant from several kiloelectron volts to several megaelectron volts for all absorbers and is more noticeable than photoelectric absorption for absorbers with small Z, such as organic materials.

Figure 5-2 shows plots of the components of the linear attenuation coefficients for an organic scintillator (anthracene) and inorganic scintillator [sodium iodide NaI(Tl)] frequently used as phosphors in scintillation detectors. For anthracene the photoelectric effect can be neglected as compared with the Compton interaction for $E_\gamma > 60$ KeV, whereas for sodium iodide the influence of photoelectric absorption is noticeable up to $E_\gamma \cong 1$ MeV. For instance, when $E_\gamma = 1$ MeV, the ratio of the linear attenuation coefficients of the two is still substantial and is $\tau/\sigma = 0.05$.

Table 5-2

α	2	3	4	5	6	7	8	9	10
$F(\alpha)$	0	0.078	0.21	0.36	0.56	0.75	0.90	1.1	1.3

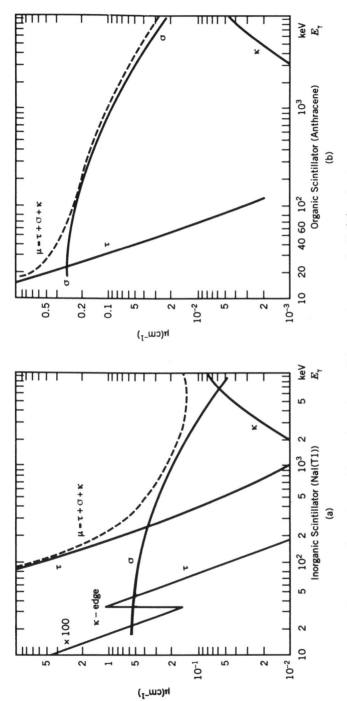

Figure 5-2 Dependence of linear absorption coefficients on the energy for NaI(Tl) and anthracene.

5-2 PRINCIPLES OF RADIATION DETECTION AND DETECTORS [2, 3, 4]

5-2-1 General Characterizations of Detectors

Spectrometric detectors can be divided into two groups. The first group includes pulse ionization chambers as well as proportional and semiconductor counters. The operating principle of these detectors is based on the use of the ionizing phenomenon of the radiation. The particle or the quantum produces in the sensitive volume of the detector a certain number of ion pairs N that is proportional to the energy E. With the aid of electrodes of definite configuration, an electric field of intensity W is produced in the sensitive volume. The ions formed after passage of the particle are collected by the corresponding electrodes, thereby charging the interelectrode capacitance C. In this case, as in the proportional counter, for example, the transfer of the primary charge can be accompanied by some amplification. If the leakage of the charge during the time of its collection can be neglected, then the capacitance becomes charged to a voltage Q/C or Nq/C, where $Q = Nq$ is the charge of the ion. The amplitude of the voltage pulse obtained in this manner is proportional to the energy of the particle causing the ionization; that is, $V = qE/\varepsilon C$, since $N = E/\varepsilon$ where ε is the energy needed for the generation of an electron-ion pair.

The second group is comprised of scintillation detectors based on the excitation of the molecules of the medium when the investigated radiation passes through it. For some substances the intensity of the electromagnetic radiation emitted by the excited molecules is proportional to the energy lost by the particle during the deceleration process. The scintillating substance, comprising the sensitive volume of the scintillation counter, can be in any state—solid, liquid, or gaseous. The scintillations produced in the sensitive volume are registered by a photomultiplier tube (PMT) and are converted into a current pulse in the collector or anode circuit. Under certain conditions a linear relation is maintained between the charge gathered on the output capacitance of the photomultiplier anode and the energy of the decelerated particle.

As was already indicated, spectrometric detectors should possess, regardless of the method used to convert the energy of the investigated particle into an electric pulse, the following two properties: linearity and sufficiently high resolution. It is also necessary that the sensitive volume of the detector be matched to the type of incident radiation. The ranges of the particles whose energies are measured should fit well within the limits of the volume. It is desirable that the time of conversion of the particle energy into a pulse amplitude be small; in other words, the detector should be fast in response to the incident particle or quanta.

The conversion linearity commonly depends on the type of registered radiation. Thus, for example, scintillation counters with sodium iodide, cesium iodide, anthracene, or stilbene crystals, which have a perfectly satisfactory linearity over a wide energy range with respect to electrons, are noticeably nonlinear in the detection of heavy particles. However, if the range of the measured energy is not too wide (e.g., from 4 to 7 MeV for alpha particles), then the conversion can be regarded as linear within its limits. It is then said that the detector has limited linearity of conversion with respect to the given type of radiation. Some of the modern semiconductor detectors have better characteristics, for example, the pulse amplitude is linearly proportional to the energy for electrons, heavy particles, fission fragments, and gamma quanta.

5-2-2   Resolution of Detectors [1, 2]

The process of converting the particle energy into a pulse amplitude follows a certain probability law that depends on the type of detector. Individual stages of this process—namely ionization or excitation, gas amplification in a proportional counter, or amplification of the primary electron beam in a photomultiplier—represent a particle-interaction sequence that obeys probability laws. Therefore, even if the energies of the particles to be detected are the same, the corresponding pulses at the output of the detector have different amplitudes—or, as is customarily stated, the amplitudes are distributed in accordance with some probability laws. More specifically the form of the amplitude distribution often follows a Gaussian-like distribution,

$$p_E(v) = \frac{1}{\sqrt{2\pi\sigma^2}} \exp\left(-\frac{1}{2}\frac{(v - v_0)^2}{\sigma^2}\right) \tag{5-10}$$

where $p_E(v)$ is the probability distribution of the voltage amplitude which we have assumed to be proportional to the energy of the registered particle, v_0 is the mean value of the amplitude, and σ is the standard deviation.

This distribution has the form of a peak centered at $v = v_0$, the width of which is characterized by a parameter σ. If two lines of the investigated radiation E_1 and E_2 are so close that the distance between the corresponding amplitude peaks v_{01} and v_{02} is essentially smaller than σ, then the spectrometer with such a detector cannot distinguish these two lines because of its insufficient resolving power.

The measure of detector resolution in spectrometry is, however, usually defined as the total width δ of the peak at the level of half the maximum of the distribution, known as *full width at half maximum* (fwhm). The relation between this fwhm and given distribution parameter σ is expressed by

$$\delta(\text{fwhm}) = 2\sqrt{2\ln 2}\,\sigma \cong 2.36\sigma \tag{5-11}$$

The resolution η is usually defined as the ratio of δ to the mean amplitude

v_0, expressed in percent as

$$\eta = \frac{\delta}{v_0} 100\% = 236 \frac{\sigma}{v_0} \%$$ (5-12)

It should be noted that in addition to the statistical character of the conversion of energy into an amplitude, the resolution is also influenced by the inhomogeneity of the detector material, leakage of current and imperfection in charge collection, among other things. In the detector it therefore is necessary to check these factors and be sure that they are smaller than the total variance σ^2.

The amplitude distribution parameter δ plays an important role in the determination of the requirements imposed on the analyzing apparatus. The drift of the threshold devices or the noise of the analyzer should be appreciably smaller than the measured value of δ (i.e., the intrinsic line width of the detector). The resolution and other spectrometric characteristics of several detectors, namely, pulsed ionization chambers, proportional counters, semiconductor detectors, and scintillation detectors, will be studied next.

5-2-3   A Pulsed Ionization Chamber

A pulsed ionization chamber is a hermetically sealed vessel filled with gas in which two electrodes produce a strong electric field. The electrodes can be plane, cylindrical, or spherical. The particles whose energies are being measured ionize the gas contained in the cavity or chamber between the electrodes. The charges produced upon ionization are gathered by the electrodes, thereby charging the capacitance of the chamber to a definite potential, the value of which is then measured.

Let us consider the conversion of the energy of a particle into a voltage pulse using, as an example, the plane ionization chamber shown in Fig. 5-3(a). The negative electrode is usually the substrate on which a thin layer of the radioactive compound is usually deposited. Assume that a fast charged particle (e.g., an alpha particle) is emitted from a thin source at the substrate so that its range fits well within the volume of the chamber. During deceleration $N = E/\varepsilon$ pairs of ions will be produced along the track of the particle (ε is the specific energy consumed in the production of a pair of ions for a specific gas or filling medium).

The ions, moving in the filed of the chamber to the electrodes, produce a current in the chamber circuit. The elementary current due to the motion of each individual ion is

$$I = \frac{q\mu W}{V}$$
$$= q\mu \frac{l'}{d}$$ (5-13)

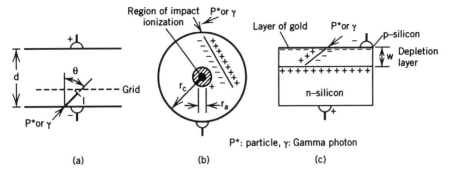

Figure 5-3 Passage of a particle through (a) an ionization chamber, (b) a proportional counter, and (c) a semiconductor detector. P^* and γ denote the particle and gamma photon, respectively.

where d is the distance between the electrodes, l' is the distance between the point where the charge is situated and the positive electrode, V is the potential difference between the electrodes of the chamber, W is the field intensity at the point where the charge is situated at the given instance, μ is the velocity of ion in motion, and q is its charge. On moving from the point of its production to the electrode, the ion charges the capacitance of the chamber by an amount $\Delta Q = q\,\Delta V/V$, where ΔV is the potential difference between the place of production of the ion and the electrode.

If we assume that the ions are distributed along the track uniformly (this, strictly speaking, is incorrect since the ionization losses are larger at the end of the track), then the charges that are brought by the positive and negative ions, for a track arrangement such as the one shown in Fig. 5-3(a), are equal to

$$Q_- = qN\left(1 - \frac{1}{2}\frac{l}{d}\cos\theta\right)$$

$$= qN\left(1 - \frac{1}{2}\frac{l}{d}\right)\Big|_{\theta=0} \tag{5-14}$$

$$Q_+ = qN\frac{l}{2d}\cos\theta$$

$$= qN\frac{l}{2d}\Big|_{\theta=0} \tag{5-15}$$

where d is distance between the electrodes of the chamber and l is the track length. The total charge then becomes $Q = Q_+ + Q_- = qN$, and the potential V to which the capacitance of the chamber is charged is $V = qN/C$, and is not dependent on the orientation of the track. As long as $N = E/\varepsilon$ and

$V = qE/C\varepsilon$, the conversion of the energies is linear. However, complete charge collection is guaranteed only if the time of motion of the slowest positive ions is smaller than the discharge time of the capacitor through the load resistance R, which is connected in the anode circuit of one of the electrodes (i.e., $RC \gg d/\mu_+$). This requirement often limits the speed of the chamber. For example, when the time of gathering or collection time of the positive ions is in the range of 100 μsec (d/μ_+), as a rule of thumb, the overall counting rates will be limited in the range of 10 to 100 pulses per second only.

To increase the speed of the pulse chamber, usually only the negative charges (electrons) are collected. They are more mobile than the heavier positive ions and the collection time of the electron component is usually on the order of 1 μsec. To ensure nearly complete collection of the electrons but exclude the slow ionic component, the time constant of the charging circuit is chosen such that $d/\mu_+ > RC \gg d/\mu_-$ (i.e., $RC \cong 10$ μsec). In this case the pulse amplitude is

$$v_e = \frac{Q_-}{C} = \frac{qN}{C}\left(1 - \frac{l/2}{d}\cos\theta\right) \qquad (5\text{-}16)$$

As seen earlier, the signal v_e depends not only on the ionization (energy) but also on the relative dimensions of the length of the track, and further both on the distance between electrodes and the angle of emission of the particle or the track. If no collimation is used and the angle of particle emission is arbitrarily between 0 and $\pi/2$, then the corresponding variation of the pulse amplitudes will be $\Delta v_e = (l/2)qN/dC$, and the relative scatter will be $\Delta v_e/v_e \cong (l/2d)$. The scatter or amplitude variation can be decreased or eliminated by several means.

One of the methods of reducing the scatter is to reduce the ratio $(l/2)/d$ by increasing the distance d between the electrodes. However, to maintain the constant field intensity, it becomes necessary to take into account the voltage on the electrodes especially on their surface so as to reduce the influence of the edge effects. Reduction in the length of the track by increasing the gas pressure is not always possible. If high gas pressure conditions are created, recombination of the ions will be facilitated, thereby introducing an additional error in the measurement of the total ionization.

A better result is obtained by using a third electrode in the chamber, a grid that screens the gathering electrode from the region of direct ionization. The distance between the grid and the radioactive compound is somewhat larger than the mean free path of the particles with maximum energy in the gas, and a positive potential is applied to the grid so as to draw in the electrons between the grid and the gathering electrode. So long as the electrons move between the negative electrode and the grid, no current is induced in the circuit of the gathering electrode or positive electrode, owing to the screening effect of the grid. When the electrons move between the grid and the collecting electrode, they pass through an identical potential difference and the collected charge is equal to qN. This is equivalent to making $l = 0$ in Eqs. (5-14) and (5-15).

In practice, one also uses chambers of cylindrical or spherical form. In these cases the electrons in the chambers are collected on a central positive electrode (filament or sphere). Most of the ionization is carried out, however, in the region where the potential gradients are small. Since the main part of the induced charge is connected with the motion of the electrons in the region of strong field near the central electrode where the electric field is strongest, paths traversed by all the electrons appear practically identical. This ensures consistancy of the amplitudes, independent of the direction of motion of the particle.

The amplitude of the pulse is also influenced by the presence of impurities of electronegative gases, such as oxygen, in the filling gas. As a result of the large cross section for the capture of electrons by the molecules of such gases, some of the electrons "stick" to the heavy molecules of the electronegative gas during the course of their motion to the collecting electrode. The mobility of the resultant negative ion is much lower than that of the electron. Consequently the electron is unable to participate in collection of the charge. The "sticking" phenomenon sharply decreases the amplitude of the signal and leads to an additional spread of the pulse amplitudes. Thus, for example, when working with gases N_2 or Ar_2, one observes that an impurity of 0.05% oxygen reduces the amplitude of the signal by almost one-half compared to that of pure gases.

The influence of oxygen impurities can be reduced considerably by using a mixture of 96% to 98% nitrogen and 2% to 4% argon. In such a gas mixture the electron energies correspond to the minimum capture cross section, and the "sticking" effect becomes small.

In addition to the problems already noted, considerable errors, particularly in the detection of heavy particles, can be introduced by ion recombination such as column-type recombination—for example, recombination among ions of a single track. Different probabilities of recombination for different tracks, introduce additional scatter in the pulse amplitudes. When the density of ionization by heavy particles (protons, alpha particles, fission fragments) is large, it is necessary to use sufficiently powerful electric fields to reduce the errors due to recombination to a minimum.

Pulse chambers are usually employed to measure the energies of heavy particles, most frequently alpha particles. The measurement of fission-fragment energies is made complicated by the high ionization density of the gas and the intense recombination. Let us calculate the output parameters of a signal from the chamber used to detect alpha particles. The probable amplitude of the output voltage pulse is, in the case of complete charge collection, $v_0 = qE/C\varepsilon$. Substituting in the values $q = 1.6 \times 10^{-19}$ coulomb, $C = 20$ pF, and $\varepsilon = 30$ eV, we obtain

$$v_0(\text{mV}) = 0.27E \text{ (MeV)} \tag{5-17}$$

For example, pulses corresponding to 5 MeV alpha particles have an amplitude of approximately 1.3 mV.

The variance of the amplitude distribution can be determined by assuming that N obeys a Poisson distribution. Then the mean-square deviation is $\sigma = \sqrt{N}$. A more rigorous analysis taking into account the basic ionization phenomenon of gas molecules shows that $\sigma = \sqrt{FN}$, where $F = 0.3$ to 0.5 and is known as the *Fano factor*. For alpha particles with energy E, we have a fwhm resolution of $\delta = 2.36\sqrt{FE/\varepsilon}$. Consequently the resolving power of the chamber is $\eta = (\delta/v_0)100\% = 236(\sqrt{F\varepsilon}/\sqrt{E})\%$. If we substitute the values $\varepsilon = 30 \times 10^{-6}$ and $F = 0.4$, η becomes

$$\eta = \frac{0.85}{\sqrt{E}}\% \tag{5-18}$$

where E is in MeV. Such a characteristic dependence of the resolution on the energies of the detected particles is common to all detectors and reflects the statistical character of the conversion of particle energy into the measurable electrical parameters.

5-2-4 Proportional Counters

When the voltage on the electrodes of an ionization chamber is increased, the electrons moving in the electric field can acquire, over the length of the free path, a velocity such that impact ionization becomes possible, thereby increasing the number of electrons reaching the positive electrode compared with the number of electrons initially formed by the ionizing particle. This is called *gas multiplication*. Usually proportional counters have a cylindrical form, as shown in Fig. 5-3(b). This makes it possible to obtain a high potential gradient near the filament at the center with a relatively small voltage U applied to the electrodes, since the field intensity in a cylindrical counter is inversely proportional to the distance from the center as given by

$$W(r) = \frac{1}{r}\frac{U}{\ln(r_c/r_a)} \tag{5-19}$$

where r is the radial coordinate at the point where the intensity is measured and r_c and r_a are the radii of the cathode cylinder and anode filament, respectively.

Another important advantage of cylindrical proportional counters is the weak dependence of the coefficient of gas multiplication M on the trajectory of the particle in the counter. This is explained by the fact that impact ionization is concentrated in a small region near the anode, which is a thin wire electrode, while primary ionization occurs over the entire volume of the counter. Therefore all the primary electrons can be considered more or less under equal conditions before they reach the region of impact ionization.

Let us examine the operation of the counter. We introduce the parameter α which determines the multiplication of the primary electrons as they move toward the collecting electrode. The value of α is equal to the number of secondary electrons produced over a unit distance (e.g., 1 cm) of path by a primary electron in a constant field. For a parallel-path counter, if the primary ionization N_0 occurred at a distance x_0 from the anode or collecting electrode, the number of secondary electrons produced in a layer Δx is equal to $\Delta N = N(x)\alpha\,\Delta x$. Consequently the number of electrons reaching the collector is equal to $N = N_0 \exp(\alpha x_0)$, and the coefficient of gas multiplication $M = N/N_0 = \exp(\alpha x_0)$. From the latter expression we see that the coefficient of gas multiplication depends strongly on the localization of the primary ionization.

In a cylindrical counter the field is not constant but is a function of the radius. Therefore direct integration of the differential relation given above is not possible, since α is a function of the radial position r; that is, $\alpha = \alpha(r)$. To determine the coefficient of gas multiplication, we separate the volume of the counter into several sufficiently thin cylindrical layers of thickness Δr in such a way that within the limits of each layer the field can be regarded as constant. Then the multiplication in an elementary layer at a distance r from the center is assumed to be $m(r, r + \Delta r) = \exp[\alpha(r)\,\Delta r]$. The overall coefficient of gas multiplication is obviously equal to the product of the coefficients of all the elementary layers, and when $\Delta r \to 0$, we have $M \to \exp[\int_r^{r_a}\alpha(r)\,dr]$. Here r is the radius of the layer in which the primary ionization takes place. However, α differs from zero only in a narrow region near the anode wire. Therefore the integral in the exponent is a function of the upper limit only, and consequently $M = f(r_a)$. The consistancy of the amplification coefficient ensures linearity of the conversion of the primary ionization, and therefore also of the particle energy, into an output voltage pulse.

Sometimes this linearity may be violated. For example, in the presence of impurities of electronegative gases, the dependence of the coefficient of gas multiplication M on the radius can be influenced by the different probability of electrons "sticking" to the heavy molecules in regions with weak and strong fields. As a result the reduction in the number of electrons reaching the regions of impact ionization from the regions that are remote from the filament turns out to be stronger than the reduction in the number of electrons from the regions near the filament. Therefore the working media employed are usually inert gases: argon, krypton, and xenon. The same difficulties arise in measuring the energy of heavy ionizing particles, for example, alpha particles or protons, owing to the high density of ions created where they ionize the gas. Recombination of the ions at the cathode is much stronger in this case than in the regions close to the anode where the high field intensity prevents recombination.

The range of the coefficients of gas multiplication is quite wide, from unity to 10,000. However, when working with low gas multiplication coefficients (up to several hundred), the mechanism of operation considered above is the principal one, and when $M > 1,000$, secondary cascades—caused by ultraviolet radiation and by bombardment of positive ions with the cathode which produces electrons at the cathode—come into play.

Impact ionization of the gas molecules is accompanied by their excitation with subsequent de-excitation and the emission of ultraviolet photons. Owing to the photoelectric effect of these ultraviolet photons at the cathode, the photons can knock out secondary photoelectrons. This begins a second cascade. The probability of the photoelectric effect can be neglected, however, with an increase of gas multiplication. In this case the avalanches become so intense that the number of secondary electrons overwhelm the photoelectric effect of the ultraviolet photons at the cathode. Let γ be the probability of excitation of a molecule with emission of an ultraviolet photon, λ be the probability that the photon knocks out a photoelectron from the cathode, and N_0 be number of ion pairs produced by the charged particle in the volume of the counter (primary ionization). Then, because of impact ionization, the first avalanche reaching the anode (filament) will contain $N_0 M_0$ electrons. The de-excitation of the excited molecules brings to the anode $(N_0 M_0) \gamma \lambda M_0$ electrons. As a result of the subsequent avalanches, the total number of electrons collected at the anode is

$$N = N_0 M_0 + N_0 M_0^2 \lambda \gamma + N_0 M_0^3 (\lambda \gamma)^2 + \cdots = \frac{N_0 M_0}{1 - M_0 \lambda \gamma} \quad (5\text{-}20)$$

Thus the actual gas multiplication coefficient becomes

$$M = \frac{N}{N_0} = \frac{M_0}{1 - M_0 \lambda \gamma} \quad (5\text{-}21)$$

As seen from Eqs. (5-20) or (5-21), a proportional counter acts like an amplifier with positive feedback. When $M_0 \to \lambda \gamma \cong 10^4$, the gas multiplication increases rapidly and become unstable. Therefore, to obtain high gain with stable gas multiplication, one frequently adds to the filling inert gas a small amount of polyatomic gas such as methane or isopentane. The molecules of the polyatomic gas effectively absorb the ultraviolet photons and dissociate into simpler radicals, without emitting any photons.

Proportional counters are usually used in the spectrometry of soft beta or gamma radiation. Depending on the construction of the counter, the gas employed, and the pressure, the upper limit of the measured energies is from 20 to 100 keV. For the probable amplitude of the proportional counter, if only the electronic component of the pulse is collected, an empirical expression is given by (for $C = 20$ pF).

$$v_0 \text{ (mV)} \cong 0.13 ME \text{ (MeV)} \tag{5-22}$$

Thus, for electrons with energy $E = 0.03$ MeV and $M = 500$, we have $v_0 \cong 2$ mV.

The resolving power of a proportional counter is determined by the fluctuations of the primary ionization N_0 and of the gas multiplication M

$$\left(\frac{\sigma_{v_0}}{v_0} \right)^2 = \left(\frac{\sigma_{N_0}}{N_0} \right)^2 + \left(\frac{\sigma_M}{M} \right)^2 \tag{5-23}$$

where σ_{v_0}, σ_{N_0}, and σ_M are the mean square deviations of the distribution of v_0, N_0, and M, respectively. Calculations show that $\sigma_M / M = 1/\sqrt{N_0}$. After substituting the expression $\sigma_{N_0} = \sqrt{N_0 F}$ into Eq. (5-23), assuming as before that $F = 0.4$, we obtain $(\sigma_{v_0}/v_0)^2 = 1.4/N_0$. Finally, the expected energy resolution becomes

$$\eta = \frac{1.5}{\sqrt{E \text{ (MeV)}}} \% \tag{5-24}$$

where N_0 is assumed $N_0 = E/\varepsilon$. For example, the resolving power of the detector, when used to measure the energies of 30 keV electrons, is about 9%.

5-2-5 Semiconductor Detectors [2]

In the last two decades, there has been explosive development in the areas of semiconductor detectors of various kinds. In the case of semiconductor detector the transformation of the particle energy into electric pulses occurs in the junction region of semiconductor material, such as, silicon and germanium.

Silicon Detectors
Early semiconductor detectors were mostly of a planar silicon diode type. In most of the p-n junction silicon detectors, the useful region or the ionization chamber is located on the very surface of the detector. There are several methods for constructing such junction semiconductor detectors. We shall note the most widely used method only. The method consists of sputtering on

a n-silicon crystal with p-type or donor material (e.g., phosphorus). Following the subsequent heat treatment, the donor atoms diffuse inside the n-type crystal and form a thin layer of p-type conductivity.

We will discuss one example of the method that consists of sputtering a thin film of a noble metal (e.g., gold) on a well-polished n-type silicon crystal surface. On the surface a layer of p-type silicon will be formed. Such junctions are usually called *surface-barrier junctions*, and they are the most commonly used silicon junctions in semiconductor detectors for particle detection.

In these types of silicon semiconductor detectors, the partial densities of the electrons in the n-region and the holes in the p-region predominate, so there is a tendency toward opposed diffusion of the carriers (i.e., the holes in the p-region diffuse into the n-region while the electrons in the n-region diffuse into the p-region). As a result the n-region turns out to be positively charged and the p-region negatively charged, thus producing a potential barrier on the boundary preventing further diffusion of the carriers.

The layer in which the sharp change in the potential occurs contains practically no mobile carriers, since they are transferred under the influence of the electric field into the region with corresponding conductivity. This layer is therefore called the *depletion layer*, and its conductivity is equal to the conductivity of the pure semiconductor.

If one applies an external voltage to a p-n junction (the positive terminal of the source to the n-region and the negative to the p-region), the height of the barrier increases. The thickness of the depletion layer also increases, and consequently almost all the voltage appears on the depletion layer. Since the thickness of the depletion layer is usually on the order of ten microns in the silicon surface barrier detector even with an external voltage of only 10 V, the potential gradients produced in the depletion layer are on the order of $\Delta U / \Delta x \cong 10^4$ (V/cm). Consequently, if electron-hole pairs are produced in the depletion layer due to the incident particles or quanta, then the charge carriers created are directed by the field and are carried into the regions with suitable conductivity or respective electrodes (i.e., electrons to the positive electrode via the n-silicon layer and holes to the negative electrode or p-layer).

Thus the depletion layer in a semiconductor detector is analogous to the working volume of the ionization chamber. When a charged particle passes through the depletion layer [Fig. 5-3 (c)], electron-hole pairs are produced along its track. The carriers produced move under the influence of the strong field of the junction toward its boundaries. If N pairs were produced, then the capacitance of the detector is charged by qN and a potential to be developed across the capacitor becomes $v = qN/C$. The thickness of the depletion layer w is analogous to the distance between the plates in an ordinary chamber, and the voltage U applied to the detector determines the field intensity in the depletion layer. Since the mobility of the electrons and of the holes in the silicon at room temperature differ merely by a factor of 2

Table 5-3

Bias Voltage U \ Specific Resistance ρ \ Parameters	Parameters	100 (ohms/cm)	500 (ohms/cm)	5,000 (ohms/cm)	10,000 (ohms/cm)
100 V	w (microns)	$50\ \mu m$	$110\ \mu m$	$350\ \mu m$	$\sim 500\ \mu m$
100 V	C_0 (pF/cm^2)	220 pF/cm^2	95 pF/cm^2	30 pF/cm^2	10 pF/cm^2

($\mu_e = 1200$ cm^2/V-sec and $\mu_h = 500$ cm^2/V-sec), charge collection is relatively fast. This makes the semiconductor detector superior to the ordinary ionization chamber, where the mobilities of the ions and electrons usually differ by two orders of magnitude.

Like gas-filled chambers, semiconductor detectors have a capacitance, whose value per cm^2 is $C_0 = k/4\rho w$, where k is the dielectric constant of silicon equal to 12 and w is the thickness of the depletion layer. The thickness of the depletion layer is determined to a considerable degree by the specific resistivity of the material and by the voltage applied to the junction

$$w = \sqrt{A10^{-9}\rho(U + U_0)} \qquad (5\text{-}25)$$

where A is a constant ($A = 1$ for p-silicon and $A = 2.5$ for n-silicon), ρ is the specific resistivity in ohm-cm, U_0 is the potential barrier for the external voltage which is equal to 0.5 V, and U is the external voltage applied to the junction. In Table 5-3 the values of w and C_0 for crystals of n-silicon with different specific resistivities ρ and for different bias voltages are given as an illustrative example.

It is usually difficult to obtain sufficiently pure silicon with high specific resistivity. Therefore the material employed at the present time has a specific resistivity at best on the order of 10,000 ohm-cm, corresponding to a capacitance of some 10 pF/cm^2 for a voltage of 50 to 100 V. A further increase in the working voltage, in an attempt to reduce the capacitance, however, increases the reverse leakage current and thereby increases the internal noise of the detector.

The linearity of the conversion of the energy of the registered particles into an amplitude is based, as in the case of gas-filled detectors, on the consistancy of the average energy ε consumed in the production of an electron-hole pair, but it differs greatly from that of the gas-filled detector by approximately an order of magnitude smaller for semiconductor detectors;

this amounts to approximately 3.6 eV for silicon. Therefore, a better resolution is attained in a semiconductor detector than in the pulse chambers.

A characteristic feature of semiconductor detectors is also the independence of the value of ε not only on the energy but also on the mass and charge of the particles. This is due to the powerful electric field acting in the depletion layer, and also the small charge collection time of the carriers (< 10 nsec), making their recombination loss small. Therefore silicon semiconductor detectors are the best suited for the spectrometry of heavy particles. For the correct measurement of the energy, however, the thickness of the junction must be larger than the range of the measured particles. In addition the thickness of the surface "dead" layer must be as small as possible compared to the range. The range of alpha particles with an energy 5 MeV in silicon is approximately 20 μm, so a detector made of silicon with a specific resistivity of 500 ohm-cm at a base voltage $U = 100$ V is sufficient for measurement. The thickness of the "dead" layer for the best diffusion junctions is insignificant (< 0.1 μm).

Spectrometry of beta particles entails difficulties because beta electrons with an energy of merely 100 keV have a range of approximately 150 μm in silicon. The improvement in the characteristics is limited by the fact that in order to make detectors with a sufficiently thick junction, pure or high-resistivity silicon is necessary (see Table 5-3). The pulse amplitude at the output of the detector, assuming total collection of the charge on the capacitance, is

$$v_0 = \frac{q}{\varepsilon C_0 S} E \tag{5-26}$$

where S is the area of the detector in cm^2. If one uses silicon with $\rho = 500$ ohm-cm and a bias voltage $U = 100$ V, then $C_0 = 95$ pF and v_0 (mV) $=$ $(0.3/S)E$ (MeV). For alpha particles with energy $E = 5$ MeV and for a detector of area $S = 0.25$ cm^2, we have $v_0 = 6$ mV. The resolving power of the detector is determined by the dispersion of the number of pairs of carriers formed in individual acts of interaction of the particles with the detector. Assuming, as before, that the mean square deviation is $\sigma = \sqrt{N}$, we obtain for the resolving power an equation $\eta = 236/\sqrt{N}$, or after substituting $N = E/\varepsilon$ ($\varepsilon = 3.6$ eV),

$$\eta = \frac{0.5}{\sqrt{E \text{ (MeV)}}} \% \tag{5-27}$$

For alpha particles with energy $E = 5$ MeV, the resolution amounts to approximately 0.2%. For complete utilization of such a high-resolution detector, it is necessary to impose on the corresponding apparatus rather stringent requirements with respect to stability of the amplification and noise. The number of channels of the analyzing circuit should be very large (several thousand), or else an insufficient number of channels would make it necessary to employ an amplifier with variable bias or a biased amplifier just to enlarge the spectrum of interest.

Surface-barrier-type semiconductor detectors are convenient in that they call for a low supply voltage for the bias on the junction. It is usually around 10 to 50 V. In addition the dependence of the amplitude of the input signal on the bias voltage is considerably less than, for example, that of proportional and scintillation counters. This reduces appreciably the requirement for a highly stable supply voltage.

A shortcoming of most junction detectors is their small working surface area and extremely thin depletion layer, which manufactured at the present time, amounts to several tenths of a square centimeter and less than a millimeter, respectively. If junction could be developed with a large area, they would have poor spectrometric characteristics because of the increase in capacitance and subsequent deterioration of the signal to noise ratio. The latter reduces the resolution of the detector.

Germanium Lithium Drifted Detectors for Gamma Rays [2]

Silicon spectrometers become less favorable when the incident quanta are in the form of X-rays or gamma-rays or when their energy increases due to the poor photoelectric-to-Compton ratio in silicon. For the high-energy X-rays or gamma rays with energies above 100 keV, the germanium lithium (Ge(Li)) spectrometers are more useful. For instance, the resolution of a good planar Ge(Li) detector 6 mm thick with a thin entrance window using an amplifier and preamplifier system would be on the order of 850 eV fwhm or $\eta = 0.123\%$ for the 661.6 keV gamma ray line from a ^{137}Cs source; a resolution hundreds of times better than scintillation counters [e.g., NaI(T1) has approximately 8% to 9% fwhm resolution for the 661.6 keV gamma rays].

A typical experimental spectrum for the 661.6 keV gamma rays obtained from a thin window planar type Ge(Li) detector is shown in Fig. 5-4(a). The resolution obtained here should be compared with that of a NaI(T1) scintillator to be shown later. For high-efficiency gamma ray detection, relatively large volume coaxial Ge(Li) detectors are more common. However, this large detector increases noise relative to the small-volume planar detector due to the increased capacitance of the device, resulting in increased noise from the preamplifier, increased leakage current from the large volume, poor charge collection, and an uncompensated p-type core and a thick lithium-doped n^+ window. A typical spectrum for 661.6 keV gamma rays in a large-volume true coaxial detector is shown in Fig. 5-4(b).

The absolute efficiency of large-volume Ge(Li) gamma ray detectors are not as easy to establish as those for NaI(T1) scintillators, for example. The reason for this is that the size and shape of the uncompensated p-type core has a major effect both on the total efficiency and on the peak-to-total or peak-to-Compton ratio for the detector. It is now usual practice to quote the efficiency of a Ge(Li) detector as a percentage of that for the 1.33 MeV

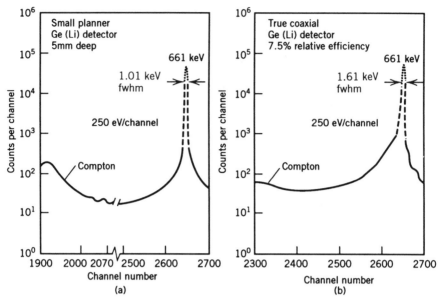

Figure 5-4 Gamma ray spectra obtained from germanium (lithium drifted) detectors. (a) A spectrum obtained from a small planar Ge(Li) detector. (b) A spectrum obtained from a relatively large true coaxial Ge(Li) detector.

gamma ray from ^{60}Co for a 76.2 mm (diameter) × 76.2 mm (long) NaI(T1) (~ 3″ × 3″) detector with the source placed 250 mm from the face of the scintillation detector. Ge(Li) detectors with efficiencies of up to 20% of the NaI(T1) crystal mentioned above can now be obtained. It is usual to calibrate the Ge(Li) detector with known gamma ray standard sources.

5-2-6 Scintillation Detectors [6]

High-detection efficiency, large amplitude of output signals, and high speed make scintillation detectors—or as they are frequently called, *scintillation counters*—an indispensable tool for many spectrometric experiments. A scintillation counter usually consists of a scintillating phosphor and a photo-multiplier, which are coupled together with an optical contact. The fast charged particle or gamma ray passing through the scintillator loses part of its energy to the excitation of a molecule, which then returns to the ground state, emitting optical photons. It is obvious that the intensity of each scintillation is proportional to the energy lost by the particle or gamma ray in the phosphor. For phosphors it is generally found that there is a good degree of correlation between the amount of light flashes generated and the particle energy. Naturally this calls for linearity of conversion of the intensity of the scintillation into current pulses in the collector circuit.

Let us consider in detail the process of transforming the particle energy into a photomultiplier current pulse. Let the range of the particle fit entirely in the scintillator, and let the total number of optical photons n_0, emitted upon de-excitation of the excited luminescence centers be $n_0 = kE/E_{ph}$. In this expression E_{ph} is the average energy of the photons and k is the conversion efficiency of the scintillator—that is, the part of the particle or gamma energy converted into the energy of optical photon. The conversion efficiency is a most important characteristic of the scintillator from the point of view of its spectrometric properties. For the energy conversion to be linear, it is necessary that the quantity k not depend on the energy; only then will the number of converted photons be proportional to the particle energy. In addition, as will be shown below, to obtain the best amplitude resolution, the value of k should be as large as possible.

Among the n_0 photons arriving at the photocathode, only $n = g_0 n_0$ will produce the photoelectrons which will be further multiplied in the PM tube (g_0 is the coefficient that takes into account the losses of the part of the photons due to the geometrical coupling to the photomultiplier). If we also take into account the probability of the photon knocking out a photoelectron from the cathode of the photomultiplier Q, which is often known as the quantum efficiency of a photomultiplier, the number of electrons emitted by the photocathode will turn out to be $N_0 = Qn = kg_0 QE/E_{ph}$. Subsequently the primary flux of electrons is multiplied by the secondary emission on the dynodes of the photomultiplier. The total multiplication factor or coefficient of a PMT is then equal to m^l, where l is the number of dynodes of the photomultiplier and m is the average secondary emission or multiplication coefficient of each dynode. Consequently the total number of electrons in the collector or anode circuit of the photomultiplier, in the case of an incident particle of energy E, is $N = kg_0 Q m^l E/E_{ph}$. For N to be proportional to the energy, it is necessary that all the coefficients entering into the last expression be independent of the particle energy. With the exception of the conversion efficiency, they are connected either with the geometry of the light collection or with the parameters of the photomultiplier, such as the multiplication coefficient, and therefore they do not depend on the energy. The conversion efficiency, however, depends on the scintillator material, the type of incident particles, and their energy. There are at present no universal spectrometric scintillation detectors. However, for any specific spectrometric purpose, various detectors can be used successfully.

The most widely used scintillators are alkali-halide crystals activated with thallium, namely NaI(Tl) and CsI(Tl), and also the organic crystals of anthracene and stilbene [6]. Currently higher-stopping power or high atomic number inorganic scintillators are in active use, such as bismuth germinate also known as BGO ($Bi_4 Ge_3 O_{12}$) [10], and barium flouride, also known as BaF_2 [11].

The conversion efficiency of these scintillators when the scintillators are excited by fast electrons is practically independent of the energy in the range

Table 5-4

Phosphor	NaI(T1)[a]	CsI(T1)[a]	BGO[a]	Anthracene[b]	Stilbene[b]
ε (keV)	0.65	0.8	—	1.3	2.0
λ (keV)$^{1/2}$	7	8	14	10	12.5

[a] Inorganic scintillators.
[b] Organic scintillators.

from 0.01 to 10 MeV. If the scintillator is bombarded with heavy charged particles, the conversion efficiency drops with decreasing energy, particularly for the organic crystals. The dependence of the conversion efficiency on the energy is strong; the larger the mass of the particle, the larger the scintillations produced. Alkali-halide phosphors usually exhibit a higher linearity with heavy particles. Thus, for example, for protons with energy higher than 1.5 MeV and for alpha particles with energy higher than 4 MeV, the conversion efficiency is practically constant. To ensure the linearity of conversion of the energies, it is necessary to calibrate the spectrometer beforehand in order to set its zero.

For an estimate of the practical parameters of the scintillation detectors, it is convenient to introduce a quantity $\varepsilon = E/N_0 = E_{ph}/kg_0 Q$; this is the average energy needed for a photoelectron to be knocked out from the cathode of the photomultiplier for a given particle. This quantity is the analogue of the average energy needed for production of a pair of ions in ionization detectors. An exact calculation of the value of ε is difficult. Other conditions being equal, ε is determined by the conversion efficiency. In Table 5-4 are given the values of ε, which were obtained by processing the experimental data for several different phosphors.

The amplitude of the pulse at the output of the scintillation counter is

$$v_0 = \frac{qm^l}{C\varepsilon}E \quad \text{or} \quad \frac{qM}{C\varepsilon}E \tag{5-28}$$

where M is the total electron multiplication factor (i.e., $M = m^l$).

The average secondary-emission coefficient or dynode multiplication factor m is usually equal to 3 to 4 at optimum voltage on the photomultiplier, and the number of dynodes for the majority of modern multipliers is 10 to 13. Letting $m = 3.5$ and $l = 11$ ($M = 10^6$), $C = 20$ pF, $\varepsilon = 0.65$ keV (for sodium iodide) for the calculation, we obtain v_0 (V) $\cong 10E$ (MeV). For electrons with an energy of 1 MeV, the probable amplitude of the pulses is approximately 10 V, which is many times the amplitude of the pulses from detectors of other types.

The resolving power of scintillation counters is determined by N_0, the fluctuations of its amplification coefficient M, and the magnitude of the statistical fluctuations of the primary electron stream from the photocathode of the photomultiplier. Assuming, as before, that the elementary acts leading to the formation of the primary flux and its amplification obey a probability law, we can use the Poisson distribution for the determination of the fluctuations on each stage of this process. Then the mean square deviation of the number of electrons reaching the first dynode is $\sigma_1 = \sqrt{fN_0}$, and that for the second dynode is $\sigma_2 = \sqrt{fN_0 m}$, and so on, where f is the collection factor of the photoelectrons for the first dynode from the cathode of the input electron-optical system. The relative dispersion of the output electron flux is therefore

$$\left(\frac{\sigma}{N}\right)^2 = \left(\frac{\sigma_1}{fN_0}\right)^2 + \left(\frac{\sigma_2}{fN_0 m}\right)^2 + \cdots + \left(\frac{\sigma_l}{fN_0 m^l}\right)^2 = \frac{1}{fN_0} + \cdots + \frac{1}{fN_0 m^{l-1}}$$

(5-29)

Equation (5-29) can also be written as

$$\left(\frac{\sigma}{N}\right)^2 = \frac{1}{fN_0} \frac{(1/m)^l - 1}{(1/m) - 1} \cong \frac{1}{fN_0} \frac{m}{m-1}, \qquad l \gg 1 \qquad (5\text{-}30)$$

Then the resolving power of the counter is

$$\eta = 236 \sqrt{\frac{1}{fN_0} \frac{m}{m-1}} \ \% \qquad (5\text{-}31)$$

Substituting $m = 3.5$, $N_0 = E/\varepsilon$, and $f = 1$ into this expression, we obtain

$$\eta = \frac{\lambda}{\sqrt{E \ (\text{MeV})}} \ \% \qquad (5\text{-}32)$$

where $\lambda = 8.8\sqrt{\varepsilon}$. The values of λ calculated for different phosphors appear in the second row of Table 5-4. The resolution of the gamma radiation line corresponding to photoelectric absorption in a sodium iodide crystal of quanta from the isotope ^{137}Cs, which has an energy of 661.6 keV, amounts to about 8.5%.

The resolution obtained in practice frequently exceeds the indicated value. The deterioration in resolution can be attributed, for example, to the inhomogeneity of the distribution of the activator over the volume of the crystal and to the poor optical contact between the crystal and the photomultiplier. The uneven sensitivity of the photocathode, the loss of charge in the input electron-optical system $(f < 1)$, and a low coefficient of secondary emission also cause a reduction in the resolving power. It is further worthwhile to note that the photomultiplier gain depends strongly on the voltage applied to the photomultiplier, especially on dynodes, and follows the equation

$$\frac{\Delta M}{M} \cong l\frac{\Delta U}{U} \tag{5-33}$$

where ΔU and U are the voltage fluctuation and total voltage applied to the PM tube, respectively. To stabilize the gain, it is necessary to maintain the supply voltage at a constant with a high degree of stability. Thus, for the gain to be stable within better than 1%, the high voltage must be kept constant to within 0.1% or better for both the anode and the dynode.

5-3   PULSE SHAPES OF THE DETECTORS [12]

In the preceding section we have discussed the detector properties connected with the amplitude characteristics, linearity, and resolution. The time characteristics were not considered, and for simplicity it was assumed that the entire charge is collected on the detector capacitance. In many cases of practical importance, however, the time characteristics of the process wherein the particle energy is converted into a current or voltage pulse (which determines the waveform of such a pulse) play a primary role. These cases include spectrometry under fast coincidence detection, under increased pulse repetition frequencies, and pulse shape discrimination. In the design of apparatus intended for the solution of the above-mentioned problems, it is often necessary to have information concerning the forms and shapes of the detected pulses. To this end, we will study in this section information on the forms and shapes of current and voltage pulses at the outputs of the spectrometric detectors studied previously.

5-3-1   General Equation

All detectors can be regarded with good approximation as being generators of current pulses. The physical basis of this fact is that the amplitude of the pulses produced across the detector load is, as a rule, so small compared with the supply voltage that the collection or the coefficient of amplification of the charge (in proportional and scintillation counters) remains practically constant during the development of the pulse.

The equivalent circuit of the output of the detector constitutes a parallel RC network, whose capacitance is equal to the sum of the capacitance of the detector, the input capacitance of the preamplifier, and the capacitance of the wiring (connecting leads) often called *stray capacitance*. The ohmic resistance R, which is connected in the detector circuit, not only delivers a constant potential to one of the detector electrodes but serves also to discharge the capacitor C so as to avoid the accumulation of charge. The load resistance R is not chosen arbitrarily. If the amplitude of the voltage pulses at the output of the detector is small, then to reduce the noise and to improve the signal to noise ratio, the value of R must be chosen to be sufficiently large (several times 10 kiloohms) such that the time constant is $RC \cong 1$ μsec to 1 msec. Large RC time constants, such as 1 msec, make operation of the detector at high-pulse repetition frequencies difficult. When operating with scintillation counters, the noise of the amplifier is, as a rule, not as important as in the case of semiconductor detectors, for example. The tendency is to make R smaller, so as to eliminate the superposition or pileup of signals and the associated errors during the subsequent amplitude analysis.

For the analysis of the integrated charge we introduce the following notation:

$i(t)$ = output pulse of detector current

$i_R(t)$ = current component flowing in the resistance R

$i_C(t)$ = current component charging the capacitor C

Let us set up Kirchhof's equations for the output RC circuit, which is given by

$$i_R(t) + i_C(t) = i(t) \qquad \text{(currents)}$$

$$i_R(t)R = \frac{1}{C} \int i_C(t) \, dt \qquad \text{(voltages)} \qquad (5\text{-}34)$$

Differentiating the second equation with respect to t and substituting it $[i_C(t) = RC(di_R(t)/dt)]$ into the first equation, we obtain

$$\frac{di_R(t)}{dt} + \frac{i_R(t)}{\tau} = \frac{i(t)}{\tau} \qquad (5\text{-}35)$$

where $\tau = RC$. The solution of this equation can be written in the form

$$i_R(t) = \frac{1}{\tau} e^{-t/\tau} \int_0^t i(t') e^{-t'/\tau} \, dt' \qquad (5\text{-}36)$$

The corresponding voltage pulse is simply

$$v(t) = i_R R = \frac{1}{C} e^{-t/\tau} \int_0^t i(t') e^{-t'/\tau} \, dt' \qquad (5\text{-}37)$$

The physical meaning of this formula is particularly clear if we assume that τ greatly exceeds the duration of the detector current pulse T_p. Then the integrand function $[i(t')e^{-t'/\tau}]$ is equal to $i(t)$, and the integral is equal to the charge accumulated on the capacitor up to the instant t. When $t \gg T_p$, we have $v(t) = (Q/C)\exp(-t/\tau)$; that is, the signal decreases exponentially from its maximum value $v_m = Q/C$ to zero with a time constant τ.

We will henceforth denote $\int_0^t i(t')e^{-t'/\tau}\,dt'$ by $Q(t)$. When $\tau \gg T_p$, the value of this integral is equal to the charge gathered on the capacitance up to the instant t.

5-3-2 Pulse Shape of an Ionization Chamber

Based on the above current and voltage pulse, let us consider a parallel-plate ionization chamber with a grid and introduce the following notation:

t_1 = time of motion of the electrons from the cathode to the grid

T = time of motion of the electrons from the grid to the collector

$t_2 = t_1 + T$ = time of motion of the electrons from the cathode to the collector

$T_\theta = l\cos\theta/u_1$ = time delay of the arrival of the electrons at the extreme ends of a track of length l to the collector at an angle θ to the field direction

u_1, u_2 = speeds of the electrons from the cathode to the grid and from the grid to anode, respectively

The elementary current of each electron moving in the space between the grid and the collector is $i = qu_2(W/U) = qu_2(1/d) = q/T$, where W and U are the field intensity and voltage, respectively.

If at the instant $t = 0$, an alpha particle passes through the working volume (cathode-grid) with an angle θ, producing N pairs of ions along a track length l, then the current pulse flowing through the chamber can be expressed as [see Fig. 5-5(a)]

$$i(t) = \begin{cases} 0 & \text{for } 0 \le t \le t_1 - T_\theta \\[2mm] \dfrac{Nq}{T}\dfrac{t-(t_1-T_\theta)}{T_\theta} & \text{for } t_1 - T_\theta \le t \le t_1 \\[2mm] \dfrac{Nq}{T} & \text{for } t_1 \le t \le t_2 - T_\theta \quad (5\text{-}38) \\[2mm] \dfrac{Nq}{T}\left[1 - \dfrac{t-(t_2-T_\theta)}{T_\theta}\right] & \text{for } t_2 - T_\theta \le t \le t_2 \\[2mm] 0 & \text{for } t_2 \le t \end{cases}$$

Henceforth, for simplicity in the calculations, we will assume that $t_2 \ll \tau$ and that $\int_0^t i(t')e^{-t'/\tau}\,dt' \cong \int_0^t i(t')\,dt'$. Then $v(t) = [Q(t)/C]\exp(-t/\tau)$, where

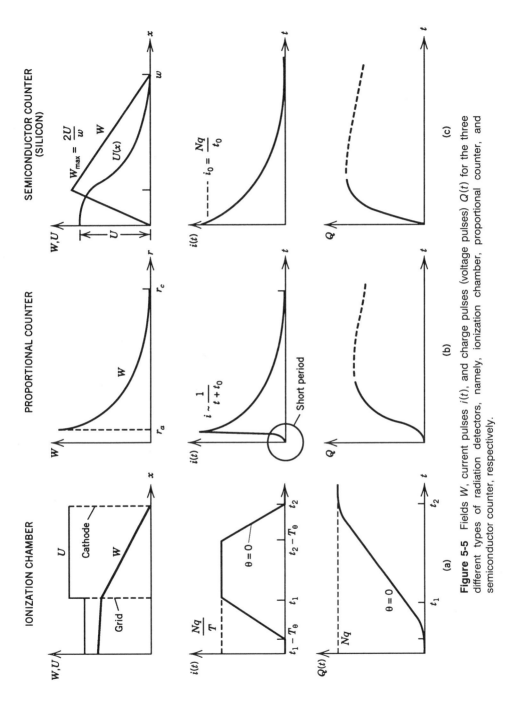

Figure 5-5 Fields W, current pulses $i(t)$, and charge pulses (voltage pulses) $Q(t)$ for the three different types of radiation detectors, namely, ionization chamber, proportional counter, and semiconductor counter, respectively.

137

$Q(t)$ is the fraction of the charge collected on the capacitor of the chamber at the instant t. Integration of the current on individual intervals leads to the following results:

$$Q(t) = \begin{cases} 0 & \text{for } 0 \le t \le t_1 - T_\theta \\[2mm] \dfrac{1}{2}\dfrac{Nq}{T}\dfrac{[t - (t_1 - T_\theta)]^2}{T_\theta} & \text{for } t_1 - T_\theta \le t \le t_1 \\[2mm] \dfrac{1}{2}\dfrac{Nq}{T}T_\theta + \dfrac{Nq}{T}(t - t_1) & \text{for } t_1 \le t \le t_2 - T_\theta \\[2mm] \dfrac{1}{2}\dfrac{Nq}{T}T_\theta + \dfrac{Nq}{T}(T - T_\theta) & \\[2mm] \quad + \dfrac{Nq}{T}\{[t - t(t_2 - T_\theta)]\} & \\[2mm] \quad - \dfrac{1}{2T_\theta}[t - (t_2 - T_\theta)]^2 & \text{for } t_2 - T_\theta \le t \le t_2 \\[2mm] Nq & \text{for } t_2 \le t \end{cases}$$

(5-39)

Figure 5-5(a) shows the shape of the charge or voltage pulse for an angle of the ion column relative to the field direction $\theta = 0$ and, $T_\theta = T/2$. A characteristic feature is the presence of a finite delay in the growth of the signal relative to the instant of passage of the particle through the working volume of the counter. If collimation is used, limiting the direction of the motion of the particles from the cathode to the collector (anode) by a narrow solid angle about $\theta = 0$, it is possible to reduce the time spread. There is no amplitude spread, however, due to different emission directions if $\tau \gg t_2$. For a field intensity of 800 to 1000 (V/cm) in the chamber, at a gas pressure of 760 mm Hg, the velocity of the electrons in the chamber is $u \cong 10^6$ cm/sec, and the scale of the time intervals t_1 and t_2 (determining the duration of the leading front and falling edge of the current pulse) is on the order of a microsecond. Therefore in most cases the choice of a time constant $\tau \cong 10$ μsec ensures almost complete collection of the charge. When τ is decreased, the exponential factor in the integrand differs from unity, and values of the integral would vary and result in dispersion of amplitudes of the pulses.

5-3-3 Pulse Shape of a Proportional Counter

The elementary current occurring when a charge q moves in a field intensity of W the current pulse produced by two electrodes on which a voltage U is applied, as shown in Fig. 5-5(b)—is equal to $i = quW/U$, where u is the velocity component of the charge in the direction of the field and W is the electric field. For a cylindrical geometry we have $W(r) = (1/r)[U/\ln(r_c/r_a)]$ and $u \to u_r$ with $u_r = \mu W$ (μ is the mobility of the charge). The particle incident into the counter produces a column of ions along its path. The electrons begin to move toward the filament or collector under the influence of the field. When the electrons due to the primary ionization move, a small current of short duration will flow in the circuit of the counter [see the i pulse in Fig. 5-5(b)]. However, a major current component arises only after multiple secondary impact ionization. As discussed earlier, this occurs near the anode, where the field intensity is large. In this region there will be multiple secondary impact ionizations, and the primary electron charge will suddenly become large. However, there is no instantaneous increase in current as the result of the electron charge carriers produced near the filament because they are too close to the anode (filament), which has a positive potential and therefore collects only electrons.

Instead, further increase in the current is due to the displacement of the ions from the anode electrode to the cathode, which is a much larger distance, by the positive ions. Since all the ions are localized near the anode, their contribution is the major part of the total current and also occurs in the same time as the electron collection. This current can be written in the form

$$i = \frac{Nq\mu_i U}{[\ln(r_c/r_a)]^2} \frac{1}{r^2} \tag{5-40}$$

where N is the total number of secondary pairs of ions and μ_i is the mobility of the heavy or positive ions. It must be noted that despite the low mobility of the ions, the growth in the current is very rapid, owing to the strong dependence of the current on the radial coordinate of the ions. At small r, the derivative $di/dr \approx 1/r^3$ is quite high, so the initial part of the growth amounts to less than a microsecond, as seen from the current pulse shown in Fig. 5-5(b).

Let us find the dependence of the current due to the ionic charge on the time where the following relations are assumed: (see relation $u_r = u_i W = u_i[U/\ln(r_i/r_1)]1/r$);

$$u_i = \frac{dr_i}{dt} = \frac{\mu_i U}{\ln(r_c/r_a)} \frac{1}{r}$$

$$\int_{r_a}^{r} r \, dr = \int_0^t \frac{\mu_i U}{\ln(r_c/r_a)} dt \tag{5-41}$$

Then from Eq. (5-41) we obtain

$$r^2 - r_a^2 = \frac{2\mu_i U}{\ln(r_c/r_a)} t \tag{5-42}$$

Obviously the total charge collection time T can be obtained by setting $r = r_c$:

$$T = \frac{\ln(r_c/r_a)}{2\mu_i U} r_a^2 \left(\frac{r_c^2}{r_a^2} - 1 \right) = t_0 \left(\frac{r_c^2}{r_a^2} - 1 \right) \tag{5-43}$$

where we have introduced the notation $t_0 = [\ln(r_c/r_a)/2\mu_i U]r_a^2$. Using Eq. (5-42), it is then possible to write $r^2 = [2\mu_i U/\ln(r_c/r_a)](t + t_0)$. Then the equation for the current pulse given by Eq. (5-40) becomes

$$i(t) = \frac{Nq}{2\ln(r_c/r_a)} \frac{1}{t + t_0} \tag{5-44}$$

When $t \gg T$, the charge pulse $Q(t)$ becomes

$$Q(t) = \int_0^t i(t') \, dt' = \frac{Nq}{2\ln(r_c/r_a)} \ln\left(\frac{t}{t_0} + 1 \right) \tag{5-45}$$

If $t = T$, $Q(t)$ becomes

$$Q(t) = Nq \tag{5-46}$$

Figure 5-5(b) shows the current and voltage pulses of a proportional counter for $T = 10^{-3}$ sec and $r_c/r_a = 10^3$. Although the contribution of the primary ionization electrons to the total charge can be neglected if the multiplication coefficients of the counter are sufficiently large, this portion of the pulse delay is not negligible and often equals a fraction of a microsecond depending on the trajectory of the detected particle.

With a time constant τ ($\cong RC$) comparable to the collection time constant T, it is necessary to take into account the exponential term under the integral sign. However, in as much as the result of the integration cannot be expressed in the form of one of the elementary functions, it is sometimes convenient to use the first-order approximation result:

$$Q(t) \cong \frac{Nq}{2\ln(r_c/r_a)} \left[\ln\left(\frac{t}{t_0} + 1 \right) + \frac{t}{\tau} \right] \tag{5-47}$$

where t/τ is the first-order approximation of $e^{-t/\tau} = 1 - t/\tau$.

Complete collection of the ionic charge occurs within a time interval of 100 μsec to 1 msec, where as the collection time of the electronic charge is on the order of 1 μsec. To obtain sufficiently high speed, a resistive load circuit in the order of 100 to 1000 kilohms with a capacitance of 20 pF is commonly used, and the resulting time constant of $\tau = 1$ to 10 μsec can easily be obtained. The voltage pulse is then mainly due to the electronic charge and can be shortened. The voltage pulse can be expressed by $v(t) \cong [Q(t)/C]\exp(-t/\tau)$. This electronic charge collection is more widely used than the total charge collection despite the somewhat smaller voltage pulse obtainable by collecting only the electronic charge.

5-3-4 Pulse Shapes of Semiconductor Detectors

Silicon Detectors

In the silicon detector the charge collection phenomena are almost analogous to the gas-filled ionization chamber with only slight differences. An important factor for the determination of the waveform of the pulse of a semiconductor detector is the inhomogeneity of the field within the junction which represents the depletion layer and has a maximum near the boundary of the n-silicon [if the main crystal was originally p-silicon (note this is the case of p-silicon as a base material); see Figs. 5-3(c) and 5-5(c)]. If we assume that all the carriers are produced in the region of the maximum field, then we can write the equation of the current of the hole component only (neglecting the electronic component since the maximum field is on the boundary of the n-silicon) as

$$i(t) = \frac{Nq}{U}\mu_p W_{max}^2 \exp\left(\frac{-2\mu_p W_{max} t}{w}\right) \tag{5-48}$$

where μ_p is the mobility of the holes, W_{max} is the value of the field at the maximum, U is the voltage applied to the junction, and $2\mu_p W_{max}/w = \mu_p W_{max}^2/U = 1/t_0$. The normalization condition $\int_0^\infty i(t)\,dt = Nq$ is satisfied in this case, since for a linearly decreasing field we have $W_{max} = 2U/w$, where w is the width of the entire junction.

Let us estimate the time constant of the decay in the current pulse for $U = 10$ V and $w = 50$ μm:

$$t_0 = \frac{w}{2\mu_p W_{max}} = \frac{w^2}{4\mu_p U} = \frac{(50 \times 10^{-4})^2}{4 \times 500 \times 10} \cong 1 \text{ nsec} \tag{5-49}$$

where μ_p of silicon is assumed to be 500 cm^2/sec.

The equation for the pulse can be rewritten in the form $i(t) = (Nq/t_0)\exp(-t/t_0)$. Substituting this expression in the right-hand side of the general expression for the voltage pulse, we obtain

$$Q(t) = \frac{Nq}{t_0} \int_0^t e^{(-t'/t_0)} e^{(-t'/\tau)} \, dt' \tag{5-50}$$

When τ has a value less than 100 nsec, we have

$$Q(t) = Nq \left[1 - \exp\left(-\frac{t}{t_0} \right) \right] \tag{5-51}$$

Therefore, provided complete charge collection is made the equation for the voltage pulse has the form

$$v(t) = \frac{Nq}{C} (1 - e^{-t/t_0}) e^{-t/\tau} \tag{5-52}$$

Note that the last exponential term $e^{-t/\tau}$ is the signal decay due to the circuitry with RC time constant τ. The amplitude of the pulse is $V_m = Nq/C$, and the time necessary to reach a level of 99% of the maximum value is approximately $5t_0$, that is, on the order of 10 nsec.

If the electron-hole column is located not in the region of the maximum field but arbitrarily, the waveform of the current pulse becomes more complicated than a simple exponential decrease. However, even in this case it is characterized by a short duration, $Nq[1 - \exp(-t/t_0)]$. The relative scatter in the leading fronts of the pulses of a semiconductor detector for different track orientations of the detected particles from the depletion layer is also small.

Ge(Li) Detectors

Ge(Li) detectors differ slightly from the Si surface-barrier-type detectors discussed above, and they follow two different shapes depending on the type of detector configuration: for example, planar type or coaxial type. Although Ge gamma ray detectors yield excellent energy resolution, the best time resolution obtained is still not as good as that available with scintillation counters. If amplifier noise were the only limitation, timing with Ge could be very precise, particularly at high energies. Unfortunately, timing accuracy is seriously degraded by pulse shape variations, which depend on the location of the interaction in the depletion volume of the detector and on the detector geometry. In planar detectors the rise time is found to vary by about a factor of two, and in coaxial detectors the variation is even greater because of the nonuniform electric field. If one neglects carrier velocity saturation effects, the rise time and signal shapes for the two detector geometries can be classified as either planar or coaxial.

Planar Germanium Detectors   For the planar Ge(Li) case the charge collection times of the electrons and holes are given by

$$t_e = \frac{x_0}{\mu_e W}$$

$$t_h = \frac{x - x_0}{\mu_h W} \qquad (5\text{-}53)$$

where the μ_e and μ_h are the mobilities of the electrons and holes at 77°K,
respectively, and W is the electric field. The charge collection pulse shape
then becomes

$$Q(t) = Nq\left\{\left(\frac{x_0}{x}\right)[t - (t - t_e)H(t - t_e)] + \left(\frac{x - x_0}{x}\right)\right.$$

$$\left. \times [t - (t - t_h)H(t - t_h)]\right\} \qquad (5\text{-}54)$$

where N is the number of the charges ionized, q is the electronic charge,
$H(t - t_e)$ and $H(t - t_h)$ are the delayed unit step functions associated with
electrons and holes, and x and x_0 are the distances shown in Fig. 5-6 (a),
respectively.

Coaxial Ge(Li) Detectors   For the case of the coaxial double open-ended
detector, the corresponding charge collection times are observed

$$t_e = \frac{\ln(r_2/r_1)}{2\mu_e U}(r_2^2 - r_0^2)$$

$$t_h = \frac{\ln(r_2/r_1)}{2\mu_h U}(r_0^2 - r_1^2) \qquad (5\text{-}55)$$

Charge collection pulse shape then becomes

$$Q(t) = \frac{Nq}{2\ln(r_2/r_1)}\left\{\ln\left[1 + \frac{r_2^2 - r_1^2}{r_0^2}\left(\frac{t}{t_e}\right)\right] - \ln\left[1 - \frac{r_2^2 - r_1^2}{r_0^2}\left(\frac{t}{t_h}\right)\right]\right\}$$

$$(5\text{-}56)$$

where r_1, r_2, and r_0 are the detector radii shown in Fig. 5-6 (b), and U is the
applied voltage on the detector.

Calculated charge pulse shapes based on Eqs. (5-54) and (5-56) are shown
in Figs. 5-6 (a) and (b) on the assumption that electron and hole mobilities μ_e
and μ_h are equal and that, in the case of the coaxial detector, the electric

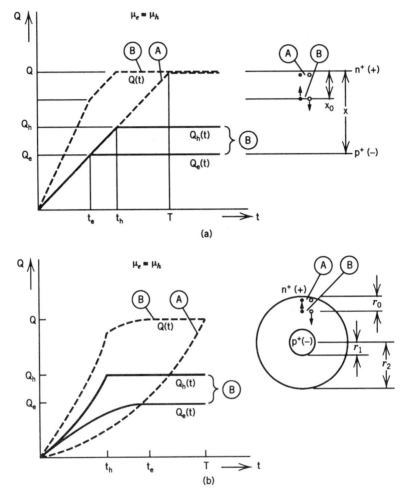

Figure 5-6   Charge pulse shapes for the planar and coaxial Ge(Li) semiconductor detectors. On the right side of each charge pulse, positions of the electrons and hole pairs created are indicated. ● and ○ are the electrons and holes.

field has a $1/r$ dependence. Figure 5-6 also assumes an infinitely fast charge amplifier.

5-3-5   Pulse Shapes of a Scintillation Counter

When a particle or quanta passes through the phosphor of a scintillation counter, a chain of excited phosphor molecules is produced along its track. Let the total number of excited molecules be $n_0 = kE/E_{\text{ph}}$. They will subsequently go into the ground state and emit optical photons in accordance

Table 5-5

Phosphor	NaI(T1)[a]	CsI(T1)[a]	BGO[a]	Anthracene[b]	Stilbene[b]
t_0 (μsec)	0.25	0.8	0.3	0.036	0.006

[a]Inorganic scintillator.
[b]Organic scintillator.

with the decay law similar to that of radioactive decay with a time constant t_0 (t_0 is the average lifetime of the excited molecule). The number of optical photons emitted by the phosphor per unit time is $dn/dt = (n_0/t_0)\exp(-t/t_0)$. If we assume that the photomultipler is an ideal electron multiplier in terms of time, then the electron beam striking the photomultiplier collector will follow the original photon emission decay; that is, $dN/dt = (N_0/t_0)e^{-t/t_0}$ with N_0 being the number of electrons arriving at the anode.

Thus, the current pulse at the output of a scintillation counter can be written in the form $i(t) = q(dN/dt) = (N_0 q e^{-t/t_0})/t_0$ where the time constant t_0, the falloff time constant of the current, is determined by the de-excitation or decay time constant of the phosphor and amounts to approximately a microsecond or less for the many spectrometric phosphors such as NaI(T1), or CsI(T1) and BGO, which are generally considered as the scintillators of maximum conversion efficiency. The values of t_0 for the most widely used phosphors are given in Table 5-5.

As in the case of the silicon semiconductor detector [see Eq. (5-50)], if there is a wide scatter in the values of t_0 for the given phosphors, one should consider the different ratios of τ and t_0. For this purpose we find the values of the integral as

$$Q(t) = \frac{Nq}{t_0} \int_0^t e^{-t'/t_0} e^{t'/\tau} \, dt' = \frac{Nq}{t_0} \frac{1}{[(1/\tau) - (1/t_0)]} [e^{-t/t_0} e^{-t/\tau} - 1]$$

$$(5-57)$$

The voltage pulse will then become

$$v(t) = \frac{Nq}{C} \frac{q}{(t_0/\tau) - 1} (e^{-t/t_0} - e^{-t/\tau}) e^{-t/\tau} \qquad (5-58)$$

If $\tau \gg t_0$, then, as in the case of semiconductor detectors, the voltage pulse becomes

$$v(t) = \frac{Nq}{C} (1 - e^{-t/t_0}) e^{-t/\tau} \qquad (5-59)$$

If we set $t = t_M \cong t_0 \ln(\tau/t_0)$, corresponding to the time at which the voltage pulse becomes its maximum value v_M, the maximum value v_M is given by

$$v_M = \frac{Nq}{C} \qquad (5\text{-}60)$$

This condition is usually realized in gamma ray spectrometry with the aid of organic crystals of anthracene and stilbene at $\tau \geq 1$ μsec. If $\tau \approx t_0$, then

$$v(t) = \frac{Nq}{C} \frac{t}{\tau} e^{-t/\tau} \qquad (5\text{-}61)$$

The maximum voltage is obtained at $t = t_M = \tau$ and v_M becomes

$$v_M = \frac{1}{e} \frac{Nq}{C} \qquad (5\text{-}62)$$

Thus, owing to the incomplete gathering of the charge due to the too short integration time, the amplitude of the pulse is reduced to a value 2.7 times smaller than the amplitude of the pulse corresponding to the total charge collection or integration. A similar ratio of t_0 and τ can occur if crystals such as CsI(Tl) and NaI(Tl) are used with $\tau = 1$ to 0.3 μsec.

Sometimes, for the registration of fast coincidences, the photomultiplier is loaded with a small resistance, as small as 50 to 100 ohms, so that $\tau \ll t_0$. The voltage pulse then duplicates the wave form of the current pulse

$$v(t) = \frac{Nq}{C} \frac{\tau}{t_0} e^{-t/t_0} = i(t) R \qquad (5\text{-}63)$$

The amplitude of the signal is, in this case, τ/t_0 times smaller than in the case of complete collection of the charge.

It must be noted that when amplitude decreases as τ decreases, the relative variation of the amplitudes of the pulses will increase. This is due to the fact that the charges stored at the load circuit (RC network) fluctuates from pulse to pulse. If $\tau \gg t_0$, then almost complete collection of the charge takes place and the best resolution is obtained. When $\tau < t_0$, the resolution deteriorates owing to the incomplete collection of the charge.

REFERENCES

1. R. L. Chase. *Nuclear Pulse Spectrometry*. New York: McGraw-Hill, 1961.
2. G. Knoll. *Radiation Detection and Measurement*. New York: Wiley, 1979.
3. R. D. Evans. *The Atomic Nucleus*. New York: McGraw Hill, 1955.

4. K. Siegbahn. α, β, *and γ ray Spectroscopy*. Amsterdam: North Holland, 1968.

5. E. Segre. *Nuclei and Particles*. New York: W. A. Benjamin, 1965.

6. J. B. Birks, *Scintillation Counters*. London: Pergamon, 1960.

7. W. Hendee, *Medical Radiation Physics*. Chicago: Year Book Medical Publishers, 1970.

8. H. E. Johns and J. R. Cunningham. *The Physics of Radiology*. Springfield, IL: Charles C. Thomas, 1953.

9. D. Halliday. *Introductory Nuclear Physics*. New York: Wiley, 1950.

10. Z. H. Cho and M. R. Farukhi. *J. Nucl. Med.* 18: 840–844 (1977).

11. M. Laval. *Nucl. Instr. Meth.* 206: 169–176 (1983).

12. Z. H. Cho and R. L. Chase. Comparative study of the timing techniques currently employed with Ge detectors. *Nucl. Inst. Meth.* 98:335 (1972).

6

X-RAY COMPUTERIZED TOMOGRAPHY

6-1 BASIC CONCEPTS AND IMAGE RECONSTRUCTION

X-ray CT is a product of X-ray technology with advanced computer signal processing, and is capable of generating a cross-sectional display of the body. It is, in fact, the origin of the entire CT evolution which began in the early 1970s [1, 2].

The basic principle of the X-ray CT involves X-ray generation, detection, digitization, processing, and computer image reconstruction. X-rays passing through a body are attenuated at different rates by different tissues. The attenuated X-rays are then collected by the detectors and converted to digital numbers or data by the analog to digital converters (ADCs). The digital data are fed into a computing device for image reconstruction.

Generally the pencil-beam-type X-ray is simply scanned along a line at a given direction or view. To achieve several different angles of perspective or projection data, the scanning is repeated at each given angular view by simply rotating both the X-ray tube and detectors.

6-1-1 Basic Physical Principles

Contrast Mechanism and Projection Data

The photon density that emerges when a narrow beam of monoenergetic photons with energy E_0 and intensity I_0 passes through a homogenous absorber of thickness x can be expressed as [3]

$$I = I_0 \exp\left[-\mu(\rho, Z, E_0)x\right] \tag{6-1}$$

where μ, ρ, and Z are the linear attenuation coefficient, density of the

148

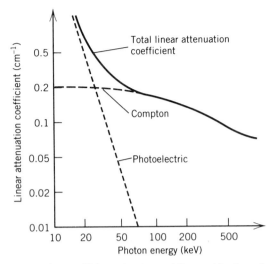

Figure 6-1   Linear attenuation coefficient of water and the contribution of each interaction to the total attenuation of X rays as a function of the energy.

absorber, and atomic number, respectively. In the energy region where most commercial X-ray CT systems are being engaged for medical tomography ($\cong 70$ keV), two types of interactions are dominant, namely photoelectric absorption and Compton scattering.

In photoelectric interaction the X-ray photon is completely absorbed by transferring all of its energy to an electron. In Compton scattering, on the other hand, scattered X-rays undergo both a directional and energy change. Figure 6-1 depicts the interactions of the X-rays with water. It shows the contribution of each photon interaction mechanism to the linear attenuation coefficient as a function of energy. If the absorber is not homogeneous, $\mu(\rho, Z)$ is simply a space-variant function dependent on the distributions of the material. By directing a monochromatic X-ray beam in the y direction, for instance, the output X-ray intensity $I(x)$ can be written as

$$I(x) = I_0(x)\exp\left[-\int\mu(x, y)\,dy\right] \qquad (6\text{-}2)$$

where I_0 and $\mu(x, y)$ are the incident X-ray intensity and X-ray attenuation coefficient, respectively. For example, by taking the logarithm and rearranging Eq. (6-2), one can obtain projection data $p(x)$:

$$p(x) = -\ln\left[\frac{I(x)}{I_0(x)}\right]$$

$$= \int\mu(x, y)\,dy \qquad (6\text{-}3)$$

where $p(x)$ is equivalent to a simple integration or summation of the total attenuation coefficients along the X-ray path (i.e., y direction). Equation (6-3) in a digital form becomes

$$p(x) = \sum_{i=1}^{i=N} \mu_i(x, y), \qquad N = 1, 2, \ldots, N \qquad (6\text{-}4)$$

Equation (6-4) represents the summation of the attenuation coefficients of N-pixels along a given X-ray path.

In X-ray CT the contrast is associated with the different attenuation coefficients of the material involved. Since each set of projection data represents the integral value of the attenuation coefficients along the path, the projection data taken at different views are the basic for tomographic image reconstruction. An example of a ray for the case of a single beam of $N = 4$ is illustrated in Fig. 6-2(a). In practice, a radiation source scans

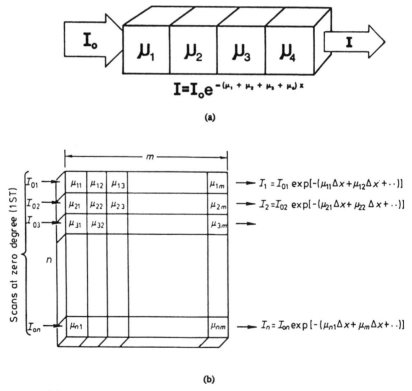

(a)

(b)

Figure 6-2   (a) A simplified X-ray beam I_0 attenuated through a pixel and results of the attenuated beam I. (b) A two-dimensional matrix of linear attenuation coefficients of the image. Attenuated beam intensities for the corresponding rows (i.e., $I_1, I_2, \ldots$) are shown at the right.

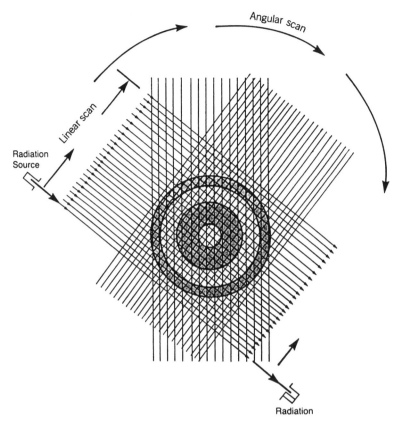

Figure 6-3 Parallel beam linear and angular scannings. Line-integral data sets from different angles measuring the amount of radiation passing through the body along each ray are the basic data sets to be used for image reconstruction. Each ray here represents the line-integrals along the path.

linearly along an object at a given view ϕ, and after completion of a linear scan, the source and detector pair rotate a small angle $\Delta\phi$ and repeat the linear scan until the completion of 180° or 360° rotation. For the parallel-beam data collection scheme, a total of 180°/N scans with an angular increment of $\Delta\phi$ is collected for a scan angle of 180°. An example of a complete 2-D attenuation coefficient matrix and examples of attenuated beam intensities for a set of rows at $\phi = 0°$ are shown in Fig. 6-2(b). A basic form of the linear and angular scannings is illustrated in Fig. 6-3. For the final image reconstruction in an image matrix of $N \times N$, each beam is backprojected in the image matrix with some form of spatial or spatial frequency domain filtering. Again, an example of the beam $p_\phi(x')|_{\phi=45°}$ backprojected onto the image matrix is illustrated in Fig. 6-4. As discussed in Chapter 3,

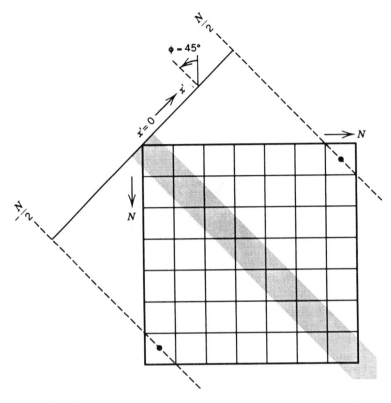

Figure 6-4 Total X-ray beam attenuation is determined (after taking logarithms) by the sum of the amounts attenuated by each square block of tissue. Note here that the line-integral is in strict sense a strip-integral with a width equivalent to the width or height of each pixel or rectangle in the matrix.

projection data $p_\phi(x')$ generally can be written as

$$p_\phi(x') = \int f(x, y)\, dy' \qquad (6\text{-}5)$$

where $f(x, y)$ is an image function, and x' and y' are the rotated coordinates given by

$$x' = x \cos \phi + y \sin \phi$$
$$y' = -x \sin \phi + y \cos \phi \qquad (6\text{-}6)$$

6-1-2 Contrast Mechanisms

Basic atomic and density modulation in X-ray transmission imaging has been studied by a number of investigators and interested readers should study the references [4, 5, 6]. When a multienergetic or polychromatic X-ray passes through a sample characterized by various attenuation coefficients quantized in Δx on a grid, the exit beam may be expressed as (e.g., see Fig. 6-2).

$$I_i = \int_{E_1=0}^{E_2=E_{max}} I_{0i}(E)\exp\left(-\sum_{ij}\mu_{ij}(E)\,\Delta x\right)dE \qquad (6\text{-}7)$$

where $I_{0i}(E)$ is the energy-dependent initial photon intensity of the ith beam and $\mu_{ij}(E)$ is the linear attenuation coefficient of the jth element at the ith beam. Equation (6-7) is usually simplified to a monoenergetic case and reduced to

$$I_i = I_{0i}\exp\left[-(\mu_{11}\,\Delta x + \mu_{12}\,\Delta x + \cdots + \mu_{1n}\,\Delta x)\right] \qquad (6\text{-}8)$$

The three-dimensional image reconstruction algorithms applied for most of the transmission scanners assume monoenergetic beams for convenience, although the validity of such an assumption warrants detailed discussion. In general, they assume a "most probable energy" or "effective energy," a term somewhat ambiguous in practice. Since linear attenuation coefficients are strongly energy dependent, any energy spread eventually leads to the averaging of linear attenuation coefficients which is naturally a resolution-degrading factor in transmission tomography.

Contrast due to Atomic Number and Electron Density with a Monoenergetic Photon Source [7, 8]

For simplicity, let us first review contrast and modulation effects arising from atomic number and electron density in the case of monoenergetic photons. The linear attenuation coefficient μ, which is the sole measurable quantity from an object, can be decomposed into two main components: one arising from the photoelectric effect, μ_p, and the other due to the Compton effect μ_c, expressed in units of cm^{-1} as

$$\mu_p = K_1\frac{\rho n_0 \tilde{Z}^{m-1}}{E^{3.1}} \qquad (6\text{-}9)$$

$$\mu_c = K_2\left\{\frac{1+\beta}{\beta^2}\left(\frac{2(1+\beta)}{1+2\beta} - \frac{\ln(1+2\beta)}{\beta}\right) + \frac{\ln(1+2\beta)}{2\beta} - \frac{(1+3\beta)}{(1+2\beta)^2}\right\}$$

$$= K_2\rho n_0 f(E) \qquad (6\text{-}10)$$

where K_1 and K_2 are constants, ρ is the density (g/cm³), n_0 is the electron density per gram (number of electrons/g), $\tilde{Z}$ is the effective atomic number, E is the energy of the incident photon, m is an empirical constant chosen to be 4.4 for biological materials at energies below 150 keV, and β is $E/511$

with E in keV. The effective atomic number $\tilde{Z}$, for compound materials such as water and human tissue, can be readily calculated from [4]

$$\tilde{Z} = \left(\lambda_1 Z_1^{3.4} + \lambda_2 Z_2^{3.4} + \cdots + \lambda_n Z_n^{3.4} \right)^{1/3.4}$$

$$= \left(\sum_1^n \lambda_i Z_i^{3.4} \right) \qquad (6\text{-}11)$$

with

$$\lambda_i = \frac{P_i Z_i / A_i}{\sum_{j=1}^n P_j Z_j / A_j} \qquad (6\text{-}12)$$

where P_i is the percentage weight, Z_i is the atomic number, and A_i is the atomic weight of the element i. Equations (6-9), (6-10), and (6-11) are the formulas that can be used for the calculation of $\tilde{Z}$ hence the attenuation coefficients of the compound materials.

As can be seen from Eqs. (6-9) and (6-10), the differences in attenuation coefficients arise mainly from two factors, namely the effective atomic number $\tilde{Z}$ of the material in the low-energy region (which is nearly a fourth power of the effective atomic number) and the electron density (ρn_0) effect at high energy (over 50 keV), which is mostly in the region of Compton interactions. The overall modulation is then the accumulation of these two. It should be pointed out that for some biological materials it is conceivable that the photoelectric effect modulation and the Compton effect modulation may enhance or degrade each other, thereby canceling out the overall modulation effect. For a material having lower Z but a higher density (or strictly speaking ρn_0) than another material, the overall modulation effect between the two may be positive or negative depending on the energy. At a certain critical energy, the modulation may be zero. Nevertheless, the modulation effect changes rapidly with respect to energy because of the strongly energy dependent ($E^{3.4}$) photoelectric effect, though at higher energies (above 50 keV) the change is somewhat more gradual because the Compton effect prevails and $f(E)$ is a weakly energy-dependent function. Both theoretical calculations and experimental results, as shown in later sections, strongly support the notion that the atomic number modulation dominates in the lower energy region while the electron density dependent modulation prevails at higher energies.

Attenuation Coefficient Averaging Effect and Contrast Degradation with a Polychromatic Bremsstrahlung X-ray Source

Simple modulation or contrast mechanisms discussed in the previous section apply readily in the case of monoenergetic sources: This simple picture may, however, change drastically, for example, if we use an X-ray tube that produces Bremsstrahlung X-rays. As can be seen from Eqs. (6-7) through (6-10), evaluating linear attenuation coefficients by transmission becomes more complex when multienergetic or polychromatic sources are used. Let's restate Eq. (6-7) with the additional fact that the atomic number and electron density dependent linear attenuation coefficients are also a function of energy (i.e., it can then be rewritten in a discrete form) as

$$I_i(\tilde{E}) = \sum_{k=1}^{n} I_{0i}(E_k)\exp\left(-\sum_j \mu_{ij}(\tilde{Z}, \rho, E_k, n_0)\,\Delta x\right) \quad (6\text{-}13)$$

where $\tilde{E}$ is the effective energy to be defined and

$$\sum_j \mu_{ij}(\tilde{Z}, \rho, E_k, n_0) = \sum_j \left[\mu_{pj}(\tilde{Z}, \rho, E_k, n_0) + \mu_{cj}(\rho, E_k, n_0)\right] \quad (6\text{-}14)$$

Equation (6-14) is the total linear attenuation coefficient represented in two parts, namely the photoelectric (μ_{pj}) and Compton(μ_{cj}) effects as a function of n_0, ρ, $\tilde{Z}$, and E_k. Note here that the variables i and j still represent the jth element at the ith beam but that the variable k represents the discrete energy or energy range where they are evaluated within an incident photon energy spectrum. For the sake of simplicity, let us assume in Eq. (6-13) that $\Delta x = 1$ and that $\sum_j \mu_{ij}(\tilde{Z}, \rho, E_k, n_0)\,\Delta x = \mu_j(\tilde{Z}, \rho, E_k, n_0)$. Then, if such a multienergetic beam is used to measure the linear attenuation coefficient of an unknown material, it can be evaluated effectively as

$$\tilde{\mu}_i(\tilde{Z}, \rho, \tilde{E}, n_0) = \ln\left[\frac{\sum_{k=E_{\min}}^{E_{\max}} I_{0i}(E_k)}{I_i(\tilde{E})}\right] = \ln\left[\frac{I_{0i}(\tilde{E})}{I_i(\tilde{E})}\right] \quad (6\text{-}15)$$

where $\sum I_{0i}(\tilde{E})$ is the total incident photon flux and thus $\tilde{\mu}$ is numerically equal to a μ value at a hypothetical monoenergetic energy $\tilde{E}$, which we will call "effective energy," and the resulting attenuation coefficient is called the "effective attenuation coefficient $\tilde{\mu}$." The general approach was to define this effective energy $\tilde{E}$ for a reference material, such as water, at a fixed thickness and assume that $\tilde{E}$ will remain constant for other materials. However, this will introduce error, as we will show, since the effective energy is different for different materials of the same thickness. Suppose that we know $\tilde{\mu}$ and $\tilde{E}$ of a known reference material (e.g., water) of thickness $(l - \Delta x)$, and suppose that we have a compound material with a mixture of water l and unknown (Δx). Then it is easy to show that the number of transmitted photons through such a compound material having total thickness l is

$$
\begin{aligned}
I_i(\tilde{E}) &= \sum_k I_{0i}(E_k)\exp\left[-\mu_x(E_k)\,\Delta x\right]\exp\left[-\mu_w(E_k)(l - \Delta x)\right] \\
&= \sum_k I_{0i}(E_k)\exp\left[-\mu_w(E_k)l\right]\exp\left\{-\left[\mu_x(E_k) - \mu_w(E_k)\right]\Delta x\right\} \\
&= I_{0i}(\tilde{E})\exp\left[-\tilde{\mu}_w(\tilde{E}_w)l\right]\exp\left\{-\left[\tilde{\mu}_x(\tilde{E}_x) - \tilde{\mu}_w(\tilde{E}_w)\right]\Delta x\right\} \quad (6\text{-}16)
\end{aligned}
$$

Then, provided that we are at an energy region where $[\tilde{\mu}_x(\tilde{E}_x) - \tilde{\mu}_w(\tilde{E}_w)]$ is fairly constant, Eq. (6-16) can be rewritten as

$$\lim_{\tilde{E}_x \to \tilde{E}_w} I_i(\tilde{E}) = I_{0i}(\tilde{E})\exp\left[-\tilde{\mu}_x(\tilde{E}_x)l\right]\exp\{-\Delta\mu\,\Delta x)\}$$

$$= I'_{0i}\exp(-\Delta\mu\,\Delta x) \tag{6-17}$$

where $I'_{0i} = I_{0i}(\tilde{E})\exp[-\tilde{\mu}_w(\tilde{E}_w)l]$ and $\Delta\mu = \tilde{\mu}_x(\tilde{E}_x) - \tilde{\mu}_w(\tilde{E}_w)$. When we also assume that $\tilde{E}_x \approx \tilde{E}_w$, then $\tilde{\mu}_x(\tilde{E}_w)$ can be expressed simply as

$$\tilde{\mu}_x(\tilde{E}_w) = \Delta\mu + \tilde{\mu}_w(\tilde{E}_w) \tag{6-18}$$

Now we have replaced the unknown $\tilde{E}_x$ by the known value of $\tilde{E}_w$. Equation (6-17) is clearly true when a monoenergetic source is employed; that is, $\tilde{E}_x = \tilde{E}_w$. Error, however, will occur due to the fact that $\Delta\mu$ is not $\tilde{\mu}_x(\tilde{E}_w) - \tilde{\mu}_w(\tilde{E}_w)$ but rather $\tilde{\mu}_x(\tilde{E}_x) - \tilde{\mu}_w(\tilde{E}_w)$. Thus the $\Delta\mu_{\text{error}}$ is

$$\Delta\mu_{\text{error}} = \tilde{\mu}_x(\tilde{E}_x) - \tilde{\mu}_x(\tilde{E}_w) \tag{6-19}$$

The error is a strong function of energy and the associated energy spectrum. It is easy to see that the error is again zero for the monoenergetic photon case, $\tilde{E}_x = \tilde{E}_w$. As will be shown in the later sections, an advantage may be gained by using a reference material such as water, depending on the energy of the photons, when a multienergy source is used. Error arises when we use a reference material because we assume that the same multienergetic source will yield a fixed effective energy and we interpret the unknown μ_x as the sum of the difference $\Delta\mu$ and the reference, again at the effective energy of the reference for a given path length. For all practical approaches, the error can be neglected and can effectively be used to compensate the energy-dependent attenuation coefficient averaging effect. A good example is the definition of an effective energy of 73 keV for the early CT scanner for 120 kV$_p$ operation and the above argument is applied for the fixed-length water bath, and $\Delta\mu$ is interpreted and evaluated based on $\tilde{\mu}_x(\tilde{E}_w) - \tilde{\mu}_w(\tilde{E}_w)$ [4, 6].

6-1-3   Beam Hardening

As discussed in the previous section, X-ray beams generally used in X-ray CT are not monoenergetic and have a finite spectrum. When this polychromatic X-ray beam passes through a material, X-rays of different energy k in the spectrum undergo different amounts of attenuation, and as a result the output energy spectrum differs from the input spectrum. In other words, lower-energy X-rays are attenuated more heavily than higher-energy X-rays. This trend is accentuated if the path length is large or if a material possesses components of a high atomic number. The consequence of the X-ray path length dependent nonuniform attenuation of the polychromatic X-ray beam is called the beam-hardening effect. It produces a visible artifact in the final reconstructed image. The original EMI utilized compensatory measures to deal with the beam-hardening effect, namely a water bag as a compensator by surrounding the head so that the total path lengths of the X-rays were the same for all projections. Another method often used is to preharden the X-ray beam by passing it through an aluminum or copper filter so that the output X-ray beam is made more monoenergetic before being passed through the body.

6-1-4   X-ray Source

Two types of X-ray sources are currently used in X-ray CT. The first simple type is the fixed-anode X-ray tube, in which the anode is cooled by oil and is continuously energized. A typical focal spot size of this type is about 2 mm × 16 mm on a 20° angle tungsten target. The relatively small heat dissipation capability associated with this type of tube limits the amount of photon flux generation, resulting in a statistically noisy image. The other more widely used X-ray tube is the rotating-anode X-ray tube. This type of tube allows for more photon flux because it has a much greater heat capacity.

6-1-5   Detectors

X-ray photons are collected by radiation detectors of various kinds, including a scintillation crystal coupled with a photomultiplier tube (PMT). In general, the output of the detectors are electrical signals that are proportional to the incident X-ray energy or fluence. The most important parameters to be considered in the selection of detectors for X-ray CT are efficiency, response time (or afterglow), and linearity. Efficiency refers to the absorption and conversion efficiency of the incident X-rays to electrical signals. Linearity refers to the dynamic range of the detector response. Response time refers to the speed with which the detectors can detect X-ray photons and recover in order to detect the next photon. This is determined by the afterglow, one of the important characteristics of detector materials for X-ray CT application. Detector types currently in use for X-ray CT can be divided into two classes: scintillation detectors and gas ionization detectors.

Scintillation Detector
As discussed in Chapter 5, scintillation crystals such as NaI(T1) and CsI(T1) produce flashes of light as they absorb X-ray photons. The light is then converted to electrical signals by subsequent electronics. Two types of scintillation detector systems are commonly used in X-ray CT: the scintillation crystal-photomultiplier coupled detector and the scintillation crystal-photodiode coupled detector.

Table 6-1   Characteristics of detectors used in X-ray CT

Type	Advantages	Disadvantages
NaI(T1)-PMT	High-detection efficiency 100% at 70 keV (1-in. crystal)	Afterglow Restricted dynamic range Low packing density Hygroscopic
CaF$_2$-PMT	No afterglow	Low-detection efficiency (62% with 1 in. thick)
BGO-PMT	No afterglow High-detection efficiency Nonhygroscoic	Low-light output
CsI(T1)-Photodiode	Good spectral match with available PMTs High-detection efficiency (94.5% at 120 keV with 5 mm thick)	
Xenon gas ionization detection	Simple and compact No afterglow High-resolution capability	Low efficiency Possible instability Slow response time

Scintillation Crystal-Photomultiplier Coupled Detector   Light produced in the crystal is coupled to the photocathode of a PMT. In the PMT, photoelectrons are generated from the photocathode as the light strikes it. These electrons are then multiplied through a series of cascaded dynodes in which electron multiplication processes take place. Each dynode produces more electrons than incident electrons. The multiplied or amplified electrons then constitute output signals in the form of a charge or current. This charge is the indicator of the energy and fluence of the incident X-ray photons on the scintillation crystal. An overall gain of a few million is common in most PMTs. The detector crystals used are generally the scintillating phosphors of high absorption with small afterglow. Among the popular scintillation crystals, BGO (bismuth germanate) and CaF$_2$ are the most often used scintillators (see Table 6-1).

Scintillation Crystal-Photodiode Coupled Detector   The performance of the crystal-photodiode type of detector, which was developed more recently than its counterpart, has been found to be satisfactory. A typical scintillation crystal-photodiode detector is comprised of a CsI(T1) scintillation crystal coupled to a p-n junction photodiode, and a subsequent preamplifier follows for the low-level signal amplification. As in the case of the scintillator-PMT coupled detector, the incident X-ray photon is converted to visible light in the scintillation crystal, which then falls into the pn junction photodiode. Generated electron-hole pairs are then collected at the junctions. Since the generated current is usually weak, a low-noise preamplifier is generally required. The voltage output is proportional to the energy and fluence of the X-ray incident on the detector (see Table 6-1).

Gas Ionization Detector

Some commercial X-ray CT systems use gas ionization detectors. To improve the detector efficiency, xenon gas is pressurized to as high as 20 atm in a long chamber to maximize detection efficiency. It consists of tungsten plates, which serve as anodes for electrons and gas chambers. When X-ray photons are incident on the detector cell or gas chamber, the gas is ionized. This ionized gas provides a current that is directly proportional to the X-ray photon energy and fluence.

The advantages of the gas ionization detector are high spatial resolution capability and simplicity. In addition the compact detector assembly can be made on a large scale by packing a few hundred equivalent detector elements that have detector widths as narrow as 1 mm. The disadvantage of the ionization detector, even with highly pressurized gas, is the low detection efficiency. Characteristics of each detector are briefly described in Table 6-1.

6-1-6 Data Acquisition and Reconstruction Algorithms

At each view, detector signals from the detector system are converted to digital pulses by the ADC. These signals are collected by the computer via signal processing electronics for image reconstruction. The steps of the view angle between successive views are normally on the order of 1° or less, and a few hundred views are usually taken from each tomographic slice. After the entire projection data sets (i.e., line-integral projection data for all views) are obtained, image reconstruction takes place. The time required for image reconstruction can usually be made relatively short in comparison to data acquisition time by using, for instance, special-purpose computer peripherals, such as array processors or backprojectors. Details of the image reconstruction algorithms applicable to X-ray CT are given in Chapter 3.

6-2 SYSTEM CONFIGURATION AND EVOLUTION

Basic system configuration of a typical X-ray CT system currently in use is shown in Fig. 6-5. A 16- to 32-bit minicomputer system equipped with a dedicated backprojector is normally used for data acquisition, signal processing, system control, and image display. Although remarkable progress has been made in all aspects of X-ray CT since it was introduced in 1972 by Hounsfield at EMI, the most significant changes have been made in the area

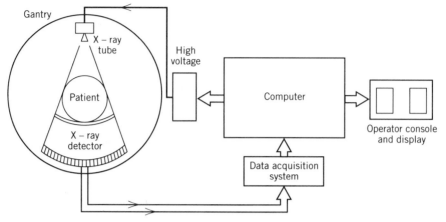

Figure 6-5   Basic system configuration of X-ray CT.

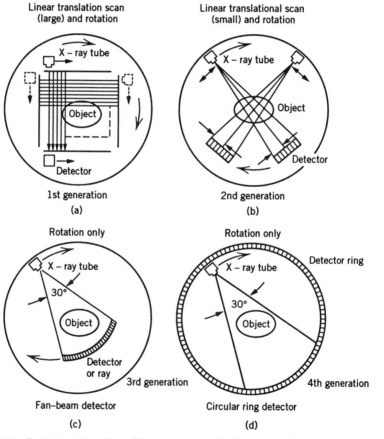

Figure 6-6   Evolution of the X-ray CT systems from the first to fourth generation scanners.

of data acquisition. These stages of progress are often classified into "generations." Since 1972 X-ray CT has evolved from the first generation to the fourth and possibly the fifth generation, which includes the latest developments in dynamic scanners.

6-2-1 First Generation

The first generation of X-ray CT naturally entailed the first EMI scanner developed by Hounsfield. This scanner used a single pencil beam and a single detector, which translated and rotated synchronously. There was translational motion across the object being scanned, and at the end of each translational motion an incremental 1° rotation followed in preparation for the upcoming scanning. This procedure is depicted in Fig. 6-6 (a). The collection of a set of projection data needed for tomographic image reconstruction of a slice usually took several minutes.

6-2-2 Second Generation

The design of the second generation CT incorporated a small-angle fan-beam X-ray and an array of multiple detectors. Since the diverging fan beams passing through the patient increased data collection channels, the number of angular rotations required could be reduced. Therefore the scan time in this second generation scanner was shortened substantially; the nominal scan time was approximately 20 sec. The second-generation scanner still entailed translational motion as well as rotational motion in order to cover the object fully. Figure 6-6 (b) illustrates the configuration of the second-generation CT scanner.

6-2-3 Third Generation [9]

In the third generation the fan-beam angle was widened, thereby allowing the fan to cover the entire object to be scanned. Each projection path is defined by a matching detector, which can be either a small and narrow scintillation detector slab or a segment of a gas ionization chamber. Because the entire object is covered or encompassed, no translational movement is required. Therefore both the X-ray tube and the detector array need only simple rotational motion around a fixed axial center. The entire 360° is usually scanned for whole data collection. The scan time can be as short as 1 to 3 sec. The major drawback of this configuration is that the effects of the drift of the detectors are cumulative, so artifacts appear in the reconstruction image. Figure 6-6(c) shows the configuration of the third-generation CT scanner. Almost all third-generation scanners use pulsed X-ray sources in order to take advantage of significant dead time between successive views.

6-2-4 Fourth Generation

The construction of a stationary circular ring detector array is probably the ideal choice for a rotating X-ray source. A striking analogy is the circular ring PET scanners of various types developed during the 1970s. This stationary ring is the most distinct feature of the fourth-generation X-ray CT. The X-ray source rotates, but the detector array does not. A wide-angle fan-beam X-ray encompasses the entire patient, and 600 or more stationary detectors form a circular ring array. With this kind of configuration, detector drift is not cumulative and therefore can be corrected. The advantages of this system are similar to those of the third-generation systems, but the main drawback of the third-generation systems, the drift effects, have been eliminated since detector drifts no longer accumulate over successive views. The fourth-generation systems are generally more expensive due to the large number of scintillation detectors and PMTs are employed. Figure 6-6(d) shows a schematic diagram of the fourth-generation X-ray CT scanner. The speed of fourth-generation scanners allows for the synchronized rotational motion with physiological signals such as that obtained from electrocardiograph (ECG) when the imaging of moving organs is required [10].

6-2-5 Dynamic Scanners

Ultrafast scanners are required for the imaging of moving organs, such as the heart. Typical systems of this kind are the dynamic spatial reconstructor (DSR) and cardiovascular CT (CV CT). These can be categorized as the fifth-generation X-ray CT scanners.

Dynamic Spatial Reconstructor

The development of the DSR at the Mayo Clinic was completed in 1982 [11]. It can produce real-time images of body organs in motion. The DSR comprises 28 X-ray sources with 28 opposing X-ray imaging detectors, which are image intensifiers coupled with X-ray detector phosphors mounted in the same gantry. The physical size of components and the required radiation flux determine the number of X-ray sources and imaging detectors. As many as 240 images of adjacent slices with a thickness of 1 mm can be made from a cylindrical volume that is 38 cm in diameter and 24 cm long. A complete volume scan is achieved in 0.01 sec after each of the 28 X-ray sources is pulsed in succession (for 0.34 msec). These scans can be repeated 60 times per second. A high temporal resolution image can be obtained with 28 angles of view recorded in 0.01 sec while the gantry is kept stationary. For stationary objects, however, high-spatial and high-density resolution images can be produced using all 240 views for reconstruction. Trade-offs between temporal, spatial, and density resolution can be made by selecting the appropriate subsets from the projection data. Figure 6-7 depicts a schematic diagram of the DSR scanner.

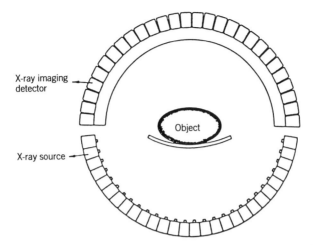

Figure 6-7   First dynamic scanner DSR developed at the Mayo Clinic [11].

Cardiovascular CT

The CV CT system was proposed and developed by Boyd et al. [12] with the same goal in mind but with a more compact and physically integrated design than that of the first DSR. The heart of the CV CT is the electron beam scan tube and stationary scintillation crystal-photodiode coupled detector array. An accelerated and focused electron beam is deflected by a computer-controlled bending magnet to be swept along a 210° curved tungsten target ring. Four target rings are swept serially to obtain a multiple-section examination. Approximately 30° of the fan-shaped sector of the X-ray beam generated at the tungsten target is detected by the detector array for image reconstruction. The detector array comprises two to four detector layers of a half-ring. A simple scan produces two to four side-by-side tomographic slices; a total of eight to sixteen slices can be produced to cover a region approximately 9 to 18 cm wide by sweeping four targets in succession. Two to four adjacent tomographic slices can be obtained in 50 msec, and eight to sixteen slices can be obtained in 200 msec if four targets are swept serially. Although the basic principles of X-ray CT have not changed since they were introduced, the scanning scheme, speed, and resolution of X-ray CT have improved substantially. At the same time each stage of X-ray CT development has brought about new applications and widened the scope of X-ray CT. X-ray CTs of different forms are now utilized in many diverse fields, including the inspection of tires on the production line and the detection of defects in nuclear reactor cores.

Although scanning speed has evolved from minutes to a few milliseconds, making possible dynamic scans of moving organs such as the heart, the search for better and higher contrast and spatial resolution with shorter and shorter imaging time is expected to continue. The growth of applications of X-ray CT to the fields other than medical imaging is also anticipated [13].

REFERENCES

1. G. N. Hounsfield. *Br. J. Radiol.* 46:1016 (1973).
2. Z. H. Cho (ed). Special issue on physical and computational aspects of 3-dimensional image reconstruction. *IEEE Trans. Nucl. Sci.* NS-21 (1974).
3. Z. H. Cho, I. Ahn, C. Bohm, and G. C. Huth. *Phys. Med. Biol.* 19:511 (1974).
4. Z. H. Cho, C. M. Tsai, and G. Wilson. *Phys. Med. Biol.* 20:879 (1974).
5. M. E. Phelps, E. J. Hoffman, and M. M. Ter-Pogossian. *Radiology* 117:573 (1975).
6. E. C. McCullough, H. L. Baker, O. W. Houser, and D. F. Reese. *Radiology* 111:709 (1974).
7. J. Weber and Z. D. J. Van Den Berg. *Br. J. Radiol.* 42:378 (1969).
8. A. Charlesby, *Atomic Radiation and Polymers*, International Series of Monographs on Radiation Effects in Materials, vol. 1. Oxford: Pergamon, 1960, p. 335.
9. G. E. Brochure, 1975.
10. L. A. Shepp and J. A. Stein. Simulated reconstruction artifacts in CT. In *Reconstruction Tomography in Diagnostic Radiology*. Baltimore: University Park Press, 1977.
11. R. Robb, E. Ritman, and E. H. Wool. *IEEE Trans. Nucl. Sci.* NS-26:2713 (1979).
12. D. P. Boyd, R. G. Gold, J. R. Quinn, and R. Sparks. *IEEE Trans. Nucl. Sci.* NS-26:2724 (1979).
13. Z. H. Cho. *Computerized Tomography*, *Encyclopedia of Physical Science and Technology*, vol. 3. San Diego: Academic Press, 1987, pp. 508–541.

7

NUCLEAR TOMOGRAPHIC IMAGING—SINGLE PHOTON EMISSION COMPUTED TOMOGRAPHY

Nuclear medical imaging, or "nuclear medicine" as it is popularly called, is based on detecting nuclear radiation emitted from the body after introducing a radiopharmaceutical inside the body to tag a specific biochemical function. The radiopharmaceutical may emit photons in the form of X-rays or gamma rays, or alternatively, it may emit positrons (which immediately annihilate to produce two 511 keV photons). As long as the photons emanating from the radionuclide have sufficient energy to escape from the human body in significant numbers, images can be generated that portray the *in vivo* distribution of the radiopharmaceutical. For example, Tc-99m, the most commonly used radionuclide in nuclear medicine, decays to its normal ground state with a half-life of 6.03 h by primarily emitting a gamma ray at 140.5 keV (which is easily detectable) and has been incorporated into a variety of radiopharmaceuticals to tag specific biochemical functions *in vivo* in virtually every human organ. Similarly F-18 flurodeoxyglucose, an analog of glucose tagged with F-18 (a positron emitter with a half-life of 109 min), is widely used to image glucose metabolism *in vivo*.

In general, nuclear medical imaging may be divided into three categories:

1. Conventional or planar imaging
2. Single photon emission computed tomography or SPECT
3. Positron emission tomography or PET

Planar imaging and SPECT are described in this chapter, and PET is described in the next chapter.

7-1   CONVENTIONAL OR PLANAR IMAGING

In the conventional mode the three-dimensionally distributed radiopharmaceutical is imaged onto a planar or two-dimensional surface, producing a projection image. Imaging of this type received its impetus from the scintillation camera invented by Hal Anger in the late 1950s [1]. These cameras, which use a large NaI (T1) crystal coupled to an array of photomultiplier tubes to record the distribution of gamma-emitting radiopharmaceuticals, are in wide clinical use and can be found in virtually every nuclear medicine facility around the world.

The principle components of a scintillation camera are depicted in Fig. 7-1. Photons deposit energy within the scintillation crystal by a photoelectric or a Compton scattering interaction. A small portion ($\sim 10\%$) of the deposited energy is converted into visible light photons of approximately 3-eV energy. These visible light photons (also called the *light flash* created by the "scintillation event") are guided toward the photocathodes of an array of photomultiplier tubes where they are converted to electrons, multiplied, and finally converted into an electrical signal at the anode of each photomultiplier tube. The amplitudes of the anode signals from each anode are then examined by analog or digital positioning circuitry to estimate the x, y coordinates of the scintillation event on the crystal. A mechanical collimator attached to the NaI crystal relates the x, y coordinates of each event on the scintillation crystal to the x, y coordinates of a two-dimensional projection image of the object [2, 3]. The collimator is usually made out of a plate of lead or a similar high atomic number substance, such as tungsten, in which a

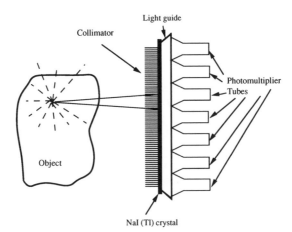

Figure 7-1   A simplified diagram of a scintillation camera. A small portion of the radiation emitted from a point source within the object is able to transmit through a few apertures to reach the NaI(Tl) crystal.

large array of apertures are drilled, as shown in Fig. 7-1. The purpose of the collimator is to mechanically confine the direction of incident photons reaching the scintillation crystal and thereby to localize the site of the emitting sources. If the apertures of the collimator are all parallel to each other, as shown in Fig. 7-1, the collimator is then called a *parallel-hole* collimator. Most clinical examinations are conducted with the parallel-hole collimator because it provides the ideal combination of resolution and sensitivity for most regions of the body with no geometrical distortion. In some applications the apertures may be angulated to form converging- or diverging-hole collimators. This feature provides certain advantages in imaging relatively small regions (converging collimator) or relatively large regions (diverging collimator) with appropriate magnification or minification of the images [3]. Alternatively, just one or a limited number of holes may be used to form a *pinhole* collimator which is particularly useful in imaging very small regions or small organs such as the thyroid gland [3].

The operating principle of a scintillation camera can be summarized by the following chain of events:

1. Photons emitted isotropically from within the subject are mechanically collimated by an appropriate collimator.
2. The collimated radiation is incident on the NaI(Tl) crystal at "point" (x, y) giving rise to visible light or scintillation in a small region surrounding (x, y).
3. The scintillation light is guided toward the photocathodes of the photomultiplier tubes optically coupled to the NaI(Tl) crystal. Since light spreads while traversing the thickness of the crystal, the photocathodes view a small disc of light (rather than an ideal point source), quantified in terms of a light spread function.
4. The scintillation light is divided among the bank of photomultiplier tubes in proportion to its proximity to each tube.
5. Each tube converts the light it receives to a voltage pulse at its anode. Thus the height of the output pulse from each tube is proportional to the total light received by each tube's photocathode.
6. The pattern of voltage pulses from each tube are fed to analog or digital positioning circuitry to determine uniquely the location, that is, the x and y coordinates of each scintillation event on the crystal.
7. The output from each tube is summed to produce a net signal proportional to the total energy deposited in the crystal by the scintillating event. This signal is referred to as the "z signal."
8. Pulse height discrimination is applied to the z signal to retain only those events where the total energy deposited in the crystal lies within a prescribed energy window. This procedure enables a reduction of counts from photons that have undergone a Compton scatter event

inside the subject before interacting with the scintillation crystal. Reduction in the Compton scattered portion of the incident radiation is an important issue in quantitative emission imaging and is discussed in detail in the next section under SPECT.

9. The (x, y) coordinates of each count passing the pulse height discrimination are stored to produce a projection image where the projection axis is normal to the plane of the collimator.

The performance of a scintillation camera can be characterized in terms of its resolution and sensitivity and nonlinearities therein. The resolution R of scintillation imaging is mainly determined by the intrinsic resolution of the camera R_i and the resolution of the collimator R_c. The net resolution may be obtained from a quadrature addition of these two factors:

$$R^2 = R_i^2 + R_c^2 \qquad (7\text{-}1)$$

7-1-1 The Intrinsic Resolution

The intrinsic resolution indicates the ability of the camera to pinpoint the location at which the incoming photon interacts with the scintillation crystal. Although the total number of photomultiplier tubes affects the intrinsic resolution—generally the more tubes there are, the better the intrinsic resolution—there are some fundamental limitations to improving the intrinsic resolution set by the statistical variability in the generation of the scintillation light by photons of a given energy. For example, let us consider an event occurring exactly midway between two phototubes. Let us say that $N = 100$ light photons are generated by a photon of energy E. Ideally then each tube should receive 50 light photons every time a primary photon of energy E is absorbed in the crystal. From simple statistical considerations, however, the total number of light photons produced by subsequent events can fluctuate by $\pm \sqrt{N}$, or 10 in this example. Thus the light photons received by the two tubes can divide as 60–50 or 40–50 instead of the ideal 50–50 division. Consequently the output voltage from each tube will fluctuate, even when all interactions take place at exactly the same (x, y) position on the crystal, leading to an intrinsic resolution limitation. Since N is a linear function of the incident energy E, contributions to the intrinsic resolution due to statistical factors are a function of $1/\sqrt{E}$, with the resolution improving at higher energies. Further limitations arise from the following effects:

First, due to the finite thickness of the crystal, the scintillation light spreads during its traversal of the crystal. As shown in Fig. 7-2, the scintillation light can be modeled as a cone whose vertex lies at the point of interaction. The diameter of the base of this cone at the exit surface of the NaI crystal depends on the thickness of the crystal and determines the width

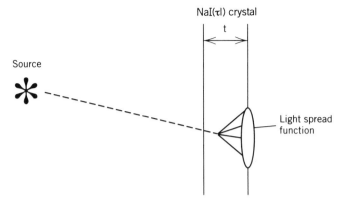

Figure 7-2 Diagram of how the scintillation light spreads as it propagates through the thickness *t* of the NaI(Tl) crystal.

of the light spread function. Since the photomultiplier tubes view the base of the cone and not its vertex, there is an inherent limitation to the resolution, which depends on the accuracy of locating the vertex of the cone from its base. (In practice the depth of the interaction is ignored. However, there is some research underway to estimate the depth of the interaction from a knowledge of the shape of the light spread function [4], which should lead to improvements in the intrinsic resolution).

Second, a Compton scattering interaction within the crystal followed by a photoelectric absorption at some distance from the first interaction produces

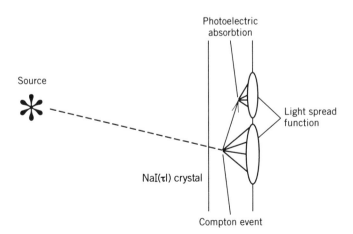

Figure 7-3 Diagram of how a Compton scattering event followed by a photoelectric absorbtion within the NaI(Tl) crystal produces a distorted light spread function.

a distorted light spread function, as depicted in Fig. 7-3, leading to an error in the localization of the first interaction point. Combining the contributions from the above-mentioned factors, the intrinsic resolution of currently used scintillation cameras containing 37 or 61 photomultiplier tubes lie in the 3- to 5-mm range.

7-1-2 Collimator Resolution

Contributions to the resolution from the collimator, however, can be much larger, making the collimator resolution R_c the main factor. R_c depends on the design of the collimator (the shape, diameter, and length of the apertures) and the distance of the region being imaged from the collimator. R_c may be defined in terms of a point spread function from the expression

$$R_c = \frac{d(l + b)}{l} \qquad (7\text{-}2)$$

In this expression d and l are the diameter and length of an aperture within the array of apertures, and b is the distance of the point source from the outer surface of the collimator. Details of various collimator designs and their resolution and sensitivity characteristics are given in several publications, for example, Anger [3]. Typically the collimator resolution is ~ 1 cm at a distance of 10 cm from the collimator.

7-1-3 Nonlinearities

The response of each of the photomultiplier tubes in a scintillation camera is dependent on (x, y). In other words, the response is spatially variant and is a function of the interaction point on the scintillation crystal. For example, if a point source is moved across the photocathode of one tube, from one end to the other, the response varies nonlinearly across the entire surface of the photocathode. Consequently, if a large flat source, called a *flood source*, is imaged by a scintillation camera, the image is not uniform but shows point-to-point fluctuations more than that caused by count statistics. In addition the resolution is nonuniform across the face of the scintillation camera, producing "pincushion" and "barrel" distortions. In other words, straight lines appear to be distorted, either bowing inward or outward [5].

The intensity nonuniformities may be corrected by imaging a flood source with good statistics and then normalizing subsequent images with the flood-source image. Correction for resolution distortions is more difficult and requires generation of a "lookup" table to correct the resolution on a point-by-point basis. Also digital schemes based on a maximum likelihood estimation of the point of interaction on the scintillation camera have been proposed to improve the intrinsic resolution and reduce nonlinear distortions [6, 7].

The performance of scintillation cameras is also limited by the count rate since events producing pulse pileup (a second interaction occurring before the scintillation light from the first event has decayed to a negligible level) either distort the positioning circuitry and the resolution or are not counted, resulting in a dead time. The counting rate of the initial scintillation cameras was restricted to about 50,000 counts per second (or cps). Currently the usable count rate is in the 100,000–200,000 cps range though some special cameras are specified to operate at rates as high as 500,000 cps. An alternative to conventional cameras is the concept of the small modular scintillation camera. Each camera is designed to operate at a relatively high count rate of about 200,000 cps [7]. Since counts are now divided among N modules, where each module can count at a high rate, the net counting rate for an area equal to a conventional scintillation camera is very high and can reach 1,000,000 cps. Modular cameras are particularly useful in SPECT, as described below.

7-2 SINGLE PHOTON EMISSION COMPUTED TOMOGRAPHY (SPECT)

Conventional planar imaging techniques suffer from artifacts and errors due to superposition of underlying and overlying objects that interfere with the region of interest. The techniques of CT discussed earlier can be used to obviate the superposition problems and provide an *in vivo* quantitative estimate of the distribution of gamma emitting radionuclides in three dimensions. The emission CT approach, called *SPECT*, is based on detecting individual photons emitted at random by the radionuclide to be imaged. As described earlier, a mechanical collimator is used to localize the gamma emitting activity along a narrow region similar to the "ray sum" generated in X-ray CT. Collimation is achieved by restricting the acceptance angle as depicted in Fig. 7-1. A simple calculation (see Fig. 7-4) shows that the solid angle is extremely small, with only 0.015% of the emitted radiation transmitted through the apertures of a typical parallel-hole collimator onto the scintillation crystal. Thus the intrinsic sensitivity of SPECT based on conventional collimation is very low. Nevertheless, SPECT has found widespread use because it provides a unique modality to study noninvasively the relationships of anatomic structure to biochemical function in vivo, using readily available gamma-emitting radiopharmaceuticals.

Historically Kuhl and Edwards [8] were the first to demonstrate transaxial reconstruction of gamma emitting radionuclides in 1963 by using a simple backprojection of profile data acquired from multiple angles using a rectilinear scanner. Simple backprojection, however, is not quantitative. Budinger and Gullberg [9] were the first to attempt quantitative SPECT by rotating a patient in front of a stationary scintillation camera and applying reconstruction algorithms based on an iterative or a filtered backprojection approach.

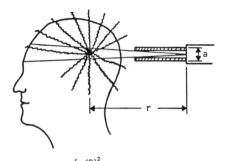

Figure 7-4 Localization of the activity by a mechanical aperture. Collimation is based upon restricting the acceptance angle. The solid angle Ω is very small.

$$\Omega = \frac{\pi(a/2)^2}{4\pi r^2}$$

$a = 0.5$ cm, $r = 10$ cm

$\Omega = 0.015\%$

There are, however, some difficult engineering problems in accurately maintaining a fixed center of rotation while rotating a patient. Since a subpixel error in the center of rotation can lead to severe imaging artifacts, the preferred approach in SPECT is to rotate the scintillation camera around the patient, as described below.

7-3 ROTATING SCINTILLATION CAMERA

Keyes et al. [10], Jaszczak et al. [11], and Singh et al. [12] were among the first investigators to conduct SPECT studies with a rotating scintillation camera. The concept is depicted in Fig. 7-5. Projection data in terms of ray sums are

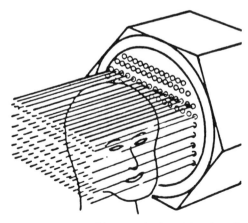

Figure 7-5 A conceptual depiction of how projection data at a given angle of view are acquired from multiple planes by a gamma camera equipped with a parallel-hole collimator.

acquired at a given angle of view but over multiple planes simultaneously with a conventional scintillation camera. The camera is then rotated around the subject in steps of $\Delta\theta$ covering the full 360° range. In some situations, such as imaging the heart with a low-energy emitter like Tl-201, an 180° scan is preferred to a full 360° rotation. Recently a three-headed scintillation camera system has been developed to improve the sensitivity of head or body imaging [13]. The three-headed triangular system can perform four revolutions per minute in a continuous data acquisition mode, in theory enabling a 5-sec temporal resolution. In practice, however, the temporal resolution is limited by photon statistics to about 30 sec, which is still much better than the several minute temporal resolution practically achievable by a single rotating scintillation camera.

The reconstruction problem is schematically depicted in Fig. 7-6. Referring to Fig. 7-6, let

A_i = activity contained in the ith voxel

$P^{k,\theta}$ = profile data at angle θ, that is, the sum of activity or ray sum along the kth ray at angle of view θ

$f_i^{k,\theta}$ = fractional volume of the ith element that is contained within the kth ray

μ_i = the attenuation coefficient of the ith element corresponding to the energy of the emitted photon

$l_i^{k,\theta}$ = length of the portion of the kth ray that is contained within the ith element [The attenuation suffered by the kth ray while traversing the ith element is therefore $\exp(-\mu_i l_i^{k,\theta})$]

$\exp[-\sum_j \mu_j l_j^{k,\theta}]$ = attenuation factor for radiation originating from the ith element. (The index j denotes elements lying along the kth ray between the ith element and the boundary of the object nearest the detector.)

The acquired ray sums can then be expressed by

$$P^{k,\theta} = \sum_{i \in k,\theta} f_i^{k,\theta} A_i \exp\left[-\sum_j \mu_j l_j^{k,\theta}\right] \qquad (7\text{-}3)$$

Reconstruction involves estimating A_i which can be carried out using direct algorithms based on an appropriate filtering technique or an iterative algorithm, as discussed previously in Chapters 3 and 4. It should be noted that there are several problems unique to SPECT that are not encountered in X-ray CT, which makes the reconstruction problem inconsistent, leading to errors in quantitation. These problems are related to (a) variation of spatial resolution or line spread function and sensitivity as a function of distance from the collimator, (b) lack of an accurate method to correct for attenuation [note that the attenuation term in Eq. (7-3) is absent in X-ray CT

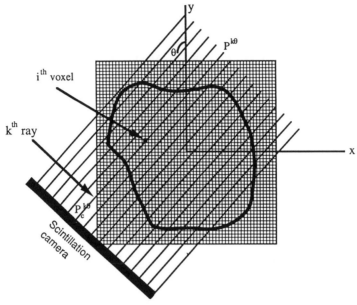

Figure 7-6 The geometry for acquiring projection data at any angle θ. $P^{k\theta}$ is the kth ray sum at angle θ and $P_c^{k\theta}$ is its conjugate ray sum at angle $\theta + \pi$.

reconstruction], and (c) scatter of gamma radiation within the subject. These issues have been discussed by several investigators (e.g., Singh et al. and Jaszczak [12, 14]) and a brief review of the various correction approaches is given below.

7-3-1 Line Spread Function (LSF) and Sensitivity Variation

The results of an experiment to measure and demonstrate the variation in the line spread function using a line source of Tc-99m and a conventional 40-cm diameter scintillation camera are presented in Fig. 7-7 [12]. The line profiles shown here were generated by moving the source away from the collimator in 2-cm steps, and measurements were performed in air as well as in water. The increase in the width of the line spread function profile is apparent in Fig. 7-7. The figure also shows that forming the arithmetic mean of counts from conjugate views (i.e., summing data recorded 180° apart) minimizes the variation in the line spread function with depth. After conjugate summing, a uniform line spread function of 1.4 cm, with variations on the order of 10%, was obtained in this example for a source immersed in water and located 20 cm from the collimator. A uniform line spread function can also be generated from a geometric mean of conjugate views [15]. Clearly, although the line spread function varies with depth, simple techniques can be used to reduce the variation to about 10%.

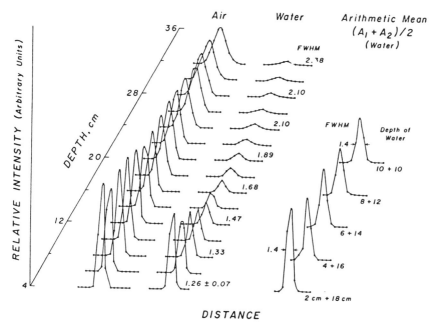

LSF FOR 3 mm SOURCE OF ^{99m}Tc

Figure 7-7 Variation of the line spread function with distance from collimator in air and water (source 3 mm in diameter, Tc-99m). At far right are line spread functions as arithmetic means of conjugate depth data for a 20-cm water-filled object. Note that these conjugate functions are approximately uniform, with full width at half maximum of 1.4 cm. (From ref. [12]).

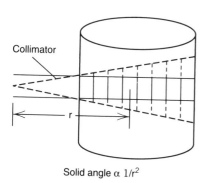

Solid angle α $1/r^2$

Volume of activity viewed α r^2

Figure 7-8 Diagram of how the decrease in the solid angle is compensated by the volume of activity viewed to produce uniform sensitivity with depth.

The sensitivity variation with depth is not that critical because the solid angle for acquiring counts from a given region decreases roughly as the inverse square of distance from the emitting source to the detector, whereas the sensitive area (i.e., the region from which counts are acquired by a given collimator aperture) increases roughly as the square of this same distance. Thus, as illustrated in Fig. 7-8, the variation of sensitivity with depth (not considering attenuation of radiation within the object) may be neglected to a first approximation as long as the activity is uniformly distributed within voxels along a ray sum [12].

It should be noted that the above approaches are approximate. Accurate modeling studies for the line spread function as a function of depth have been performed by several investigators (e.g., Tsui et al. [16], Zeng and Gullberg [18]) for incorporation in iterative reconstruction algorithms to increase the quantitation accuracy in SPECT.

7-3-2 Attenuation and Scatter Correction

Emitted gamma radiation interacts with the body by photoelectric absorption and Compton scattering processes, producing a significant attenuation in the primary beam at energies used in SPECT. Since attenuation depends on the properties of the medium interposed between the point of origin of the photons and the object boundary, it is necessary to know the distribution of attenuation coefficients corresponding to the energy of the emitted radiation within the object and the source distribution in order to accurately compensate for attenuation. Since the source distribution is unknown, obtaining an exact solution to the attenuation correction problem is theoretically very difficult. Several approaches that yield approximate solutions are discussed in this subsection. Besides the attenuation caused by photoelectric events, Compton scattering of the emitted photons within the object introduces another error in the acquired data. Because of the finite energy resolution of the detection system, many of the scattered photons are indistinguishable from the primary photons and are recorded under the photopeak. Since the scattered photons originate mostly from regions outside the spatial region defined by the collimator line spread function (LSF), counts produced by the scattered photons cause blurring and a reduction of contrast in the image. The blurring function generally depends on the three-dimensional source activity and attenuation coefficient distribution within the object. Although the effects of scattered photons are not as prominent as attenuation losses [19], corrections for scatter are necessary in order to obtain the higher quantitation accuracy possible in SPECT.

Several methods, depending on the type of image reconstruction algorithm, have been proposed to correct for attenuation in SPECT. An outline of eight of the earlier methods has been given by Budinger and Gullberg [9]. In general, iterative reconstruction algorithms represent a relatively straightforward approach to correct for nonuniform attenuation by incorporating a map of known or measured attenuation coefficients into the weighting factor for each pixel [9]. At the present time, however, iterative algorithms are considered to be much slower than the direct methods based on Fourier filtering or convolve-and-backproject-type approaches. Iterative algorithms are therefore not commonly used in clinical SPECT.

Existing attenuation correction techniques for filtered backprojection algorithms generally approximate the source or attenuation distribution to arrive at a tractable solution. For example, Chang [20] has proposed a method where corrections are made to the image by dividing each pixel value with the average attenuation for that pixel. Several methods, which may be classified as weighted backprojection, have also been proposed whereby an analytical expression is derived for the filtered backprojection after including an exponential weighting of the projection data [21–24]. Bellini et al. [25] have proposed a similar approach in Fourier space after performing an arithmetic mean of conjugate views. Tanaka et al. [26] have suggested a method for reducing noise propagation in the weighted backprojection algorithm. With the exception of the first weighted backprojection attenuation correction algorithm proposed by Singh et al. [12], all of the earlier weighted backprojection approaches mentioned above assumed a uniform attenuation coefficient for the object and are thus expected to produce errors in imaging regions such as the human thorax which exhibits large variations in attenuation. Recently maps of attenuation coefficients have been incorporated in some of the approaches given above to account for nonuniform attenuation, particularly in myocardial imaging [27]. In the weighted backprojection version proposed by Singh et al. [12], a map of the object's attenuation coefficients is used to apply a weight at each pixel at each angle of view during the backprojection step. Typical experimental results obtained from this technique using a large object containing nonuniform activity and attenuation are discussed later in this chapter.

Several techniques have also been suggested to remove the contribution of scattered photons in SPECT. Since scattered photons add counts, the simplest solution would be to undercorrect for attenuation [28]. Obviously this approach is not quantitative, since it ignores the dependence of scattered photons on the three-dimensional source and attenuation distribution. A second approach relies on a Monte Carlo computation of scattering from a model of the source and attenuation distribution [29]. However, this method is computationally tedious and is limited by the accuracy of the model [30]. Another approach, based on deconvolving an average scatter line spread function [31] also suffers from errors due to the nonuniformities in the object [32]. An alternative approach relies on collecting counts in two energy windows—a photopeak window and a scatter window at a lower energy—and subtracting either a fraction of counts in the scatter window from the photopeak window [33] or a fraction of the reconstructed image corresponding to counts within the scatter window from the reconstructed image corresponding to counts acquired in the photopeak window. Subtracting data before reconstruction, however, has some theoretical advantages because it removes (or reduces) the inconsistencies in the reconstruction algorithm that may be introduced by the spatially variant scatter function. Subtracting data instead of images also reduces the net images to be reconstructed by a factor of two.

A novel two-window technique for scatter correction where counts are subtracted before reconstruction has been described by Singh and Horne [34]. The technique is based on using a high-energy germanium (Ge) detector as an estimator of the scattered photons that would be recorded by the scintillation camera. Details of the techniques have been described in [34, 35]. As an illustration of the scatter and attenuation problems, a brief overview of the Ge detector based approach for scatter correction and the weighted backprojection method for attenuation correction are given below.

Attenuation Correction

The filtered backprojection algorithm may be expressed by the equation [36]

$$A_i = \sum_{k,\theta} \left(P^{k,\theta}\right)^* f_i^{k,\theta} \, \Delta\theta \tag{7-4}$$

where $(P^{k,\theta})^*$ represents the filtered ray sum and $\Delta\theta$ is the angular increment. $f_i^{k,\theta}$ is a weighting factor defined earlier. Attenuation correction is accomplished by using an additional weighting factor $f_{i1}^{k,\theta}$ in Eq. (7-4) given by

$$f_{i1}^{k,\theta} = \frac{1}{\exp\left[-\sum_j \mu_j l_j^{k,\theta}\right]} \tag{7-5}$$

When conjugate views are formed to correct for nonuniformities in the collimator line spread function, the ray sum in Eq. (7-3) is modified to

$$P_2^{k,\theta} = 0.5\left[P^{k,\theta} + P_c^{k,\theta}\right] \tag{7-6}$$

where $P_c^{k,\theta}$ denotes the ray sum for the conjugate view. The filtered backprojection algorithm now yields

$$A_{i1} = \sum_{k,\theta} \left(P_2^{k,\theta}\right)^* f_i^{k,\theta} \, \Delta\theta \tag{7-7}$$

where $(P_2^{k,\theta})^*$ is the filtered ray sum after conjugate summing. The additional weighting factor for attenuation correction is now given by

$$f_{i2}^{k,\theta} = \frac{1}{\exp\left(-\sum_j \mu_j l_j^{k,\theta}\right) + \exp\left(-\sum_j \mu_j l_j^{k,\theta}\right)_c} \tag{7-8}$$

Incorporating the additional weighting factor, the attenuation corrected pixel value A'_i is given by

$$A'_i = \sum_{k,\theta} \left(P_2^{k,\theta}\right)^* f_i^{k,\theta} f_{i2}^{k,\theta} \, \Delta\theta \tag{7-9}$$

Equation (7-9) was used to implement the attenuation correction technique for SPECT imaging of a nonuniform test object described later. Note that $f_{i2}^{k,\theta}$ is not separable from other terms in the summation in Eq. (7-9). If it is separated (incorrectly), Eq. (7-9) becomes

$$A'_i = A_{i1} \sum_{k,\theta} \frac{1}{\left[\exp - \left(\Sigma_j \mu_j l_j^{k,\theta}\right) + \exp\left(-\Sigma_j \mu_j l_j^{k,\theta}\right)_c\right]} \tag{7-10}$$

Equation (7-10) is equivalent to the attenuation correction scheme proposed by Chang [20]. Thus Chang's methods represents a mathematically approximate version of Eq. (7-9). As an example of the conjugate summing and attenuation correction approach, we describe next the results of a test-object study and a study to image acute myocardial infarction (AMI) in dogs [12].

Test-Object Study

A 20 cm diameter cylinder containing three 0.95-cm diameter cylinders in one row, three 1.9-cm diameter cylinders in another row, and one relatively large 4.3-cm diameter cylinder placed near the top of the cylindrical cross section was imaged. All cylinders were filled with water containing 10 μCi/cc of Tc-99m. The activity in the background surrounding these cylinders was varied to achieve 5:1, 10:1, and 15:1 uptake to background ratios in all cylinders. The object was rotated in front of a large-field-of-view (LFOV) scintillation camera equipped with a parallel-hole collimator. The views were recorded in 6° angular increments over 360°. Attenuation correction was performed using the weighted backprojection method discussed above [12] with a constant attenuation of 0.15 cm^{-1}.

The reconstructed transaxial images with 1.4-cm slice thickness and 63 $\times$ 63 pixels with a pixel size of 7 $\times$ 7 mm are shown in Fig. 7-9. A section lying above the background is also shown for comparison. The following conclusions were drawn from these and several other test object studies [12]:

1. The spatial resolution in the reconstructed image (or the system's response function) is uniform to about 10%. A uniform full width at half maximum (FWHM) of 1.8 cm was produced in the transaxial image using a parallel-hole collimator whose line spread function was about 1.4 cm in the conjugate mean measurement.

2. The reconstructed size of an activity distribution is, to a first approximation, a quadrature addition of the true size and the system's response function.

SPATIAL AND CONTRAST RESOLUTION
IN EMISSION RECONSTRUCTION IMAGES
Effect of Background Activity
(Ratio "Hot Spot" : Background)

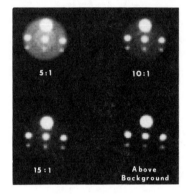

Figure 7-9 Attenuation-corrected reconstructions of 20-cm diameter test object containing rows of cylinders 0.95 and 1.90 cm in diameter, and one 4.30-cm cylinder. All cylinders contained water with 10 μCi / cc of Tc-99m. The surrounding background water contained 2, 1, or 0.67 μCi / cc, as noted by the ratios. At bottom right is the section lying above the background tank. Reconstructions are on a 63 $\times$ 63 grid with a 7 $\times$ 7 mm pixel size. (From ref. [34]).

3. The reconstructed activity within cylinders of equal size is independent of location.

4. The reconstructed activity is a nonlinear but monotonic function of size. Since the true size of an activity distribution can be determined, the relative value of activity uptake can be quantitated with a "lookup" table which relates size to true uptake.

Myocardial Infarct Imaging with Dogs

Dogs with surgically induced acute myocardial infarct (AMI) were imaged with the gamma camera in steps of 6° around 360° following an intravenous injection of Tc-99m pyrophosphate. Data were collected for 100–150 sec at each angle of view with a 15 mCi injection. Transmission cross-sectional images were obtained with a cone-beam X-ray CT scanner described by Sturm et al. [37]. Transmission images provide the map of attenuation coefficients required for making attenuation corrections in the emission images as well as a view of anatomical structures not seen in the emission images. Hence one can study the interrelationship between anatomy and biochemical function from a set of corresponding emission and transmission images.

A set of emission and transmission transaxial cross sections is shown in Fig. 7-10 for a dog whose left anterior descending (LAD) artery was ligated.

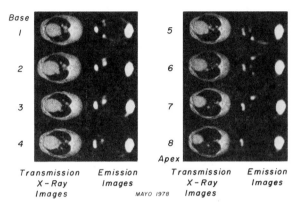

COMPUTED TOMOGRAPHIC IMAGING OF
DISTRIBUTION OF $^{99m}TC-PYROPHOSPHATE$
(Dog #1, 12 kg, Ligation of LAD Coronary Artery)

Figure 7-10 Eight corresponding emission and transmission reconstructed levels through thorax of dog with infarct (ligation of the left anterior artery). X-ray transmission images at the left show structure; emission transaxial images at right are corrected for attenuation using values from transmission images. Section 14 mm thick, spacing 7 mm (overlapping), extending from base to apex of heart. Note location and extent of Tc-99m pyrophosphate uptake into the infarct, as well as into ribs, sternum, and spine. (From ref. [34]).

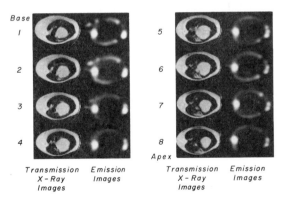

COMPUTED TOMOGRAPHIC IMAGING
OF DISTRIBUTION OF $^{99m}TC-PYROPHOSPHATE$
(Dog #6, 20 kg, Control Without Ligation of Coronary Artery)

Figure 7-11 Same as Fig. 7-10 for control dog. No uptake is seen in the myocardium.

Uptake in the infarcted region is clearly visualized in addition to the sternum, ribs, and the backbone. The transaxial images obtained with a control dog who underwent a same operation are shown in Fig. 7-11. No uptake is seen in the myocardium. It was found that the size of the infarcted region as determined from the SPECT images was highly correlated with histological estimates [12]. These studies thus demonstrate the potential of SPECT in quantifying the three-dimensional extent, shape, and uptake of activity within an organ or a region of the body.

Scatter Correction

Corrections for scatter are becoming increasingly important as higher quantitation accuracy is sought in SPECT. A novel scatter correction technique utilizing a Ge detector is described here in order to illustrate the general concepts of scatter correction. A collimated 5-mm × 5-mm × 6-mm Ge detector with an energy resolution of 1 keV fwhm at 140 keV was used to collect 24 samples around 360° of the energy spectrum emanating from the large test object depicted in Fig. 7-12 [34]. The spectrum from a point source in air provided a scatter-free reference. Each spectrum contained a fixed number of counts (10 K) within a 140 ± 1 keV window, thereby normalizing for attenuation effects.

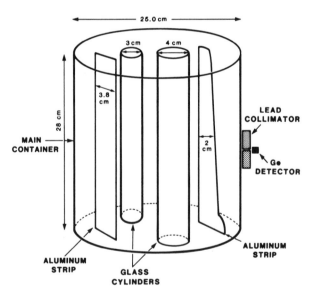

Figure 7-12 The test object from which the emitted primary and scattered photons were recorded with a collimated Ge detector. The main container was filled to a height of 26 cm with water containing a uniform distribution of ^{99m}Tc and the inner glass cylinders were filled with a higher concentration of ^{99m}Tc. The aluminum strips were used to attain a nonuniform distribution of attenuation within the object. (From ref. [34]).

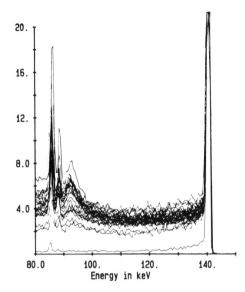

Figure 7-13 The emitted radiation's energy spectra, acquired with the Ge detector from 24 positions around the test object. The 140-keV primary peak is shown at the right. The two peaks at the left are the K_β X rays of lead (at ~ 85.0 keV and 87.3 keV). The K_α X rays of lead appear further left and are not shown. A twenty-fifth scatter-free reference spectrum, obtained from a ^{99m}Tc point source in air, is shown at the bottom. Each spectrum contains 10 K counts within a 140 ± 1 keV window. The spectra shown here have been normalized for the change in detection efficiency of the 6-mm-thick Ge detector as a function of energy. (Reproduced with permission from *J. Nucl. Med.* 28(12):1853–1860, 1987).

A few of these spectra are shown in Fig. 7-13, which clearly show variations in the scattered photon emission as a function of detector position. These spectra were then convolved with a Gaussian function equivalent to 15% fwhm energy resolution at 140 keV. The purpose of this convolution was to estimate data that would be collected with a typical scintillation camera.

By comparing the convolved test-object spectra with the scatter-free reference spectrum, contributions from the primary and scattered photons could be separated in each spectrum, and it was possible to develop an optimization technique for scatter subtraction under a given count-statistics situation. Details are given in [34, 35]. Briefly, using i as an index of the 24 samples, if C_i represents counts within a specified photopeak window and B_i counts within a scattered window, the corrected counts X_i are given by

$$X_i = C_i - aB_i \qquad (7\text{-}11)$$

where a is a scaling factor. For given windows and for count-statistics (which are based on the number of counts recorded under the photopeak window), the value of a can be optimized [34].

Figure 7-14 shows the optimum values of a for a range of photopeak and scatter windows when 100 counts are recorded in the photopeak window, which is equivalent to acquiring 100 counts per 5×5 mm pixel in a scintillation camera image. The windows were then optimized by maximizing the SNR after scatter correction. The signal was defined as the mean value of the ensemble photopeak counts after subtraction, and the noise was defined as the standard deviation of the fluctuations therein. A plot of the SNR as a

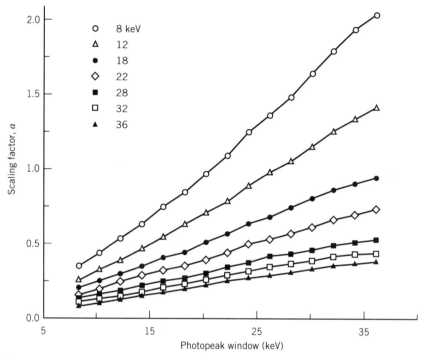

Figure 7-14 A plot of optimum *a* values as a function of photopeak and background (scatter) windows. (From reference [35]. Reproduced with permission from *IEEE Trans. Nucl. Sci.* NS-35, No. 1, 767 – 771, 1988. © 1988 IEEE).

function of window sizes for the 100 count-statistics case is shown in Fig. 7-15. The optimum settings suggested by the figure are a 28-keV photopeak window centered at 140 keV and a 32-keV contiguous scatter window ranging from 93 to 125 keV. From Fig. 7-14 the optimum value of *a* for this setting is 0.37.

To evaluate the correction techniques, a SPECT study of a 25-cm diameter × 26-cm tall plastic cylinder containing a nonuniform activity and attenuation distribution (see Fig. 7-12) was used. The cylinder was filled with water containing 0.2 μCi/cc of Tc-99m. Immersed in it were two plastic cylinders of diameters of 3 cm and 4 cm containing 2.0 μCi/cc and 5.0 μCi/cc of Tc-99m, respectively, two 25-cm long × 2-mm thick aluminum strips (one 3.8-cm wide and the other tapered to a width of 2.0 cm at its midpoint), and a 3-cm diameter × 6-cm tall bottle filled with water containing no activity. A midlevel transaxial cross section of the test object is shown in Fig. 7-16. The test object was rotated in 80 equangular steps around 360° in front of a conventional scintillation camera (parallel-hole collimator) with 15% fwhm energy resolution at 140 keV.

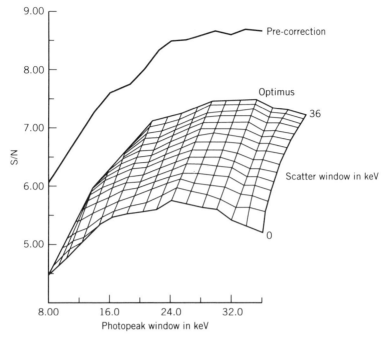

Figure 7-15 SNR as a function of photopeak and scatter window, indicating an optimum at the 28-keV photopeak window and at the 32-keV scatter window. Pre-correction SNR as a function of photopeak window is also shown. (From reference [35]).

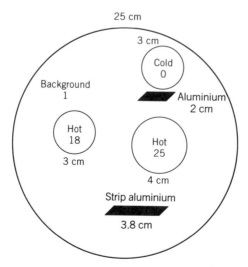

Figure 7-16 A midlevel cross section of the test object. (From reference [35]).

Complete projection data were acquired on a 64×64 grid (pixel size, 0.56 cm) from each of the three windows described below. The first window was a 28-keV wide photopeak window centered at 140 keV, the second a 32-keV wide scatter window ranging from 93 to 125 keV. After adding two adjacent rows, approximately 100 counts per pixel were obtained in the photopeak projection images with 50 sec acquisition. The count statistics thus correspond approximately to the 100-count case shown in Figs. 7-14 and 7-15. The acquisition time was increased in proportion to the half-life of Tc-99m to maintain initial conditions. SPECT images were reconstructed using a standard Shepp and Logan filter [38].

Results of SPECT imaging with the test object are shown in Fig. 7-17. The left column in Fig. 7-17 shows, from top to bottom, respectively, the midlevel transaxial image with no corrections, with attenuation correction using an attenuation coefficient of 0.15 cm^{-1} for water and 0.39 cm^{-1} for aluminum, and with attenuation and scatter correction using $a = 0.1$. The middle and right columns show the attenuation and scatter-corrected images with $a = 0.2$, 0.3, and 0.4, respectively (middle column), and $a = 0.5$, 0.7, and 0.9, respectively (right column).

These images were evaluated with respect to contrast recovery in the 4-cm hot region and the SNR (mean/standard deviation) in the background portion. In addition, as a gauge of quantitative accuracy, the rms error in the background portion of each image was computed with respect to a noise-free simulated image containing the known relative activity distribution.

A plot of the contrast, defined as the ratio of the peak value in the 4-cm hot spot to the mean value of the background, is shown in Fig. 7-18 for the two scatter windows as a function of a. The value of a that produces the correct contrast of $25.0(\pm 1.2)$ is 0.36 from Fig. 7-18 for the 28-keV wide scatter window and 0.45 for the 18-keV scatter window. The value of a for the 28-keV window is in excellent agreement with theory, which predicts $a = 0.37$. The experimental value with the 18-keV window, however, is

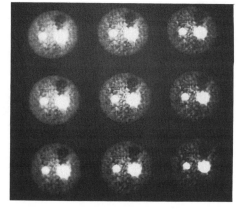

Figure 7-17 Attenuation and scatter-corrected images with 28-keV photopeak window and 32-keV scatter window, as a function of the scaling factor a. The first, second, and third columns correspond to a values ranging from 0.1 to 0.3, 0.4 to 0.6, and 0.7 to 0.9 respectively. (From reference [35]).

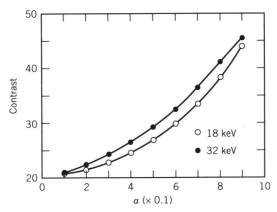

Figure 7-18 A plot of the contrast in the 4-cm hot region as a function of the scaling factor a using the 32-keV and 18-keV scatter windows, respectively. The correct contrast of 25 is recovered at $a = 0.36$ and 0.45, respectively, for the two scatter windows. (From ref. [35]).

approximately 36% lower than the theoretical value of 0.71. No suitable reason for this discrepancy can be given at the present time. It is noteworthy that with no attenuation or scatter correction, the contrast is 11.9, which is more than a factor of 2 below the correct value. With attenuation correction alone, the contrast improves to 19.6, which is about 21% lower than the true value. The relative significance of the attenuation and scatter correction procedures might be appreciated from these numbers.

The SNR in the background of the reconstructed images is plotted in Fig. 7-19. The SNR shows a small degradation with increasing a, which is expected from statistical effects as more counts are subtracted from the photopeak counts. Two points are noteworthy here: (1) the SNR for the value of a that produces the correct contrast with the 32-keV scatter window is slightly better than the SNR at the corresponding value with the 18-keV scatter window, which is in accordance with the scatter correction optimization procedure (see Fig. 7-15), and (2) the SNR values in Fig. 7-19 are much lower than those in Fig. 7-15, which is probably due to additional noise introduced by nonuniformities in the scintillation camera and propagation of noise in the image reconstruction algorithms.

A plot of the rms error in the background portion of the reconstructed images with respect to a simulated noise-free image of the test object is shown in Fig. 7-20. The simulated image was generated using relative activity values shown in Fig. 7-16 and Gaussian smoothing in accordance with the spatial resolution of the SPECT images. Negative values in the reconstructed images, which are normally set to zero, were retained for the rms computation. The rms plot shows a minimum at $a = 0.36$ for the 32-keV window,

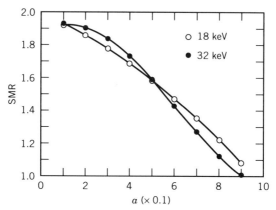

Figure 7-19 A plot of the SNR in the background of the reconstructed images as a function of the scaling factor a for the two scatter windows mentioned in Fig. 7-18. (From ref. [35]).

which is identical to the value for recovering the correct contrast, as seen in Fig. 7-18. The minimum rms error for the 18-keV window is at $a = 0.55$, and is now in relatively better agreement with theory. Using the rms values as an indicator of quantitation, scatter correction using the 32-keV window followed by attenuation correction produces a minimum rms error of 11.4%, whereas the same procedure produces a minimum rms error of 17.0% with the 18-keV scatter window. These results demonstrate the superiority of the

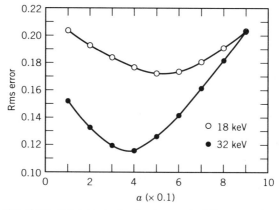

Figure 7-20 A plot of the rms error in the background of the reconstructed images as a function of the scaling factor a. Minima are produced at $a = 0.36$ and 0.55, respectively, for the two scatter windows mentioned in Fig. 7-18. (From ref. [35]).

32-keV scatter window over the 18-keV scatter window and are consistent with results shown in Fig. 7-15.

7-4 CONE-BEAM SPECT WITH CONVENTIONAL SCINTILLATION CAMERA

Convergent-beam collimators in SPECT, when compared to parallel collimators, offer the potential for improved sensitivity and resolution for imaging of relatively small organs such as the brain and the heart. These advantages are obtained by using the magnifying properties of convergent-beam collimators to better utilize the available crystal area on a standard rotating gamma camera. Collimators of this type were originally proposed and developed by Jaszczak for brain imaging [39]. These ideas were later applied to heart imaging by Gullberg [40].

The earliest convergent collimators were configured as a stack of fan-beam collimators, one for each transaxial plane. This arrangement leads to improved sensitivity transaxially but not axially. To obtain the best sensitivity, the collimator should be convergent in both the axial and transaxial directions. This is achieved using a cone-beam geometry.

While convergent-beam collimators offer significant improvements in sensitivity and resolution, they present a much more difficult reconstruction problem than their parallel and fan-beam counterparts. We can classify the two main approaches to the reconstruction of cone-beam SPECT images as direct and iterative. The direct methods are based on an inversion formula derived from the formulation of the problem in terms of line integrals through the desired image. Although these methods do not take account of important factors such as attenuation, detector response, and noise, the algorithms provide reconstructions in a relatively short time. For this reason they are generally preferred in clinical settings. The iterative methods are able to include a full statistical model for the data and may directly include all of the above factors. This improvement in the modeling, and consequently in image quality, is achieved at significantly increased computational costs. In this section we will consider at length both of these approaches.

The image reconstruction problem for cone-beam SPECT has important differences than that for the parallel and fan-beam systems. In both of the latter cases the reconstruction problem has been widely investigated, and the closed form filtered backprojection reconstruction algorithms are well known. These methods, originally developed for X-ray CT are easily adapted to the SPECT problem. However, the cone-beam reconstruction problem remains an area of active research, primarily because, to date, a fast and accurate reconstruction algorithm has still not been available.

The major difference between cone-beam and parallel systems and the fan-beam system is that in the latter case rotating the gamma camera once around the patient provides a full set of projections, from which theoretically the image can be exactly reconstructed. In contrast, rotation of a cone-beam-collimated gamma camera around the patient does not provide sufficient data to exactly reconstruct the image. The conditions under which an image could be reconstructed from its cone-beam projections were studied in some depth by Smith [41] and Tuy [42]. A sufficient condition for reconstruction is that the curve traced out by the cone vertices as the data are collected should be such that all planes that pass through the object also cut this curve. Thus, for example, a pair of orthogonal circles around the object [43], a circle and perpendicular line [44], and a spiral [45] are examples of curves from which theoretically the object can be recovered exactly. Closed-form solutions for curves satisfying the above properties have been proposed [42, 46]; however, numerical implementations are computationally very expensive, and to date these methods have not been used on clinical data. Alternative approximate reconstructions for geometries for which exact inverses exist have been studied with the aim of fast implementation [43–45].

Although the circular geometry does not possess the invertibility property of the geometries discussed above, the ease of data collection using a standard SPECT system with a converging collimator make this the most practical cone-beam arrangement. The earliest attempts at reconstruction for this geometry were applied to data collected from the X-ray CT dynamic spatial reconstruction (DSR) machine [37]. These methods made the assumption that the data were a set of stacked fan-beam projections rather than truly cone beam. Reconstructions based on this assumption are reasonable for transaxial slices in planes adjacent to the plane in which the circular orbit lies, but they deteriorate rapidly away from this plane. Probably the most important contribution to reconstruction from cone-beam data is the method of Feldkamp et al. [47]. Using a heuristic argument, Feldkamp was able to extend the fan-beam-filtered backprojection method to develop a reconstruction algorithm for cone-beam data that requires one-dimensional filtering of the cone-beam data followed by a weighted 3-D backprojection. The algorithm performs nicely, in practice, particularly when the radius of the circle is large compared to the support of the object [48]. This is the reconstruction method that is currently in clinical use. However, the Feldkamp method does produce reconstruction artifacts, and considerable research effort is still directed at finding better solutions to this problem.

Iterative reconstruction methods in SPECT are based either on a formulation in terms of a large set of linear equations, such as ART (algebraic reconstruction technique), or on a statistical model for the data, such as the EM (expectation maximum) algorithm for maximum likelihood estimation. In both cases the major computational requirements are the calculation of forward- and backprojections. While these operations differ for parallel and cone-beam geometries, the mathematical details of the algorithms are independent of the data collection geometry. Therefore cone-beam images can be reconstructed using the iterative algorithms described in chapter 4. In practice, iterative reconstruction is currently used in most clinical settings for the following reason. Cone-beam tomography is a truly 3-D imaging modality—that is, the problem cannot be decomposed into a set of 2-D reconstruction problems, as can the parallel problem, and thus the computational cost involved in performing multiple forward- and backprojections is prohibitive.

7-5 RING, CYLINDRICAL, AND SPHERICAL SPECT SYSTEMS

A great variety of specialized SPECT systems utilizing a ring [49, 50], cylindrical [51], or spherical [52] geometry have appeared in the literature since the early Mark IV brain scanner developed by Kuhl et al. [53]. These systems are designed to reduce the distortions caused by rotating scintillation cameras due to the motion of the bulky camera head [54] and to improve the resolution and sensitivity under specific imaging situations.

For example, a SPECT system (called ASPECT) based on a single NaI cylindrical crystal and a rotating collimator has been recently designed. An initial version of this instrument, designed for head imaging, has been described in [51] to image an approximately 20-cm diameter region within a 22-cm diameter × 9-cm tall cylindrical field of view. The temporal resolution is now limited by the sensitivity and rotational period of the collimator. ASPECT, however, is a technologically complex instrument with very little flexibility in the detection geometry or the field of view. Other recent systems that provide much more flexibility utilize a ring of detectors or a ring of modular cameras [50, 55]. The modular multiple-slice systems are based on using small scintillation camera modules, where each module is composed of either a 10-cm × 10-cm planar scintillation crystal backed by four photomultiplier tubes [55] or a bank of 3-mm wide × 12.5-mm thick × 15-cm long NaI(Tl) bars coupled to 20 photomultiplier tubes [50].

As an alternative to the multiple photomultiplier tube modular scintillation cameras, a new generation of dynamic SPECT instruments based on the position-sensitive photomultiplier tube (PSPMT) has been proposed recently [52, 56]. Two systems, one for body imaging and the other for head imaging, have been investigated. Either cone-beam collimators (head imaging) or stacked fan-beam collimators (body imaging) are used to view the region to be imaged completely from many angular directions simultaneously. The system for head imaging has a spherical geometry [52] and is based on 19 PSPMTs 13 cm in diameter, with each PSPMT coupled to a diverging-hole collimator to cover a 22-cm diameter spherical field of view completely in a stationary mode. The collimator is attached to a 1.25-cm thick NaI(Tl) crystal on each PSPMT and designed to utilize the inner 10 cm linearly sensitive portion of the photocathode. At a distance of 10 cm from the collimator, the system resolution—including collimator line spread function (LSF) and intrinsic resolution of the PSPMT (assumed to be 4 mm fwhm)—is computed to be 1.2 cm [52]. Although the system resolution is approximately 20% worse

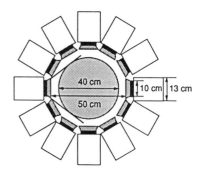

Figure 7-21 Conceptual design of a body ring SPECT system comprising 12 PSPMT cameras, each equipped with a fan-beam collimator. (From ref. [57]).

than that achievable with a parallel-hole collimator (0.98 cm) or a converging collimator (0.95 cm), the diverging collimator is considered essential to achieve a total coverage of the entire 22-cm diameter spherical object from all angular positions simultaneously. If a converging or a parallel-hole collimator were used under these conditions, peripheral regions of the object would enter or leave the field of view as a function of view angle, creating artifacts in the reconstructed images.

The conceptual design of a SPECT system for imaging the thorax or abdominal regions is shown in Fig. 7-21. A ring comprising 12 PSPMT cameras surrounds the body section to be imaged. The diverging cone-beam collimator used for the head imager, however, is not suited to body imaging, since it will result in regions leaving and entering the field of view as a function of view angle. Instead, a stacked fan-beam collimator that can provide complete coverage of a 40-cm diameter × 7.6-cm thick region of the body is used. Since the photocathode of the PSPMTs is circular, the stacked fan-beam collimator is coupled to a smaller inner region on the crystal, lying between two 7.6 cm apart chords, as shown in Fig. 7-22. Thus the stacked fan-beam collimator will provide maximum sampling at the central level (corresponding to the 10-cm inner diameter of the crystal) and decreasing

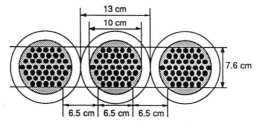

Figure 7-22 Arrangement of the stacked fan-beam collimators to sample a 7.6-cm-thick body region. (From ref. [57]).

sampling along the vertical axis of the cylindrical region. Accordingly the spatial resolution will be best for the central slice and degrade slowly in slices along the vertical axis of the imaged cylindrical region. With a stacked fan-beam collimator, 12 views of the object are obtained simultaneously. One small rotation, corresponding to half the separation between each PSPMT, provides 24 views; this is adequate for dynamic imaging. The fan-beam collimator has a focal length of 12.3 cm for the central row and 8.3 cm for the rows that correspond to the top or bottom of the field of view. Including the appropriate magnification factors of the collimator, the system resolution at a distance of 20 cm from the collimator is computed to be 2.1 cm for the central row and 2.8 cm for the top or bottom rows.

The circular shape of the photocathode and the masked nonlinear regions near the edges of the photocathode imply that the sensitivity of the body ring SPECT will be less than that of an ideal continuous ring or cylindrical crystal design. The sensitivity of the PSPMT SPECT to image a 7.6-cm thick body region is approximately 65% of a continuous cylindrical crystal. However, compared to a continuous cylindrical design, a PSPMT-based system provides great flexibility in choosing optimum geometries (e.g., circular vs. elliptical), changing configurations to focus onto a selected region (e.g., the heart, by tilting some of the cameras) and mixing different collimators to achieve better resolution.

7-6 SPECT WITH LIMITED ANGULAR SAMPLING

An alternative to a rotating gamma camera, a rotating frame of detectors, or a ring of detectors is to use a system that provides angular sampling over a limited angular range. Such systems, in general, are used for longitudinal SPECT, whereas the complete angular sampling systems are used for transaxial SPECT. A variety of longitudinal tomography systems have been developed in the past few years. These are based on coded apertures, the slant-hole collimator, and a seven-pinhole collimator.

7-6-1 Coded Apertures

The first coded aperture system was developed by Barrett [57]. It utilizes a Fresnel zone plate collimator instead of the conventional collimator used with a gamma camera. The scintigraphic image is decoded to produce tomographic images by using an appropriate Fourier transformation. This decoding may be accomplished with a laser beam after transferring the image onto film. Many other different apertures, including nonredundant and uniformly redundant pinhole arrays, annuli, and rotating slits, have been investigated [58–60]. Although the coded aperture method has high sensitivity, it produces several artifacts and has not found general use. Rogers et al. [61] have developed another coded aperture method in which data are time modulated by moving a plate containing a known sequence of apertures in front of the bare crystal of a gamma camera, and longitudinal tomograms have been reconstructed for small organs such as the heart with lateral resolution of about 0.5 cm and depth resolution that varies from 1 cm at 4 cm to about 4 cm at 12 cm with such systems.

A fundamental problem of multiplexed coded aperture imaging (i.e., coded apertures where different projections are allowed to superpose and are then separated or demultiplexed based on the design of the apertures) is that noise propagates during the decoding stage [62]. The SNR in the reconstructed images is a strong function of the degree of multiplexing and thus depends on the source distribution and the design of the apertures. In general the SNR drops rapidly as the size of the object within which the activity is distributed increases, thus limiting the use of this approach in practice.

7-6-2 Slant-Hole Collimator

In the slant-hole method a parallel-hole collimator with slanted holes is rotated with respect to the face of a gamma camera. Projections from different angles are obtained and then combined to produce longitudinal tomographs. Several commercial systems of this type are currently available. The collimator may be divided into two [63] or more sectors to obtain simultaneous views from a smaller region. Again, the performance is limited by the size of the region being imaged. Also the depth resolution is poor [62].

7-6-3 Seven-Pinhole Collimator

A collimator with 7 pinholes was first investigated by Vogel et al. [64] to obtain 7 nonoverlapping projection images of the heart. Longitudinal tomographic sections of the heart were reconstructed from these seven views. Although this method is simple to implement and has no moving parts, the images are not quantitative and are strongly influenced by geometry, as demonstrated by Budinger [62]. It further appears that this method is only suited for myocardial imaging.

7-7 ELECTRONICALLY COLLIMATED SPECT

The technique of electronic collimation, first proposed by Singh et al. [65] in 1977 for SPECT, represents an alternative to conventional mechanical collimation for localizing gamma emitters. As mentioned earlier, most SPECT studies are currently performed with a rotating scintillation camera equipped with a parallel-hole or a similar multiple-hole mechanical collimator. As is clear from Fig. 7-4, mechanical collimation suffers from a fundamentally low sensitivity, since only a small fraction of gamma rays emitted from the object are transmitted through the apertures to produce counts. Furthermore, if the energy of the emitted radiation exceeds about 250 keV, the combination of the required septal thickness, length, and diameter of the apertures for effective collimation deteriorate the resolution, uniformity, and sensitivity to the point where it becomes almost impractical for imaging. Thus only a limited number of radioisotopes with gamma energies in the 70–200 keV range have been utilized effectively in nuclear medicine and many potentially useful radionuclides either have not been considered or are imaged under suboptimal conditions.

Although the SPECT systems based on a ring of stationary detectors [49], stationary cameras [50] or a single cylindrical NaI(Tl) crystal [51] with a rotating collimator discussed above overcome the mechanical stability and field uniformity problems associated with the rotating scintillation camera, the basic limitations of sensitivity and high-energy imaging remain similar to a conventional SPECT system. Also, dynamic studies are now constrained by the collimator motion.

To overcome these fundamental drawbacks of a mechanical collimator, an electronically collimated SPECT instrument based on detecting a sequential interaction of the emitted gamma rays with two position- and energy-sensitive detectors has been designed by Singh [66, 67]. Counts in electronic collimation are acquired in a coincidence counting mode between two detectors (det1 and det2) from those gamma rays, which scatter from det1 onto det2 after depositing a measurable energy in det1. From the physics of Compton scattering, each coincident count originates from activity lying somewhere on a hollow cone whose vertex, axis, and angle are known with an accuracy depending on the position and energy resolution of the detectors. Localization of activity (i.e., collimation) is thereby achieved electronically upon hollow cones traversing the object. Since each coincident count generally identifies a different hollow cone, a very large number of intersecting conical surfaces are generated in a study from which the three-dimensional activity distribution can be reconstructed [68–74].

The design and basic characteristics of an electronically collimated system comprising a 33×33 array of small germanium (Ge) detectors as det1 and an uncollimated conventional scintillation camera as det2 are described in [66, 73]. The basic concept of electronic collimation is illustrated in Fig. 7-23. Considering a single element from the det1 array and an on-axis point source shown in Fig. 7-23, the coincident counts on det2 will form circles with radii proportional to the scattering angle and the separation between det1 and det2. Off-axis point sources, however, will not trace circles but elliptical or partial elliptical profiles representing an intersection of a tilted hollow cone with the planar det2 surface. Thus the point spread function (PSF) at a specified scattering angle, defined in terms of the coincident count profile on det2, is spatially variant, and the coincident counts from an object at a given scattering angle can be represented as a convolution of the cone-beam projection of the object (where the cone-beam projection is the same as a

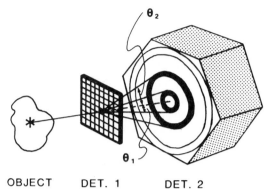

Figure 7-23 A depiction of the concept of electronic collimation based on detection of gamma rays scattered from an array of Ge detectors (det1) onto an uncollimated scintillation camera (det2). Counts are recorded in coincidence between det1 and det2 for events where a small amount of the emitted photon's energy is deposited in det1 and the remaining energy is absorbed in det2. The energy deposited in det1 determines the angle at which gamma rays are scattered from the Ge detector (θ_1 or θ_2 in the figure). (From reference [75]).

pinhole projection image) with a spatially variant psf [66]. Consequently the cone-beam projection of the object can be recovered by deconvolving the psf as a function of the known scattering angles. The deconvolution operation is greatly facilitated by mapping the coincident counts on a spherical surface centered on the det1 element under consideration [70].

After deconvolution a cone-beam projection of the object is obtained from each element of det1. Since det1 is composed of a large number of elements, on the order of 1000, a large number of cone-beam projections from multiple angles of view are obtained simultaneously. These cone-beam projections from multiple angles of view can then be used to reconstruct a three-dimensional image of the object [73]. Although the design of the original electronically collimated system called for a single 33 × 33 Ge array [66], representing a limited angular sampling instrument, later designs have considered orthogonal and cylindrical geometries to achieve 180° and 360° angular sampling, respectively [75]. Thus a totally stationary cylindrical scanning instrument for SPECT might be realized with electronic collimation.

REFERENCES

1. H. O. Anger. Scintillation camera. *Rev. Sci. Instrum.* 29:27 (1958).
2. H. O. Anger. Scintillation camera with multichannel collimators. *J. Nucl. Med.* 5:515–531 (1964).
3. H. O. Anger. In *Instrumentation in Nuclear Medicine*, vol. 1, G. J. Hine, ed. San Diego: Academic Press, 1967, pp. 485–552.

4. J. G. Rogers, R. Harrop, P. E. Kinahan, N. A. Wilkinson, and G. H. Coombes. Conceptual design of a whole body PET machine. *IEEE Trans. Nucl. Sci.* NS-35:680 (1988).

5. In *Physics in Nuclear Medicine*, J. A. Sorenson and M. E. Phelps, eds. New York: Grune & Stratton, 1980, pp. 283–302.

6. C. Burnham, J. Bradshaw, D. Kaufman, D. A. Chesler, C. W. Stearns, and G. L. Brownell. One dimensional scintillation cameras for positron ring detectors. *IEEE Trans. Nucl. Sci.* NS-32:889 (1985).

7. T. D. Milster, L. A. Selberg, H. H. Barrett, A. L. Landesman, and R. H. Beacat III. Digital position estimation for the modular scintillation camera. *IEEE Trans. Nucl. Sci.* NS-32:748 (1985).

8. D. E. Kuhl and R. Q. Edwards. *Radiology* 80:653–662 (1963).

9. T. F. Budinger and G. T. Gullberg. Three-dimensional reconstruction in nuclear medicine emission imaging. *IEEE Trans. Nucl. Sci.* NS-21:2 (1975).

10. J. W. Keyes, Jr., N. Orlandea, W. J. Heetderks, P. F. Leonard, and W. L. Rogers. *J. Nucl. Med.* 18:381–387 (1977).

11. R. J. Jaszczak, P. H. Murphy, D. Huard, and J. A. Burdine. *J. Nucl. Med.* 18:373–380 (1977).

12. M. Singh, M. J. Berggren, D. E. Gustafson, M. K. Dewanjee, R. C. Bahn, and E. L. Ritman. Emission computed tomography and its application to imaging of acute myocardial infarction in intact dogs using Tc-99m pyrophosphate. *J. Nucl. Med.* 20:50 (1979).

13. C. Lim, S. Gottschalk, R. Walker, R. Schreiner, F. Valentino, C. Pinkstaff, J. Janzo, J. Covic, A. Perusek, J. Anderson, K. I. Kim, D. Shand, K. Coulman, S. King, and D. Styblo. Triangular SPECT system for brain and body organ imaging: Design concept and preliminary imaging results. *IEEE Trans. Nucl. Sci.* NS-32:741 (1985).

14. R. J. Jaszczak. Tomographic radiopharmaceutical imaging. *Proc. IEEE* 76:1079–1094 (1988).

15. D. B. Kay and J. W. Keyes. First order corrections for absorption and resolution compensation in radionuclide Fourier tomography. *J. Nucl. Med.* 16:540–541 (1975).

16. B. M. W. Tsui, H. B. Hu, D. R. Gilland, and G. T. Gullberg. Implementation of simultaneous attenuation and detector response correction in SPECT. *IEEE Trans. Nucl. Sci.* 35:778–783 (1988).

17. B. M. W. Tsui, and G. T. Gullberg. The geometric transfer function for cone and fan beam collimators. *Phys. Med. Biol.* 35:81–93 (1990).

18. G. L. Zeng and G. T. Gullberg. Three dimensional iterative reconstruction algorithms with attenuation and geometric point response corrections. *IEEE Trans. Nucl. Sci.* 38:693–702 (1991).

19. B. E. Oppenheim. Scatter correction for SPECT. *J. Nucl. Med.* 25:928–929 (1984).

20. L. T. Chang. A method for attenuation correction in radionuclide computed tomography. *IEEE Trans. Nucl. Sci.* NS-25:638–643 (1978).

21. O. J. Tretiak and P. Delaney. The exponential convolution algorithm for emission computed axial tomography. In *Review of Information Processing in Medical*

Imaging, A. B. Brill and R. R. Price, eds. Oak Ridge National Laboratory Report ORNL/BCCTIC-2:266–278, 1978.

22. G. T. Gullberg and T. F. Budinger. The use of filtering methods to compensate for constant attenuation in single-photon emission computed tomography. *IEEE Trans. Biomed. Eng.* BME-28:142–157 (1981).

23. K. F. Kim, R. P. Tewarson, Y. Bizaris, and R. W. Rowe. Inversion for the attenuated Radon transform with constant attenuation. *IEEE Trans. Nucl. Sci.* NS-31:538–542 (1984).

24. T. Timitani. A deconvolution function for single photon emission computed tomography with constant attenuation. *IEEE Trans. Nucl. Sci.* NS-33:505–510 (1986).

25. S. Bellini, M. Piacentini, C. Cafforio, and F. Rocco. Compensation of tissue absorption in emission tomography. *IEEE Trans. Acoustics, Speech and Signal Processing* ASSP-27:213–218 (1979).

26. E. Tanaka, H. Toyama, and H. Murayama. Convolution image reconstruction for quantitative single photon emission computed tomography. *Phys. Med. Biol.* 29:1489–1500 (1984).

27. D. R. Gilland, R. J. Jaszczak, T. G. Turkington, K. L. Greer, and R. E. Coleman. Quantitative SPECT imaging with Indium-11. *IEEE Trans. Nucl. Sci.* NS-38:761–766 (1991).

28. R. J. Jaszczak, R. E. Coleman, and F. R. Whitehead. Physical factors affecting quantitative measurements using camera based single photon emission computed tomography (SPECT). *IEEE Trans. Nucl. Sci.* NS-28:69–80 (1981).

29. S. D. Egbert and R. S. May. An integral-transport method for Compton-scatter correction in emission computed tomography. *IEEE Trans. Nucl. Sci.* NS-27:543–548 (1980).

30. J. W. Beck, R. J. Jaszczak, R. E. Coleman, C. F. Starmer, and L. W. Nolte. Analysis of SPECT including scatter and attenuation using sophisticated Monte Carlo modeling methods. *IEEE Trans. Nucl. Sci.* NS-29:506–511 (1982).

31. B. Axelsson, P. Msaki, and A. Israelsson. Subtraction of Compton scattered photons in single-photon emission computerized tomography. *J. Nucl. Med.* 25:490–494 (1984).

32. P. Bloch and T. Sanders. Reduction of the effects of scattered radiation on a sodium iodide imaging system. *J. Nucl. Med.* 14:67–72 (1972).

33. R. J. Jaszczak, K. L. Greer, C. E. Floyd, and R. E. Coleman. Improved SPECT quantification using compensation for scattered photons. *J. Nucl. Med.* 25(8):893–900 (1984).

34. M. Singh and C. Horne. Use of germanium detector to optimize scatter correction in SPECT. *J. Nucl. Med.* 28:1853–1860 (1987).

35. M. Singh, C. Horne, D. Maneval, J. Amartey, and R. Brechner. Non-uniform attenuation and scatter correction in SPECT. *IEEE Trans. Nucl. Sci.* NS-35:767–771 (1988).

36. R. A. Brooks and G. Di Chiro. Principles of computer assisted tomography (CAT) in radiographic and radioisotopic imaging. *Phys. Med. Biol.* 21:689–732 (1976).

37. R. E. Sturm, E. L. Ritman, S. A. Johnson, M. A. Wondrow, D. I. Erdman, and E. H. Wood. *Proc. San Diego Biomedical Symposium* 15:181–188 (1976).

38. L. A. Shepp and B. F. Logan. The Fourier reconstruction of a head section. *IEEE Trans. Nucl. Sci.* NS-21:21–43 (1974).

39. R. J. Jaszczak, K. L. Greer, C. E. Floyd, and R. E. Coleman. *IEEE Trans. Nucl. Sci.* NS-35:644–648 (1988).

40. G. T. Gullberg, G. L. Zeng, P. E. Chrintian, et al. Information processing in medical imaging. *XIth IPMI Conf.*, 1990.

41. B. D. Smith. *IEEE Trans. Med. Imag.* MI-4:14–25 (1985).

42. H. K. Tuy. *SIAM J. Appl. Math.* 43:546–552 (1983).

43. R. Clack, G. L. Zeng, Y. Weng, et al. *Phys. Med. Biol.* 37 (1992).

44. G. L. Zeng and G. T. Gullberg. *Phys. Med. Biol.* 37 (1992).

45. X. Yan and R. Leahy. *Phys. Med. Biol.* 37:1–14 (1992).

46. P. Grangeat. *Mathematical Methods in Tomography*. Lecture Notes in Mathematics. Berlin: Springer-Verlag, in press.

47. L. A. Feldkamp, L. C. Davis, and J. W. Kress. *J. Opt. Soc. Am.* 1:612–619 (1984).

48. X. Yan and R. Leahy. *IEEE Trans. Med. Imag.* MI-10:462–472 (1991).

49. W. Chang, B. M. Tsui, Z. Tian, et al. Design and investigation of a modular focused collimator based multiple detector ring system for SPECT imaging of the brain. *SPIE* 671:200–205 (1986).

50. W. L. Rogers, N. H. Clinthorne, L. Shao, et al. SPRINT II: A second generation single photon ring tomograph. *IEEE Trans. Med. Imag.* 7:291–297 (1988).

51. S. Genna and A. P. Smith. The development of ASPECT, an annular single crystal brain camera for high efficiency SPECT. *IEEE Trans. Nucl. Sci.* NS-35:654–658 (1988).

52. M. Singh, R. Leahy, R. R. Brechner, and X. Yan. Design and imaging studies of a position sensitive photomultiplier based dynamic SPECT system. *IEEE Trans. Nucl. Sci.* NS-36:1132–1137 (1989).

53. D. E. Kuhl, R. Q. Edwards, A. R. Ricci, et al. *Radiology* 121:405–413 (1976).

54. W. L. Rogers, N. H. Clinthorne, B. A. Harkness, K. F. Koral, and J. W. Keyes. Field-flood requirements for emission computed tomography with an Anger camera. *J. Nucl. Med.* 23:162–168 (1982).

55. T. D. Milster, L. A. Selberg, H. H. Barrett, et al. A modular scintillation camera for use in nuclear medicine. *IEEE Trans. Nucl. Sci.* NS-31:578–580 (1984).

56. M. Singh, R. Leahy, K. Oshio, R. R. Brechner, and X. Yan. *IEEE Trans. Nucl. Sci.* NS-37:1321–1327 (1990).

57. H. H. Barrett. Fresnel zone plate imaging in nuclear medicine. *J. Nucl. Med.* 13:382 (1972).

58. W. L. Rogers, K. S. Hans, L. W. Jones, and W. H. Beierwaltes. Application of a Fresnel zone plate to gamma-ray imaging. *J. Nucl. Med.* 13:612 (1972).

59. R. G. Simson and H. H. Barrett. Coded-aperture imaging. *Imag. Diagnostic Med.* (S. Nudelman, ed.):217 (1980).

60. L. Renaud, M. L. G. Joy, and D. L. Gilday. Fourier multiaperture emission tomography. *J. Nucl. Med.* 20:1986 (1979).

61. W. L. Rogers, K. F. Koral, R. Mayans, et al. Coded aperture imaging of the heart. *J. Nucl. Med.* 21:371 (1980).

62. T. F. Budinger. Physical attributes of single photon tomography. *J. Nucl. Med.* 21:579 (1980).

63. O. Nalcioglu, M. E. Morton, and N. Milne. *IEEE Trans. Nucl. Sci.* NS-27:430–434 (1980).

64. R. A. Vogel, D. L. Kirch, M. T. LeFree, et al. *J. Nucl. Med.* 19:648–654 (1978).

65. M. Singh, D. E. Gustafson, M. J. Berggren, B. K. Gilbert, and E. L. Ritman. Physics of electronic collimation for single photon transaxial tomography. *Med. Phys.* 4:350 (1977).

66. M. Singh. An electronically collimated gamma camera for single photon emission computed tomography. Part I: Theoretical considerations and design criteria. *Med. Phys.* 10:421–427 (1983).

67. M. Singh and D. Doria. An electronically collimated gamma camera for single photon emission computed tomography. Part II: Image reconstruction and preliminary experimental measurements. *Med. Phys.* 10:428–435 (1983).

68. M. Singh and D. Doria. Computer simulation of image reconstruction with a new electronically collimated gamma tomography system. *SPIE* 273:192–200 (1981).

69. D. Doria and M. Singh. Comparison of reconstruction algorithms for an electronically collimated gamma camera. *IEEE Trans. Nucl. Sci.* NS-29:447–451 (1982).

70. R. Brechner and M. Singh. Reconstruction of electronically collimated images obtained from single gamma emitters using a spherical system of coordinates. *IEEE Trans. Nucl. Sci.* NS-33:583–586 (1986).

71. R. Brechner, M. Singh, and R. Leahy. Computer simulated studies of tomographic reconstruction with an electronically collimated camera for SPECT. *IEEE Trans. Nucl. Sci.* NS-34:369–373 (1987).

72. T. Hebert, R. Leahy, and M. Singh. Maximum likelihood reconstruction for a prototype electronically collimated single photon emission system. *SPIE* 767:77–83 (1987).

73. M. Singh and D. Doria. Single photon imaging with electronic collimation. *IEEE Trans. Nucl. Sci.* NS-32:843–847 (1985).

74. T. Hebert, R. Leahy, and M. Singh. 3-D ML reconstruction for an electronically collimated single photon emission imaging system. *J. Opt. Soc. A,* 7:1305–1313 (1990).

75. M. Singh and R. R. Brechner. Experimental test-object study of electronically collimated SPECT. *J. Nucl. Med.* 31:178–186 (1990).

8

TOMOGRAPHIC NUCLEAR MEDICAL IMAGING—POSITRON EMISSION TOMOGRAPHY

Although the potential of positron imaging was recognized as early as the 1950s, actual tomographic mode imaging began only after X-ray CT was developed in 1972. Positron emission tomography is an interesting example of a joint effort of many disciplines, including chemistry, and computer science. PET requires short-lived cyclotron-produced radionuclides. These radionuclides are suitable for radiopharmaceuticals that can be administered into the human body and for instrumentation that can detect the annihilation photons and process the signals to provide images of their activity distribution. Small cyclotrons are now available for use in many medical facilities, and great advances in the chemical synthesis of radiopharmaceuticals have also been made. In short, there has been a phenomenal growth in PET instrumentation research and development in recent years, resulting in a few system designs that are potentially capable of imaging with a resolution as high as 2 to 3 mm fwhm. This chapter will discuss the physical and instrumentational aspects of PET, namely some of its basic principles, the various physical factors affecting its performance and computational models, design considerations, and the evolution of types of PET in recent years.

8-1 BASIC PRINCIPLES OF POSITRON EMISSION TOMOGRAPHY (PET)

8-1-1 Positron Emitters and Physics [1 – 9]

Positron-emitting radionuclides possess several important and unique physical properties that make the PET a unique imaging device. Its most impor-

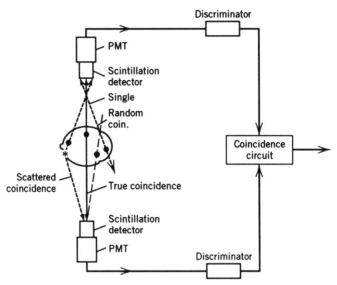

Figure 8-1 Principle of coincidence detection. True coincidence (solid line), singles and random coincidence (broken line) , and scattered coincidence (dashed line)are indicated.

tant property is the directionality or collinearity of the simultaneous emission of two photons by the annihilation process. In other words, when a positron is emitted and combines with a nearby electron, two photons are generated. These two annihilation photons, each with an energy of 511 keV($= m_e c^2$), are generated simultaneously (simultaneity) and travel in opposite directions, nearly 180° back to back (collinearity). The near collinearity of the two annihilation photons makes it possible to identify the annihilation event or the existence of positron emitters through the detection of two photons by two detectors posed exactly in opposite sides within a short time (i.e., within 10^{-8} sec or less). This is usually achieved by a coincidence detection circuit, which records an event only if both detectors sense annihilation photons simultaneously (solid lines in Fig. 8-1). Because the two detectors record coincidence events only from a volume of space defined by a column or strip joining the two detectors, a relatively uniform collimation characteristic is observed compared with SPECT, where the activity volume seen by the detector is mainly determined by the physical collimation. For this reason coincidence detection is also called "electronic collimation." The total number of coincidence events detected by a given pair of detectors constitutes a measure of the integrated radioactivity (i.e., line-integral projection data) along the strip joining the two detectors. From a complete set of line-integral projection data obtained from a large number of detectors at different views surrounding the entire object, the activity distribution within the slice or

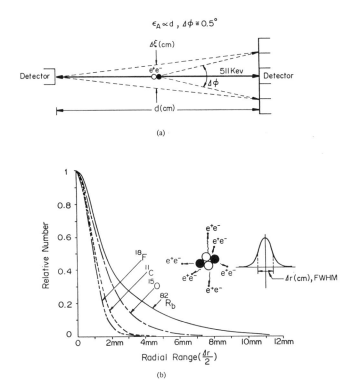

Figure 8-2 (a) Angular uncertainty effect of annihilation of positron on the resolution; (b) effects of range on resolution for different positron-emitting isotopes obtained experimentally in water with a high-resolution coincidence system.

volume can be measured quantitatively using the reconstruction algorithms discussed in the previous chapter (see Chapters 3 and 4).

The accuracy of the spatial localization of a positron emitting radionuclide through the coincidence detection procedure is, however, limited by two physical properties of positron annihilation: (1) the angular uncertainty arising from the fact that the two annihilation photons are not exactly collinear and (2) the uncertainty of the annihilation position of the emitted positrons (i.e., uncertainty due to the positron ranges), as shown in Fig. 8-2 (a) and (b). The second property is strongly dependent on the kinetic energy of the emitted positron (see also Table 8-1) for a given radionuclide. The combined effect of the two properties introduces a fundamental uncertainty in locating the sources of the positrons (i.e., radionuclides). This uncertainty, depending on the radionuclides used on the separation distance of the two detectors, is typically 2 to 3 mm fwhm. This value is accepted as the lower limit of the resolution that can be achieved by positron tomogra-

Table 8-1   Values of variables for some positron-emitting radionuclides

Positron-Emitting Isotopes	$^{11}_{6}C$	$^{13}_{7}N$	$^{15}_{8}O$	$^{18}_{9}F$	$^{82}_{38}Sr(^{82}_{37}Rb)$
Maximum energy (MeV)	0.959	1.197	1.738	0.633	3.148
Most probable energy (MeV)	0.326	0.432	0.696	0.2025	1.385
Half-life (min)	20.3	10.0	2	109.7	1.3
Path length (for electron of same maximum energy in water) (cm)	0.498	0.535	0.822	0.239	1.561
Radial range in water $(Exp)^a$ fwhm/2 (cm)	0.111	0.142	0.149	0.102	0.169

phy. Despite these inherent spatial resolution limits, PET has the highest resolution, as well as sensitivity, of any other nuclear imaging devices due to its electronic collimation capability.

8-1-2   Advantages of PET

Perhaps the greatest advantage of PET over other nuclear imaging systems is electronic collimation, which virtually allows each detector to see the entire object. The sensitivity (photon collection capability) gain is greater than that of the SPECT because of the increased detection solid angle resulting from the electronic collimation. Two other distinct advantages of PET, enabled by electronic collimation, are the uniformity of resolution and sensitivity over the entire object. The uniform sensitivity stems from the fact that the combined attenuation factor of annihilation photon detections by a detector pair is the same along the strip or column defined by a detector pair regardless of the position of the annihilation. This allows us to accurately compensate the attenuation suffered within the object. This is again an advantage of PET over SPECT.

Another advantage of PET over other nuclear imaging systems is the physiological aspect of the many available positron-emitting radionuclides, which are usually radionuclides of low atomic number. Among these radionuclides, ^{11}C, ^{13}N, ^{15}O, and ^{18}F are the most often used radionuclides in PET, and they have a strong physiological affinity to the human body. These nuclides also have short physical half-lives (^{11}C = 20.34 min, ^{13}N = 9.96 min, ^{15}O = 2.05 min, ^{18}F = 110 min), so they facilitate effective imaging with minimal dosages to the patient (see Table 8-1). It should be noted that since ^{11}C, ^{13}N, and ^{15}O are the three major components of the molecules in living matter, these radionuclides are closely related to the metabolic processes in human physiology.

8-2 PHYSICAL FACTORS AFFECTING SYSTEM PERFORMANCE

8-2-1 System Geometry

Later, when we discuss system development, we will explain more fully how the PET system has evolved from a planar shape to a spherical shape. Since the development of X-ray CT, influenced by the tomographic concept, various PET systems have been developed. The first of its kind to be introduced was the PETT-I (positron emission transaxial tomography). This system employed a hexagonal shape with which both translational linear and rotational scannings could be conducted. Circular system development subsequently allowed both linear and angular scannings without translational motion. Improved sensitivity and multilayer imaging could be achieved by using multiple rings in a cylindrical arrangement or spherical arrangement

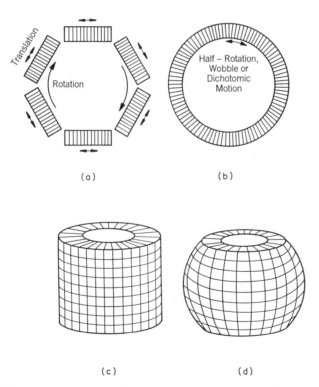

(a)   (b)

(c)   (d)

Figure 8-3   (a) Hexagonal geometry with translational and rotational motions; (b) circular ring geometry. In this scheme the entire ring could be stationary or move along the circular path or wobble. (c) Multilayer cylindrical system which consists of multiples of ring detector arrays; (d) multilayer spherical system which consists of multiples of ring detector arrays. The spherical system with collimators focused onto the center maximizes the sensitivity at the center.

with trunctions at both ends of the sphere. Simplified illustration of the several PET systems are shown in Fig. 8-3.

8-2-2 Detectors [10, 11, 12]

The spatial resolution of the positron camera depends on the width of the detection channel and the sampling interval. The former sets the resolution limit obtainable with the system provided that the sampling requirement or the Nyquist sampling criterion is met. The detection channel can be characterized by the detector aperture or response function and can be determined through simple ray tracing. For a detector pair the resolution function can be represented by a triangular response curve with a fwhm approximately equal to half of the detector's width. The aperture function approaching the detector becomes gradually trapezoidal and ultimately becomes rectangular at a position immediately adjacent to the detector face (for a rectangular detector).

In most PET instruments a standard gamma ray detector design is chosen for the detector assembly. It consists of a PMT and a scintillation crystal coupled together. Several scintillation crystals used in the past are being recommended for PET design. In the early 1970s NaI(T1) was the most commonly used scintillation detector for PET, even though it was comparatively inefficient in high-energy 511 keV photon detection. Recent developments in scintillation detectors include BGO (bismuth germanate), which has led to a substantial improvement in detection efficiency compared with existing scintillators such as NaI(T1) [10]. The nonhygroscopic nature of BGO crystal facilitates a more compact detector assembly, or better packing of even narrower crystals in an array, thereby further improving overall sensitivity as well as system resolution. Most of the recent advances in high-resolution PET systems were made possible by the use of detectors made of a narrow slabs (width) of BGO, some of them as narrow as 4–5 mm

Table 8-2 Properties of the typical detector materials used in positron emission tomographs

Detector Material	NaI(TI)	BGO	CsF	BaF$_2$
Density (g/cm^3)	3.67	7.13	4.64	4.89
Linear attenuation coefficient at 511 keV (cm^{-1})	0.34	0.92	0.44	4.47
Scintillation decay time (nsec)	250	300	5	0.8
Emission wavelength (nm)	410	480	390	225
Energy resolution in fwhm at 511 keV (%)	> 7	> 10	23	13

enabling a resolution of 2–3 mm fwhm. It should be cautioned, however, that a narrow width detector that is less than a certain critical size or width will reduce detection efficiency drastically [11].

Two other crystals have recently been considered for PET applications, specifically CsF and BaF$_2$, both of which have good timing characteristics. These crystals provide excellent time resolution, thereby making it possible to reduce the coincident time window and perhaps even to adopt time-of-flight (TOF) tomography [12]. The physical properties of the most common detector materials mentioned here are listed in Table 8-2.

8-2-3   Sampling [13, 14, 15]

Since narrow detector width will reduce detection efficiency and will increase intercrystal scatter and penetration, thereby degrading the resolution, the detector widths are usually kept at a certain size, which of course limits both the resolution and the sampling. For a given detector size or width, maximum resolution in linear sampling can be achieved by satisfying the Nyquist sampling criterion; that is, the sampling distance in linear sampling must be less than half the desired spatial resolution. This sampling distance in a ring PET design is therefore one-fourth of the detector width. In addition there is the angular sampling requirement to be satisfied. As is intuitively clear, the angular sampling requirement can easily be met in the circular ring PET design, while the linear sampling requires some additional considerations [5].

In the polygonal geometry, such as the hexagonal PET system developed in the early days, the desired linear sampling can easily be achieved by introducing translational motions [Fig. 8-4 (a)]. In the circular ring system, however, improving the linear sampling has been difficult due to the fixed detector array. Several sampling schemes have been developed and proposed to overcome this inherent difficulty. For example, wobbling motion [13] has been proposed and widely used [Fig. 8-4 (b)]. More recently, a few new sampling schemes suitable for the circular ring system have also been developed, such as dichotomic sampling [14] [Fig. 8-4 (c)].

Although the wobbling scheme is one of the most commonly used sampling scheme in the circular ring systems, it is generally believed that the samples obtained through this method are usually neither uniform nor equally spaced. To obtain more uniform and equally spaced samples with minimal redundancy for a given number of motions, alternatives such as the dichotomic sampling or its variations appear to be useful [see Fig. 8-4 (c)]. The dichotomic scheme employs two half rings (from which the term "dichotomic" is derived) that are rotated back and forth to obtain finely sampled parallel or fan data sets. By this method any desired sampling can be obtained with a minimal number of scan stops. Another method to avoid insufficient linear sampling in circular ring PET was the "positology" proposed by Tanaka [15].

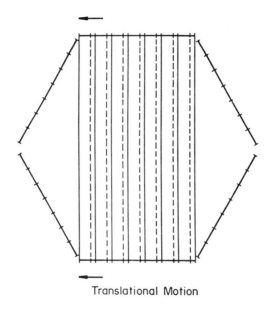

Translational Motion

(a)

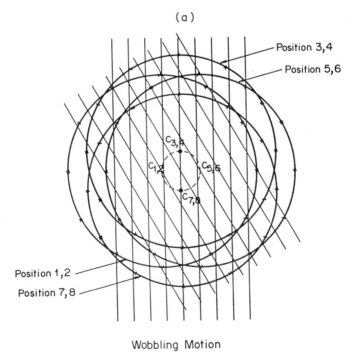

Wobbling Motion

(b)

Figure 8-4 Sampling motions. (a) Hexagonal geometry with translational and rotational motions; (b) wobbling motion applied to circular ring systems. In this scheme the entire ring moves in a circular path (small track of circle shown at the ring center); this is 2-D motion. (c) Dichotomic sampling applied to circular ring system. In this scheme the ring is separated into two halves that move back and forth.

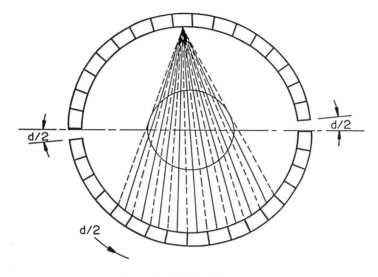

Dichotomic Motion (Rotation)

(c)

Figure 8-4 *(Continued)*

8-2-4 Sensitivity

Sensitivity in PET is defined as the capability of detecting the true coincidences (solid line in Fig. 8-1) with a given amount of radioactivity. Sensitivity has conventionally been measured with a phantom of a certain diameter (e.g., ~ 20 cm) filled with a uniform activity concentration ρ, where ρ is usually given in units of $\mu\text{Ci}/\text{cm}^3$ ($1\mu\text{Ci} = 37{,}000$ disintegrations/sec). By considering several factors—including the activity in the field of view, the self-attenuation of gamma rays within the phantom, the solid angle subtended by the detector array, and the detection efficiency of the array—an empirical formula of the true coincidence counts that represents one of the sensitivity measures of a PET system is derived and given by

$$C_T = \frac{k\rho\alpha\eta^2 h^2 d^2}{D} \qquad \left(\frac{\text{counts}}{\text{sec}} \cdot \frac{\mu\text{Ci}}{\text{cm}^3}\right) \qquad (8\text{-}1)$$

where k is a constant equivalent to 14,500, α is the probability of neither annihilation photon scattering within the object volume, η is the detector efficiency (including the detector packing ratio) and h, d, and D are the thickness of the slice to be imaged, the diameter of the phantom, and the ring or system diameter, respectively, measured in centimeters.

If the system contains two or more detector rings, then coincidences can be measured between the detectors in the different rings (coincidences between the planes that are more or less perpendicular to the axis) to form an intermediate cross-slice imaging plane. Sensitivity is higher in the cross-slice plane due to the fact that each cross-slice plane involves twice as many detectors as opposed to the slice planes without interlayer crossing. This idea can be extended to cross plane imaging in the multilayer system of 3 or more rings. The latter eventually will lead to what is known "septaless" volume imaging.

8-2-5   Random (or Accidental) Coincidences

One of the sources of background noise in PET images is random or accidental coincidences resulting when two unrelated annihilation photons are emitted from two independent sources and are detected within the time window of the coincidence resolving time τ (e.g., dashed lines in Fig. 8-1). Random coincidences produce a background haze over the field of view in the reconstructed image and are therefore highly undesirable.

For a uniform distribution of activity, a formula for the random count rate per ring has been established:

$$C_R = \tau f C_s^2 \qquad \left(\frac{\text{counts}}{\text{sec}} \cdot \frac{\mu\text{Ci}}{\text{cm}^3} \right) \qquad (8\text{-}2)$$

where C_s is the single count rate for the entire ring, τ is the coincidence resolving time, and f represents the coincidence fraction of a given phantom (which is the ratio of the number of detectors in a fan to the total number of detectors in the ring, each of which is in coincidence with any one of the detectors on the opposite side). The value of f for a ring system is given by

$$f = \left(\frac{2}{\pi} \right) \sin^{-1} \left(\frac{d}{D} \right) \qquad (8\text{-}3)$$

where d and D are the object diameter and system diameter, respectively.

Since both the single and true coincidence rates are proportional to the amount of activity, it is apparent from Eq. (8-2) that the random coincidence rate is proportional to the square of the single count rate. For the reduction of the random coincidences, it is important to minimize the single counts or activity in the object as well as the coincidence resolving time. Since single counts can arise from both in-slice as well as out-of-slice annihilation events, they can be suppressed by limiting the detection channels by some form of slice collimation. It is common practice to reduce out-of-slice annihilation events by using annular-shaped interdetector ring collimators or septa (more detailed discussions will be given in the following sections). The low-energy threshold can also be raised so that the maximum rejection of scattered single events can be achieved.

Random coincidences can be corrected by software or postprocessing. Two simple procedures for doing so are the use of a delayed coincidence measurement with the same coincidence time window and the other is the estimation (the random coincidences) by use of the single count rate of Eq. (8-2). By the same token, random coincidences can be reduced by reducing the activity, that is, reducing the single count rate.

8-2-6 Scatter Coincidences

Scatter coincidences occur when one or both annihilation photons are scatter, yet they are detected in coincidence because the scattered photon energy is higher than the preset threshold energy (broken line in Fig. 8-1). This scatter coincidence tends to give incorrect positional information, thus broadening the line spread function with a long tail. As will be discussed, the scatter coincidences are usually more difficult to correct than the random coincidences. Various attempts to reduce the scatter coincidences have had only limited success.

Since the scatter coincidences are prompt in time, just like true coincidences, and especially since the small angle scatterings are difficult to differentiate by energy from those of the unscattered photons, they cannot be as easily reduced or eliminated as random coincidences. Because of their prompt nature, trying to differentiate between scatter and true coincidence simply by reducing the time window is not effective. In addition the energy losses in small angle scatters are so small that it is also difficult to differentiate between them through energy windowing. In the multilayer ring system, scatter can be eliminated with tighter interslice collimation; nevertheless, some loss of observable volume or some reduction in the number of interdetector ring slices will occur.

8-2-7 Attenuation Correction

The attenuation correction is one of the most important as well as advantageous characteristics of the PET scanner compared to other imaging modes such as SPECT. Various correction schemes have been developed in the past. One of the simplest and crudest for correcting the attenuation is the use of geometrical shapes—namely finding the edge contours and then using the contour information to find the attenuation length of each projection or line integral for the subsequent correction. In this method attenuation coefficients are customarily assumed to be constant within the boundary. A more accurate method is to use the transmission scan information obtained through an external positron source surrounding the patient. This technique often suffers from statistical noise, thereby making the attenuation correction less effective unless a statistically sufficient amount of data are taken. The correction can also be made by using X-ray CT data in a procedure similar to that of the external positron source such as the ring source, but one should be aware that the attenuation coefficients obtained are different from those of 511 keV photons.

8-3 COMPUTATIONAL MODELS OF THE TRUE, SCATTER, AND RANDOM COINCIDENCES [16]

In this section numerical analyses of the true, scatter, and random counts are given to quantitatively estimate those values under different circumstances. Although the present model uses the spherical detection scheme of a multilayer PET, the formulas and the basic concept can easily be reduced to single layer and multilayer systems of different forms, such as the cylindrical multilayer system.

8-3-1 True Coincidences

The true coincidence is the only information useful for image reconstruction unless more sophisticated scatter ray tracing techniques or other exotic techniques are employed. Theoretically true coincidence is a function of a number of parameters—namely source volume, activity intensity, source medium, and physical instrumentation—while scatter and random coincidences are more dependent on the collimator or septum structure, activity volume, source medium, source intensity, and coincidence circuit timing window, for example. Computational models of true coincidences will be formulated, first for the general case and then for the specific cases of both spherical and cylindrical geometries. The latter will be computed to show the advantages of the spherical geometry over the cylindrical shape in limited volume imaging, especially for high-resolution mode imaging where the system detection efficiency is of prime importance.

Let the true coincidence count rate between two arbitrarily selected layers L_1 and L_2 be denoted as $C_T(L_1, L_2)$ which is given by (see Fig. 8-5)

$$C_T(L_1, L_2) = m_f \int_{-R_{obj}}^{R_{obj}} dc_T(L_1, L_2; x) \qquad (8\text{-}4)$$

where m_f is a multiplication factor depending on the condition of the two layers (i.e., whether they are in-plane or cross-plane), R_{obj} is the radius of the object under investigation, and dc_T is the fractional true coincidence.

More specifically, the fractional true coincidence count rate $dc_T(\cdot)$ is the true coincidence arising from the source volume between L_1 and L_2 at x and is given by

$$dc_T(L_1, L_2; x) = \psi a A_{tt} G \eta^2 p^2 \, dV_{sos} \qquad (8\text{-}5)$$

where ψa is the disintegration rate per unit volume, A_{tt} is the attenuation

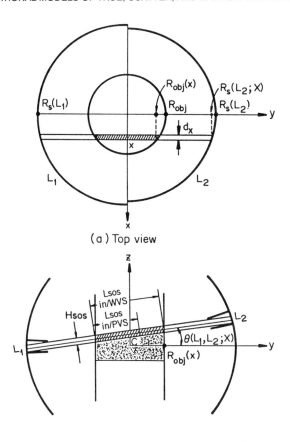

(a) Top view

(b) Cross section

Figure 8-5   Illustration of true coincidence events between arbitrary layers L_1 and L_2.

factor, G is the geometrical efficiency, ηp is the detection efficiency for incident photons determined by the detector efficiency η and the packing ratio p, and dV_{sos} denotes an infinitesimally small source volume.

As is shown in Fig. 8-5(a), the calculation is now simplified to the simple integration of a part of a plane along x, even in the case of a cross-plane, as indicated in the figure. For the numerical calculation dV_{sos} is given as

$$dV_{\text{sos}} = H_{\text{sos}} L_{\text{sos}} \, dx \qquad (8\text{-}6)$$

where H_{sos} and L_{sos} are the values geometrically defined in Fig. 8-5(b) and will vary as a function of the inclination of the source volume element defined by L_1 and L_2 and the length of the annular collimators, and dx is the width of the source volume element. The source volume height H_{sos} can be calculated by first projecting the edge points of the related annular collimators in the ray (or θ) direction and finding the difference between the minimum upper point and the maximum lower point.

L_{sos} is the length of the source volume element which differs for the two cases; one for the partial volume sensitivity (PVS) calculation and the other for the whole volume sensitivity (WVS) calculation. L_{sos} for the WVS calculation is given as

$$L_{sos} = \frac{2R_{obj}(x)}{\cos \theta(L_1, L_2; x)} \tag{8-7}$$

where $R_{obj}(x) = \sqrt{R_{obj}^2 - x^2}$, and $\theta(L_1, L_2; x)$ is the angle between the horizontal plane and the volume element. $\theta(L_1, L_2; x)$ is given by

$$\theta(L_1, L_2; x) = \tan^{-1}\left\{\frac{|Z(L_1) - Z(L_2)|}{R_s(L_1; x) + R_s(L_2; x)}\right\} \tag{8-8}$$

where $R_s(L_i, x) = \sqrt{R_s^2(L_i) - x^2}$, and $R_s(L_i)$ and $Z(L_i)$ are the radius and z position of the layer L_i, respectively, as indicated in Fig. 8-5(a). L_{sos} for the PVS case can also be calculated based on Eq. (8-7) and an additional examination of the length in the predefined partial volume as indicated in Fig. 8-5(b).

It should be noted, however, that the attenuation factor A_{tt} used in Eq. (8-5) is equal for both the PVS and WVS cases and is given by a simple exponential; that is, $A_{tt} = \exp(-\mu l_{A_{tt}})$, where $l_{A_{tt}} = L_{sos}$ in Eq. (8-7). The geometrical efficiency denoted by G is the polar angle dependent geometrical reduction factor which is a maximum at $\theta = 0$ (i.e., the maximum for the horizontal plane), and elsewhere G is defined as

$$G = \frac{1}{2}\xi_T\left[\frac{1}{2}\cos \theta(L_1, L_2; x)\right] \tag{8-9}$$

where $\xi_T/2$ is the polar acceptance angle seen from the center of the source volume element and $(\cos \theta)/2$ is a reduction factor arising from the rotation transform.

Equation (8-4) can now be rewritten as

$$C_T(L_1, L_2) = \frac{m_f}{2}\int_0^{R_{obj}} \psi a \eta^2 p^2 \exp(-\mu l_{A_{tt}}) H_{sos}\xi_T \cos \theta(L_1, L_2; x) L_{sos} \, dx \tag{8-10}$$

Equation (8-10) can be used for both the PVS and WVS cases and can be further simplified to

$$C_T(L_1, L_2) = \frac{K_T}{2}\int_0^{R_{obj}} \exp(-\mu l_{A_{tt}}) G_1 \cos \theta(L_1, L_2; x) L_{sos} \, dx \tag{8-11}$$

where K_T is a constant (i.e., $K_T = m_f \psi a \eta^2 p^2$) that is determined by the detector system and the activity distribution, and G_1 is another geometrical factor that is entirely dependent upon the length of the annular collimator and is defined as

$$G_1 = H_{\text{sos}} \xi_T \qquad (8\text{-}12)$$

For the WVS case, Eq. (8-11) can be further simplified, using Eq. (8-7), to

$$C_T(L_1, L_2) = K_T \int_0^{R_{\text{obj}}} \exp(-\mu l_{A_{tt}}) G_1 R_{\text{obj}}(x)\, dx \qquad (8\text{-}13)$$

8-3-2 Scatter Coincidences (Single Scatter)

In a positron tomography system, scatter coincidences can also occur and produce noise or bias in the reconstructed image. In such a case it is assumed that one of the annihilation gamma photons suffers scattering while the other is unscattered and detected, resulting in a scatter coincidence that behaves like a true coincidence. The promptness of scatter coincidences makes their discrimination from the true events inherently difficult, and they can be prevented only by physical collimation such as annular collimators or septa. Since two-photon scatter and double-scatter coincidences are rare, it is sufficient to calculate only one-photon scatter or single-scatter coincidences to demonstrate the effect of scatter and compare the relative counts of single-scatter coincidences with the true ones.

Let us denote the single-scatter coincidence count rate between two arbitrary layers L_1 and L_2 as

$$C_{SC1}(L_1, \tilde{L}_2) = \int_V c_{SC1}(L_1, \tilde{L}_2; x, y, z)\, dV \qquad (8\text{-}14)$$

where V is the volume that contributes to the single-scatter coincidence count $C_{SC1}(L_1, \tilde{L}_2)$, $c_{SC1}(L_1, \tilde{L}_2; x, y, z)$ is the single-scatter coincidence count resulting from a volume element $dV = dx\,dy\,dz$ positioned at (x, y, z), and $\tilde{L}_2$ (or $\tilde{L}_1$) denotes the layer where scattered photons are detected. The single scatter coincidence count $c_{SC1}(L, \tilde{L}_2; x, y, z)$ arising from a volume element dV can be given by combining the probability functions which are related to the two annihilation photons ν_1 and ν_2' as

$$c_{SC1}(L_1, \tilde{L}_2; x, y, z) = \psi a \left[\frac{1}{2} \cos \theta(L_1; x, y, z) \right] P_{\nu_1} P_{\nu_2'} \qquad (8\text{-}15)$$

where P_{ν_1} and $P_{\nu_2'}$ are the probabilities of detecting the unscattered photon ν_1 in layer L_1 and the scattered photon ν_2' in layer L_2, respectively (see Fig. 8-6), and angle $\theta(L_1; x, y, z)$ is the polar angle between the direction of the unscattered photon ν_1 and the direction of the layer L_1. This angle is

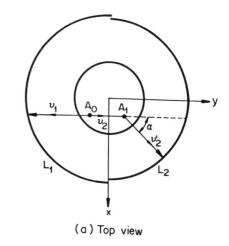

(a) Top view

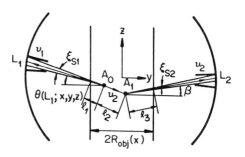

(b) Cross section

$A_0 = (x, y, z)$; annihilation position

$A_1 = (x_1, y_1, z_1)$; scatter position

Figure 8-6 Diagram of single-scatter coincidence events. For the photons annihilated at point A_0, one is detected by layer L_1 without scatter and the other is detected by layer L_2 with single scatter at A_1.

calculated similarly to the one defined previously and is given by

$$\theta(L_1; x, y, z) = \tan^{-1}\left[\frac{|z - Z(L_1)|}{y + R_s(L_1; x)}\right] \tag{8-16}$$

The detection probabilities of the two photons v_1 and v_2' are

$$P_{v_1} = \exp(-\mu l_1)\xi_{S1}\eta p, \tag{8-17}$$

and

$$P_{v_2'} = \int_y^{R_{obj}(x)} \exp(-\mu l_2) P_s P_{as} \, dy_1 \tag{8-18}$$

where $l_1 = [R_{obj}(x) + y]/\cos \theta(L_1; x, y, z)$ is the distance traveled by the unscattered photon ν_1 in the object, ξ_{S1} is the polar acceptance angle of the unscattered photon ν_1 relative to layer L_1, $l_2 = (y_1 - y)/\cos \theta(L_1; x, y, z)$ is the distance between the source point $A_0(x, y, z)$ and the scatter point $A_1(x_1, y_1, z_1)$, P_s is the probability of scatter per unit length, and P_{as} is the detection probability of the scattered photon ν'_2 by layer L_2. The probabilities P_s and P_{as} are

$$P_s = \frac{\mu}{\cos \theta(L_1; x, y, z)} \tag{8-19}$$

and

$$P_{as} = \int_{-\alpha_m}^{\alpha_m} d\alpha \exp(-\mu l_3) g_f \xi_{S2} \eta_1 p \cos \beta \tag{8-20}$$

where α_m is the maximum allowed scatter angle directed toward the layer L_2 direction which is determined by the low-energy setting of the discriminator, $\exp(-\mu_1 l_3)$ represents the probability of no scatter from the scatter point $A_1(x_1, y_1, z_1)$ to the object boundary, l_3 is the attenuation length of the scattered photon ν'_2, g_f is the normalized Klein-Nishina formula, ξ_{S2} is the polar acceptance angle of the scattered photon ν'_2 ($\xi_{S2} \cos \beta \, d\alpha$ represents an infinitesimal detection solid angle), and $\eta'p$ is the detection efficiency of the scattered photon ν'_2. More specifically, l_3 is given by

$$l_3 = \frac{-x_1 \sin \alpha - y_1 \cos \alpha + \sqrt{R_{obj}^2 - (x_1 \cos \alpha - y_1 \sin \alpha)^2}}{\cos \beta} \tag{8-21}$$

In conjunction with l_3, angles related to the scattered photon ν'_2 are defined and denoted as α and β together with the photon scatter angle ζ, where α is the span angle along the layer L_2 and β is the polar angle between the direction of the scattered photon and the horizontal plane. The polar angle β and the Klein-Nishina formula used in the calculation are given by

$$\beta = \tan^{-1} \left[\frac{|z_1 - Z(L_2)|}{x_1 \sin \alpha + y_1 \cos \alpha - \sqrt{R_s^2(L_2) - (x_1 \cos \alpha - y_1 \sin \alpha)^2}} \right] \tag{8-22}$$

and

$$g_f = \frac{[1 + \gamma(1 - \cos \zeta)](1 + \cos \zeta) + \gamma^2(1 - \cos \zeta)^2}{\lambda_0(\gamma)[1 + \gamma(1 - \cos \zeta)]^3} \tag{8-23}$$

where $\gamma = E_i/E_0$, $E_0 = 511$ keV, and $\lambda_0(\gamma)$ is the normalizing factor. The low-energy threshold E_{th} and the maximum allowed scatter angle α_m are related by

$$\alpha_m = \cos^{-1}\left[\frac{(2 - E_0/E_{th})}{\cos(\beta - \beta_0)}\right]$$ (8-24)

where $\beta_0 = \beta|_{\alpha=0}$. The single-scatter coincidence count rate given in Eq. (8-14) can now be rewritten as

$$C_{SC1}(L_1, \tilde{L}_2) = K_{SC1}\int_{-R_{obj}}^{R_{obj}} dx \int_{-R_{obj}(x)}^{R_{obj}(x)} dy \int_{-\infty}^{\infty} dz \int_{y}^{R_{obj}(x)} dy_1 \int_{-\alpha_m}^{\alpha_m} d\alpha \, I_{SC1}$$ (8-25)

where

$$K_{SC1} = \frac{1}{2}\psi a \mu \eta \eta_1 p^2$$ (8-26)

and

$$I_{SC1} = \xi_{S1}\xi_{S2} \cos \beta g_f \exp\left[-\mu(l_1 + l_2) - \mu l_3\right]$$ (8-27)

For the opposite case of Eq. (8-25), that is, $C_{SC1}(\tilde{L}_1, L_2)$, the single-scatter coincidence count rate where ν_1 is scattered and ν_2 unscattered can be calculated in a similar way. The total single-scattered coincidence between the two layers L_1 and L_2 is therefore given by

$$\begin{aligned}
C_{SC1}(\tilde{L}_1, \tilde{L}_2) &= m_f\left[C_{SC1}(L_1, \tilde{L}_2) + C_{SC1}(\tilde{L}_1, L_2)\right] \\
&\cong 2m_f C_{SC1}(L_1, \tilde{L}_2) \\
&\cong 2m_f C_{SC1}(\tilde{L}_1, L_2)
\end{aligned}$$ (8-28)

where m_f is a multiplication factor mentioned earlier [see Eq.(8-4)].

Although in theory it is possible to eliminate these scatter coincidences by energy discrimination, the energy spread of the detectors available today does not allow one to discriminate scatter coincidences from true coincidences, especially for the small-angle scatters. Annular interlayer collimators or septa for the multilayer ring or spherical PET system therefore should be designed to meet the scatter rejection capability while allowing maximum object volume coverage and sensitivity.

8-3-3 Random Coincidences

Another limiting factor in imaging with PET systems is the true to random-coincidence ratio resulting from the finite resolving time of the coincidence circuits, primarily due to the inherent timing uncertainty of the detectors. Estimation of random coincidences and eventual correction of those random coincidences are one of the most important topics in PET. Random coincidences may be estimated by actual observation, indirect measurement by time shift, or by using a predetermined coincidence resolving time together with the measured single count rates [5]. The latter is often adopted in complex PET systems in which single counts can be measured easily by time sampled count rates obtainable from each detector [8, 16].

The random coincidence count rate between two arbitrarily selected layers L_1 and L_2 is given by

$$C_R(L_1, L_2) = 2m_f \tau f C_{SG0}(L_1) C_{SG0}(L_2) \qquad (8\text{-}29)$$

where τ is the coincidence resolving time, $f = (2/\pi)\sin^{-1}(R_{\text{obj}}/R_s)$ represents the coincidence fan fraction which is the ratio of the number of detectors formed by a fan to the total number of detectors in a layer, and $C_{SG0}(L_1)$ and $C_{SG0}(L_2)$ are the unscattered single count rates of layers L_1 and L_2, respectively.

As is seen from Eq. (8-29), the random coincidence count rate can be reduced by either reducing the coincidence resolving time τ or the single count rate $C_{SG0}(L_i)$, or both. It should be noted, however, that the random count rate is proportional to the square of the single count rate. Random coincidence is therefore usually considered to be a minor problem in low count rate situations but it rapidly becomes a major source of noise with an increase in the single count rates or the source activity in the object.

Clearly, it is important to reduce the single counts as much as possible, such as by reducing the activity volume seen by the detectors through collimators. Collimators of annular shape are usually employed in a ring system to restrict the activity volume only to the slice seen by the detectors in a ring. In the conventional multilayer system, annular collimators or septa are also used between ring layers, primarily to reduce the volume seen by the detectors. These ring systems, where each is virtually an isolated ring, give images each of which is limited to the corresponding slice only. Although an annular collimator arrangement in a multilayer ring system ideally fulfills the reduction requirements of the random and scatter coincidences, it does not allow one to take advantage of the 4π radiation of photons in positron tomography, thereby essentially reducing the sensitivity by not utilizing all the available photons. To solve this problem, a spherical PET (S-PET) has been proposed [16]. In this scheme suitably sized annular collimators are all focused onto the center of the sphere,* thereby achieving nearly 4π detection while keeping random and scatter coincidences to a minimum.

The random count rate can be analyzed for various types of PET, namely spherical or cylindrical by calculating the single (unscattered only) count

---

*For low activity, collimators or septa can be eliminated alltogether.

rates. Subsequently true-to-random ratios for the spherical rather than cylindrical PET systems can be estimated. For simplicity assume that the scattered single count rate is relatively small so that the single count rate defined here represents only unscattered singles. Then the total single count rate detected by a layer L can be given by

$$C_{SG0}(L) = \int_V c_{SG0}(L; x, y, z) \, dV \qquad (8\text{-}30)$$

where $c_{SG0}(L; x, y, z)$ is the single count rate obtained by layer L originating from an activity volume element $dV = dx \, dy \, dz$ and is given by

$$c_{SG0}(L; x, y, z) = 2\psi a A'_{tt} G' \eta p \qquad (8\text{-}31)$$

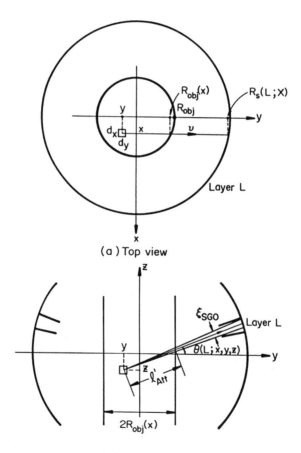

(a) Top view

(b) Cross section

Figure 8-7 Diagram of unscattered single events detected by layer L. Counts of singles are important for the calculation of the random coincidences.

In Eq. (8-31), A'_{tt} and G' are the attenuation coefficient and geometrical efficiency, respectively, and are given by (see also Fig. 8-7)

$$A'_{tt} = \exp(-\mu l'_{A_{tt}})$$ (8-32)

and

$$G' = \frac{1}{2} \cos \theta(L; x, y, z) \xi_{SG0}$$ (8-33)

The $\cos \theta(L; x, y, z)/2$ factor given in Eq. (8-33) is again the reduction factor arising from the rotation transform, and ξ_{SG0} is the polar acceptance angle as defined in Fig. 8-7 (b).

The total single count rate therefore can be obtained by integrating $c_{SG0}(L; x, y, z)$ over the entire volume seen by the detectors in a layer L. Equation (8-30) can be written as

$$C_{SG0}(L) = K_{SG0} \int_{-\infty}^{\infty} dz \int_{-R_{obj}}^{R_{obj}} dx \int_{-R_{obj}(x)}^{R_{obj}(x)} dy \exp(-\mu l'_{A_{tt}}) \xi_{SG0} \cos \theta(L; x, y, z)$$

(8-34)

where $K_{SG0} = 2\psi a \eta p$. The single count rate obtained by Eq. (8-34) can then be used for the calculation of the random coincidence count rate by using Eq. (8-29).

8-4 SOME DESIGN CONSIDERATIONS OF THE HIGH-RESOLUTION PET

8-4-1 Resolution and Sensitivity as a Function of Detector Size and System Geometry [17]

As we have already noted, design of high-resolution PET requires small or narrow-width detectors. With narrow-width detector arrays, however, the detection efficiency is reduced due to the escape of high-energy photons, both unscattered and scattered, to the outside of the detector volume or to the adjacent crystals. For narrow-width crystals spillage to adjacent crystals can be the major factor responsible for degrading resolution as well as sensitivity. An example of the sensitivity variation of a BGO crystal as a function of the size (i.e., the width of the crystal) is calculated for several different photon incident angles (incident angle relative to the normal to the detector face) and the results are shown in Fig. 8-8. Ultimately there exists a physical limit to the further development of a high-resolution system using narrow-width crystals. If the crystal width is narrow, annihilation photons can easily penetrate several adjacent crystal layers, especially when the incident angles are large. A partial remedy for the problem of obliquely incident

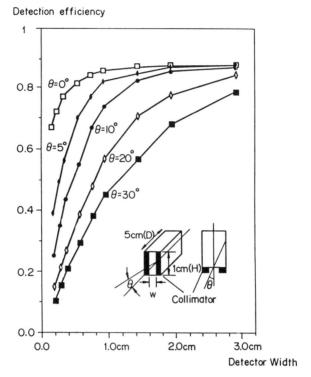

Figure 8-8 Detection efficiency of a single BGO crystal as a function of detector width w for several different photon incident angles.

photons is to enlarge the system ring diameter so that the incident angle of the annihilation photons relative to the detector face becomes less oblique. Although spillage to the adjacent detectors due to the scattered photons in the narrow-width crystal system still remains, an increase in the system diameter would ease the spillage problem arising from the obliquely incident photons. Consequently there appear to be two different approaches in PET system design to resolve the spillage and penetration problems of obliquely incident photons: (1) a system with a few large crystals with a small aperture collimation and small system diameter and (2) a system with a large number of narrow-width crystals with a large system diameter. In this context we define a critical angle θ_c that is the angle with which the incident 511 keV photons would pass through or penetrate to the next crystal no more than 20%. To be specific, we note that θ_c^l an θ_c^s are the critical angles for a large crystal and a small (narrow-width) crystal, respectively.

In the first case a small (narrow-width) crystal system with a large system diameter reduces the obliquity effect, thereby reducing the photon spillage. However, it will also reduce the solid angle of each unit detector, thereby reducing the sensitivity. The sensitivity loss of each unit detector, as well as the overall system sensitivity, can be demonstrated by a simple comparison of two extreme cases. As a first step, it is evident that the system diameter should be varied to meet the critical angle requirement; that is, the narrower the width of the crystal size, the larger is the system diameter. For example, in a 4-cm width BGO crystal system, which is considered to be a large crystal system (with a few large detectors with aperture collimation), the minimum system diameter that will satisfy the critical angle requirement is 26 cm. On the other hand, for a 5-mm BGO crystal system, which is considered to be a small or narrow-width crystal system, the ideal minimum system diameter to meet the critical angle requirement is 204.8 cm. However, to obtain a 2.5-mm fwhm intrinsic resolution with the large crystal system, a small-size collimating aperture [5 mm (W) × 10 mm (H)] should be used in the face of each crystal, resulting in a substantial loss of sensitivity.

The sensitivity improvement of the large crystal system, however, can be appreciated by increase of solid angle. Therefore, a simple comparison of the two systems would be of interest, namely, a large crystal detector system with small system diameter having aperature collimation (5 mm × 10mm) compared to a narrow-width crystal system with a large system diameter. In this idealized situation a unit detector solid angle improvement of a factor (Ω) of 62 is obtained for the large crystal system. If one includes the efficiency gain (ε^2) of 3.02 for each large crystal detector pair due to the detection volume increase, the unit detector pair sensitivity gain ($\varepsilon^2\Omega$) becomes as large as 187 compared with the narrow-width crystal. This large individual detector gain, however, will be counter balanced when compared to narrow width detector systems, since the overall system sensitivity is also related to the number of crystals, a semiquantitive calculation of the total system sensitivity as a function of crystal width is shown in Fig. 8-9. This calculation includes the sensitivity loss due to the system diameter increase based on the critical angle requirement. As can be seen in Fig. 8-9, a large sensitivity loss is observed when narrow crystals are used due to the loss in unit crystal detection efficiency. To illustrate the overall sensitivity more quantitatively, the system sensitivity is calculated by estimating the true coincident count per ring for a given activity in the object, which is given by

$$C_t = \kappa \eta^2 n_D n'_D \Omega \tag{8-35}$$

where κ is a constant which includes the source activity for a given phantom and attenuation, ε is the detection efficiency of a unit detector, n_D and n'_D are the total number of crystals and the number of crystals in a fan formed by the object or the region of interest, respectively, and Ω is the coincidence solid angle. Equation (8-35) can be used for a comparison of the narrow-width crystal system versus the large crystal system, by noting that

$$C_{t_i} = \kappa \eta_i^2 n_{D_i} n'_{D_i} \Omega_i, \qquad i = 1, 2 \tag{8-36}$$

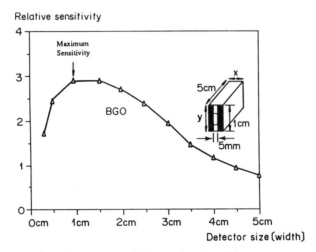

Figure 8-9 Overall system sensitivity as a function of detector width for BGO.

where 1 and 2 refer to the narrow-width crystal system and the large crystal system, respectively. Equation (8-36) further assumes that a fixed-size collimating aperture is placed at the front face of each detector for the large crystal system so that the coincident volume fractions seen by the unit crystal pair in the two systems are identical.

Let us calculate the sensitivity of each system and observe the results. First, the ratio of the geometrical factors S_1 (i.e., the ratio of the coincidence solid angles Ω_i for the unit detector of the two systems in the above examples) can be given by

$$S_1 = \frac{a/R_{s_1}^2}{a/R_{s_2}^2} = \frac{R_{s_2}^2}{R_{s_1}^2} \tag{8-37}$$

where a is the detector surface area, and R_{s_1} and R_{s_2} are the system radii of the narrow-width crystal and large crystal systems, respectively. Note that the detector surface area a for the large crystal system is the area exposed to annihilation photons through the collimating aperature. It is obvious that S_1 greatly favors large crystal systems, as far as individual detectors are concerned. Second, the other factor influencing the overall sensitivity is the fan fraction of the systems. This fraction involves the number of detectors in each fan and is given by

$$S_2 = \frac{n_{D_1} n'_{D_1}}{n_{D_2} n'_{D_2}} \cong \frac{n_{D_1}^2 \tan^{-1}(R_{o_1}/R_{s_1})}{n_{D_2}^2 \tan^{-1}(R_{o_2}/R_{s_2})} \Bigg|_{R_{o_1} = R_{o_2}} \tag{8-38}$$

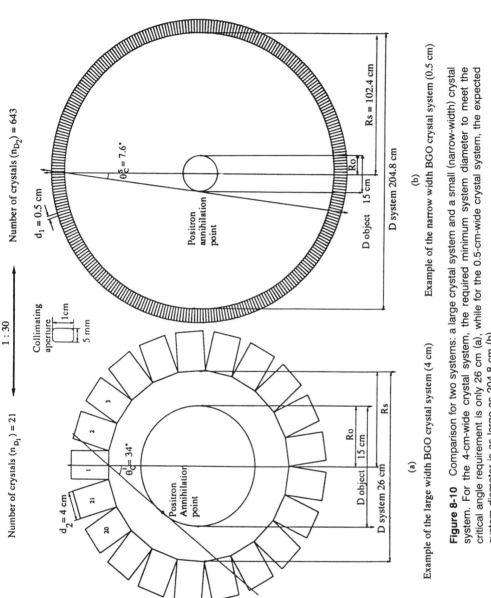

Number of crystals $(n_{D_1}) = 21$ 1 : 30   Number of crystals $(n_{D_2}) = 643$

$d_1 = 0.5$ cm

Collimating aperture

1 cm

5 mm

$\theta_c^s = 7.6°$

Positron annihilation point

$R_s = 102.4$ cm

R_0

D object 15 cm

D system 204.8 cm

(b)

Example of the narrow width BGO crystal system (0.5 cm)

$d_2 = 4$ cm

$\theta_c^l = 34°$

Positron Annihilation point

R_0

R_s

D object 15 cm

D system 26 cm

(a)

Example of the large width BGO crystal system (4 cm)

Figure 8-10 Comparison for two systems: a large crystal system and a small (narrow-width) crystal system. For the 4-cm-wide crystal system, the required minimum system diameter to meet the critical angle requirement is only 26 cm (a), while for the 0.5-cm-wide crystal system, the expected system diameter is as large as 204.8 cm (b).

225

where R_{o_1} and R_{o_2} are the radii of the objects for both the narrow-width and the large crystal systems and should be identical (i.e., $R_{o_1} = R_{o_2}$). For example, S_2 is found to be on the order of 100 in favor of the narrow-width crystal system ($w = 0.5$ cm). This large S_2 is naturally an important advantage for the narrow-width crystal system and demonstrates a very serious sensitivity loss for the large crystal system mainly resulting from the aperture collimation. Third, the narrow-width crystal system has a substantial disadvantage compared to the large crystal system in the individual detection efficiency. The ratio of the coincidence detection efficiency per detector pair can be given as

$$S_3 = \frac{\eta_1^2}{\eta_2^2} \qquad (8\text{-}39)$$

where η_1 and η_2 denote the individual detection efficiencies of a narrow-width crystal and a large crystal, respectively. The overall sensitivity ratio of the two systems therefore is

$$S = S_1 S_2 S_3. \qquad (8\text{-}40)$$

As seen from Fig. 8-9, the overall system sensitivity S, the ratio of the two systems, becomes a maximum for BGO when the detector size is in the range of 1 to 2 cm, and S approaches unity. This is an important result, since it is generally believed that the sensitivity loss of the large crystal system with a small collimating aperture will be so large that the total system sensitivity of the large crystal system will be smaller than that of the narrow-width crystal system with a large number of detectors. Considering the sensitivity gains of the large crystal system over that of narrow width crystal system discussed above and the scattered photon penetrations that would further degrade the resolution in the case of a narrow-width crystal system, a large detector system has an advantage for very high-resolution imaging of small objects such as brain imaging. In addition, a large-width crystal is again favored over a small crystal due to the small angular uncertainty effect associated with the small diameter of the large crystal system [see Fig 8-2(a)].

For a high-resolution PET system, photon spillage should be as small as possible so that the resolution is determined solely by the detector intrinsic resolution and not by other effects, such as the intercrystal penetration, especially due to obliquely incident photons. In Fig. 8-10 an illustrative comparison of the two systems is given, namely a large crystal system with relatively few crystals compared to a narrow-width crystal system with a large number of crystals.

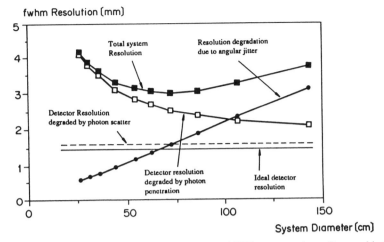

Figure 8-11 Resolution limits of a narrow-width crystal PET system using a 3-mm-wide BGO crystal detector array.

8-4-2 Resolution Limits of the Narrow-Width Crystal Detector Array

As discussed earlier, resolution degradation due to intercrystal penetration affects both the resolution and sensitivity in a narrow-width crystal system. These effects are more pronounced when the system diameter is made small. The overall resolution as a function of system diameter for a narrow-width crystal system using a 3-mm width BGO crystal array is plotted in Fig. 8-11. It is interesting to note that the detector resolution degraded by photon scatter is relatively small in BGO, but the resolution degradation due to the intercrystal penetration appears large, especially when the system diameter is small. It is therefore important to limit the penetration effect, especially for very high resolution imaging aiming for better than 2- to 2.5-mm fwhm resolution using narrow-width crystals. The alternative technique to prevent resolution degradation due to intercrystal penetration is the larger crystal approach. To further elaborate on this issue, computer simulation results for the two systems with the same system diameter (25-cm diameter) are shown in Fig. 8-12. As expected, the resolution degradation for the narrow-width crystal system is substantial. For example, resolution elements as large as 5-mm diameter spots are not resolved with the narrow-width crystal system. In contrast, the large crystal system resolves all the resolution elements well down to the 2-mm diameter circles with uniform sensitivity. These comparisons obviously suggest an alternative design criteria for high-resolution PET design in conjunction with the sensitivity issue, especially for a small ring diameter system such as the brain PET.

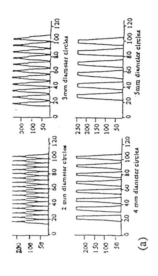

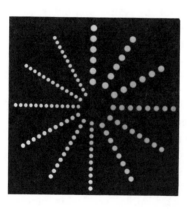

(a)

Figure 8-12 (a) A computer-generated resolution phantom and its cut view resolutions. The diameter of the phantom is 15 cm with groups of circular hot spots having spot diameters of 2, 3, 4, and 5 mm, respectively, with the same separation distances, 2, 3, 4, and 5 mm, respectively. (b) The resolution response of the above phantom for a PET system using a narrow-width crystal array ($3 \times 10 \times 50$ mm BGO) with a system diameter of 25 cm. (c) The resolution response of the above phantom for a PET system using large crystal ($2 \times 2 \times 5$ cm BGO) with the same system diameter ($D = 25$ cm).

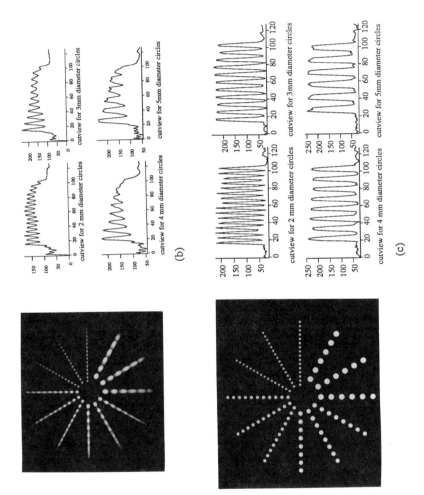

(b)

(c)

Figure 8-12 (Continued).

229

8-5 VARIOUS POSITRON EMISSION TOMOGRAPHIC SYSTEMS

There have been continuous efforts to develop PET imaging systems since the early 1950s. Some notable examples include the two NaI detector system developed in the early 1950s, the 32 discrete NaI(T1) detector systems developed in 1962, and the PC-I with two banks of detectors (127 detectors per bank) developed at Massachusetts General Hospital (MGH) in 1972. Although these systems can be utilized for tomographic imaging, they remained quasi-tomographic machines until the introduction of the X-ray CT in 1972.

The first two tomographic systems developed following the introduction of Hounsfield's X-ray CT were the PETT (positron emission transaxial tomography) I-III series designed by a Washington University group [3, 4, 6] and CRTAPC (circular ring trans-axial positron camera) designed by a group at UCLA [5]. Another circular ring system was developed later by a group at UC Berkeley [7]. In the PETT design, a hexagonal detector array was employed, and both translational and rotational motions were utilized for sampling, while the CRTAPC remained virtually stationary. Following these developments, PET instruments have rapidly progressed through the development of various new detectors and geometries. For example, system geometry has evolved from planar to hexagonal type, from hexagonal to circular ring type, from single ring to multiple ring, and so on. Detector materials have evolved from NaI(T1) to BGO, CsF, and BaF_2. The time-of-flight technique has also been introduced recently although with only marginal success [12].

It is most interesting to observe how the system geometry has evolved in the last several decades. The system geometry (the arrangement of detector arrays) is the most basic design choice because it determines fundamental system performance. The system geometries can be categorized into three basic types: planar, polygonal, and circular ring. To cover the imaging volume in the axial direction, multiple ring systems have been proposed in which several rings are stacked upon one another. They provide high total sensitivity and offer $2N - 1$ (N is the number of rings) image slices simultaneously when the annular collimators or interring septa are used.

The recent trend appears to be toward more generalized circular ring types of various forms. The advantages of the circular ring geometry are uniformity, high sensitivity due to a high packing fraction, and high angular sampling capability or near-stationary characteristic of the system. With small-size detectors the requirement for angular as well as linear sampling can easily be met, thereby allowing systems to remain stationary if needed. Many present systems do not require any rotation or movement for improving angular sampling. However, linear sampling has been a limiting factor in the circular ring system. Various solutions to this problem have also been suggested, as described in the previous section. It is also worth noting that more recent trends are in the direction of volume imaging, either through a cylindrical multilayer ring type or through a spherical concept without inter-slice annular collimators or septa.

8-5-1   Planar System [1, 2]

The planar type consists of two detector planes (made of either discrete crystal arrays or position sensitive devices, such as the Anger camera or multiwire proportional chambers (MWPC)) facing each other. A set of projection data can be obtained by rotating the dual planes around the patient, from which a series of image slices covering a sufficient axial volume can be reconstructed. A disadvantage of this type is the requirement for angular rotation.

MGH systems (PC-I, PC-II) by Brownell et al. [1, 2] and their commercial versions (TCC 4200) fall into the category of discrete crystal arrays.

8-5-2   Polygonal System [3, 4, 6]

Systems such as PETT III and PETT IV by Ter-Pogossian [3, 6] and ECAT and NeuroECAT by Phelps et al. [4] fall into this category. With the exception of the octagonal-shaped NeuroECAT, the other three are hexagonal. In this type of system, coincidence detection channels are formed between those banks opposing each other so that efficiency is usually limited, particularly toward the periphery of the image. An advantageous feature of the hexagonal system is the relatively simple translational and rotational sampling motions which easily satisfy the requirements of uniform linear and angular samplings.

8-5-3   Circular Ring and Cylindrical Systems [5, 7, 8, 9]

A natural extension of the polygonal PET system is the circular ring geometry which provides uniformity as well as natural symmetry. The first circular ring PET system was conceived and developed by Cho et al. at UCLA in 1975. Various other circular ring systems have been developed subsequently at Berkeley [9], Stockholm [13], and Montreal [11], and by various commercial firms. Some of the problems associated with insufficient linear sampling associated with ring systems have been resolved by incorporating new sampling schemes, such as the wobbling and the dichotomic sampling schemes [20]. A natural extension of the ring system was the multilayer cylindrical system developed, for instance, by CTI (Computer Tomography Inc.) [18] and the spherical system by Columbia University [16, 19].

8-5-4   Spherical-PET System [16, 19]

To increase the overall sensitivity and for direct volume imaging, a spherical shape for the PET system appears to be the natural choice. The first extensive spherical-PET (S-PET) design and preliminary study were carried out at Columbia University in the early 1980s and the design was initially intended for high-resolution imaging, namely a resolution of ~3 mm fwhm. To support this high resolution, it is imperative to maximize system sensitivity without impairing the true-to-random as well as true-to-scatter coincidence ratios. For this purpose a spherical geometry requires slice collimators focused onto the system center and the use of high stopping power detectors, such as BGO (with a detector width as narrow as 4–5 mm). Special PMTs such as the rectangular PMT recently developed by Hamamatsu (the R2404) and a new dichotomic sampling scheme have also been incorporated into the system [20]. In the field of image reconstruction, a true three-dimensional reconstruction (TTR) algorithm has also been utilized (see Chapter 4) [21].

8-5-5 Time-of-Flight System [11]

Ideally, if the exact difference of the flight times of the two annihilation photons can be measured, the exact position of the annihilation can be located, allowing us to determine or map the activity distribution. The time-of-flight (TOF) concept in PET therefore appears to be useful in low-resolution PET systems, where additional TOF information can be of value in enhancing the resolution and improving the signal-to-noise ratio of the image. To obtain any significant improvement, however, the time resolution should be substantially better than 100 psec. This is usually difficult to achieve through existing detectors and associated electronics. However, the recent development of a few fast scintillation crystals, such as CsF and BaF_2, is encouraging [12].

REFERENCES

1. G. L. Brownell, C. A. Burnham, and J. A. Correia. *Med. Radioiso. Scintigraphy* 1:313 (1973).
2. G. L. Brownell, J. A. Correla, and R. G. Zamenhof. In *Recent Advances in Nuclear Medicine*. J. H. Lawrence and T. F. Budinger (eds.) 5:1 (1978).
3. M. M. Ter-Pogossian, M. E. Phelps, and E. J. Hoffman. *Radiology* 114:89 (1975).
4. M. E. Phelps, E. J. Hoffman, N. A. Mullani, and M. M. Ter-Pogossian. *J. Nucl. Med.* 16:210 (1975).
5. Z. H. Cho, J. K. Chan, and L. Eriksson. *IEEE Trans. Nucl. Sci.* 23:613 (1976).
6. M. M. Ter-Pogossian. *J. Nucl. Med.* 19:635 (1978).
7. T. F. Budinger, S. E. Devenzo, and G. T. Gullberg. *J. Comput. Assist. Tomogr.* 1:133 (1977).
8. Z. H. Cho, L. Eriksson, and J. Chan. *Proceedings of Workshop on Reconstruction Tomography*, San Juan, M. M. Ter-Pogossian et al. eds., 393, 1977, University Park Press.
9. T. F. Budinger, S. E. Derenzo, G. T. Gullberg, and R. H. Huesman. *IEEE Trans. Nucl. Sci.* 26:2742 (1979).

10. Z. H. Cho and M. R. Farukhi. *J. Nucl. Med.* 18:840 (1977).

11. C. Nahmias, D. B. Kenyon, and E. S. Garnett. *IEEE Trans. Nucl. Sci.* 27:529 (1980).

12. N. A. Mullani, D. C. Ficke, and M. M. Ter-Pogossian. *IEEE Trans. Nucl. Sci.* 27:572 (1980).

13. C. Bohm, M. Kesselberg, and L. Erikson. *IEEE Trans. Nucl. Sci.* 33:1078 (1986).

14. Z. H. Cho, H. S. Lee, and K. S. Hong. *J. Nucl. Med.* 25:901 (1984).

15. E. I. Tanaka, N. Nohara, T. Tomitani, and M. Endo. *J. Comput. Assist. Tomogr.* **6**:350 (1982).

16. Z. H. Cho, K. S. Hong, and S. K. Hilal. *Nucl. Inst. Meth. Physics Research* 225:422 (1984).

17. Z. H. Cho, S. C. Juh, R. M. Friedenberg, W. Bunney, M. Buchsbaum, and E. Wong. *IEEE Trans. Nucl. Sci.* 37:842–850 (1990).

18. M. E. Casey and R. Nutt. *IEEE Trans. Nucl. Sci.* 33:460 (1986).

19. H. B. Min, J. B. Ra, K. J. Jung, S. K. Hilal, and Z. H. Cho. *IEEE Trans. Nucl. Sci.* 34:332 (1987).

20. Z. H. Cho, K. S. Hong, J. B. Ra, and S. Y. Lee. *IEEE Trans. Nucl. Sci.* 28:94 (1981).

21. Z. H. Cho, J. B. Ra, and S. K. Hilal. *IEEE Trans. Med. Imag.* 2:6 (1983).

MAGNETIC RESONANCE IMAGING

9

NUCLEAR MAGNETIC RESONANCE PHYSICS AND INSTRUMENTATION

NMR (nuclear magnetic resonance) is a phenomenon of magnetic systems that possesses both a magnetic moment and an angular momentum. The term *resonance* implies that the system is in tune with its natural magnetic frequencies; that is, the gyroscopic precession frequency of the magnetic moment of the nuclei when they are in an external static magnetic field. In other words, the application of radio waves with frequencies corresponding to the natural magnetic resonance frequencies of the magnetic system will resonate the magnetic system. Most common nuclei used for NMR fall into the radio frequency range of our communication system. Therefore the externally applied radio waves are often termed as *radio frequency* (rf) in NMR. In an NMR scanner or MR imager we select a region or an area in a sample and observe the spatial distribution of the nuclear spins by addition of the spatial field gradients and corresponding rf signals.

The advantages of NMR CT are, among others, its nonhazardous nature, high-resolution capability, potential for chemically specified imaging, capability of obtaining anatomic cross-sectional images in any direction, high tissue contrast by T_1 or T_2 (relaxation time differentiation), and flow-related imaging capabilities, such as angiography. Although it has some disadvantages, such as the inherently long data acquisition time due to the relaxation times of the spin system and the low signal-to-noise ratio (SNR), NMR imaging is rapidly becoming a major diagnostic modality because of its many, already mentioned, advantages. Moreover the NMR imager is gradually overcoming many problems once thought difficult to solve, such as time-consuming data acquisition and inherently low sensitivity. For example, high-speed imaging methods and high-field NMR using superconducting magnets allow us to image the human brain in times as short as 50 msec.

The history of "NMR imaging" goes back to the early 1970s. At that time both Lauterbur [1] and Damadian [2] proposed that NMR spectroscopic techniques could be applied to human imaging just like X-ray CT and demonstrated that these techniques could be applicable to diagnostic purposes similar to those of X-ray CT. In 1978 Andrew et al. [3] have shown a very high resolution NMR image of a lemon, demonstrating that NMR imaging could indeed show the details of the human anatomy with equal or better resolution than the existing X-ray CT. Subsequent images obtained by Moore et al. [4] and Holland et al. [5] definitively proved that NMR tomography is indeed capable of performing diagnostic imaging. In this chapter the basic physics of NMR phenomenon essential for NMR imaging or MRI (Magnetic Resonance Imaging) as well as related instrumentation will be studied.

9-1 PHYSICAL BASES OF NMR

Since the NMR phenomenon was discovered in 1946 [6], the NMR technique has advanced greatly, and its applications have grown immensely. It has become an indispensable analytical tool in chemistry and physics. The foundation and the basic physical properties of NMR are now well known.

All materials, whether organic or inorganic, consist of nuclei, which are protons, neutrons, or a combination of both [7]. Nuclei that contain an odd number of protons, neutrons, or both in combination, possess a nuclear "spin" and a "magnetic moment." Most of the materials are also composed of several nuclei, and the most common nuclei which have magnetic moments are ^{1}H, ^{2}H, ^{7}Li, ^{13}C, ^{19}F, ^{23}Na, ^{31}P, and ^{127}I. Although some materials are composed mostly of nuclei with an even number of protons and neutrons, thereby possessing no spin or magnetic moment, they often contain some nuclei with an odd number of protons or neutrons. They are therefore also subjects of NMR imaging. For this reason NMR is applicable to most solid- and liquid-phase materials. Among the many hundreds of known stable nuclei, more than 100 possess a spin or a magnetic moment.

When a given material is placed in a magnetic field, randomly oriented nuclei experience an external magnetic torque that tends to align the nuclei either in a parallel or an antiparallel direction in reference to the applied magnetic field. The fraction of magnetized nuclei aligned in either direction (parallel or antiparallel to the applied magnetic field) is dependent on the strength of the magnetic field and thermal agitation. Therefore magnetization is limited by the strength of the main magnetic field as well as the temperature. The magnetization fraction, however, is relatively small at room temperature and therefore has been the main limiting factor for the sensitivity of NMR imaging. Some of the nuclei, when they are under the magnetic field, rotate or precess like gyroscopes or spinning tops precessing around the direction of the gravitational field. The rotating or precessional frequency of

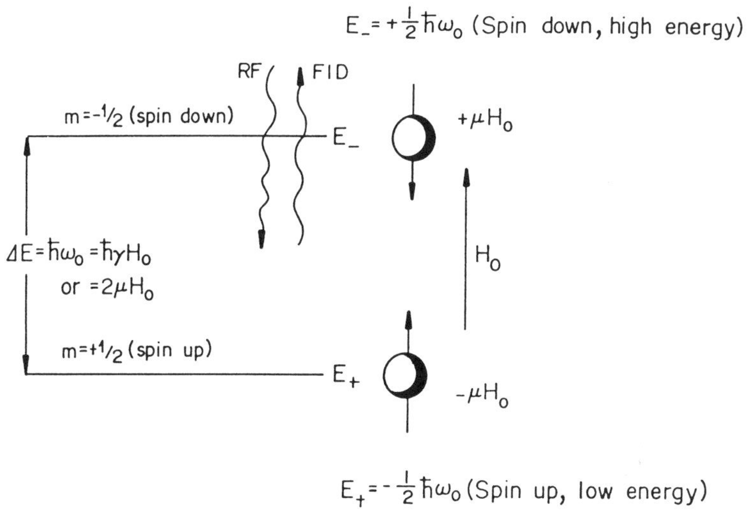

$$E_- = +\frac{1}{2}\hbar\omega_0 \text{ (Spin down, high energy)}$$

Figure 9-1 Stationary states of a proton spin in a constant magnetic field H_0.

$$E_+ = -\frac{1}{2}\hbar\omega_0 \text{ (Spin up, low energy)}$$

the spins is usually called the *Larmor precession frequency* or simply the *Larmor frequency*, and it is proportional to the magnetic field strength.

The alignment of the nuclear spins to the direction of the applied magnetic field leads the spins into two energy states: namely, $+\mu H_0$ (antiparallel to H_0) and $-\mu H_0$ (parallel to H_0) corresponding to the high- and the low-energy states, respectively [7, 8], where μ and H_0 are the nuclear magnetic moment and the applied magnetic field, respectively. This situation is depicted in Fig. 9-1. Note that the spin-dependent energy state E_m is given by

$$E_m = -m\hbar\gamma H_0$$

or

$$E_m = -m\hbar\omega_0 \tag{9-1}$$

where m is the spin quantum number that corresponds to $+\frac{1}{2}$ or $-\frac{1}{2}$ for protons, $\hbar$ is the Planck's constant, and γ is gyromagnetic ratio. Due to the fact that at thermal equilibrium the distribution of spins in those two energy states follows Boltzmann's law, the lower-energy state always has a larger population of spins than the higher-energy state. However by irradiation with an external electromagnetic radiation of energy ΔE equivalent to $2\mu H_0$, those protons in the lower-energy state or $-\mu H_0$ tend to be excited to the higher-energy state (i.e., the $+\mu H_0$ state). This energy is usually supplied by application of an rf signal to the system in the form of an rf magnetic field H_1. After cessation of the rf magnetic field H_1, the excited protons tend to return to their low-energy state by emitting a well-defined rf frequency (i.e., the same frequency as the applied rf). This emission of rf signals is then picked up by an rf coil placed near the excited object. This signal is called a *free induction decay* (FID) signal and is the central part of NMR and NMR imaging. With the emission of NMR signals, the spin system returns to the low-energy state by spin relaxation mechanisms such as spin-lattice and spin-spin relaxations.

Usually two relaxation mechanisms are associated with these excited nuclear spins: the transverse or spin-spin relaxation known as the T_2 relaxation, and the longitudinal or spin-lattice relaxation known as the T_1 relaxation. Both of these relaxations and their respective relaxation times (T_1 and T_2) are quite sensitive to the molecular structures and the environments surrounding the nuclei. For example, the mean T_1 values of normal tissues and those of many malignant tissues differ significantly thereby allowing us to differentiate malignant tissue from normal tissues. A similar tendency is observed for the T_2 values. The imaging capabilities of these two important parameters, T_1 and T_2, together with the spin densities and the flow-dependent phase information of the objects, make NMR imaging a unique, versatile, and powerful technique in diagnostic imaging. Let us now review a few of the fundamental processes in NMR and related topics involved in NMR imaging.

Although many features of the NMR phenomena can be understood only by quantum mechanical considerations, fortunately a number of properties can be visualized by means of a classical treatment. Let us consider a magnetic moment μ in the presence of a magnetic field $\mathbf{H}_0$. Figure 9-2 (a) depicts the spins precessing in two energy states: at a low-energy state (spins parallel to the field $\mathbf{H}_0$) and at a high-energy state (spins antiparallel to the

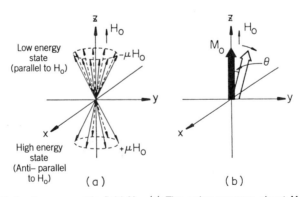

Figure 9-2 Spins in a magnetic field $\mathbf{H}_0$. (a) The spins precess about $\mathbf{H}_0$ in two energy states. More spins are usually aligned in the direction of $\mathbf{H}_0$ at room temperature. (b) The net spin magnetization vector $\mathbf{M}_0$ is given by $\mathbf{M}_0 = \Sigma\mu$. Note that at thermal equilibrium $\mathbf{M}_0$ is along $\mathbf{H}_0$. This spin magnetization can be rotated or flipped at angle θ by addition of an external magnetic field such as short duration rf pulse.

field $\mathbf{H}_0$). All the spins or magnetic moments precess about $\mathbf{H}_0$ either in a parallel or an antiparallel direction at the same frequency. Since the Boltzmann distribution favors the lower-energy state, at equilibrium there are more nuclei aligned parallel to the direction of $\mathbf{H}_0$, and the net magnetization vector $\mathbf{M}_0$, which is the vector sum of the μ's, is also oriented along the positive z-axis, as shown in Fig. 9-2(b). In other words, even though the individual spins may undergo complicated motions, the net magnetization $\mathbf{M}_0$ is the one that can be measured and actually observed. When the net magnetization vector $\mathbf{M}_0$ is at an angle θ to $\mathbf{H}_0$, the net energy of the system is given by [7–10]

$$E = -\mathbf{M}_0 \cdot \mathbf{H}_0 = -M_0 H_0 \cos \theta \qquad (9\text{-}2)$$

Note that the spin system is in its lowest energy state when $\mathbf{M}_0$ is completely in parallel with $\mathbf{H}_0$. The magnitude of the net magnetization at equilibrium is given by

$$M_0 = \frac{N(-\gamma \hbar)^2 H_0 I(I + 1)}{3kT_0} \qquad (9\text{-}3)$$

where N is the number of spins, γ is the gyromagnetic ratio, I is the spin quantum number,* k is Boltzmann's constant, $\hbar$ is Planck's constant, and T_0 is the object temperature. As is seen in Eq. (9-3), the signal strength which is proportional to M_0 can be increased by increasing the field strength H_0 or lowering the object temperature T_0.

The dynamic aspects of NMR can be understood both by observing the spin precession and by solving the differential equation of motion known as the *Bloch equation*, which is given by [6]

$$\frac{d\mathbf{M}_0}{dt} = \gamma \mathbf{M}_0 \times \mathbf{H}_0 \qquad (9\text{-}4)$$

The resulting spin precession follows the Larmor precession frequency

$$\boldsymbol{\omega}_0 = -\gamma \mathbf{H}_0 \qquad (9\text{-}5)$$

which is unique to each nucleus. The minus sign indicates a clockwise precession with a positive γ as a reference. Note that Eqs. (9-4) and (9-5) are based on the laboratory frame; that is, the spins are rotating in reference to a set of fixed cartesian coordinates, x, y, and z.

---

*The spin quantum number I provides information of the number of available states the spin quantum number m can have in Eq. (9-1), and is given by $(2I + 1)$. For example, if $I = \frac{1}{2}$, m has two states, namely $m = +\frac{1}{2}$ and $m = -\frac{1}{2}$.

9-1-1   Rotating Frame and Effective Field

Let us assume that the magnetization vector $\mathbf{M}_0$ has three basic components:

$$\mathbf{M}_0 = M_x \hat{\mathbf{x}} + M_y \hat{\mathbf{y}} + M_z \hat{\mathbf{z}} \tag{9-6}$$

where $\hat{\mathbf{x}}$, $\hat{\mathbf{y}}$, and $\hat{\mathbf{z}}$ are the unit vectors for the cartesian coordinates x, y, and z. By taking time derivative, Eq. (9-6) can be written as

$$\frac{d\mathbf{M}_0}{dt} = \left(\frac{\partial M_x}{\partial t} \hat{\mathbf{x}} + \frac{\partial M_y}{\partial t} \hat{\mathbf{y}} + \frac{\partial M_z}{\partial t} \hat{\mathbf{z}} \right) + \left(M_x \frac{\partial \hat{\mathbf{x}}}{\partial t} + M_y \frac{\partial \hat{\mathbf{y}}}{\partial t} + M_z \frac{\partial \hat{\mathbf{z}}}{\partial t} \right) \tag{9-7}$$

The time derivatives of the directional unit vectors represent rotational angular frequencies: $\partial \hat{\mathbf{x}}/\partial t = \boldsymbol{\omega} \times \hat{\mathbf{x}}$, $\partial \hat{\mathbf{y}}/\partial t = \boldsymbol{\omega} \times \hat{\mathbf{y}}$, and $\partial \hat{\mathbf{z}}/\partial t = \boldsymbol{\omega} \times \hat{\mathbf{z}}$. With these results and Eq. (9-6), Eq. (9-7) can be written as

$$\frac{d\mathbf{M}_0}{dt} = \frac{\partial \mathbf{M}_0}{\partial t} + \boldsymbol{\omega} \times \mathbf{M}_0 \tag{9-8}$$

By rewriting Eq. (9-8), the partial derivative $\partial \mathbf{M}_0/\partial t$ is given by

$$\frac{\partial \mathbf{M}_0}{\partial t} = \frac{d\mathbf{M}_0}{dt} - \boldsymbol{\omega} \times \mathbf{M}_0 \tag{9-9}$$

Equation (9-9) is the rotating frame representation of the magnetization $\mathbf{M}_0$. By knowing that $d\mathbf{M}_0/dt = \gamma \mathbf{M}_0 \times \mathbf{H}$, the rotating frame magnetization can be written as

$$\frac{\partial \mathbf{M}_0}{\partial t} = \gamma \mathbf{M}_0 \times \mathbf{H} - \boldsymbol{\omega} \times \mathbf{M}_0$$

$$= \gamma \mathbf{M}_0 \times \mathbf{H} + \gamma \mathbf{M}_0 \times \frac{\boldsymbol{\omega}}{\gamma}$$

or

$$\frac{\partial \mathbf{M}_0}{\partial t} = \gamma \mathbf{M}_0 \times \left(\mathbf{H} + \frac{\boldsymbol{\omega}}{\gamma} \right) \tag{9-10}$$

In Eq. (9-10) we have used the vector product relation of $\boldsymbol{\omega} \times \mathbf{M}_0 = -(\mathbf{M}_0 \times \boldsymbol{\omega})$. Equation (9-10) resembles Eq. (9-4) except that $\mathbf{H}_0$ is now replaced by $(\mathbf{H} + \boldsymbol{\omega}/\gamma)$. If we assume that the magnetization is rotating around $\mathbf{H}_0$ in the laboratory frame as we have in Eq. (9-4), then Eq. (9-10) suggests that the magnetization now rotates around $(\mathbf{H} + \boldsymbol{\omega}/\gamma)$, which is termed as the effective field:

$$\mathbf{H}_{\text{eff}} = \mathbf{H} + \frac{\boldsymbol{\omega}}{\gamma} \tag{9-11}$$

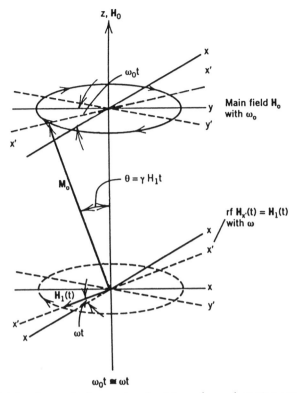

Figure 9-3 Rotating frame of reference to a fixed frame (x, y, z) rotating around the z or z' axis. The coordinates (x', y', z') rotate about the z-axis with the angular frequency ω and $\omega_0 \geq \omega$. The rotating coordinates are related to the fixed coordinates (x, y, z) as $x' = x \cos \omega t + y \sin \omega t$, $y' = -x \sin \omega t + y \cos \omega t$, and $z' = z$, respectively. Maximum insertion of energy occurs only when $\omega_0 t \approx \omega t$.

Let us now consider an rf signal of frequency ω applied along the x'-axis, as shown in Fig. 9-3. The applied rf field $\mathbf{H}_{x'}(t)$ has two components: one with the same rotational direction as the magnetization and the other with the opposite direction:

$$\mathbf{H}_{x'}(t) = \mathbf{H}_1(t) + \mathbf{H}_1^*(t) \tag{9-12}$$

where $\mathbf{H}_1(t)$ and $\mathbf{H}_1^*(t)$ are given by

$$\mathbf{H}_1(t) = H_1(\hat{\mathbf{x}} \cos \omega t - \hat{\mathbf{y}} \sin \omega t)$$
$$\mathbf{H}_1^*(t) = H_1(\hat{\mathbf{x}} \cos \omega t + \hat{\mathbf{y}} \sin \omega t) \tag{9-13}$$

If $\mathbf{H}_1(t)$ is the field that has the same directional rotation as the magnetization then $\mathbf{H}_1^*(t)$ is the field that has the opposite directional rotation. Under the circumstances it is conceivable that $\mathbf{H}_1(t)$ has the maximum effect on the magnetization, especially when the frequency ω is close to ω_0. When an rf field is applied, the effective field therefore becomes

$$\mathbf{H}_{\text{eff}} = \mathbf{H} + \frac{\omega}{\gamma} + \mathbf{H}_1(t) \tag{9-14}$$

Considering the fact that $\mathbf{H}$ and ω/γ are both along the z-axis while $\mathbf{H}_1(t)$ is along the rotating x'-axis frame, Eq. (9-14) can be written as

$$\mathbf{H}_{\text{eff}} = \left(H - \frac{\omega}{\gamma} \right) \hat{z}' + H_1 \hat{x}' \tag{9-15}$$

In NMR, even if ω the rotating frequency of the applied rf field $\mathbf{H}_1(t)$ is set to ω_0 the Larmor frequency, the frequency of the rotating frame could be different due to an inhomogeneity or chemical shift; consequently ω/γ in the fictitious field does not cancel H and leaves a small component $(\gamma H - \omega)$, which in effect appears as an effective field in the z-direction in combination with the rf field H_1 and is given by

$$\begin{aligned}
|\mathbf{H}_{\text{eff}}| &= \left[\left(H - \frac{\omega}{\gamma} \right)^2 + H_1^2 \right]^{1/2} \\
&= \frac{1}{\gamma} \left[(\gamma H - \omega)^2 + \gamma^2 H_1^2 \right]^{1/2}
\end{aligned} \tag{9-16}$$

This situation is illustrated in Fig. 9-4.

From Eq. (9-16) it is also noticed that when $\mathbf{H} = \mathbf{H}_0$, and therefore $-\gamma \mathbf{H}_0 = \omega_0$ and the rf signal frequency is the same as the resonance frequency ω_0, $|\mathbf{H}_{\text{eff}}|$ simply becomes $\mathbf{H}_1$; that is, when the system is in complete resonance, the only field is the rf field $\mathbf{H}_1(t)$. Equation (9-16) therefore simplifies to

$$\begin{aligned}
|\mathbf{H}_{\text{eff}}| &= \frac{1}{\gamma} \Omega \\
&= \frac{1}{\gamma} \Omega \bigg|_{\omega = \omega_0} = H_1(t)
\end{aligned} \tag{9-17}$$

where

$$\Omega = \left[(\omega_0 - \omega)^2 + (\gamma H_1)^2 \right]^{1/2} \bigg|_{\omega = \omega_0} = \gamma H_1(t) \tag{9-18}$$

Ω is therefore the frequency of the magnetization precessing around $\mathbf{H}_{\text{eff}}$. From this, we notice that when $\omega = \omega_0$, the $\mathbf{H}_{\text{eff}}$ axis becomes the x'-axis; therefore the entire magnetization rotates around the x'-axis. In an extension

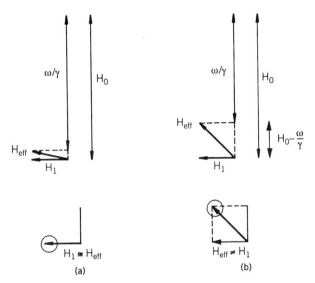

Figure 9-4 In a rotating frame, the magnetization vectors precess around the $\mathbf{H}_{eff}$ vector in the form of a cone with angular frequency $\gamma\mathbf{H}_{eff}$. (a) Represents a case of near resonance, $\omega \cong \omega_0$. (b) When the external rf is in off-resonance, $\omega \neq \omega_0$ or $\omega_{H_1} \neq \omega_0$, where ω_{H_1} is the frequency of externally applied rf pulse.

of this concept (i.e., when $\omega \cong \omega_0$), the effective field $\mathbf{H}_{eff}$ becomes effectively $\mathbf{H}_1(t)$; therefore the magnetization rotates around the $\mathbf{H}_1(t)$ field axis and leads to the interesting conclusion that rf irradiation for a certain period τ_p leads to a rotation of the magnetization M_0 about the x'-axis, as shown in Fig. 9-5. The rotational frequency and therefore the angle of rotation can be given as

$$\Omega = \omega_1 = \gamma H_1(t) \qquad (9\text{-}19)$$

and

$$\theta = \gamma \int_0^{\tau_p} H_1(t) \, dt$$

$$= \gamma H_1 \tau_p \quad \text{(rad.) if } H_1(t) = H_1 \text{ for } 0 \le t \le \tau_p \qquad (9\text{-}20)$$

where τ_p is the rf pulse duration. Equation (9-20) is known as the *flip angle*, or the amount of rotation, and it is simply the time integral of the applied rf signal. For example, when H_1 is applied along the x'-axis for a pulse period τ_p, the spin or magnetization $\mathbf{M}_0$ rotates or flips an angle θ from the z'-axis toward the y'-axis (see Fig. 9-5). In general, θ is set at $\pi/2$ or π, depending on the mode of excitation and the type of NMR experiment. In the simplest

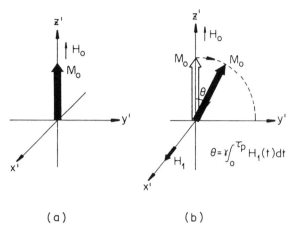

(a)   (b)

Figure 9-5 The spin magnetization in the rotating frame with and without an rf. pulse. (a) The spin magnetization $\mathbf{M}_0$ in the absence of the rf pulse. (b) The spin magnetization $\mathbf{M}_0$ flips with the application of the rf field $\mathbf{H}_1(t)$. The flip angle θ of the magnetization is given by $\theta = \gamma \int_0^{\tau_p} H_1(t)\, dt$, where $H_1(t)$ is the time-varying rf field intensity and τ_p is the length of the rf pulse. The angle θ is usually set to 90° or 180°.

case $\theta = \pi/2$ is used to observe the maximum transverse component of magnetization.

9-1-2 Relaxation Times

After the rf pulse $H_1(t)$ is turned off, the rotating spin magnetization induces a current on the pickup coil surrounding the object and dissipates nuclear spin energy through neighboring spins and lattices. One of the relaxation processes, known as *longitudinal relaxation* or T_1 relaxation leads to thermal equilibrium, that is, realigns the spins or the magnetization along the original H_0 field direction. The relaxation time associated with this process is known as the spin-lattice relaxation time or T_1. At the same time the transverse component of the magnetization also relaxes or disperses the nuclear spins, thereby dephasing the spins that were once coherent (i.e., the spins become incoherent in phase, thereby resulting in no observable signal). This relaxation is a decay process occurring through the spin-spin interactions, and the decay time associated with this process is known as the *spin-spin relaxation time* or T_2.

In addition to the inherent spin-spin relaxation mentioned above, there are other dephasing due to such as the magnetic field inhomogeneity and added field gradients in the case of imaging. As will be discussed later, in NMR imaging, magnetic field gradients are deliberately added to resolve the spatial distribution of the spin density. These gradients produce shifts or an increase or decrease of the resonance frequency in the object within a certain frequency band, resulting in a phase incoherence that eventually makes the composite sinusoidal signal decay even more rapidly than the inherent transverse relaxation time T_2. The effective transverse relaxation time T_2^* resulting from this field inhomogeneity is given as

$$\frac{1}{T_2^*} = \frac{1}{T_2} + \frac{\gamma \Delta H}{2} \tag{9-21}$$

where ΔH is the field inhomogeneity, in this case it represents the maximum deviation of the magnetic field over the region of interest. When a field gradient is added to resolve the spatial distribution of the spin density, T_2^* is further reduced to T_2^{**} as given by

$$\frac{1}{T_2^{**}} = \frac{1}{T_2^*} + \gamma GR \tag{9-22}$$

where G (in gauss per centimeter) is the gradient field strength and R (in centimeters) is the object radius. In imaging therefore the composite sinusoidal signal, which is decaying with an effective transverse relaxation time T_2^{**}, is detected with a phase-sensitive detector. The signal detected in this way is similar to a decaying demodulated AM (amplitude modulated) signal.

Concurrently, as mentioned before, the longitudinal or spin-lattice relaxation forces the spins to realign in the original H_0 (or z) direction; that is, the spins return to the low-energy state or the state of thermal equilibrium. Usually the longitudinal relaxation time T_1 is larger than the transverse relaxation time T_2; therefore the recovery of the excited spins to the equilibrium state is mainly governed by the longitudinal relaxation. We may consider the recovery of the z-component of the magnetization as an exponential recovery process by T_1 as is given by

$$M_z = M_0 \left[1 - \left(1 - \frac{M_z'}{M_0} \right) \exp\left(\frac{-t}{T_1} \right) \right] \tag{9-23}$$

where M_z' is the z-component of the magnetization at the initial stage of relaxation. As mentioned earlier, the transverse magnetization also dephases or decays concurrently with the longitudinal magnetization and follows a simple exponential form, which is given by

$$M_{x,y} = M_{x,y}(0) \exp\left(\frac{-t}{T_2} \right) \tag{9-24}$$

where $M_{x,y}(0)$ is the transverse magnetization at $t = 0$ or the initial value.

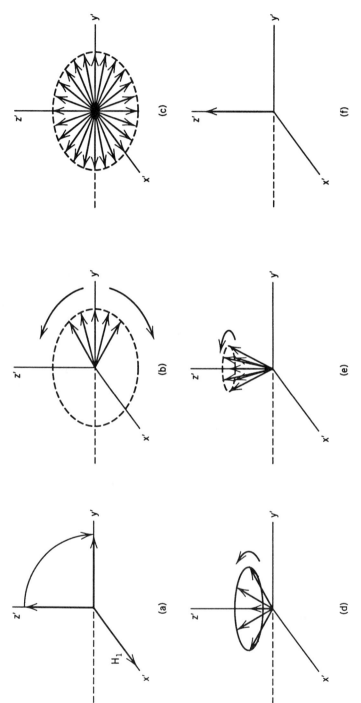

Figure 9-6 Sequential behavior of the spin relaxation processes. (a) The spin magnetization is flipped by an rf pulse $\mathbf{H}_1$. (b) The spins undergo dephasing due to the spin-spin relaxation and field inhomogeneity. (c) When fully dephased the FID signal decays to zero as the spins lose phase coherency. (d), (e), and (f) represent T_1 spin relaxation processes which lead to the recovery of the spins to the original equilibrium state via the spin-lattice relaxation process.

These two relaxation processes work simultaneously and vary greatly depending on the characteristics of the materials and the environmental conditions. For instance, in the case of tissue that is in field strengths of 1 to 20 kG, T_1 and T_2 are on the order of 0.5 sec and 50 msec, respectively. In Fig. 9-6 the sequential behaviors of these two concurrently occurring relaxation processes are illustrated. In general, T_1, T_2, T_2^*, and T_2^{**} have the following relationship:

$$T_2^{**} \leq T_2^* \leq T_2 \leq T_1 \qquad (9\text{-}25)$$

When the above two relaxation mechanisms are considered, the Bloch equations related to each relaxation mechanism are given by [7–10]

$$\frac{dM_z}{dt} = \gamma (\mathbf{M}_0 \times \mathbf{H}_0)_z - \frac{M_z - M_0}{T_1} \qquad \text{for the longitudinal or } T_1 \text{ relaxation}$$

$$(9\text{-}26a)$$

and

$$\frac{dM_{xy}}{dt} = \gamma (\mathbf{M}_0 \times \mathbf{H}_0)_{xy} - \frac{M_{xy}}{T_2} \qquad \text{for the transverse or } T_2 \text{ relaxation}$$

$$(9\text{-}26b)$$

where $(\cdot)_z$ and $(\cdot)_{xy}$ represent the z- and xy-components of the magnetization, respectively. Equation (9-26) indicates that the magnetization components M_z and M_{xy} are two independent processes related separately to the corresponding relaxation times T_1 and T_2.

9-1-3 Spin Echoes

Several forms of spin-echo techniques play many important and essential roles in data acquisition for NMR. The following basic forms of spin-echo are among the most widely used techniques in NMR and NMR imaging: the Hahn spin-echo technique [11], the Carr-Purcell and Meiboom-Gill (CPMG) technique [12, 13], and the stimulated echo techniques [11, 21]. An example of the Hahn spin-echo technique is given in Fig. 9-7. This sequence is known as the $90_{x'} - \tau - 180_{x'}$ or the $(\pi/2)_{x'} - \tau - \pi_{x'}$ sequence. As is seen, a 90° rf pulse with a suitable length is applied along the direction of the x'-axis; then the magnetization vector **M** rotates or flips to the y'-axis. Soon after the flip, the spins start dephasing over the time due to the field inhomogeneity or the added field gradients, or both. A subsequent 180° pulse applied along the x'-axis rotates the spins an additional 180° around the x'-axis, as shown in Fig. 9-7(c). From this point on, the spins start rephasing by continuing the same directional precessions. This process is completed at $t = 2\tau$, at which point the spins are all rephased. An important property of this spin echo

250

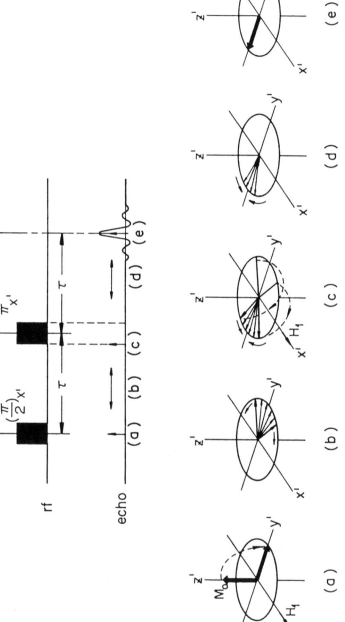

Figure 9-7 The Hahn spin-echo sequence, $90^\circ_{x'} - \tau - 180^\circ_{x'}$ or $(\pi/2)_{x'} - \tau - \pi_{x'}$. (a) The spin is rotated 90° by an rf pulse. (b) The spins are being dephased after a 90° rotation by an rf pulse. (c) When a 180° pulse is applied along the x'-axis. (d) The spins are being rephased after a 180° rotation. (e) A spin echo is generated along the $-y'$-axis by completion of the spin rephasing. Note here that the polarity of the magnetization is now altered; the magnetization has moved to the negative side of the y'-axis.

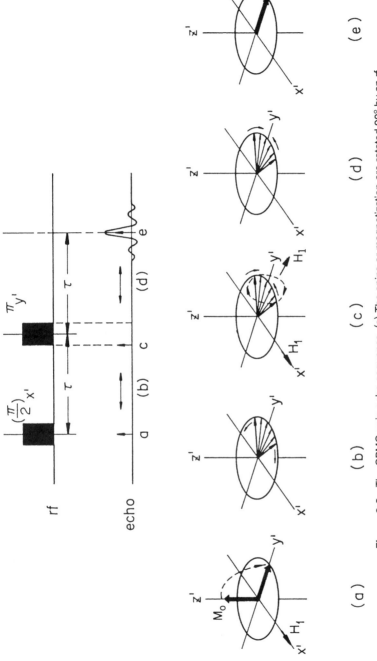

Figure 9-8 The CPMG spin-echo sequence. (a) The spins or magnetization are rotated 90° by an rf pulse. (b) The spins start dephasing immediately, after the 90° rf pulse. (c) When 180° rf pulse is applied along the y'-axis. Spins are rotated 180° around y'-axis. (d) The spins start rephasing and will be refocused. (e) A spin echo is generated along the y'-axis. Note here that the polarity of the magnetization stays at the same positive side of the y'-axis.

251

(often called the *rf spin echo*, not to be confused with the gradient spin echo) is that all the dephased spins due to the field inhomogeneity or the gradient are all rephased along the negative y'-axis. The dephasing of the magnetizations due to the T_2 relaxation, however, remains; that is, the T_2 dependent signal attenuation or decay still exists. Therefore, the decay due to T_2 relaxation is not recovered. Note here that the Hahn spin-echo reverses the polarity of the output signal.

Another interesting spin-echo technique widely used in NMR is the CPMG (Carr-Purcell and Meiboom-Gill) spin-echo sequence. It is identical to the Hahn echo except that a 180° pulse is now applied along the y'-axis, instead of the x'-axis, so that the spins flip around the y'-axis (see Fig. 9-8). Both the Hahn and CPMG techniques are widely used in all phases of NMR and NMR imaging to overcome several adverse effects that often arise in experimental situations, such as the field inhomogeneity and the effects of the gradient pulse rise time. Note here that in the case of the CPMG spin echo, the phase or the polarity of the signal is not altered as in the case of the Hahn echo technique where the polarity is reversed (i.e, the CPMG echo does not change the output signal polarity).

9-1-4 Stimulated Echoes

A stimulated echo can be obtained by a direct extension of the spin-echo techniques discussed previously. In the preceding sections we have illustrated the spin-echo formation as a result of the application of two rf pulses, namely 90° and 180° rf pulses. A stimulated echo, however, is formed by successive application of the three 90° or $\pi/2$ rf pulses, as shown in Fig. 9-9. Figure 9-10(a–f) shows the corresponding vector diagrams of the spin magnetizations at the various time marks.

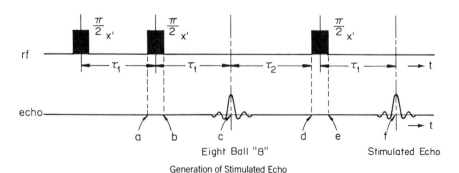

Generation of Stimulated Echo

Figure 9-9 The pulse sequence for the formation of the spin echo (eight ball) and the stimulated echo. *a, b, c, d, e,* and *f* are the time marks related to Fig. 9-10.

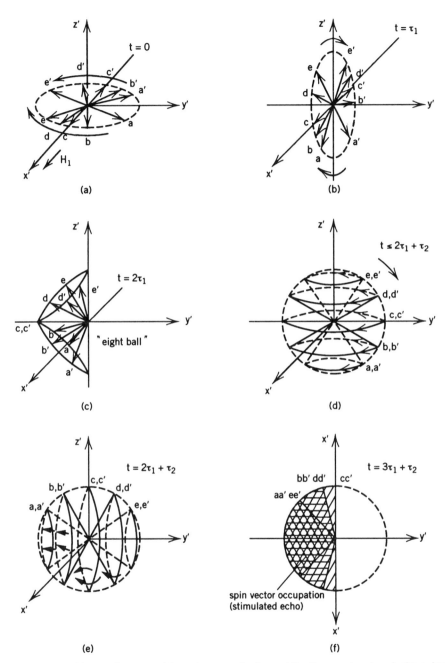

Figure 9-10 Vector diagrams of the spin magnetizations at the time marks given in the pulse sequence shown in Fig. 9-9.

In the case of stimulated echo formation, first, a 90° flip of the magnetiza-tion is achieved in the same manner as the Hahn spin-echo. After the 90° flip, spins will experience a spin dephasing by T_2 relaxation as well as field inhomogeneity. After a second 90° rf pulse, the spins that are dephased in the transverse plane are flipped onto the $x'z'$-plane, as illustrated in Fig. 9-10(b). Once the spins are in the $x'z'$-plane, the spins will experience transverse precession, and rephasing of the spin magnetizations will occur at time τ_1 after the second rf pulse. It is believed that at this point in time, rephasing of the spins resembles the numerical character "8," as shown in Fig. 9-10(c). This may be considered as a conventional spin echo and is often called "*eight ball.*" After the formation of the "eight ball," the spins will continue dephasing [see Fig. 9-10(d)]. Finally, the application of the third 90° rf pulse will rotate the spins another 90°, as shown in Fig. 9-10(e). Note here that there are similarities in spin distributions between Figs. 9-10(a) and (e). The only difference between Fig. 9-10(a) and 9-10(e) is that the spins $(a, a'), (b, b'), \ldots$ are now dispersed onto the circles, indicated by $(a, a'), (b, b'), \ldots$ in Fig. 9-10(e) in the opposite direction (i.e., the negative y'-direction). Thus, at time τ_1 after the third rf pulse, the spins in Fig. 9-10(e) are likely to be refocused similar to the Hahn spin-echo sequence. The echo generated in this manner is called the *stimulated echo*.

In the time period between the second and third rf pulses, the stimulated echo experiences only T_1 relaxation instead of T_2 relaxation, provided that $T_1 \gg T_2$; a nearly full echo is obtained at a time of $t = \tau_1$ after the third 90° rf pulse. It is interesting to note that because of this T_1 relaxation, even if the time period between the second and third rf pulses is expanded, the echo signal obtained at the time $t = 3\tau_1 + \tau_2$ or τ_1 after the third 90° rf pulse has not suffered any additional T_2 decay compared with the conventional $90_{x'} - \tau - 180_{x'}$ Hahn spin-echo technique. In other words, the same goal is achieved with three rf pulses as for the conventional Hahn spin-echo, but without additional T_2 decay. This third rf pulse is found to have many applications, including the selection of an additional slice for localization [22, 23]. Here we must notice that the stimulated echo signal is not as large as that of the conventional spin echo such as the $90_{x'} - \tau - 180_{x'}$ Hahn spin-echo. If the flip angles of the three rf pulses are α_1, α_2, and α_3, re-spectively, and if a very long repetition time is assumed for full T_1 recovery of the spins, the signal obtained by the stimulated echo is given by $(M_0/2) \sin(\alpha_1)\sin(\alpha_2)\sin(\alpha_3) \times \exp(-2\tau_1/T_2) \times \exp\{-(\tau_1 + \tau_2)/T_1\}$ [11, 21]. Thus the maximum obtainable signal at $\alpha_1 = \alpha_2 = \alpha_3 = 90°$ with $(\tau_1 + \tau_2) \ll T_1$ is still only one-half of that of the conventional spin echo provided that τ_1 is kept the same for both the stimulated echo and the conventional spin echo.

9-1-5 NMR Imaging

Conventional NMR applied in chemistry requires a magnetic field of high homogeneity (i.e., as uniform as possible) in order to reduce the spatially dependent field variations or corresponding frequency variations due to the chemical shift. As will be detailed in the following chapters on imaging techniques, a field gradient or a set of gradients is deliberately added to resolve the spatial distribution of spins by Fourier encodings. The basic form of the signal obtained from 3-D Fourier transform NMR imaging (which is known as FID or echo) can be expressed as [14, 15, 16]

$$s(t) = M_0 \iiint_{-\infty}^{\infty} \rho(x, y, z) \exp\left\{ -i\gamma \int_0^t [xG_x(t') + yG_y(t') + zG_z(t')] \, dt' \right\} dx \, dy \, dz$$

$$(9\text{-}27)$$

where $\rho(x, y, z)$ is the 3-D spin density distribution and $G_x(t)$, $G_y(t)$, and $G_z(t)$ are the time-dependent field gradients along the x-, y-, and z-axes, respectively. In Eq. (9-27) the effects of the T_1 and T_2 relaxation times are not included. The generated FID or echo is in effect a Fourier transform-domain representation of the spatially distributed spin density. From this basic form of the 3-D equation, many imaging algorithms can be derived, as will be shown in the following chapters.

9-2 ELECTRONICS AND INSTRUMENTATION FOR NMR IMAGING

A typical NMR tomographic imaging magnet and system designed for human imaging are shown in Figs. 9-11(a) and (b). In this figure, a split-solenoidal-type magnet and NMR imaging system are shown. The sample is surrounded by an rf coil and a gradient coil set [see Fig. 9-11(b)]. The more detailed configuration of the rf and the gradient coils is shown in Fig. 9-12 and may be different depending on the design, but the basic concept will be similar for the majority of NMR imaging systems.

9-2-1 Radio Frequency Coils

A NMR rf coil assembly has two primary functions: excitation of nuclear spins and detection of the resulting nuclear spin precession. During excitation the rf coil serves as a transducer that converts rf power into the transverse rf magnetic field B_1 or $H_1(t)$ in the imaging volume. Therefore high-transmission efficiency means that the coil delivers maximum B_1 to the sample volume with a minimum of rf power. During reception the rf coil also acts as a transducer that converts the precessing nuclear magnetizations into electrical signals that are suitable for further signal processing. High-detection efficiency for the reception mode then corresponds to minimal degradation of the inherent signal-to-noise ratio of the sample in the volume. A well-designed rf coil should be highly efficient as a transmitter as well as a receiver. For imaging it is also desirable that both the excitation and

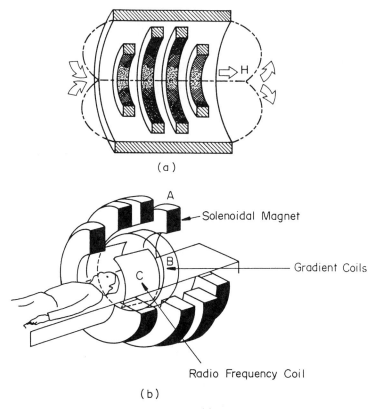

(a)

(b)

Figure 9-11 A sketch of an NMR tomograph: (a) A typical split-solenoid resistive magnet; (b) the physical arrangement of the central part of an NMR CT system. *A* is the main magnet of a split-solenoid type used in many resistive as well as superconducting magnets, *B* is a gradient coil set, and *C* is an rf coil.

reception be spatially uniform in the entire imaging volume. Unfortunately, spatial uniformity and high efficiency often cannot be obtained simultaneously. For example, if one attempts to increase the spatial uniformity, it will require a large-size rf coil, which in turn will accompany a decrease in power or a decrease in the signal-to-noise ratio.

NMR rf coils differ significantly from traditional antennas in function and characteristics. For example, a conventional rf-transmitting antenna is designed to radiate a large fraction of its output power into the far-field region, whereas the NMR rf coil requires storage of the magnetic energy in the near-field region. Although the sample material may absorb a significant part of the rf energy, only a small fraction of the rf energy is actually absorbed by the nuclear spins. Likewise the NMR receiver coil detects the rotating nuclear magnetization without extracting any significant energy from the

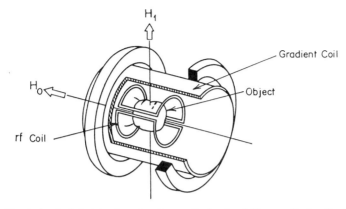

Figure 9-12   A physical sketch of an rf and a gradient coil set. The gradient coil set is usually much larger than the rf coil and also closer to the magnet inner bore.

nuclear spins. Basically the NMR rf coil is a magnetic energy storage device; therefore resonant *LC* circuits are a natural choice for magnetic energy storage.

The rf coil should also resonate at the desired operating frequency and be large enough to accommodate the imaging volume, thereby producing a homogeneous B_1 field within the imaging volume. The rf coil should also have a good filling factor for maximum sensitivity and a minimum coil resistance for reduction of the coil losses.

Currently the following types of rf coils are commonly used for imaging purposes: multiple turn solenoids, saddle types, and ring resonators of various forms. The simplest form of rf coil is a long solenoid that has a good current distribution as required for a uniform axial rf field.

Since the solenoidal rf coil is not often suitable for imaging due to geometrical considerations, a number of different resonant devices have been developed that have good transverse rf fields in a cylindrical volume. Most of the resonant devices more or less have a current density or distribution proportional to $\sin \phi$. If $\phi = 0$ corresponds to the *x*-axis, then the generated transverse field is parallel to the *x*-axis. The widely used simple approximation to $\sin \phi$ is a six-point fit, shown in Fig. 9-13(a) and is the basis of the saddle coil configuration with two equal positive currents at $\phi = 60°$ and $120°$ and two equal negative currents at $\phi = 240°$ and $300°$. The wires at $\phi = 0°$ and $180°$ can be omitted because they carry no current.

To improve the saddle coil approximation (i.e., a six-point approximation to the ideal current distribution), more conductors can be added to follow the sinusoidally weighted currents distribution as before [see Fig. 9-13(b)]. A standing wave in the one wavelength transmission line generates the needed sinusoidal current distribution. Consider a transmission line made from two

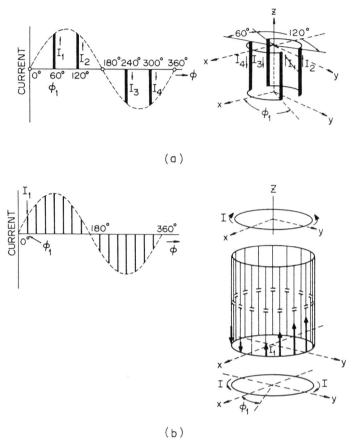

(a)

(b)

Figure 9-13 rf coils and their current distributions: (a) A commonly used saddle-shaped rf coil and current distribution; (b) a birdcage resonator coil and its current distribution.

parallel wires, each formed into a closed circle. Such a transmission line closed on itself can support standing wave resonances consisting of an integer number of wavelengths. If for the single wavelength resonance the voltage is proportional to $\sin \phi$, then the current is proportional to $\cos \phi$ in the upper circle and to $-\cos \phi$ in the lower circle. This current then will produce a transverse field along the x-axis. For practical consideration, a 2.0 tesla NMR scanner, which has a resonance frequency of 85 MHz, the one wavelength standing wave configuration would give a circle diameter of 1.18 m. This is too large and should be shortened by adding lumped-element capacitors between the two transmission lines. An rf coil based on this principle is known as "birdcage" or ring resonator [see Fig. 9-13(b)]. In this rf coil the transmission line forms the two end rings with a voltage difference across the capacitors proportional to sin ϕ. Hence the current in the capacitors is also proportional to sin ϕ. The long leads of the capacitors carry the desired approximation to a sinusoidal surface current density. This circuit is essentially a lumped-element balanced-delay line joined on itself. It can also be thought of as an N-segment low-pass filter. Each segment produces a phase shift of $2\pi/N$ at the resonator. High-pass versions of the birdcage resonator can also be built in which the capacitors are evenly spaced around both end rings, and the straight segments between the end rings are purely inductive. The birdcage resonator can incorporate a number of the design guidelines. The large number of wires can accurately simulate the desired sinusoidal surface current. The homogeneity of the rf field, therefore, is limited only by the finite length of the structure. The multiple turns of the coil are effectively wired in parallel to reduce the inductance to that of a single-turn coil. The distributed currents lower the coil losses and avoid the development of high concentrations of the magnetic field only near the conductors. Thus the uniformity of the field improves the filling factor. The lead inductance of the capacitors is fully utilized to create the desired B_1 field. The high symmetry of the resonator facilitates the use of quadrature excitation and reception, if it is desired.

Another widely used coil is the surface rf coil. Surface rf coils (or simply surface coil, as the name implies) do not enclose the sample but are instead placed on the surface of the sample material. Their greatest signal sensitivity is limited to a region close to the coil with dimensions that are comparable to the coil size. Surface coils were used initially for *in vivo* spectroscopy where their localized response permits acquisition of spectra predominantly from a particular organ or tissue of interest [17]. Surface coils are now used for imaging with improved signal-to-noise performance when only localized region imaging is of interest [18, 19, 20]. The enhanced signal strength may be used to improve image resolution by decreasing the voxel size. The simplest surface coil is a single turn circular loop of radius r, which can be tuned and matched for the desired operating frequency. This type of coil may be thought of as a very short solenoid that has an efficiency of about half of a coil that has a high filling factor and is coupled strongly to the sample. The B_1 field and the corresponding signal sensitivity for the short solenoid are highly inhomogeneous. Peak values of B_1 occur adjacent to the conductor. Along the axis of the coil, the field per unit current varies as

$$B_1 \propto \frac{1}{r\left[1 + \left(x^2/r^2\right)\right]^{3/2}} \tag{9-28}$$

where r is the radius of coil and x is the distance between the rf coil plane and the imaging point of interest.

9-2-2   Gradient Coils

Gradient coils are the new key elements added especially for NMR imaging; they used to be of no importance to conventional NMR spectroscopy. In a conventional imaging experiment, the simplest and most desirable spatial dependence for the magnetic field is a linear one. In general, three mutually orthogonal gradients $G_z = \partial B_z/\partial z$, $G_y = \partial B_z/\partial y$, and, $G_x = \partial B_z/\partial x$ are required. Note that the fields generated by these gradients are always in the z direction but vary in amplitude according to the displacment along z-, y-, and x-axis, respectively. In most imaging systems the roles of these gradients can be interchanged or combined, permitting software-controlled changes from axial to coronal, sagittal, or intermediate slice orientations. Different techniques utilize the gradients in different ways, some requiring purely static, others oscillating, and still others rapidly switched gradients. Strength and linearity needs also vary from method to method and may conflict with switching requirements. For example, a high gradient strength will need a coil system with many turns; good linearity over the sample volume will necessitate a large coil system or one with many separate elements. In both cases the result is likely to be a high-inductive system with a long switching time. Note that since substantial currents (often hundreds of amperes) are required to energize the gradient coils and since these are located within a large uniform magnetic field, quite large forces exist between the main magnet and these current-carrying conductors. Thus, for a static field B_z of 0.1 T and a current of 10 A, the force on a conductor lying normal to the field direction would be 1 newton. The supporting structure of the coil should therefore be sufficiently strong to sustain against these forces.

The most conventionally used linear gradient coils are the modified Golay-type coil for Gx and Gy [see Figs. 9-14(a) and (b)]. The Golay-type coil, as shown in Figs. 9-14(a) and (b), generates x- or y-directional gradient fields with good linearity and homogeneity. Note that the return paths are made by way of axial wires where current flows in opposite directions so as not to contribute to the field in the z-direction. The Maxwell pair shown in Fig. 9-14(c) consists of two parallel current loops with currents in opposite directions and of separation l sufficient for the volume of the object to be imaged. The direction of the gradient is along the z-axis.

9-2-3   rf Transmitter

The rf transmitter consists of a main frequency source, waveform synthesizers, a modulator, an rf amplifier and gate, rf transmission and coupling circuits, and an rf coil. To ensure coherent operation of the instrument, the rf source for the transmitter, the reference rf for the phase-sensitive detectors, and the timing for the control pulses should all ultimately be synchronized and delivered from the same master oscillator. Long-term as well as short-

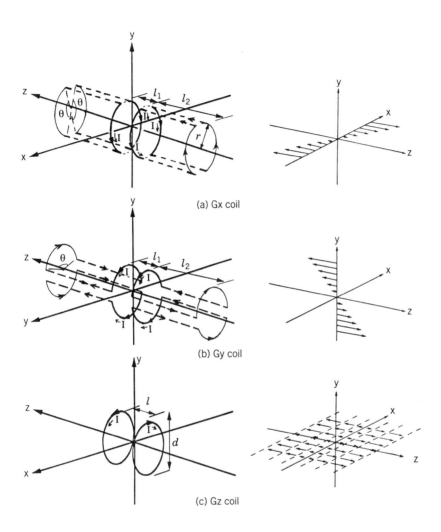

Figure 9-14 (a) An x-directional gradient coil, which is often called as the Golay coil. (b) A y-directional gradient coil, which is also a Golay type coil. (c) A z-directional gradient coil. The change of the magnetic field in the z direction is indicated by the direction and length of the arrows. This coil is called the *Maxwell pair*. In (a), (b), and (c) the optimal design parameters of coil are $\theta = 120°$, $l/d = l/2r = \sqrt{3}/2$, $l_1 = 0.78r$, and $l_2 = 2.13r$.

term stability is important and is generally less than $\sim$ 1 ppm or 0.1 ppm if the temperature is controlled (ovened).

Modulation can be achieved using double-balanced mixers (DBM) (also known as *ring modulators* or *double-balanced modulators*) which are readily available commerically. Although the modulation function can be produced directly using analog circuitry, the most of the modern flexible systems are in digital form and the necessary functions are stored digitally in the CPU or in a buffer memory from which the discrete values can be read out in sequence at a rate determined by the pulse controller. This provides a discrete, rather than a continuous, waveform with the step size governed by the voltage level corresponding to the least significant bit. After a suitable digital to analog conversion (DAC), signals from the waveform synthesizer are fed to the double-balanced mixers (DBM). The aim of the modulation is to excite a specific frequency band corresponding to a particular volume within the sample, such as a narrow slice of spins. Unfortunately, with a single channel, it is not possible to excite a single-frequency band centered at a frequency of, say, $\omega_0 + \Delta\omega/2$ (where ω_0 is the carrier); one automatically also excites the symmetric sideband at $\omega_0 - \Delta\omega$. The simplest solution is to employ single-sideband (SSB) modulation methods, which require an addition of a second rf channel in quadrature with the first. This is completely analogous to the use of rf quadrature detection methods. The practical requirements are straightforward. The rf is split into two components with a relative phase shift of 90°, using, for example, a quadrature hybrid. The circuitry of modulation is duplicated to enable modulation of the two channels which are then recombined prior to power amplification, as shown in Fig. 9-15.

To achieve the short 90° and 180° pulses that are often required in human imaging systems with their large transmitter coils, substantial peak power is required (typically several kilowatts). In most imaging applications, linear amplifiers (class A or class AB) are needed, and since these do generate noise in the "off" state, it may well prove necessary to incorporate some active gating at this stage. When in the off state, a gating circuit should isolate both the rf coil and the sensitive receiver from the transmitter rf. In Fig. 9-16 a block diagram of the receiver-transmitter system and coupler are

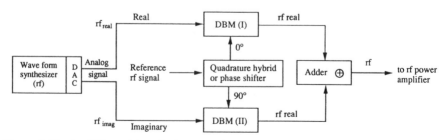

Figure 9-15 An SSB modulator in the transmitter side. DBM is the double balanced mixer.

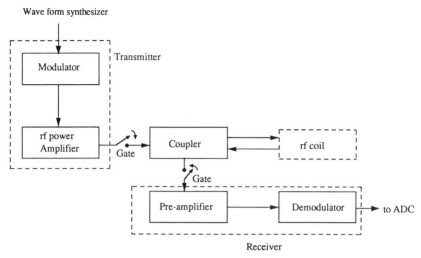

Figure 9-16   The block diagram of the receiver-transmitter system and coupler.

shown. As will be discussed further, coupler circuits often act as gates, switching between the rf transmitter amplifier and the receiver amplifier.

The rf coil, transmitter, and receiver circuits are shown in Fig. 9-17. This circuit is, in a sense, a coupler, channeling the rf power signal to the rf coil as well as routing the NMR signal to the receiver. To pick up NMR signals, an rf coil is required to interact with the spin system; that is, an rf coil must surround the sample so that current can be induced. In the upper part of Fig. 9-17, a typical transmitter tuned circuit is shown. To a first approximation, one can consider the coil L and the variable (tuning) capacitor C_2 as a parallel tuned circuit that resonates at a frequency ω_0, which is given by

$$\omega_0^2 L C_2 \cong 1 \qquad (9\text{-}29)$$

The power amplifiers are generally designed to have an output impedance of 50 Ω; that is, it delivers maximum power into a 50-Ω load. When we view the resonance circuit from the point A in Fig. 9-17, it would have a very high input impedance, since it is a parallel resonance circuit. Thus, if it were connected directly to the power amplifier, it would result in a gross mismatch in impedance and most of the power would be reflected back to the amplifier. To avoid this mismatch, the variable (matching) capacitor C_1 is inserted to tune the $C_1 L$ circuit as a series resonance circuit. This series resonance circuit is then tuned to be 50 Ω.

The crossed diodes circuits, D_1 and D_2, have the property that they will only conduct when the forward bias voltage exceeds a certain level (about 0.6 V in the case of silicon diodes). The D_1 crossed diode pair therefore

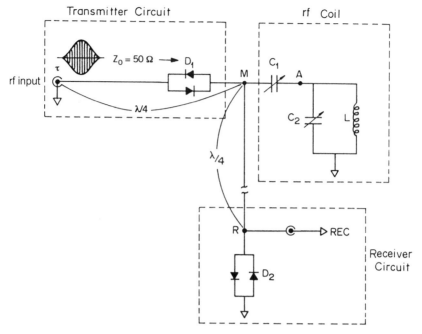

Figure 9-17 The coupler circuit around the rf coil made by a quarter wavelength ($\lambda/4$) coaxial line and diodes. The D_1 and D_2 diodes circuits are the transmitter-side rf amp blocking and high voltage receiver protection circuits, respectively. The receiver side is further protected by a $\lambda/4$ cable to minimize the transmitted signal at point R. The inductor L and the variable tuning capacitor C_2 form a parallel-tuned circuit, while the inductor L and the variable capacitor C_1 form a series-resonance circuit with an impedance of 50 Ω, which matches the 50 Ω output impedance of the transmitter.

provides a short circuit for transmitting signals to the rf coil but acts as a threshold barrier for the noise signals which are usually smaller than 0.6 V. In addition, the D_1 pair also acts as an element that cuts off the low-level signal noise originating from the amplifier. The D_2 pair, on the other hand, acts as a protection circuit against damage to the low-level preamplifier when the high-power rf signal is applied on the rf coil. They should have high-frequency characteristics such as low capacitance and also be capable of withstanding high-peak currents.

9-2-4 rf Receiver

Receiver design is crucially important because it directly determines the final image quality. The lower part of Fig. 9-17 together with the rf coil C_2L illustrates the general features of a typical receiver system. The first element in the figure is the receiver coil, which is the same coil used for transmission. The receiver coil should have the highest possible Q, since, in general, this

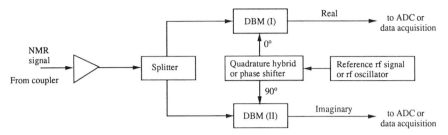

Figure 9-18 The receiver side quadrature phase-sensitive demodulator. DBM is the double balanced mixer.

will give us the best signal-to-noise ratio. To improve the sensitivity, the coil should be as small or as close to the sample as possible; in other words, it should have the highest filling factor.

The receiver should also be well isolated from the transmitter during the transmission of the rf pulse. As shown in Fig. 9-17, during the transmission phase, both sets of crossed diodes conduct; however, at the receiver side, that

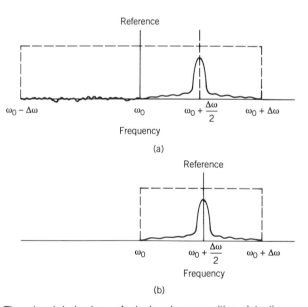

Figure 9-19 The signal behaviors of single phase-sensitive detection and quadrature phase-sensitive detection. (a) In single phase-sensitive detection, the reference frequency must be placed at one extreme of the spectrum of width $\Delta\omega$ and, since positive and negative frequencies are not distinguished, noise in the range $\omega_0 - \Delta\omega$ to ω_0 is folded onto the spectrum. (b) In quadrature phase-sensitive detection, the reference frequency is located at the center of the spectrum, allowing a filter bandwidth of only half the bandwidth employed in single phase-sensitive detection, thereby reducing noise. (Filter bandwidths are shown by broken lines.)

is, at the end of the quarter wavelength line or at the point R, the diode circuit D_2 pair effectively shortens the receiver input, thereby protecting the receiver from damage when a large voltage signal appears at the receiver input. At the transmission stage (at point M) this circuit should look like an open circuit due to the $\lambda/4$ cable between the points M and R. This assures us that all the transmitter power will be channeled to the tuned circuit. In the receiving phase the induced emf is far too small to make both diode circuits conduct, thereby effectively isolating the transmitter (D_1) as well as cutting off the signal (D_2) which would otherwise short to the ground.

Having amplified the nuclear signal to a level of perhaps a few volts, the next stage is detection, namely removal of the rf carrier. For quadrature detection, now almost universally employed, two channels are necessary. The reference rf is split into two components which are phase-shifted with respect to each other by 90°. These reference signals are used to detect the real and imaginary components of the NMR signal (see Fig. 9-18).

The advantage of using quadrature detection lies in its ability to discriminate between positive and negative frequency offsets. This allows the reference (detection) frequency to be placed in the center of the receiver frequency band, as shown in Fig. 9-19 (b), rather than placing at mid of entire frequency band as shown in Fig. 9-19 (a). This setup reduces the necessary bandwidth, thereby reduces noise.

9-2-5 Block Diagram of a NMR System

The block diagram of a typical NMR CT system is shown in Fig. 9-20 which depicts the operation of each part. The main computer generates rf and

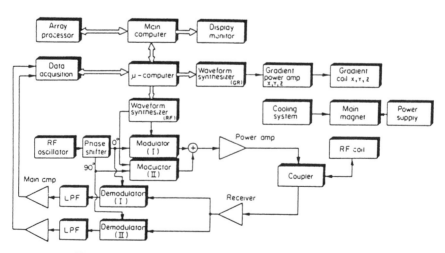

Figure 9-20 A block diagram of a typical NMR scanner system.

gradient waveforms and reconstructs images after data acquisition. The rf and gradient pulse waveforms generated in the main computer are transferred to a microcomputer and then to a waveform synthesizer where the data in the digital form are converted to the analog form. The gradient waveforms are applied to the x-, y-, and z-gradient coils after being amplified in the gradient power amplifiers. The rf waveforms from the waveform synthesizer are modulated with the rf (reference) signal or carrier in the modulator (see also Fig. 9-15), amplified through the power amplifier, and transferred to the rf coil via the coupler. The coupler circuit effectively switches on and off between the transmitting and receiving operations, as explained previously. The transmitted rf pulse excites nuclear spins in the sample. In the receiving mode, the nuclear signal is induced on the same rf coil by the precessing spins and this signal is then transferred to the receiver amplifier through the coupler. The amplified nuclear signal is demodulated with the reference rf signal and is then sent to the data acquisition part (see Fig. 9-18). Acquired nuclear signals (FIDs or echo signals) are then digitized and transferred to the main computer via the microcomputer. These data are used for the reconstruction of the image. NMR scanner systems often employ array processors for rapid image reconstruction using FFT (Fast Fourier Transform) algorithm. After reconstruction the images are displayed on a cathode ray tube (CRT).

REFERENCES

1. P. C. Lauterber. *Nature* 242:190 (1973).
2. R. Damadian. *Science* 171:1151 (1971).
3. E. Andrew, P. Bottomly, W. Hinshaw, G. Holland, and W. Moore. *Nature* 270: cover (1977).
4. W. Moore, G. Holland, and L. Kreel. *CT* 4:1 (1980).
5. G. Holland, R. Hawkes, and W. Moore. *J. Comput. Assist. Tomogr.* 4:429 (1980).
6. F. Bloch. *Rhys. Rev.* 70:460 (1946).
7. D. Shaw. *Fourier Transform NMR Spectroscopy*. New York: Elsevier Scientific, 1971.
8. T. Farrar and E. Becker. *Pulse and Fourier Transform NMR*. San Diego: Academic Press, 1971.
9. C. P. Slichter. *Principles of Magnetic Resonance*, vol. 1, M. Cardona, P. Flude, and H. J. Quessier, eds. Springer Series in Solid State Sciences. Berlin: Springer-Verlag, 1978.
10. A. Abragam. *The Principles of Nuclear Magnetism*. Oxford: Oxford University Press, 1961.
11. E. L. Hahn. *Phys. Rev.* 80:580 (1950).
12. H. Y. Carr and E. M. Purcell. *Phys. Rev.* 94:630 (1954).
13. S. Meiboom and D. Gill. *Rev. Sci. Instrum.* 29:688 (1958).

14. Z. H. Cho, H. S. Kim, H. B. Song, and J. Cumming. *IEEE Proc.* 70:1152 (1982).

15. W. S. Hinshaw and A. Lent. *IEEE Proc.* 71:338 (1983).

16. A. Kumar, D. Welti, and R. Ernst. *J. Magn. Reson.* 18:69 (1975).

17. J. J. H. Ackerman, G. H. Grove, G. G. Wong, D. G. Gadian, and G. K. Radda. *Nature* 283:167 (1980).

18. L. Axel. *J. Comput. Assist. Tomogr.* 8:381 (1984).

19. S. J. El Yousef, R. J. Duchesneau, C. A. Hubay, J. R. Haaga, P. J. Bryan, J. P. Lipuma, and A. E. Ament. *J. Comput. Assist. Tomogr.* 7:215 (1983).

20. J. F. Schenck, T. H. Foster, J. L. Henkes, W. J. Adams, C. E. Hayes, H. R. Hart, W. A. Edelstein, P. A. Bottomley, and F. W. Wehrli. *AJNR* 6:181 (1985).

21. D. E. Woessner. *J. Chem. Phys.* 34:2057 (1961).

22. J. Frahm, K. D. Merboldt, W. Hänicke, and A. Hasse. *J. Magn. Reson.* 64:81 (1985).

23. J. Frahm, K. D. Merboldt, and W. Hänicke. *J. Magn. Reson* 72:502 (1987).

10

MAGNETIC RESONANCE IMAGING: MATHEMATICS AND ALGORITHMS

Although image reconstruction in NMR imaging follows simple 2-D or 3-D Fourier transforms, projection reconstruction used in the X-ray CT can also be used in several specific applications. As will be seen in the following chapters, the NMR imaging algorithm is largely dependent on the imaging pulse sequence. Each image modeling therefore has its own image reconstruction algorithm and strategy. In this chapter the basics of the Fourier transform based and projection reconstruction based NMR image reconstruction algorithms are given together with several different forms of phase-encoded multislice imaging techniques which could be universally applicable to most imaging algorithms.

10-1 BASIC IMAGING EQUATION FROM BLOCH'S EQUATION

The Bloch equation for transverse magnetization in the presence of a linear magnetic field gradient is given by

$$\frac{dM_{xy}}{dt} = \left(i\omega_0 - \frac{1}{T_2} - i\gamma b_z \right) M_{xy} \qquad (10\text{-}1)$$

where ω_0 is the Larmor frequency, T_2 is the transverse relaxation time, γ is the gyromagnetic ratio, M_{xy} is the transverse magnetization (i.e., $M_{xy} = M_y + iM_x$), and the function b_z is defined by

$$b_z = \left(x\hat{\mathbf{x}} + y\hat{\mathbf{y}} + z\hat{\mathbf{z}} \right) \cdot \left[G_x(t)\hat{\mathbf{x}} + G_y(t)\hat{\mathbf{y}} + G_z(t)\hat{\mathbf{z}} \right]$$
$$= \mathbf{r} \cdot \mathbf{G}(t) \qquad (10\text{-}2)$$

269

where $\hat{x}, \hat{y}, \hat{z}$ are unit vectors, $\mathbf{r} = x\hat{x} + y\hat{y} + z\hat{z}$ and $\mathbf{G}(t) = G_x(t)\hat{x} + G_y(t)\hat{y} + G_z(t)\hat{z}$. In Eq. (10-1) we ignored the effects of diffusion, flow, and chemical shift. The solution of Eq. (10-1) is given as

$$M_{xy}(\mathbf{r}, t) = M_0\rho(\mathbf{r}) \exp\left[-i\gamma\mathbf{r} \cdot \int_0^t \mathbf{G}(t')\, dt'\right] \qquad (10\text{-}3)$$

where M_0 is the thermal equilibrium magnetization and $\rho(\mathbf{r})$ is the spin density function, which includes a dependence on T_1 and T_2 implicitly. In writing Eq. (10-3), we also eliminated the high-frequency or carrier term $\exp(i\omega_0 t)$ by the use of phase-sensitive detection.

The NMR signal is the integration of M_{xy} within the excited volume:

$$S(t) = \int M_{xy}(\mathbf{r}, t)\, d^3r \qquad (10\text{-}4)$$

which can be rewritten by means of Eq. (10-3) as

$$S(t) = M_0 \int \rho(\mathbf{r}) \exp\left[-i\gamma\mathbf{r} \cdot \int_0^t \mathbf{G}(t')\, dt'\right] d^3r \qquad (10\text{-}5)$$

This equation represents the NMR signal, which is often known as the FID or echo that can be measured for imaging. So far we have not specified the actual gradient wave form $\mathbf{G}(t)$. In the next several sections we will examine how this equation can be applied to a given imaging situation. Indeed NMR imaging is an interesting example of a physical Fourier transformer; in NMR imaging the NMR signal appears as the Fourier transform of $\rho(\mathbf{r})$ if a suitable change of variables is performed. The density function $\rho(\mathbf{r})$ can then be obtained by taking the inverse Fourier transform of the NMR signal $S(t)$.

10-2 FOURIER IMAGING

10-2-1 Two-dimensional Fourier Imaging

From the basic imaging equation given in Eq. (10-5), a 2-D imaging equation can be derived by replacing the spatial coordinate vector $\mathbf{r}$ with 2-D cartesian coordinates and by assuming that we are interested in imaging a slice at $z = z_0$:

$$S(t) = M_0 \iint \rho(x, y; z = z_0)$$

$$\times \exp\left\{-i\gamma(x\hat{x} + y\hat{y}) \cdot \int_0^t \left[G_x(t')\hat{x} + G_y(t')\hat{y}\right] dt'\right\} dx\, dy \qquad (10\text{-}6)$$

where $\rho(x, y; z = z_0)$ represents the 2-D spin density excited at $z = z_0$ and $G_x(t)$ and $G_y(t)$ are the x- and the y-directional time-varying gradients,* respectively.

Let us now consider Fourier-domain scanning, which uses both frequency and phase encodings. As seen from Eq. (10-6), discrete Fourier encoding can be achieved by changing the gradient amplitude (or its length):

$$S(g_x, t_y) = M_0 \iint \rho(x, y; z = z_0) \exp\left[-i\gamma(xg_x T_x + yG_y t_y)\right] dx\, dy \quad (10\text{-}7)$$

where $g_x = n\Delta G_x$ and ΔG_x is the increment of the x-gradient amplitude, and n denotes the step number of the phase encoding gradient. Equation (10-7) applies to the case of amplitude variation when the x-gradient is used for phase encoding. The pulse length can also be varied provided that the pulse amplitude is kept constant. In this case Eq. (10-6) can be rewritten as

$$S(t_x, t_y) = M_0 \iint \rho(x, y; z = z_0) \exp\left[-i\gamma(xG_x t_x + yG_y t_y)\right] dx\, dy \quad (10\text{-}8)$$

In this case $t_x = n\Delta T_x$ with ΔT_x being the increment of the x-gradient pulse length.† Figure 10-1 shows typical NMR pulse sequences for 2- and 3-D Fourier imaging. Figure 10-1(a) shows the pulse sequence for the gradient pulse amplitude variation approach corresponding to Eq. (10-7), while Fig. 10-1(b) shows the gradient pulse length variation approach corresponding to Eq. (10-8). In Eqs. (10-7) and (10-8), we assume that the y-gradient G_y is used as the readout gradient which is also known as the frequency-encoding gradient. This is distinguished from the phase-encoding gradient which in this case is the x-gradient. In Eqs. (10-7) and (10-8) the number of phase encoding steps determines the x-directional resolution, while the y-directional resolution remains constant regardless of the number of encoding steps employed. Theoretically the resolution of the latter (y) can be infinitely high. However, in most cases the resolution in the y-direction is limited by the bandwidth of the NMR data, the sampling interval, and the SNR. In practical NMR imaging the resolution is therefore largely determined by the number of phase encoding steps employed (e.g., the x-gradient in this case) provided that the signal has a sufficient SNR. Other important physical parameters involved in NMR imaging, are the spin-lattice and spin–spin relaxation times T_1 and T_2, as discussed in the previous chapter. Even though these parameters often limit the imaging time due to the requirement

---

*As will be clear, both the time-varying and amplitude-varying gradient will have the same effect on the phase encoding due to the fact that the amount of phase encoding is solely a function of the integral value of the gradients.

†Although the above two phase encoding methods can be equally used, the former [Eq. (10-7)] is more widely used due to the fact that the constant time or pulse width T_x employed in the former eliminates NMR parameter-dependent signal variations such as T_2 decay.

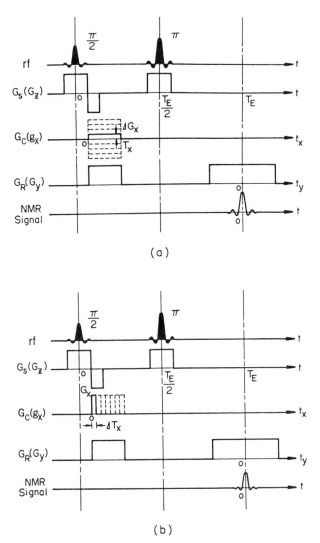

Figure 10-1   Pulse sequences for 2-D spin echo Fourier imaging. (a) The amplitude variation scheme for phase encoding (g_x), (b) the pulse length variation phase encoding scheme (t_x), and (c) the full 3-D Fourier imaging sequence. In the real experiments, the amplitude variation scheme shown in (a) is usually used. The 3-D sequence shown in (c) is a simple extension of the 2-D spin echo Fourier technique shown in (a).

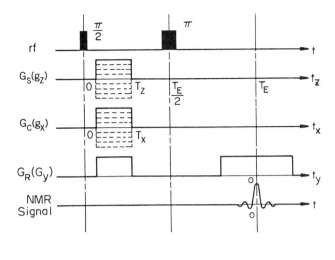

(c)

Figure 10-1 *(Continued)*

of a certain time interval to ensure sufficient recovery (especially the spin-lattice relaxation time T_1), they, together with the spin density, play an important role in the creation of NMR image contrast. On the other hand, after the initial excitation, each signal data acquisition is performed as rapidly as possible before the signal decays away due to the T_2 decay process.

Slow T_1 relaxation or the recovery of the spins to the equilibrium state forces one to use a relatively long pulse-repetition interval. To avoid the requirement of this long repetition time, method such as the multiple slice imaging using the slice-by-slice imaging technique are often used instead of single slice excitation. One can also excite the entire imaging volume with an extended phase encoding into the slice selection direction (z) as shown in Fig. 10-1(c). This method is sometimes known as direct 3-D or multislice imaging. There are some differences, however, between slice-by-slice imaging and direct multislice imaging. In the former, each excitation involves only a single slice, whereas in the latter, each excitation excites all the slices simultaneously. In the slice-by-slice technique, if a sufficiently long repetition time T_R is given and if each slice excitation time is T_S, the total number of slices N that can be imaged in a single sequence is simply related as

$$N = \frac{T_R}{T_S} \tag{10-9}$$

10-2-2 Three-dimensional Fourier Imaging

Three-dimensional Fourier imaging can be derived by a simple extension of the previously discussed 2-D case. It simply corresponds to the sequential measurement of the 3-D frequency spectrum in the presence of three orthogonal linear magnetic field gradients. The pulse sequence starts with the excitation of the whole 3-D volume by a nonselective 90° rf pulse in the absence of the gradient pulse. After the 90° rf pulse, two gradient fields $(g_z$ and $g_x)$ are applied for phase encoding. Subsequent application of a nonselective 180° rf pulse and a readout gradient pulse complete the sequence. The pulse sequence for 3-D Fourier imaging is shown in Fig. 10-1(c). The NMR signal in this case is given by

$$S(g_x, t_y, g_z) = M_0 \iiint \rho(x, y, z) \exp\left[-i\gamma(xg_xT_x + yG_yT_y + zg_zt_z)\right] dx\,dy\,dz$$

(10-10)

Equation (10-10) is a simple extension of Eq. (10-6) or Eq. (10-7) into a 3-D form. We notice that $\gamma g_x T_x$, $\gamma g_y T_y$, and $\gamma G_z t_z$ correspond to the accumulated phase of respective x, y, and z coordinates:

$$\omega_x = \gamma g_x T_x$$
$$\omega_y = \gamma G_y t_y$$
$$\omega_z = \gamma g_z T_z$$

(10-11)

Using Eq. (10-11), Eq. (10-10) can be rewritten as

$$S(\omega_x, \omega_y, \omega_z) = M_0 \iiint \rho(x, y, z) \exp\left[-i(\omega_x x + \omega_y y + \omega_z z)\right] dx\,dy\,dz$$

(10-12)

Similar to the 2-D case, the 3-D density function can be obtained by taking 3-D inverse Fourier transform of $S(\omega_x, \omega_y, \omega_z)$:

$$\rho(x, y, z) = c \iiint S(\omega_x, \omega_y, \omega_z) \exp\left[i(\omega_x x + \omega_y y + \omega_z z)\right] d\omega_x\,d\omega_y\,d\omega_z$$

(10-13)

where c is a constant. Note that $S(\omega_x, \omega_y, \omega_z) = S(g_x, t_y, g_z)$.

A slightly different version of the above technique, known as selected volume 3-D Fourier imaging, enables one to image a limited volume. In the selected volume 3-D method, the limited slice is excited by a selective rf pulse in the presence of a gradient field in the slice selection direction. Except for the selection process of a limited volume or slab by the selective

90° rf pulse in conjunction with a slice selection gradient, the data acquisition sequence is the same as for the full 3-D Fourier imaging method. The selected volume 3-D technique is useful when one is interested in imaging a limited volume or a limited number of slices of a large object [1].

10-3 PROJECTION RECONSTRUCTION

As will be seen, the application of projection reconstruction in NMR imaging is quite similar to that of X-ray CT or emission tomography and has found several important and unique applications that otherwise cannot be achieved by Fourier imaging. In this section, the principles and the implications of projection reconstruction are discussed and some useful application examples are given.

10-3-1 Two-dimensional Line-Integral Projection Reconstruction

The NMR signal corresponding to the 2-D line-integral projection at a given view θ is given by [2, 3]

$$S_\phi(t) = M_0 \int_{x'} \int_{y'} \rho(x, y)\exp(-i\gamma G_\phi x't)\, dx'\, dy' \qquad (10\text{-}14)$$

where

$$\begin{bmatrix} x' \\ y' \end{bmatrix} = \begin{bmatrix} \cos\phi & \sin\phi \\ -\sin\phi & \cos\phi \end{bmatrix} \begin{bmatrix} x \\ y \end{bmatrix}$$

and $\rho(x, y)$ and ϕ are the spin density function of the selected slice and its view angle. Figure 10-2 shows an example of pulse sequence used for the 2-D line-integral projection reconstruction using a spin-echo mode. The projection reconstruction sequence is obtained by simply replacing the time-dependent field gradient term in Eq. (10-6) with a view-angle-dependent field gradient:

$$G_\phi = G_x \cos\phi + G_y \sin\phi \qquad (10\text{-}15a)$$

and the corresponding Larmor frequency $\omega_{x'}$ by

$$\omega_{x'} = \gamma G_\phi t \qquad (10\text{-}15b)$$

Using Eqs. (10-15a) and (10-15b), Eq. (10-14) can be written as

$$S_\phi(\omega_{x'}) = M_0 \int_{x'} \int_{y'} \rho(x, y)\exp(-i\omega_{x'}x')\, dx'\, dy' \qquad (10\text{-}16)$$

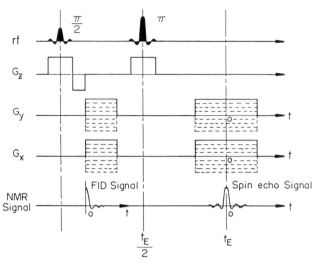

Figure 10-2 The pulse sequence for 2-D line-integral projection reconstruction. In this scheme, the z-directional gradient is used for slice selection, whereas the x- and y-directional gradients are simultaneously varied in combination to define the projection orientation according to the relation $\phi = \tan^{-1}(G_y / G_x)$. Both the FID and the spin-echo signals are illustrated.

From Eq. (10-16), the original spin density $\rho(x, y)$ can be obtained by inverse Fourier transform and backprojection as

$$\rho(x, y) = \alpha \int_0^\pi \int_{-\infty}^\infty S_\phi(\omega_{x'}) \exp(i\omega_{x'} x') |\omega_{x'}| \, d\omega_{x'} \, d\phi \qquad (10\text{-}17)$$

where α is a constant and $|\omega_{x'}|$ is Jacobian or the filter function [see Chapter 3].

An example of a unique application of projection reconstruction in NMR imaging is the magnitude method with the spin-echo technique which has been used for the correction of the phase fluctuation. Instead of the conventional spin-echo technique shown in Fig. 10-1, let us now consider a basic pulse sequence using only one 90° rf pulse, which will provide a free induction decay (FID) signal of the form given by

$$S_\phi(t) = \begin{cases} S_{\phi R}(t) + i S_{\phi I}(t), & t \geq 0 \\ 0, & t < 0 \end{cases} \qquad (10\text{-}18)$$

where $S_{\phi R}(t)$ and $S_{\phi I}(t)$ are the real and imaginary parts of the FID signal obtained by quadrature phase-sensitive detection. In this case the Fourier transform of Eq. (10-18) is given by

$$\mathcal{F}_1[S_\phi(t)] = \tfrac{1}{2}[p_\phi(x') + iq_\phi(x')] \tag{10-19}$$

where both $p_\phi(x')$ and $q_\phi(x')$ are real and imaginary components, respectively, and $\mathcal{F}_1[\cdot]$ is the 1-D Fourier transform operator. From Eqs. (10-18) and (10-19) the projection data can be obtained by taking the real part of the Fourier-transformed result.

Because of the instability of the magnet system or other instabilities (e.g., power supply instability, which amounts to 10 parts in 10^6 in some resistive magnets), the center frequency (Larmor frequency) may fluctuate at a rate of 10–100 Hz. Because of this center frequency fluctuation (or magnetic field instability), a view-angle-dependent phase shift between the FID and reference signals will cause a phase fluctuation. Equation (10-19) therefore appears as

$$\mathcal{F}_1[S_\phi(t)] = \tfrac{1}{2}[p_\phi(x') + iq_\phi(x')]\exp(i\Delta\phi) \tag{10-20}$$

Because of this phase fluctuation ($\Delta\phi$), it is difficult to obtain the phase-fluctuation-free projection data $p_\phi(x')$ alone from Eq. (10-20).

This problem can be alleviated by using the spin-echo technique, with which one can obtain a full data set both at $t < 0$ and at $t \geq 0$, where $t = 0$ corresponds to the time at the echo center. As shown below, if the full data set is obtained, it should theoretically be possible to extract the real part alone. When the spin-echo technique is used, the measured spin-echo signal $S_\phi(t)$ with a phase error $\Delta\phi$ can be written as

$$S_\phi(t) = \begin{cases} [S_{\phi R}(t) + iS_{\phi I}(t)]\exp(i\Delta\phi), & t \geq 0 \\ [S_{\phi R}(-t) - iS_{\phi I}(-t)]\exp(i\Delta\phi), & t < 0 \end{cases} \tag{10-21}$$

Since the Fourier transform of a complex-conjugate pair results in a real value, the Fourier transform of Eq. (10-21) will result in a real value with a phase delay $\exp(i\Delta\phi)$:

$$\mathcal{F}_1[S_\phi(t)] = p_\phi(x')\exp(i\Delta\phi) \tag{10-22}$$

Thus Eq. (10-22) will directly lead to a proper real value simply by taking the magnitude of Eq. (10-22):

$$|\mathcal{F}_1[S_\phi(t)]| = p_\phi(x') \tag{10-23}$$

A final image obtained by projection reconstruction using Eq. (10-23) is given by

$$\rho(x, y) = \int_0^\pi \left[p_\phi(x') * \xi(x') \right] d\phi$$

$$= \rho(r, \theta) \tag{10-24}$$

where $\theta = \tan^{-1}[y/x]$ and $*$ is a convolution operator, and $\xi(x')$ is a filter kernel, as discussed in Chapter 3.

10-3-2 Two-dimensional Fourier Imaging Based on Projection Theorem

As an alternative to the previously mentioned 2-D Fourier imaging and projection imaging, a projection-based Fourier imaging technique, which is often referred to "concentric square raster sampled Fourier imaging" will be introduced. As we have learned in Chapter 3, the projection theorem states that the Fourier transform of projection data $p_\phi(x')$ at a given view ϕ_1 is a line data in the complete set of 2-D Fourier domain data:

$$P_{\phi_1}(\omega_{x'}) = \mathscr{F}_1 \left[p_{\phi_1}(x') \right]$$

$$= F(\omega_x, \omega_y) \big|_{\phi = \phi_1} \tag{10-25}$$

where $x' = x \cos \phi_1 + y \sin \phi_1$ and is the rotated coordinate of x. Polar coordinate representation of Eq. (10-25) is also given by

$$F(\omega_{x'}, \phi_1) = F(\omega_x, \omega_y) \big|_{\phi = \phi_1} \tag{10-26}$$

where $F(\omega_x, \omega_y)$ is the complete set of 2-D Fourier domain data in cartesian coordinates.

In projection-reconstruction-based NMR imaging, Eq. (10-25) can be obtained directly from Eq. (10-14):

$$P_\phi(\omega_{x'}) = S_\phi(t) = M_0 \int_{x'} \int_{y'} \rho(x, y) \exp(-i\gamma G_\phi x' t) \, dx' \, dy'$$

$$= M_0 \int_{x'} p_\phi(x') \exp(-i\gamma G_\phi x' t) \, dx'$$

$$= M_0 \int_{x'} p_\phi(x') \exp(-i\omega_{x'} x') \, dx' \tag{10-27}$$

where $\omega_{x'} = \gamma G_\phi t$ and $G_\phi = G_x \cos \phi + G_y \sin \phi$ [see Eq. (10-15)]. A Fourier

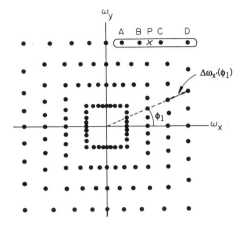

(a)

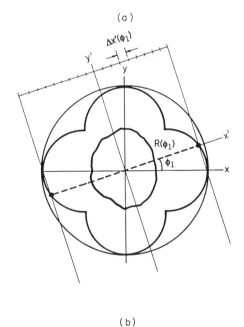

(b)

Figure 10-3 (a) Sampled points in concentric square raster scanning with variable $\Delta\omega_{x'}(\phi_1)$. These samples provide cartesian coordinate samples by simply using 1-D interpolation. (b) Spatial domain path of concentric square raster scanning. This path indicates that the sampling width with a fixed number of sample points is dependent on the view angle ϕ; that is, the largest spatial domain sampling width appears at $\phi = 0°$ and $90°$ while the smallest sampling window appears at $\phi = 45°$ and $135°$.

domain data set $F(\omega_x, \omega_y)$ in cartesian coordinates (ω_x, ω_y) is the most desirable form for 2-D Fourier domain data processing due to the readily available algorithms such as the FFT (fast Fourier transform). For this reason concentric square raster samples similar to the one shown in Fig. 10-3(a) are the desirable sampled data pattern. A characteristic of the sampling pattern shown in Fig. 10-3(a) is variable sampling in the (ω_x, ω_y) domain depending on the angle ϕ; that is, the finest sampling occurs at $\phi = 0°$ and $90°$, while the coarsest occurs at $\phi = 45°$ and $135°$. Such a sampling pattern can easily be obtained in NMR imaging simply by varying the G_ϕ. Since $\Delta\omega_{x'}(\phi) \propto 1/(\Delta x'(\phi))$ or $\Delta x' \propto 1/(\Delta\omega_{x'})$, and also $\Delta x' \propto 1/G_\phi$, it is easy to vary the sampling interval $\Delta\omega_{x'}$ by simply adjusting the G_ϕ as a function of view angle ϕ. In fact such a pattern in the Fourier domain can be obtained by varying gradient strength, as shown in Fig. 10-3(b); that is, exerts the maximum gradient at $\phi = 0°$ and $90°$, while the minimum gradient at $\phi = 45°$. Naturally concentric square raster sampling such as shown in Fig. 10-3(a) provides a well ordered set of cartesian coordinate samples which allows simple 1-D interpolation as shown; that is, sample point P can be obtained by a 1-D interpolation of the A, B, C, and D points. The advantages of this 1-D interpolation can be appreciated when it is compared with the 2-D interpolation that would be needed in the case of concentric circular raster sampled data, which is obtained by conventional projection data acquisition (compare Figs. 10-3(a) and 10-4). Concentric square raster sampling is particularly interesting in NMR imaging due to the fact that it can easily be obtained by simply changing the gradient strengths G_ϕ according to the path shown in Fig. 10-3(b).

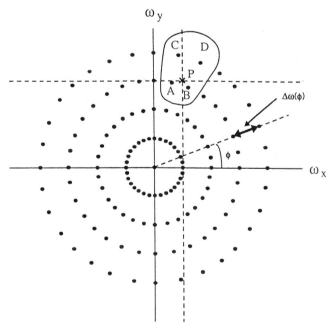

Figure 10-4 Sampled points in concentric circular raster scanning with an equal $\Delta\omega(\phi)$. To obtain cartesian coordinate samples from the concentric raster sampled data, a 2-D interpolation would be needed. For example, estimation of the point P in cartesian coordinates requires 2-D interpolation of points A, B, C, and D.

10-3-3   Three-dimensional Planar-Integral Projection Reconstruction

Like the 2-D line-integral projection reconstruction algorithm, the planar projection reconstruction (PPR) algorithm can be derived from the 2-D concept developed earlier. This approach was taken elegantly by Shepp [4] in NMR imaging and independently by others [5, 6]. In some cases the latter method [5, 6] has a computational advantage compared with the former algorithm. The new fast imaging method that we will discuss in this section is based on the latter, although the basic principles of the two methods are essentially the same (refer also to Chapter 3).

Let us first consider a spherically symmetric case. We assume that the planar-integral data are collected with uniform sampling intervals in all directions in spherical coordinates (θ, ϕ). The original image function $\rho(x, y, z)$ then can be obtained from the inverse Fourier transform of the Fourier domain planar-integral data $P(\omega_R, \theta, \phi)$ [4]:

$$\rho(x, y, z) = \left(\frac{1}{2\pi}\right)^3 \int_0^\pi \int_0^\pi \int_{-\infty}^\infty P(\omega_R, \theta, \phi) \omega_R^2 \sin\theta \exp(-iR\omega_R)\, d\omega_R\, d\theta\, d\phi$$

$$(10\text{-}28)$$

where $P(\omega_R, \theta, \phi)$ is the NMR signal obtained from NMR imaging, $\omega_R^2 \sin\theta$ is the Jacobian arising from the coordinate transformation, and R (where ω_R is the spatial frequency of R) is given by

$$R = x \sin\theta \cos\phi + y \sin\theta \sin\phi + z \cos\theta \qquad (10\text{-}29)$$

Equation (10-28) can further be simplified to

$$\rho(x, y, z) = \left(\frac{1}{2\pi}\right)^2 \int_0^\pi \int_0^\pi p_1^*(R, \theta, \phi) \sin\theta\, d\theta\, d\phi \qquad (10\text{-}30)$$

where $p_1^*(R, \theta, \phi)$ is the convolved or filtered spatial domain planar-integral projection data:

$$p_1^*(R, \theta, \phi) = \frac{1}{2\pi} \int_{-\infty}^\infty P(\omega_R, \theta, \phi) \Psi(\omega_R) \exp(-iR\omega_R)\, d\omega_R \qquad (10\text{-}31)$$

where $\Psi(\omega_R) = \omega_R^2$. It is interesting to note that $p_1^*(R, \theta, \phi)$ is equal to the second derivative of the projection data (the derivatives of Fourier transforms; see Chapter 2):

$$p_1^*(R, \theta, \phi) = -p''(R, \theta, \phi) \qquad (10\text{-}32)$$

where $p(R, \theta, \phi)$ is given by

$$p(R, \theta, \phi) = \frac{1}{2\pi} \int_{-\infty}^{\infty} P(\omega_R, \theta, \phi) \exp(-iR\omega_R) \, d\omega_R \qquad (10\text{-}33)$$

By using Eq. (10-32), Eq. (10-30) can be rewritten as

$$\rho(x, y, z) = -\left(\frac{1}{2\pi}\right)^2 \int_0^\pi \int_0^\pi p''(R, \theta, \phi) \sin\theta \, d\theta \, d\phi. \qquad (10\text{-}34)$$

Implementation of Eq. (10-28) or (10-34) requires the optimization of the filter function $\Psi(\omega_R) = \omega_R^2$. Shepp's approach to this filter function was an extension of the 2-D filter, which is given by (see also Chapter 3)

$$\Psi(\omega_R) = \left[\frac{2}{a} \sin(\omega_R)\right]^2 \qquad (10\text{-}35)$$

where a is a sampling interval of the projection data $p(R, \theta, \phi)$. The spatial domain convolution kernel $\psi(\pm a)$ derived from Eq. (10-35), the spatial frequency domain correspondence $\Psi(\omega_R)$, results in an interesting short-range convolution kernel given by

$$\psi(0) = \frac{2}{a^3}$$

$$\psi(\pm a) = -\frac{1}{a^3}$$

$$\psi(\pm a) = 0, \qquad |k| > 1 \qquad (10\text{-}36)$$

This convolution kernel is known as the *three-point filter*, and it leads to the following simple result for the convolved planar-integral projection data:

$$p_1^*(R_k, \theta_i, \phi_j) = \frac{1}{a^3}\left[2p(R_k, \theta_i, \phi_j) - p(R_{k-1}, \theta_i, \phi_j) - p(R_{k+1}, \theta_i, \phi_j)\right] \qquad (10\text{-}37)$$

where R_k is the sampling point of R at k ($k = 0, \pm 1, \pm 2, \ldots$).

There are several variations of the direct planar-integral method discussed above, such as the indirect two-stage method given in the following [7]. A brief discussion will be given on the indirect two-stage method which consists of the following two operational steps. The first step is the formation of a 2-D projection image by a filtered back projection of the planar-integral projection data set obtained at a given ϕ. This first-stage image reconstruction process is identical to that of conventional 2-D image reconstruction from the line-integral data:

$$g(r, z)_\phi = \left(\frac{1}{2\pi}\right)^2 \int_0^\pi \int_{-\infty}^\infty P(\omega_R, \theta)_\phi |\omega_R| \exp[-i\omega_R(r\sin\theta + z\cos\theta)] \, d\omega_R \, d\theta$$

$$= \frac{1}{2\pi} \int_0^\pi \int_{-\infty}^\infty p(\tau, \theta)_\phi \psi_1(R - \tau) \, d\tau \, d\theta \qquad (10\text{-}38)$$

where $R = r\sin\theta + z\cos\theta$, $r = x\cos\phi + y\sin\phi$, and $\psi_1(R)$ is the familiar one-dimensional convolution kernel used in the 2-D case. Note that $g(r, z)_\phi$ is the first-stage 2-D image that provides the line-integral projection data necessary for second-stage image reconstruction. The latter being the final image. An exemplary illustration of the two-stage reconstruction is given in Fig. 10-5.

A plane or slice perpendicular to the z-axis at a given z-value can now be reconstructed by using the images reconstructed by using the data acquired at first stage, that is, $g(r, z)_\phi$,

$$\rho(x, y; z) = \frac{1}{2\pi} \int_0^\pi \int_{-\infty}^\infty g(\tau, z)_\phi \psi_2(r - \tau) \, d\tau \, d\phi \qquad (10\text{-}39)$$

where $\psi_2(\tau)$ is again the same one-dimensional convolution kernel, as used in the 2-D case. By stacking the 2-D images obtained above, a 3-D volume image can be formed.

A more direct expression of the stacked 3-D volume image can be obtained by use of the cylindrical coordinates:

$$\rho(x, y, z) = \left(\frac{1}{2\pi}\right)^3 \int_0^\pi \int_{-\infty}^\infty \int_{-\infty}^\infty F(\omega_r, \phi, \omega_z) |\omega_r|$$

$$\times \exp\{-i[\omega_r(x\cos\phi + y\sin\phi) + z\omega_z]\} \, d\omega_r \, d\omega_z \, d\phi$$

$$= \left(\frac{1}{2\pi}\right)^3 \int_0^\pi \int_{-\infty}^\infty G(\omega_r, \phi, z) |\omega_r| \exp(-ir\omega_r) \, d\omega_r \, d\phi \qquad (10\text{-}40)$$

where $F(\omega_r, \phi, \omega_z)$ is the 3-D Fourier transform of $\rho(x, y, z)$ expressed in cylindrical coordinates and ω_r and ω_z are the spatial frequencies corresponding to r and z, respectively. Note here that we also assumed that $G(\omega_r, \phi, z) = F(\omega_r, \phi, z)$. Since $g(r, \phi, z)$ and $G(\omega_r, \phi, z)$ are related by

$$g(r, \phi, z) = \frac{1}{2\pi} \int_{-\infty}^\infty G(\omega_r, \phi, z) \exp(-ir\omega_r) \, d\omega_r$$

$$= g(r, z)_\phi \qquad (10\text{-}41)$$

Eq. (10-40) suggests that the filtered backprojection of $g(r, \phi, z)$ will finally reconstruct the 3-D volume image if the Fourier domain planar-integral

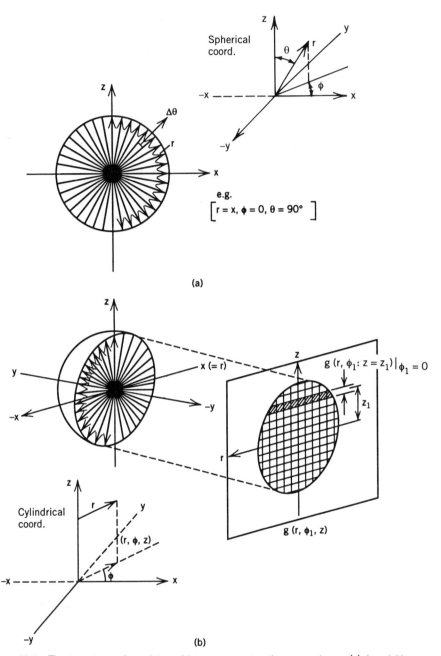

Figure 10-5 The two-stage planar-integral image reconstruction procedures: (a) Acquisition first-stage planar-integral projection data; (b) one image reconstructed from the planar-integral projection data obtained from (a) or at a given view angle ϕ_1. From this image data, various line-integral data can be derived along the z-direction and used for the final slice image reconstructions where each reconstructed slice is perpendicular to the z-axis.

projection data $F(\omega_r, \phi, \omega_z)$ exists. Since the NMR signal obtained is not in the form $F(\omega_r, \phi, \omega_z)$ but in the form $F(\omega_R, \theta, \phi) = P(\omega_R, \theta, \phi)$, first-stage reconstruction should be written in the form of spherical coordinates rather than cylindrical coordinates as given in Eqs. (10-40) and (10-41). Equation (10-41) therefore can be rewritten as

$$g(r, \phi, z) = \left(\frac{1}{2\pi}\right)^2 \int_0^\pi \int_{-\infty}^\infty P(\omega_R, \theta, \phi) |\omega_R| \exp(-iR\omega_R) \, d\omega_R \, d\theta \quad (10\text{-}42)$$

where $P(\omega_R, \theta, \phi)$ is the Fourier domain planar-integral projection data obtained at a vector or view (θ, ϕ) and $|\omega_R|$ is the Jacobian. It is now interesting to note that Eq. (10-42) explicitly indicates that $g(r, \phi, z)$ is the superposed image backprojected around θ at a given ϕ. This is the 2-D projection image that we have discussed previously in Eq. (10-38). Therefore an additional filtration and backprojection around ϕ at a given z will finally provide the reconstructed slice image:

$$\rho(x, y; z) = \frac{1}{2\pi} \int_0^\pi \int_{-\infty}^\infty g(\tau, \phi; z) \psi_2(r - \tau) \, d\tau \, d\phi \quad (10\text{-}43)$$

where $\psi_2(\tau)$ is again a one-dimensional convolution kernel and can be assumed to be the same as $\psi_1(\tau)$. Note that Eq. (10-43) is consistent with Eq. (10-39) except for slight differences in notation. An example of a reconstruction process at $z = z_1$ with $\phi = \phi_1 = 0$ and its relation to the $g(r, \phi, z)$, that is, $g(r, \phi_1; z = z_1)\phi_1 = 0$, is illustrated in Figs. 10-5(b).

10-4   ENCODING METHODS FOR MULTISLICE IMAGING

10-4-1   Encoding Matrices

To increase the SNR in NMR imaging, a large volume or multiple slices should be excited, and the nuclear signal must be collected from the large excited volume. As previously discussed, the line-integral projection data that lead to a single-slice imaging usually result in a relatively small signal, and therefore an image of relatively poor SNR. Consequently, a large amount of signal averaging is required to enhance the SNR. In some cases, the time spent in acquiring data for averaging can be better utilized for other operations such as multislice imaging [2, 8]. Three-dimensional tomography, in which one attempts to excite the entire volume, however, is found to be difficult in NMR [3, 9] because of the excessively long image data acquisition time due to the increased number of encoding steps. For example, total-volume imaging with the previously discussed PPR technique might require as much time as $N_\theta N_\phi T_R$, where N_θ and N_ϕ are the numbers of views required in spherical coordinates and T_R is the repetition time. In conventional spin-echo NMR imaging, it is found that the total data acquisition time necessary for complete data collection is on the order of an hour for total-volume imaging. However, it should be noted that each echo signal obtained at a given view with total-volume excitation is relatively large, so signal averaging is usually not required. Considering the above limitations, it is interesting to investigate the trade-off between the number of data acquisitions for averaging and the number of slices to be imaged with the multislice encoding technique using line-integral projection reconstruction.* In this multislice encoding technique, a trade-off should be made between the amount of data necessary for the imaging or a certain desired number of slices and the imaging time.

In fact, there are several useful encoding matrices that can be used in conjunction with multislice Fourier imaging or line-integral projection reconstruction. Let $M_{\phi j}(t)$ be the sum signal arising from m different slices at the jth sequence for a given view ϕ. By repeating m sequences with different encodings, m sum signals or a set of signals from which m slice images can be reconstructed will be obtained:

$$
\mathbf{M}_\phi^m(t) = \begin{bmatrix} M_{\phi 1}(t) \\ M_{\phi 2}(t) \\ \vdots \\ M_{\phi j}(t) \\ \vdots \\ M_{\phi m}(t) \end{bmatrix}
\tag{10-44}
$$

Equation (10-44) may also be written in terms of the combined sets of an ideal single-slice NMR signal arising from each slice as

$$
\mathbf{M}_\phi^m(t) = E_{mm} \mathbf{S}_\phi^m(t)
\tag{10-45}
$$

where E_{mm} is an encoding matrix and

$$
\mathbf{S}_\phi^m(t) = \begin{bmatrix} S_{\phi 1}(t) \\ S_{\phi 2}(t) \\ \vdots \\ S_{\phi j}(t) \\ \vdots \\ S_{\phi m}(t) \end{bmatrix}
\tag{10-46}
$$

$S_{\phi 1}(t), S_{\phi 2}(t), \ldots$ are the NMR signals arising from each corresponding slice;

*This technique obviously applicable to Fourier imaging.

that is, $S_{\phi 1}(t), S_{\phi 2}(t), \ldots$ represent the NMR signal from slice 1, 2, and so on. An example of the encoding matrix can be given as

$$
E_{mm} =
\begin{bmatrix}
e_{11} & e_{12} & \cdots & e_{1k} & \cdots & e_{1m} \\
e_{21} & e_{22} & \cdots & e_{2k} & \cdots & e_{2m} \\
\vdots & \vdots & & \vdots & & \vdots \\
e_{j1} & e_{j2} & \cdots & e_{jk} & & e_{jm} \\
\vdots & \vdots & & \vdots & & \vdots \\
e_{m1} & e_{m2} & \cdots & e_{mk} & \cdots & e_{mm}
\end{bmatrix}
\tag{10-47}
$$

where $|e_{jk}| \leq 1$ for $1 \leq (j, k) \leq m$, and the encoding matrix E_{mm} should be an $m \times m$ nonsingular matrix. Since $S_{\phi k}(t)$ represents the slice-resolved signal from the kth slice, the desired data or the set $\mathbf{S}_{\phi}^m(t)$ can be obtained by multiplying Eq. (10-45) by the inverse of E_{mm}:

$$
\mathbf{S}_{\phi}^m(t) = E_{mm}^{-1}\mathbf{M}_{\phi}^m(t)
\tag{10-48}
$$

where the inverse matrix E_{mm}^{-1} now represents the decoding matrix. In an optimum encoding technique the decoding matrix E_{mm}^{-1} can be represented as

$$
E_{mm}^{-1} = \frac{1}{m}E_{mm}^T
\tag{10-49}
$$

where E_{mm}^T is the transpose matrix of E_{mm}.

10-4-2 SNR Enhancement in the Encoding Technique

Keeping the above results in mind, let us now investigate the possible gain obtainable with the encoding method from an experimentally obtained NMR signal corrupted by noise. In Eq. (10-45) let us assume that a zero-mean Gaussian noise $\mathbf{n}_{\phi}^m(t)$ is added to the the ideal NMR signal $\mathbf{M}_{\phi}^m(t)$:

$$
\tilde{\mathbf{M}}_{\phi}^m(t) = \mathbf{M}_{\phi}^m(t) + \mathbf{n}_{\phi}^m(t) = E_{mm}\mathbf{S}_{\phi}^m(t) + \mathbf{n}_{\phi}^m(t)
\tag{10-50}
$$

Assuming that $n_{\phi j}(t)$ is uncorrelated with $S_{\phi k}(t)$ and also with $n_{\phi l}(t)$ for $1 \leq (j, k, l) \leq m$ and $j \neq l$, it can be shown that the mean and the covariance of $\tilde{\mathbf{M}}_{\phi}^m$ are given by [10]

$$
\mathrm{mean}\left[\tilde{\mathbf{M}}_{\phi}^m(t)\right] = E_{mm}\mathbf{S}_{\phi}^m(t)
\tag{10-51}
$$

and

$$
\mathrm{cov}\left[\tilde{\mathbf{M}}_{\phi}^m(t)\right] = \sigma^2 I_{mm}
\tag{10-52}
$$

where σ^2 is the noise variance observed in each summed or encoded NMR signal and I_{mm} is the $m \times m$ identity matrix.

In the method of least square errors, the estimates of the $\mathbf{S}_\phi^m(t)$, that is, $\tilde{\mathbf{S}}_\phi^m(t)$, should satisfy the following equation [11]:

$$\frac{\partial Q^2}{\partial \mathbf{S}_\phi^m(t)} = 0 \tag{10-53}$$

where

$$Q^2 = \sum_{j=1}^{m} \sum_{k=1}^{m} \left\{\tilde{M}_{\phi j}(t) - \text{mean}\left[\tilde{M}_{\phi j}(t)\right]\right\}[\mathbf{V}^{-1}]_{jk}\left\{\tilde{M}_{\phi k}(t) - \text{mean}\left[\tilde{M}_{\phi k}(t)\right]\right\} \tag{10-54}$$

$[\mathbf{V}^{-1}]$ in Eq. (10-54) is the inverse of the covariance matrix [see the covariance matrix given in Eq. (10-52)].

The solution of Eq. (10-53) gives the least squares estimate of $\mathbf{S}_\phi^m(t)$, which is given by [11]

$$\tilde{\mathbf{S}}_\phi^m(t) = \left[E_{mm}^{*T}\mathbf{V}^{-1}E_{mm}\right]^{-1}E_{mm}^{*T}\mathbf{V}^{-1}\tilde{\mathbf{M}}_\phi^m(t) = \left[E_{mm}^{*T}E_{mm}\right]^{-1}E_{mm}^{*T}\tilde{\mathbf{M}}_\phi^m(t) \tag{10-55}$$

where E_{mm}^{*T} is the Hermitian conjugate of the encoding matrix E_{mm}. It can be shown that the mean$[\tilde{\mathbf{S}}_\phi^m(t)]$ and the cov$[\tilde{\mathbf{S}}_\phi^m(t)]$ are given by [12]

$$\text{mean}\left[\tilde{\mathbf{S}}_\phi^m(t)\right] = \mathbf{S}_\phi^m(t) \tag{10-56}$$

and

$$\text{cov}\left[\tilde{\mathbf{S}}_\phi^m(t)\right] = \sigma^2\left[E_{mm}^{*T}E_{mm}\right]^{-1} \tag{10-57}$$

From the previous condition that $|e_{jk}| \leq 1$, the variance of each estimated signal $\tilde{S}_{\phi k}(t)$ cannot be less than σ^2/m [10]:

$$\text{var}\left[\tilde{S}_{\phi k}(t)\right] \geq \frac{\sigma^2}{m}, \qquad 1 \leq k \leq m \tag{10-58}$$

In the expression given in Eq. (10-58), the equality is valid when

$$E_{mm}^{*T}E_{mm} = mI_{mm} \tag{10-59}$$

Note here that the matrix E_{mm}^{*T} is equal to the transpose matrix E_{mm}^{T}. Together with Eq. (10-59), Eq. (10-58) indicates that the variance of the estimated NMR signal $\tilde{S}_\phi^m(t)$ for each slice (i.e., the noise variance $\tilde{\sigma}^2$ of the decoded NMR signal) is now reduced by a factor of $1/m$:

$$\tilde{\sigma}^2 = \frac{\sigma^2}{m} \tag{10-60}$$

Equation (10-60) leads to the well-known SNR-enhancement factor $\sqrt{m}$ in Gaussian random processes when the experiments are repeated m times. For m encoded multislice imaging therefore the SNR improves by a factor $\sqrt{m}$ and produces m-slice images, compared to the single-slice imaging, which produces only a one-slice image with the same improvement of the SNR (i.e., a factor of $\sqrt{m}$).

10-4-3 Some Useful Encoding Matrices

There are a number of unitary matrices that can be used for encoding in which the SNR can be enhanced. Among others, Fourier, Hadamard-like, sine, and cosine transform matrices are currently known and can be applied to the encoding techniques discussed earlier. It should be noted, however, that the application of transform matrices of some forms have less than ideal SNR enhancement (i.e., always larger than σ^2/m). In this subsection we discuss a few examples applicable to NMR imaging.

Fourier Encoding Matrix
The most widely known and often used encoding matrix is the Fourier transform matrix, whose elements are given by

$$e_{jk} = \exp\left[i\frac{2\pi}{m}(j-1)(k-1)\right], \qquad 1 \le (j, k) \le m \tag{10-61}$$

where m is the number of discrete sample points that represents the number of slices to be coded in NMR imaging. An example of a matrix for four-slice encoding (i.e., $m = 4$) can be given as

$$E_{F44} = \begin{bmatrix} 1 & 1 & 1 & 1 \\ 1 & \sqrt{-1} & -1 & -\sqrt{-1} \\ 1 & -1 & 1 & -1 \\ 1 & -\sqrt{-1} & -1 & \sqrt{-1} \end{bmatrix} \tag{10-62}$$

where F denotes the Fourier encoding while 44 represents the mm. Since this Fourier encoding matrix satisfies the condition of Eq. (10-59), the noise variance of the decoded NMR signal is reduced by a factor of $1/m$. This matrix coding can be achieved by variation of the gradient pulse amplitude similar to the Fourier imaging discussed previously [13, 14] (e.g., in the z direction) or by coding the selective rf pulse (i.e., the rf spectrum coding).

Hadamard and Hadamard-like Encoding Matrices

Hadamard encoding, whose basic form consists of 1 or -1, is often used in conjunction with selective rf pulses [2, 8, 15]. The basic form of an unnormalized Hadamard matrix is given by

$$E_{H_{2m \cdot 2m}} = \begin{bmatrix} E_{H_{mm}} & E_{H_{mm}} \\ E_{H_{mm}} & -E_{H_{mm}} \end{bmatrix} \tag{10-63}$$

where H denotes the Hadamard matrix and $E_{H_{mm}}$ is given by

$$E_{H_{mm}}\big|_{m=2} = E_{H_{22}} = \begin{bmatrix} 1 & 1 \\ 1 & -1 \end{bmatrix} \tag{10-64}$$

The element e_{jk} of the Hadamard encoding matrix $E_{H_{mm}}$ may be written as

$$e_{jk} = (-1)^{\sum_{l=0}^{n-1}\{(j-1)_l(k-1)_l\}} \tag{10-65}$$

where $n = \log_2 m$, and $(j)_l$ and $(k)_l$ are the lth bit in the binary representation of j and k, respectively. Hadamard encoding is one of the most simple and effective encoding matrices and has the property of reducing the noise variance by $1/m$.

The Hadamard-like encoding matrix, a variation of the Hadamard encoding matrix, is basically similar to the Hadamard matrix except that it has a slightly different pattern; the matrix consists of -1 along the diagonal axis and $+1$ elsewhere:

$$e_{jk} = \begin{cases} -1, & j = k \\ 1, & j \neq k \end{cases} \tag{10-66}$$

An example of $E_{HL_{mm}}$ with $m = 4$ is given by

$$E_{HL44} = \begin{bmatrix} -1 & 1 & 1 & 1 \\ 1 & -1 & 1 & 1 \\ 1 & 1 & -1 & 1 \\ 1 & 1 & 1 & -1 \end{bmatrix} \tag{10-67}$$

where HL denotes the Hadamard-like matrix. The general Hadamard-like matrix form is the same as the one given in Eq. (10-63) for $m > 4$, and the noise variance is again reduced by $1/m$.

Sine and Cosine Transform Encoding Matrices

Although the statistical gain attainable with either the sine transform or cosine transform encoding matrix is less than those attainable with the aforementioned Fourier, Hadamard, and Hadamard-like transform matrices, the sine and cosine transform matrices possess unique and interesting properties that are worth noting. The sine transform has a similar form to the Fourier transform matrix:

$$e_{jk} = \sin\left(\frac{jk}{m+1}\pi\right) \tag{10-68}$$

An example of $E_{S_{mm}}$ with $m = 4$ is given by

$$E_{S44} = \begin{bmatrix} \sin\dfrac{\pi}{5} & \sin\dfrac{2\pi}{5} & \sin\dfrac{2\pi}{5} & \sin\dfrac{\pi}{5} \\[2ex] \sin\dfrac{2\pi}{5} & \sin\dfrac{\pi}{5} & -\sin\dfrac{\pi}{5} & -\sin\dfrac{2\pi}{5} \\[2ex] \sin\dfrac{2\pi}{5} & -\sin\dfrac{\pi}{5} & -\sin\dfrac{\pi}{5} & \sin\dfrac{2\pi}{5} \\[2ex] \sin\dfrac{\pi}{5} & -\sin\dfrac{2\pi}{5} & \sin\dfrac{2\pi}{5} & -\sin\dfrac{\pi}{5} \end{bmatrix} \tag{10-69}$$

where S denotes the sine transform encoding matrix. E_{S44}^{-1} is given by

$$E_{S44}^{-1} = \tfrac{2}{5}E_{S44}^T \tag{10-70}$$

Consequently the noise variance is reduced to $\tfrac{2}{5}$ (compared with the Fourier and Hadamard encodings where variance is reduced to $\tfrac{1}{4}$):

$$E_{S44}^T E_{S44} = \left(\tfrac{5}{2}\right)I_{44} \tag{10-71}$$

The cosine transform matrix is similar to the sine transform matrix and the elements e_{jk} are given by

$$e_{jk} = \begin{cases} \dfrac{1}{\sqrt{2}}, & j = 1 \\[2ex] \cos\left[\dfrac{\pi(j-1)}{m}\left(k - \dfrac{1}{2}\right)\right], & \text{otherwise} \end{cases} \tag{10-72}$$

Table 10-1 Transform matrices for the multislice encoding technique

	Matrix E				
	Fourier (E_F)	Hadamard[a] (E_H)	Hadamard-like (E_{HL})	Sine (E_S)	Cosine (E_C)
$e_{jk} \, 1 \le j, k \le m \, (= 4)$	$\exp\left[i \dfrac{2\pi(j-1)(k-1)}{4} \right]$	$e_{jk} = (-1)^{\sum_{l=0}^{\eta-1}(j-1)_l(k-1)_l}$	$\begin{array}{l} -1, \ \text{for } j = k \\ 1, \ \text{for } j \ne k \end{array}$	$\sin\!\left(\dfrac{jk\pi}{5}\right)$	$\dfrac{1}{\sqrt{2}} \ \text{for } j = 1$ $\cos\!\left[\dfrac{\alpha}{4}(j-1)\left(k - \dfrac{1}{2}\right)\right]$ $\text{for } j \ne 1$
SNR gain $(= 4)$	$\sqrt{4}$	$\sqrt{4}$	$\sqrt{4}$	$\sqrt{\dfrac{5}{2}}$	$\sqrt{2}$
rf Pulse coding	Yes	Yes	Yes	Yes	Yes
Gradient pulse coding	Yes	No	No	No	No
Matrix characteristic $(= 4)$	$E_F^{*T} E_F = 4I$	$E_H^T E_H = 4I$	$E_{HL}^T E_{HL} = 4I$	$E_S^T E_S = \tfrac{5}{2}I$	$E_C^T E_C = 2I$

[a] $(j-1)_l$ and $(k-1)_l$ are the bit states of the binary representations of $(j-1)$ and $(k-1)$.

[b] E^T is the transpose of E, I is the identity matrix, and E^{*T} is the transconjugate of E.

292

From Eq. (10-72), a 4 × 4 cosine encoding matrix is given as

$$
E_{C44} = \begin{bmatrix} \dfrac{1}{\sqrt{2}} & \dfrac{1}{\sqrt{2}} & \dfrac{1}{\sqrt{2}} & \dfrac{1}{\sqrt{2}} \\[2mm] \cos\dfrac{\pi}{8} & \sin\dfrac{\pi}{8} & -\sin\dfrac{\pi}{8} & -\cos\dfrac{\pi}{8} \\[2mm] \dfrac{1}{\sqrt{2}} & \dfrac{1}{\sqrt{2}} & \dfrac{1}{\sqrt{2}} & \dfrac{1}{\sqrt{2}} \\[2mm] \sin\dfrac{\pi}{8} & -\cos\dfrac{\pi}{8} & \cos\dfrac{\pi}{8} & -\sin\dfrac{\pi}{8} \end{bmatrix} \qquad (10\text{-}73)
$$

where C denotes the cosine transform encoding matrix. The inverse matrix of the cosine encoding matrix E_{C44} is given by

$$
E_{C44}^{-1} = \tfrac{1}{2}E_{C44}^{T} \qquad (10\text{-}74)
$$

The resultant noise variance is $\sigma^2/2$ for a 4 × 4 matrix, and

$$
E_{C44}^{T}E_{C44} = 2I_{44} \qquad (10\text{-}75)
$$

In Table 10-1 a summary of some useful unitary transform matrices and their SNR gains is given for reference. It should be noted that each transform encoding matrix requires a specific coding technique. For example, a Hadamard or Hadamard-like encoding matrix requires rf pulse spectrum encoding, whereas Fourier encoding can be performed either by rf pulse spectrum encoding (discrete case) or gradient encoding (pulse variations). In the next section an example of the Hadamard-like encoding technique applied to the case of multislice imaging will be given.

10-4-4 Example of Hadamard-like Encoding Technique Applied to Multislice Imaging

As was mentioned earlier, the Hadamard or Hadamard-like encoding method requires rf spectrum encoding. An example of the rf pulse spectrum for the four-slice encoding technique [15] is shown in Fig. 10-6. Because of the spectrum composition, spin-echo techniques of both the Hahn and the Carr-Purcell-Meiboom-Gill (CPMG) types are needed, that is, with the Hahn spin-echo technique a negative echo signal is obtained, while with the CPMG technique a positive echo signal is obtained. At each view m different kinds of rf pulse sets are needed, each with a specific spectral composition that corresponds to the Fourier transform of the Hadamard-like sequence, as described earlier (see Fig. 10-6).

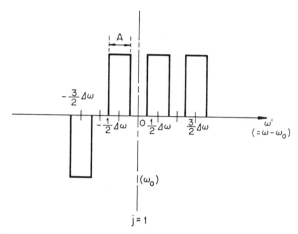

Figure 10-6 The rf pulse spectrum of the first row (i.e., $j = 1$) of Hadamard-like matrix encoding. A is the slice thickness (i.e., bandwidth), and $\Delta\omega$ is the separation distance between the slices.

Let us investigate an example of an rf pulse set using the Hahn and CPMG spin-echo techniques. First, assume that the spin echo is that of Hahn's and has an rf pulse 'spectrum of a finite bandwidth A (rectangular bandwidth) with a center frequency shift of an amount $\Delta\omega$ from ω_0 (i.e., Larmor frequency). Then, by invoking Fourier convolution theorem, its corresponding time domain rf pulse can be obtained and is given by

$$RF_H(t) = \frac{A}{2}\,\text{sinc}\left(\frac{A}{2}t\right)\cos(\omega_0 + \Delta\omega)t = SC_H(t)\cos(\omega_0 t) + SS_H(t)\sin(\omega_0 t)$$

$$(10\text{-}76)$$

where H denotes Hahn's echo, A is the bandwidth of a selected slice, and $SC_H(t)$ and $SS_H(t)$ are the modulating pulses given by

$$SC_H(t) = \frac{A}{2}\,\text{sinc}\left(\frac{A}{2}t\right)\cos(\Delta\omega t)$$

$$SS_H(t) = -\frac{A}{2}\,\text{sinc}\left(\frac{A}{2}t\right)\sin(\Delta\omega t) \qquad (10\text{-}77)$$

On the other hand, when Eq. (10-76) is replaced with the CPMG spin-echo technique, the polarity of the signal will be reversed compared with that of the Hahn echo; that is, it becomes positive. The CPMG technique simply requires a phase change of $\pi/2$:

$$RF_C(t) = \frac{A}{2} \operatorname{sinc}\left(\frac{A}{2}t\right)\cos\left[(\omega_0 + \Delta\omega)t + \frac{\pi}{2}\right]$$

$$= SC_C(t)\cos(\omega_0 t) + SS_C(t)\sin(\omega_0 t) \qquad (10\text{-}78)$$

where C denotes CPMG and $SC_C(t)$ and $SS_C(t)$ are given by

$$SC_C(t) = -\frac{A}{2} \operatorname{sinc}\left(\frac{A}{2}t\right)\sin(\Delta\omega t)$$

$$SS_C(t) = -\frac{A}{2} \operatorname{sinc}\left(\frac{A}{2}t\right)\cos(\Delta\omega t) \qquad (10\text{-}79)$$

Knowing the desired polarity of the output signal of each slice, choice of the Hahn and the CPMG spin-echo sequences can be made depending on the desired output signal polarity.

Based on the above rf pulse excitation rule, an example of the spectral composition set shown in Fig. 10-6, a first rf pulse of the set, for example, $j = 1$, can be derived and is given by

$$\begin{aligned}
{}_4RF_j(t)\big|_{j=1} &= \frac{A}{2} \operatorname{sinc}\left(\frac{A}{2}t\right)\left[\cos\left(-\frac{3}{2}\Delta\omega t\right) - \sin\left(-\frac{1}{2}\Delta\omega t\right)\right. \\
&\qquad \left. - \sin\left(\frac{1}{2}\Delta\omega t\right) - \sin\left(\frac{3}{2}\Delta\omega t\right)\right]\cos(\omega_0 t) \\
&\quad + \frac{A}{2} \operatorname{sinc}\left(\frac{A}{2}t\right)\left[-\sin\left(-\frac{3}{2}\Delta\omega t\right) - \cos\left(-\frac{1}{2}\Delta\omega t\right)\right. \\
&\qquad \left. - \cos\left(\frac{1}{2}\Delta\omega t\right) - \cos\left(\frac{3}{2}\Delta\omega t\right)\right]\sin(\omega_0 t) \qquad (10\text{-}80)
\end{aligned}$$

where j represents the row number; therefore Eq. (10-80) is the case of the first row or first rf pulse spectrum out of four sequences. Subsequent sets ${}_4RF_2(t)$, ${}_4RF_3(t)$, and ${}_4RF_4(t)$ can be generated in a similar fashion. Equation (10-80) can be written in a more compact form as

$$_4RF_j(t) = SC_j(t)\cos(\omega_0 t) + SS_j(t)\sin(\omega_0 t) \qquad (10\text{-}81)$$

where $SC_j(t)$ and $SS_j(t)$ are given by

$$SC_j(t) = \frac{A}{2} \text{sinc}\left(\frac{A}{2}t\right)\left[\sum_{k=1}^{4}\left\{\frac{e_{jk}+1}{2}C[C_k(t)] - \frac{e_{jk}-1}{2}H[C_k(t)]\right\}\right]$$

$$SS_j(t) = \frac{A}{2} \text{sinc}\left(\frac{A}{2}t\right)\left[\sum_{k=1}^{4}\left\{\frac{e_{jk}+1}{2}C[S_k(t)] - \frac{e_{jk}-1}{2}H[S_k(t)]\right\}\right]$$

$$(10\text{-}82)$$

In Eq. (10-82), e_{jk} is the encoding matrix element of the jth row with the kth column, and $C[C_k(t)]$, $C[S_k(t)]$, $H[C_k(t)]$, and $H[S_k(t)]$ are the rf pulse wave forms that will be modulated with $\cos(\omega_0 t)$ and $\sin(\omega_0 t)$ in conjunction with the CPMG and the Hahn spin-echo techniques, respectively. The values corresponding to the above cases are tabulated in Table 10-2 for $1 \le m \le 4$. In Fig. 10-7 the rf pulse waveforms $SC_j(t)$ and $SS_j(t)$ corresponding to the above example are shown for $1 \le j \le 4$.

Table 10-2 Components of the rf pulse waveforms of 4 × 4 Hadamard-like encoded multislice imaging sequences

j	$SC_j(t)$	$SS_j(t)$
1^a	$\frac{A}{2}\text{sinc}\left(\frac{A}{2}t\right)\left[\cos\left(-\frac{3}{2}\Delta\omega t\right) - \sin\left(-\frac{1}{2}\Delta\omega t\right)\right.$ $\left. - \sin\left(\frac{1}{2}\Delta\omega t\right) - \sin\left(\frac{3}{2}\Delta\omega t\right)\right]$	$\frac{A}{2}\text{sinc}\left(\frac{A}{2}t\right)\left[-\sin\left(-\frac{3}{2}\Delta\omega t\right) - \cos\left(-\frac{1}{2}\Delta\omega t\right)\right.$ $\left. - \cos\left(\frac{1}{2}\Delta\omega t\right) - \cos\left(\frac{3}{2}\Delta\omega t\right)\right]$
2	$\frac{A}{2}\text{sinc}\left(\frac{A}{2}t\right)\left[-\sin\left(-\frac{3}{2}\Delta\omega t\right) + \cos\left(-\frac{1}{2}\Delta\omega t\right)\right.$ $\left. - \sin\left(\frac{1}{2}\Delta\omega t\right) - \sin\left(\frac{3}{2}\Delta\omega t\right)\right]$	$\frac{A}{2}\text{sinc}\left(\frac{A}{2}t\right)\left[-\cos\left(-\frac{3}{2}\Delta\omega t\right) - \sin\left(-\frac{1}{2}\Delta\omega t\right)\right.$ $\left. - \cos\left(\frac{1}{2}\Delta\omega t\right) - \cos\left(\frac{3}{2}\Delta\omega t\right)\right]$
3	$\frac{A}{2}\text{sinc}\left(\frac{A}{2}t\right)\left[-\sin\left(-\frac{3}{2}\Delta\omega t\right) - \sin\left(-\frac{1}{2}\Delta\omega t\right)\right.$ $\left. + \cos\left(\frac{1}{2}\Delta\omega t\right) - \sin\left(\frac{3}{2}\Delta\omega t\right)\right]$	$\frac{A}{2}\text{sinc}\left(\frac{A}{2}t\right)\left[-\cos\left(-\frac{3}{2}\Delta\omega t\right) - \cos\left(-\frac{1}{2}\Delta\omega t\right)\right.$ $\left. - \sin\left(\frac{1}{2}\Delta\omega t\right) - \cos\left(\frac{3}{2}\Delta\omega t\right)\right]$
4	$\frac{A}{2}\text{sinc}\left(\frac{A}{2}t\right)\left[-\sin\left(-\frac{3}{2}\Delta\omega t\right) - \sin\left(-\frac{1}{2}\Delta\omega t\right)\right.$ $\left. - \sin\left(\frac{1}{2}\Delta\omega t\right) + \cos\left(\frac{3}{2}\Delta\omega t\right)\right]$	$\frac{A}{2}\text{sinc}\left(\frac{A}{2}t\right)\left[-\cos\left(-\frac{3}{2}\Delta\omega t\right) - \cos\left(-\frac{1}{2}\Delta\omega t\right)\right.$ $\left. - \cos\left(\frac{1}{2}\Delta\omega t\right) - \sin\left(\frac{3}{2}\Delta\omega t\right)\right]$

[a]An example of the 1st row ($j = 1$) is given in the text (see also the first column of Fig. 10-7), and the corresponding spectrum is shown in Fig. 10-6.

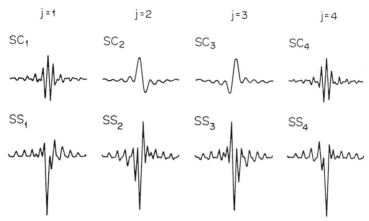

Figure 10-7 The rf pulse waveforms $SC_j(t)$ and $SS_j(t)$ for four-slice Hadamard-like encoded multislice imaging.

REFERENCES

1. Z. H. Cho, H. S. Kim, H. B. Song, and J. Cumming. *Proc. IEEE* 70:1152 (1982).
2. C. H. Oh, H. S. Kim, H. W. Park. W. S. Kim, S. W. Lee, and Z. H. Cho. *IEEE Trans. Nucl. Sci.* NS-30:1899 (1983).
3. Z. H. Cho, O. Nalcioglu, and H. W. Park. *J. Opt. Soc. Amer. A*, 4:923 (1987).
4. L. A. Shepp. *J. Comput. Assist. Tomogr.* 4:94 (1980).
5. M. Y. Chiu, H. H. Barrett, and R. G. Simpson. *J. Opt. Soc. Am.* 70:755 (1980).
6. R. Marr, C. N. Chen, and P. Lauterbur. In *Proceedings of the Conference on Mathematical Aspects of Computerized Tomography*, vol. 8, G. T. Herman and F. Natterer, eds. Berlin: Springer-Verlag, 1981, p. 225.
7. P. Lauterbur and C.-M. Lai. *IEEE Trans. Nucl. Sci.* NS-27:1227 (1980).
8. A. A. Maudsley. *J. Magn. Reson.* 41:112 (1980).
9. T. Inouye. *IEEE Trans. Nucl. Sci.* NS-26:2666 (1979).
10. D. Raghavarao. *Constructions and Combinational Problems in Design of Experiments.* New York: Wiley, 1971.
11. W. T. Eadie et al. *Statistical Methods in Experimental Physics.* Amsterdam: North-Holland, 1972.
12. W. B. Davenport. *Probability and Random Process.* New York: McGraw-Hill, 1970.
13. A. Kumar, D. Welti, and R. Ernst. *J. Magn. Reson.* 88:69 (1975).
14. H. B. Song, Z. H. Cho, and S. K. Hilal. *IEEE Trans. Nucl. Sci.* NS-29:493 (1982).
15. W. K. Pratt. *Digital Image Processing.* New York: Wiley, 1978.

MAGNETIC RESONANCE IMAGING: METHODS AND TECHNIQUES

In this chapter, we will discuss three different categories of imaging techniques, namely (1) conventional imaging, such as spin-echo sequence, (2) high-speed imaging such as the echo planar and gradient echo imagings, and (3) high-resolution imaging such as the microscropic and ultra-high resolution imagings.

11-1 CONVENTIONAL IMAGING

There are three basic NMR imaging sequences in conventional imaging: the spin-echo sequence, the inversion recovery sequence, and cardiac and respiratory gated imaging.

11-1-1 Spin-Echo Sequences of T_1- and T_2-Weighted Imaging

The spin-echo sequences of various types are the most widely used imaging techniques and their basic form consists of 90° and 180° rf pulses with a time separation of half an echo time (T_E) between the two pulses [1]. As shown in Fig. 11-1, the spin-echo signal is acquired T_E seconds after the 90° rf pulse. For 3-D imaging, this pulse sequence is repeated both in the z and y directions, provided the x-gradient is the frequency-encoding or readout gradient. In conventional spin-echo imaging the repetition time is usually longer than the echo time to allow recovery of the longitudinal magnetization or T_1 recovery. The first 90° rf pulse rotates or flips the magnetization of the spins into the transverse plane. Immediately after the 90° flip, spins in the transverse plane start the T_1 and T_2 relaxations. Although the T_1 relaxation process continues, the addition of a 180° pulse at the time of $T_E/2$ flips the spins to the opposite side, as we have seen in Chapter 9, and eventually

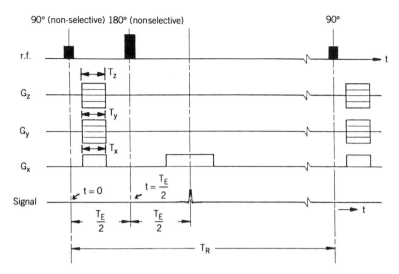

Figure 11-1 The pulse sequence for 3-D spin-echo imaging.

rephases the spins that were dephased due to the inhomogeneity during the time from $t = 0$ to $t = T_E/2$. In addition, true T_2 decay, the transverse component of the magnetization, also takes place. As we discussed in Chapter 9, the equivalent decay time due to both the T_2 relaxation and the field inhomogeneity is known as T_2^* which is given by [2]

$$\frac{1}{T_2^*} = \frac{1}{T_2} + \frac{\gamma \Delta B_0}{2} \qquad (11\text{-}1)$$

where γ is gyromagnetic ratio and ΔB_0 is the inhomogeneity of the magnetic field. It should be noted, however, that the decay of the signal because of the field inhomogeneity can be recovered by the application of a 180° rf pulse or rf spin echo, which rephases the spins that have been dephased during the period between the 90° and 180° rf pulses (i.e., the time between $t = 0$ and $t = T_E/2$). Spin dephasing due to T_2 relaxation, however, cannot be recovered. With the application of three orthogonal gradients, as shown in Fig. 11-1, the acquired echo signal can now be expressed as [3]

$$s(t, g_y, g_z) = \int_{-\infty}^{\infty} \int_{-\infty}^{\infty} \int_{-\infty}^{\infty} \rho(x, y, z) \exp\left[i\gamma(G_x x t + g_y y T_y + g_z z T_z)\right] dx\, dy\, dz$$

$$(11\text{-}2)$$

where $\rho(x, y, z)$ represents the spin density function including the T_1 and T_2 decays, G_x is the readout gradient (constant gradient during data acquisition), g_y and g_z are the phase encoding gradients in the y and z directions with varying amplitudes in steps, and T_y and T_z are the durations for the G_y and

G_z gradients, respectively. From Eq. (11-2) it can be shown that the echo signal is the 3-D Fourier transform of the spin density function. Hence the spin density function modulated by the T_1 and T_2 relaxations can be obtained by the 3-D Fourier transform of the spin-echo signal and is given by

$$\rho(x, y, z) = \rho_0(x, y, z) \left\{ \exp\left[\frac{-T_E}{T_2(x, y, z)} \right] \right\} \left\{ 1 - \exp\left[\frac{-T_R}{T_1(x, y, z)} \right] \right\}$$

$$(11\text{-}3)$$

where $\rho_0(x, y, z)$ denotes the initial values of the spin density function at a location (x, y, z) and the two terms in { } denote the T_1 and T_2 decays. In writing Eq. (11-3), the repetition time is assumed to be sufficiently larger than the T_1 relaxation time of the sample so that the signal variation due to the interpulse time fluctuation is negligible. As implied by Eq. (11-3), by suitable combination of T_E and T_R, both the image intensity and contrast can be manipulated. Among others, the three most often used and interesting imaging sequences are (1) the spin-echo sequence with short T_R and short T_E, (2) spin-echo sequence with long T_R and long T_E, and (3) the spin-echo sequence with long T_R and short T_E. Let us consider these three cases in 2-D imaging.

Short T_R and Short T_E: T_1-Weighted Imaging

With a short echo time, the T_2-dependent term in Eq. (11-3) will be unity, and Eq. (11-3) becomes

$$\rho(x, y) \cong \rho_0(x, y) \left\{ 1 - \exp\left[-\frac{T_R}{T_1(x, y)} \right] \right\}$$

$$(11\text{-}4)$$

With a short T_R, Eq. (11-4) can be further approximated as

$$\rho(x, y) \cong \rho_0(x, y) \left[\frac{T_R}{T_1(x, y)} \right]$$

$$(11\text{-}5)$$

The short T_R and short T_E sequence can therefore be considered as an imaging mode where the image intensity is inversely proportional to the longitudinal relaxation time T_1. Consequently this mode is often called T_1-weighted imaging and is one of the most frequently used pulse sequences in conventional NMR imaging.

Long T_R and Long T_E: T_2-Weighted Imaging

With a long repetition time ($T_R \gg T_1$), the T_R dependent term in Eq. (11-3) will become zero, and Eq. (11-3) in 2-D becomes

$$\rho(x, y) \cong \rho_0(x, y) \left\{ \exp\left[-\frac{T_E}{T_2(x, y)} \right] \right\}$$

$$(11\text{-}6)$$

In this mode the signal is usually large because of the long T_R. On the other hand, due to the long echo time, the image is heavily weighted by T_2; consequently the signal is reduced significantly. This mode is therefore known as T_2-weighted imaging, and the image is somewhat noisy. Nevertheless, this T_2-weighted image results in useful T_2-weighted contrasts and is found to be one of the most often used imaging methods in clinical situations.

Long T_R and Short T_E: T_1-Weighted Density Imaging

Again using Eq. (11-3), with a long T_R and a short T_E it can easily be seen that the resulting image becomes neither T_1-weighted nor T_2-weighted and tends to appear as the pure density function $\rho_0(x, y)$.

Basic Pulse Sequences

The above three basic spin-echo sequences are usually implemented in 2-D form as shown in Fig. 11-2. In the 2-D spin-echo sequence, a set of selective rf pulses is applied with a set of selection gradients. If the z-gradient is used as the selection gradient for the selection of a slice along the z direction at $z = z_0$, the acquired signal can be expressed as

$$s(t, g_y; z_0) = \int_{-\infty}^{\infty} \int_{-\infty}^{\infty} \rho(x, y; z_0)\exp\left[i\gamma(G_x xt + g_y yT_y\right] dx\, dy \quad (11\text{-}7)$$

In Eq. (11-7) we have assumed x to be the readout gradient direction. Often a short echo time with a long repetition time allows us to perform time-multiplexed multislice imaging in 2-D. This multislice imaging technique has

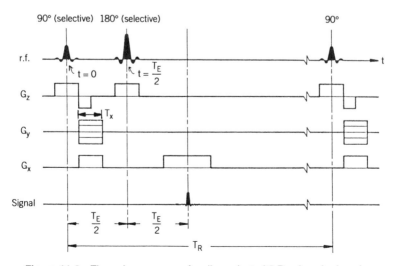

Figure 11-2   The pulse sequence for slice-selected 2-D spin-echo imaging.

become one of the standard NMR imaging techniques widely used in clinical applications.

11-1-2 Inversion-Recovery Imaging

One of the variations of the spin-echo sequence is the inversion-recovery sequence [4] shown in Fig. 11-3. In this scheme a 180° selective rf pulse is added before a normal pulse sequence to flip the magnetization vector from the $+z$-axis to the $-z$-axis. The time between the 180° inversion pulse and the beginning of the normal pulse sequence is known as the "inversion time" T_I. By adjusting this T_I, one can enhance the T_1 contrast as,

$$\rho(x, y) = \rho_0(x, y)\left\{1 - 2\exp\left[-\frac{T_I}{T_1(x, y)}\right]\right\} \qquad (11\text{-}8)$$

An interesting feature of Eq. (11-8) is that the T_1 contrast is enhanced by a factor of two compared with the conventional spin-echo sequence. As shown in Fig. 11-3, the inversion recovery and the conventional spin-echo sequences are identical except for the 180° inversion pulse that precedes the conventional spin-echo sequence. This inversion recovery sequence widens the T_1 contrast range, thereby enhancing the T_1 contrast. The drawback of inversion recovery imaging is the fact that the resulting image often contains negative values and requires reconstruction of real part (taking the real part after

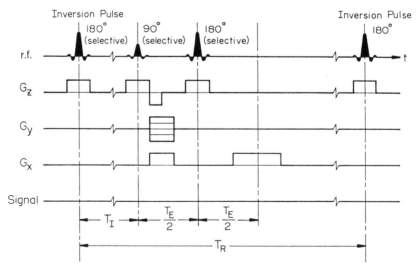

Figure 11-3 The pulse sequence for the single slice or slice-selected inversion recovery spin-echo sequence.

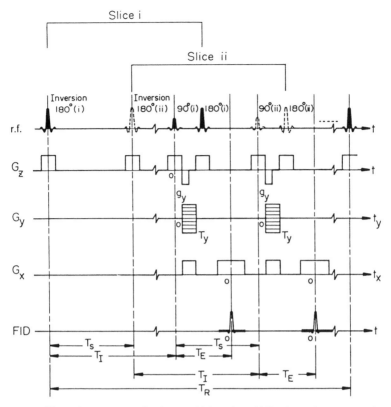

Figure 11-4 The pulse sequence for time-multiplexed, multislice inversion recovery imaging; *i* and *ii* represent the slices *i* and *ii*, respectively.

Fourier transform). Multislice imaging of the inversion recovery sequence can also be derived using the time-multiplexed technique discussed earlier. An example of the time-multiplexed, multislice inversion recovery sequence is shown in Fig. 11-4. By using this inversion-recovery sequence, for a certain material with known T_1 such as fat, one can selectively eliminate the excessive contrast arising due to fat by suitable adjustment of T_I, thereby enhancing the T_1 contrast.

11-1-3 Cardiac and Respiratory Gated Imaging

There is a need for the imaging of moving organs such as the heart or the abdomen. MRI data acquisitions are carried out line by line in the spatial frequency domain. Therefore imaging of moving organs usually introduces severe blurring or ghostlike artifacts. To eliminate the motion artifacts, the NMR imaging sequence is usually synchronized to the physiological motion

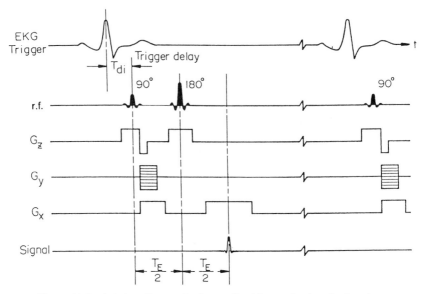

Figure 11-5   A timing diagram for the cardiac-triggered spin-echo imaging.

using ECG or respiratory monitor signals. In these cases the repetition time is set equal to the cardiac or respiratory cycle or to a multiple of one of these cycles. Typical cardiac or respiratory gated imaging sequences are shown in Figs. 11-5 and 11-6. Normally in cardiac gated imaging a synchronization pulse is derived from the ECG signal (usually the R-wave peak in the ECG signal is used as a reference), while in respiratory motion gated imaging an additional respiratory motion cycle has to be derived. This cardiac or respiratory motion signal is then used to trigger the NMR imaging pulse sequences, as shown in Fig. 11-6. The cardiac and respiratory gated imaging techniques can be extended to 3-D imaging. In normal 2-D imaging, however, the multislice imaging technique is not applicable. Instead, each slice image now represents the image of a different cardiac phase, as shown in Fig. 11-6. In the conventional spin-echo technique, where T_R is in the range of 300 to 500 msec, multiphase imaging is not usually applicable because one cardiac cycle is suitable only for one pulse sequence. The more commonly used method is the free running mode in which data collections are made in synchronization with the cardiac cycle using a short repetition time, and then the data set is rearranged later based on the recorded cardiac phase [6]. By taking 16 or more phases within a cardiac cycle, a movielike image set of a selected slice can be reconstructed. Respiratory motion synchronization can also be obtained in a similar way. In NMR both the cardiac and respiratory motion cycles can be derived by use of projection data acquisition and used for the imaging [7].

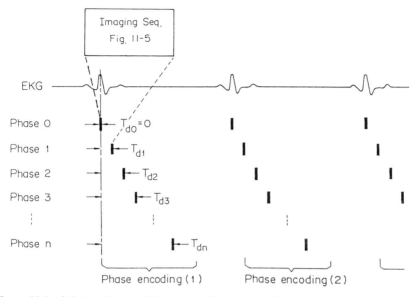

Figure 11-6   A timing diagram of the cardiac-triggered multiphase imaging pulse sequence.

11-2 HIGH-SPEED IMAGING

The term "high-speed imaging" is somewhat unclear at this time, and it is under constant development in several different directions. Nevertheless, several techniques already developed in the area of high-speed imaging can be discussed in context of their excitation modes. They may be classified as single-shot or multiple-shot imaging. In single-shot imaging one rf excitation is followed by a series of gradient pulses, thereby collecting a complete set of NMR signals. These NMR signals are created either by a series of gradient reversals or oscillations. Single-shot imaging can also be divided into two basic approaches according to the gradient waveform, namely, echo planar imaging (EPI) and spiral scan echo planar imaging (SEPI). SEPI can further be divided into circular spiral and square spiral. In the multiple-shot technique each excitation is followed by one data acquisition sequence, and this process is repeated rapidly like the conventional imaging. This technique can also be divided into two basic approaches, namely fast low angle shot (FLASH) imaging and steady state free precession (SSFP) imaging. The data acquisition times of the known single-shot imaging methods lie between 32 and 128 msec, while in multiple-shot imaging such as FLASH and SSFP the data acquisition times are substantially longer (i.e., on the order of 0.1–5 sec). As will be discussed in more detail, it is generally accepted that the image quality of the multiple-shot imaging is better than that of the single-shot imaging, although it takes a somewhat longer imaging time.

11-2-1 Single-Shot Techniques

Echo Planar Imaging

Mansfield was the first to propose the scheme now known as *echo planar imaging* (EPI). This method, in principle, allows us to obtain 2-D image data by single excitation [8]. Although the EPI technique can be extended to a 3-D form, our discussion will be limited to the 2-D case.

The originally proposed echo planar imaging pulse sequence is shown in Fig. 11-7. First, together with G_z and a 90° selective rf pulse, a slice of thickness Δz is selected. Following this preparation, an oscillating gradient G_x and a small constant gradient G_y are applied, as shown in Fig. 11-7. The effect of the oscillating gradient is simple gradient echo generation using alternating gradient reversal instead of a 180° rf pulse train. The resulting FID and echoes are shown in Fig. 11-8 and can be written as

$$f(t) = \left\{ \sum_{n=0}^{\infty} g_n(t - 2n\pi) \right\} \exp\left(-\frac{t}{T_2} \right) \qquad (11\text{-}9)$$

where $g_n(t - 2n\pi)$ is the echo signal:

$$g_n(t - 2n\pi) = s(t) \qquad (11\text{-}10)$$

As shown in Fig. 11-7, a full two-dimensional planar experiment can now be performed by using the additional gradient G_y which is much smaller in amplitude than G_x. This operation may be viewed as a trajectory in Fourier

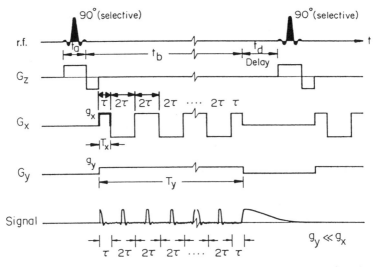

Figure 11-7 The pulse sequence of the slice-selected 2-D echo planar imaging.

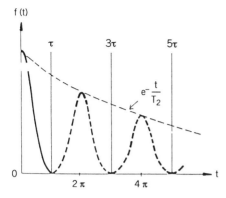

f (t)

Figure 11-8 A series of echoes produced by the alternating gradient G_x with T_2 decay in the echo signals. Because of the small, continuously applied, constant gradient G_y, each echo is coded differently.

or k-space, as shown in Fig. 11-9. This k-space illustration resembles a conventional sequence covering the k-space, except that the trajectory is tilted due to the combined application of the small G_y gradient (for phase encoding gradient in this case) and the large but short G_x gradient (for frequency encoding). The only difference compared with the conventional spin-echo sequence is that the phase encoding is continuous rather than discrete. Naturally the pulse sequence shown in Fig. 11-7 can be modified to

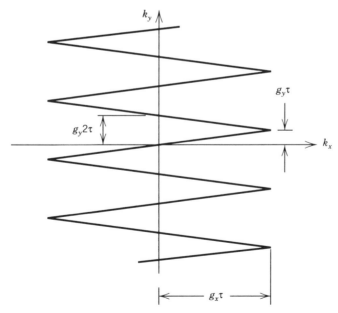

Figure 11-9 The k-domain trajectory of EPI. Trajectory represented by the dotted line is obtained by reversing the G_y in Fig. 11-7.

have discrete phase encoding by simply replacing the continuous gradient by a train of rectangular pulses.

By adjusting G_x and G_y, one can cover the entire frequency or k-space by a single 90° rf pulse excitation. As is intuitively clear, T_2 decay requires a rapidly alternating gradient pulse of a large amplitude, which is often difficult to obtain in practice. Another problem in original echo planar imaging is the poor resolution in the phase encoding direction due to the limitation in the number of phase encoding steps or the number of echoes that can be recalled due to the signal decay by T_2.

Spiral Scan Echo Planar Imaging

Some of the difficulties mentioned for the original echo planar imaging such as the resolution limits in phase encoding direction can be partially resolved by the use of a spiral scan [9]. Let us again consider well-known 2-D Fourier NMR imaging with two time-varying gradient fields as given by

$$S(t) = \int_x \int_y \rho(x, y; z_0) \exp\left\{ i\gamma \int_0^t \left[xG_x(t') + yG_y(t') \right] dt' \right\} \exp\left(\frac{-t}{T_2} \right) dx\, dy$$

$$(11\text{-}11)$$

where $S(t)$ is the NMR signal, $\rho(x, y)$ is the spin density distribution, and $G_x(t)$ and $G_y(t)$ are the time-varying gradient fields in the x and y coordinates, respectively. As is known, the exponential term $\exp(-t/T_2)$ representing the T_2 decay appears as a limiting factor in echo planar imaging and therefore is added in the equation.

By using k-space notation, Eq. (11-11) can be rewritten as

$$S(t) = \int\int \rho(x, y; z_0) \exp\left\{ i\left[k_x(t)x + k_y(t)y \right] \right\} dx\, dy$$

$$\cong S(k_x, k_y) \qquad (11\text{-}12)$$

where the vectors $k_x(t)$ and $k_y(t)$ are given by

$$k_x(t) = \gamma \int_0^t G_x(t')\, dt'$$

$$k_y(t) = \gamma \int_0^t G_y(t')\, dt' \qquad (11\text{-}13)$$

From Eqs. (11-11) and (11-12), it can easily be shown that $\rho(x, y)$ and $S(k_x, k_y)$ are again the Fourier transform pair. Note here that in Eq. (11-12) the T_2 decay term is not included for simplicity.

Unlike the original EPI, to obtain equal high-frequency cutoffs for both the x and y directions, k_x and k_y should be equal:

$$k_x(T_x) = k_y(T_y) \qquad (11\text{-}14)$$

For Mansfield's original EPI [8], the following relation should be satisfied:

$$T_y = nT_x \qquad (11\text{-}15)$$

where n corresponds to the number of echoes to be generated by the alternating gradient pulses in the x-direction.

As mentioned earlier, one of the main drawbacks of the EPI technique is the fact that the alternating gradient to be applied is a series of rectangular pulses and is often difficult to generate when the required gradient power and frequency are high. Another difficulty with this method is that the x-directional sampling in the k-domain is determined by the number of echoes that can be generated by the number of alternating gradient pulses, and is limited by the intrinsic property of NMR (i.e., T_2 decay).

To alleviate these drawbacks, another approach is proposed in which two oscillating gradient pulses are used to form a spiral scan in k-space known as *spiral scan echo planar imaging* (SEPI). In the SEPI scheme the entire frequency domain is covered uniformly by a form of spiral scan, thereby obtaining a circularly symmetric response function. Let us consider a continuous and circularly symmetric frequency or k-space scan and the necessary conditions to achieve this goal [9]. Clearly a simultaneous k-domain sinusoidal pulse pair will result in a set of circularly symmetric circles with different radii in the k-domain. Two sinusoidal pulses required for the formation of discrete circles are

$$k_x(t) = \gamma\eta_i(t)\cos \xi t$$
$$k_y(t) = \gamma\eta_i(t)\sin \xi t \qquad (11\text{-}16)$$

where $\eta_i(t)$ is the discrete amplitude as a function of time and ξ is an angular frequency yet to be determined. By slightly modifying Eq. (11-16), one can obtain a continuous, rather than discrete, spiral circle. Two sinusoidal pulses to obtain the spiral scan are

$$k_x(t) = \gamma\eta t \cos \xi t$$
$$k_y(t) = \gamma\eta t \sin \xi t \qquad (11\text{-}17)$$

From Eqs. (11-13) and (11-17), the desired time domain gradient pulse forms

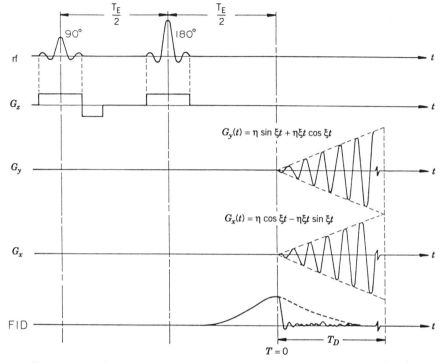

Figure 11-10   The pulse sequence for the spiral scan echo planar imaging (SEPI).

that will generate a spiral scan in the k-domain can be obtained and given by [10]

$$G_x(t) = \frac{1}{\gamma}\frac{d}{dt}k_x(t) = \eta \cos \xi t - \eta \xi t \sin \xi t$$

$$G_y(t) = \frac{1}{\gamma}\frac{d}{dt}k_y(t) = \eta \sin \xi t + \eta \xi t \cos \xi t \qquad (11\text{-}18)$$

These equations represent sinusoidal signals with linearly increasing amplitudes as a function of time (see Fig. 11-10). The resulting spiral scan will represent a close approximation of the concentric circles with which the entire frequency range of interest can be covered using uniform circularly symmetric frequency domain sampling, thereby achieving circularly symmetric resolution.

To define several necessary conditions, let us derive the k-domain functions in polar coordinates $k_r(t)$ and $k_\theta(t)$. Using Eq. (11-17) and cartesian-to-polar-coordinate transformation, $k_r(t)$ and $k_\theta(t)$ can be derived as

$$k_r(t) = \sqrt{k_x^2(t) + k_y^2(t)} = \gamma \eta t$$

$$k_\theta(t) = \tan^{-1}\left[\frac{k_y(t)}{k_x(t)}\right] = \xi t \qquad (11\text{-}19)$$

Note here that both $k_r(t)$ and $k_\theta(t)$ are explicit functions of time. As shown, both the radial and rectangular increments; that is, $\Delta k_r(t)$ and $\Delta k_\theta(t)$ are related to the sampling interval ΔT in the signal domain as

$$\Delta k_r = \gamma \eta N_\theta \, \Delta T$$

$$\Delta k_\theta = \xi \, \Delta T \qquad (11\text{-}20)$$

where N_θ is the number of samples in one complete rotation and ΔT is the time necessary to rotate an angular increment Δk_θ (see Fig. 11-11). The required k-domain radial and angular sampling rates can be defined as

$$\Delta k_r = \frac{2\pi}{2N_r \, \Delta r}$$

and

$$\Delta k_\theta = \frac{2\pi}{N_\theta} \qquad (11\text{-}21)$$

where N_r and Δr denote the number of rotations in the k-domain and the image resolution in the spatial domain, respectively. From Eqs. (11-20) and (11-21), constants η and ξ can be determined; they are given by

$$\eta = \frac{\pi}{\gamma N_\theta N_r \, \Delta T \, \Delta r}$$

$$\xi = \frac{2\pi}{N_\theta \, \Delta T} \qquad (11\text{-}22)$$

The total required image data acquisition time T_D can be equated in relation with angular incremental time ΔT, the number of rotations, and the number of samples in one complete rotation. It can also be related to the T_2 relaxation time, especially if one chooses to equate the total acquisition time

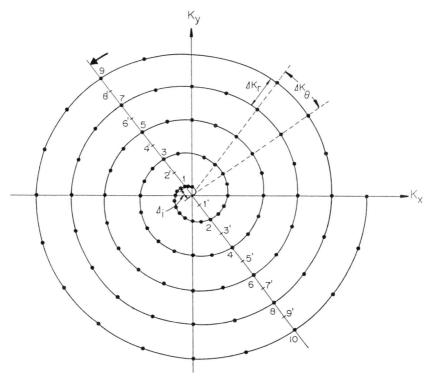

Figure 11-11   A k-domain trajectory of SEPI corresponding to the pulse sequence shown in Fig. 11-10. Note the radial and angular sampling obtainable in SEPI and conjugate symmetry filling.

to one decay time T_2:

$$T_D = N_r N_\theta \, \Delta T \cong T_2 \qquad (11\text{-}23)$$

The required maximum gradient amplitude can also be determined from the total data acquisition time T_D, and it is given by

$$G_{max} = \eta \xi T_D \qquad (11\text{-}24)$$

Using Eq. (11-23), the maximum radial frequency $k_{r_{max}}$ can also be derived:

$$k_{r_{max}} = \gamma \eta T_D = N_r \, \Delta k_r \qquad (11\text{-}25)$$

The $k_{r_{max}}$ is the determining factor for the resolution that can be attained with the spiral scan echo planar technique provided that sufficient sampling

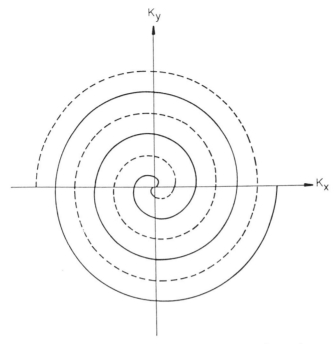

Figure 11-12 Interlaced spiral scans to improve k-domain sampling and overcome the T_2 decay and gradient requirement limitation.

is made. As seen, the resolution is explicitly related to the number of circles or rotations in a spiral scan with a given excitation. For the case of limited T_D due to T_2 at each scan, N_r or $k_{r_{max}}$ can be increased by repeated scanning. This can easily be achieved with what is called the "interlacing technique," as shown in Fig. 11-12. An additional advantage noted in conjunction with N_r is the conjugate symmetry property of the spiral scan. This property allows us to increase radial sampling by a factor of two, as illustrated in Fig. 11-11. An example of radial sampling along a radial line is shown by an arrow in Fig. 11-11; point 2′ in the figure is a conjugate symmetry of the point 2, and therefore it can be considered as a real sampled point, effectively increasing the number of sampling points. Similarly points 3′, 4′, and so on, can be obtained from point 3, 4, and so on. A typical example of SEPI in an attempt to reconstruct the image of an object of diameter 30 cm in a matrix size of 128×128 would require $N_r = 32$ (considering the conjugate filling discussed above), $\xi/2 = 300$ Hz with a sampling time interval of $\Delta T = 8$ μsec, and a total image data acquisition time of 100 msec.

Image reconstruction of SEPI involves the formation of the projection data via the Fourier transform of the k-domain data in the radial direction, as shown in Fig. 11-11. An example of the *l*th view data in the *k*-domain, which is denoted Q^l, can be written as

$$
Q^l = \left\{ S\left[l\,\Delta T + (N_r - 1)N^\theta \Delta T \right], S\left[l\,\Delta T + (N_r - 2)N^\theta \Delta T \right], \right.
$$

$$
\ldots, S(l\,\Delta T), S\left[l\,\Delta T + \frac{N_\theta}{2}\Delta T \right],
$$

$$
\left. \ldots, S\left[l\,\Delta T + (N_r - 1)N_\theta\,\Delta T + \frac{N_\theta}{2}\Delta T \right] \right\} \tag{11-26}
$$

By the projection theorem it can be shown that the Fourier transform of the *k*-domain data given in Eq. (11-26) will be the projection data $P^l(k)$ with which the convolution backprojection reconstruction can be made (see Chapter 3).

As has been mentioned, SEPI has several advantages over the original EPI, including the circularly symmetric sampling property under T_2 decay in the *k*-domain which will result in a circularly symmetric image resolution or point spread function regardless of the number of rotations in the spiral

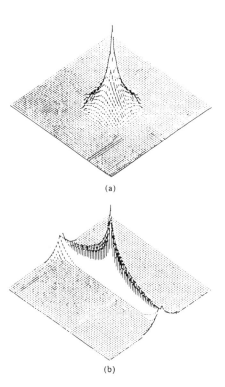

(a)

(b)

Figure 11-13 Point spread functions (PSF) of the SEPI and the original EPI shown on a log scale. The data acquisition time is assumed to be three times the T_2 relaxation time: (a) the PSF of the SEPI and (b) the PSF of the original EPI.

scans. For example, in the original EPI technique there are often noticeable asymmetric point spread functions [see Fig. 11-13(b)]. This is mainly due to the fact that the conventional EPI technique samplings in the x and y directions are not equal, especially the y-directional sampling due to the T_2 decay. In SEPI, on the other hand, perfect symmetric point spread functions can be obtained, as is seen from Fig. 11-13(a), due to the symmetric k-domain sampling. It is the number of spiral rotations N_r that is the key parameter that ultimately affects the overall system resolution in the SEPI technique. An increase of N_r by "interlacing" scanning is therefore necessary in many cases, and this is an important requirement for the high-resolution SEPI technique (see Fig. 11-12).

Square Spiral (Raster) Scan Echo Planar Imaging

To be implemented in digital computers, spiral scan echo planar imaging requires sampling data suited for cartesian coordinates in order to utilize fast Fourier transform techniques such as the FFT algorithm; in other words, spiral scan requires 2-D interpolation of the polar coordinate data to cartesian data if the computation is to be implemented in frequency domain. To alleviate such complexity, a modified form of the spiral scan known as *square spiral* or *raster scan* echo planar imaging has been suggested [11, 12]. This technique provides constant linear velocity in the k_x or the k_y direction in k-space rather than the constant angular velocity employed in the original spiral scan imaging [10, 11]. This constant linear velocity spiral k trajectory can be obtained by

$$k_x(t) = A\sqrt{t}\cos(B\sqrt{t})$$

and

$$k_y(t) = A\sqrt{t}\cos(B\sqrt{t}) \tag{11-27}$$

where A and B are the constants chosen by

$$A = \frac{1}{W}\sqrt{\frac{1}{2\pi T}}$$

and

$$B = \sqrt{\frac{1}{2\pi T}} \tag{11-28}$$

In Eq. (11-28), T is the temporal sampling interval and W is the spatial extent of the object. An example of a square spiral scan trajectory in k-space and the gradient pulses associated with the pulse sequence are shown in

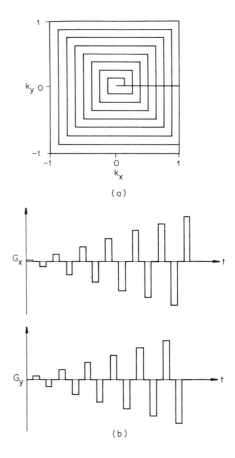

Figure 11-14 (a) The k-domain trajectory of a square spiral scan and (b) corresponding x and y gradient pulse waveforms.

Fig. 11-14. As can be seen in the figure, the samples are on a rectangular lattice or grid; therefore, simple 1-D interpolation is all that is needed to form a data set in cartesian coordinates that can be used for image reconstruction by a simple 2-D FFT.

11-2-2 Multiple Shot Techniques

Gradient Echo Imaging: FLASH (Fast Low Angle Shot) Imaging

As we have learned in the previous sections spin-echo techniques provide multiple echoes with a single rf excitation. Eventually the data collected can be used for 2-D image reconstruction. Instead of taking the multiple-echo approach with a single excitation, multiples of the single echo approach, such as the pulse sequence shown in Fig. 11-15, can also be taken. The important difference between the conventional imaging techniques and this fast sequence is the use of an rf pulse with a low flip angle. Low-angle pulses have been used in conventional NMR spectroscopy experiments in order to optimize the SNR for a given measuring time [13, 14]. However, repetition times on the order of tens of milliseconds with flip angles as low as 15° have not been used because most of the spectroscopic NMR signals normally have durations of several hundreds of milliseconds. In NMR imaging, however, long pulse duration is not needed because of the strong magnetic field gradients, which tend to reduce the signal duration of FID to a time as short as a few milliseconds. For example, using a flip angle of 15°, the signal strengths of the FID correspond to approximately 25% ($= \sin 15°$) of the maximum amplitude obtainable by a 90° pulse. In contrast to conventional imaging sequences, in fast gradient echo sequences over 90% ($= \cos 15°$) of the longitudinal magnetization remains unaffected and thus is available for immediate subsequent excitations (see Fig. 11-15). After termination of the rf pulse, the slice-selective gradient (G_z) is inverted for proper refocusing of the transverse magnetization and in-plane spatial discrimination is achieved by applying a readout gradient (G_y) and phase-encoding gradient (G_x) similar to the conventional 2-D Fourier imaging method. The readout gradient is inverted prior to the data acquisition period, leading to a so-called gradient or field echo. Immediately after acquisition of the data, the experiment is repeated. Thus the duration of the entire pulse sequence for a given phase encoding is reduced to about 10–20 msec. Note, however, that in conventional gradient echo imaging, a 90° rf flip-angle is used.

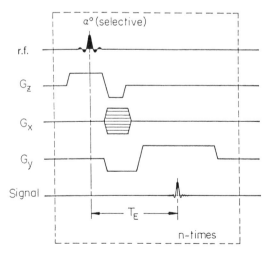

Figure 11-15 Fast low-angle shot (FLASH) imaging sequence. This method employs a slice-selective excitation pulse with a small flip angle (e.g., $\alpha \leq 15°$). The signal is detected in the form of a gradient echo after reversal of the readout gradient. This sequence is repeated n times for phase encoding.

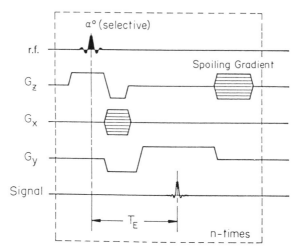

Figure 11-16 FLASH imaging sequence of Fig. 11-15 with an added spoiling gradient in the direction of the slice-selection gradient G_z. Steps employed in adding the spoiling gradient usually follow some form of random encoding steps.

In Fig. 11-15 a FLASH sequence is shown where only the phase encoding gradient is varied in the imaging experiment. A problem often encountered with this simple FLASH sequence imaging is the residual transverse magnetization. When the nth phase encoding gradient is followed by the $(n + 1)$th rf pulse, it will produce a spin echo, thus producing interfering echoes and consequently resulting in an artifact on the final image in the direction of phase-encoding. To remove this artifact, a variable spoiling gradient in the direction of the slice-selection gradient is introduced, as shown in Fig. 11-16. The spoiling gradient pulse is applied after data acquisition but prior to the next rf pulse, and may vary like a phase-encoding gradient from one phase encoding to another in a random fashion. A major reason for this spoiler is the fact that conventional constant spoiling gradients are unable to remove the effects of coherent transverse magnetizations. A variable spoiling gradient in the direction of the readout gradient would only rotate, but not eliminate, the central artifact. Thus an incremental slice-selection spoiler may be understood as a function that rotates the artifact thus redistributing the artifacts in the imaging plane uniformly.

Steady State Free Precession (SSFP) Imaging

By employing the gradient echo imaging sequence together with small flip-angle excitation, the speed of data acquisition has been improved considerably without much loss of signal-to-noise ratio even with significantly reduced repetition time. Because the signals obtained are still relatively large, it has become possible to reduce the scan time to a few seconds.

As the repetition time of the gradient echo imaging sequence becomes smaller and comparable to the spin-spin relaxation time T_2, it is believed that a large amount of the transverse spin magnetization remains and that its residual phase coherency is preserved. This residual phase coherency is believed to be responsible for the formation of another nuclear signal similar to the conventional spin-echo signal. This residual phase coherency has been fully utilized in the SSFP (steady state free precession) technique in which constant rf pulses and gradient fields are applied in rapid sequences with repetition times much shorter than those of conventional sequences so that transverse spin magnetization reaches a steady state condition [15–23]. In the presence of the conventional unipolar phase encoding gradients, however, this steady state condition cannot be reached. Therefore the conventional fast gradient echo imaging sequence may be classified in general as a non-SSFP-type. Most of the fast gradient echo imaging techniques such as FLASH can be classified as non-SSFP techniques.

Let us consider some characteristic differences between the fast SSFP gradient echo technique and the conventional non-SSFP gradient echo techniques. The main difference between the SSFP technique and the non-SSFP techniques appears to be the preservation of the phase coherency of the transverse spin magnetization; that is, phase coherency is preserved in the

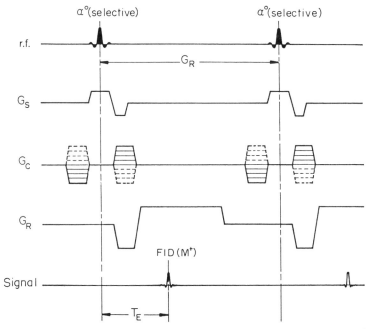

Figure 11-17   Fast SSFP pulse sequence designed for the acquisition of a FID or M^+ signal. Note here that the encoding gradient G_c is now balanced so that the total gradient is always zero within each pulse repetition interval.

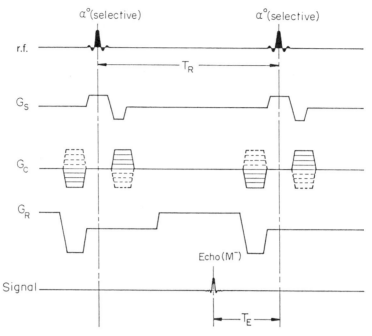

Figure 11-18 Fast SSFP pulse sequence designed for the acquisition of an echo or M^- signal. This sequence is also known as contrast enhanced fast steady state technique (CE-FAST).

former (SSFP), while the phase coherency is lost in the latter (non-SSFP) due to the presence of the variable (unipolar) phase encoding gradients. In the SSFP sequence the phase incoherency is remedied by the use of a balanced bipolar phase encoding gradient pair so that the total effective gradient becomes zero within each pulse repetition interval (see Figs. 11-17 and 11-18), thereby initating the zero phase encoding situation within a pulse repetition interval. By use of the residual phase coherency in the SSFP mode, both FID* and echo signals can be obtained in a steady state, as shown in Figs. 11-17 and 11-18. The FID signal is obtained right after the rf pulse while the echo signal is obtained just before the rf pulse. By combining the two sequences given in Figs. 11-17 and 11-18, two NMR (i.e., a FID and an echo) can be obtained simultaneously in a single SSFP sequence, as shown in Fig. 11-19. It appears that the FID obtained is mainly T_1 weighted, while the echo is T_2 weighted. The availability of a FID and an echo signal is unique and attractive aspect of the SSFP sequence because the echo signal is similar

---

*The term FID used here is not correct in the strict sense. FID is used, however, to differentiate the term from that of echo. Here FID means T_1 weighted, while echo means more T_2 weighted signal.

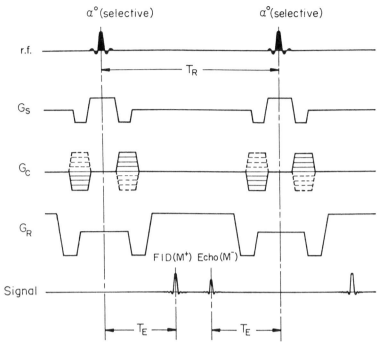

Figure 11-19   The combined fast SSFP pulse sequences of Figs. 11-17 and 11-18. With this combined pulse sequence, both the FID (M^+) and the echo (M^-) signals can be obtained simultaneously. Each image has a characteristic contrast, namely strong T_1 contrast in the FID (M^+) image and strong T_2 contrast in the echo (M^-) image.

to the T_2-weighted spin-echo signal in the conventional spin-echo sequence, which is usually difficult to obtain due to the long repetition time. We now turn to some theoretical considerations of the SSFP technique.

As is known, in conventional gradient echo imaging, the Ernst angle α_E, which is the optimal flip angle maximizing the signal amplitude under a given pulse repetition time is given by

$$\alpha_E = \cos^{-1}\left[\exp\left(\frac{-T_R}{T_1}\right)\right] \qquad (11\text{-}29)$$

where T_1 is the spin-lattice relaxation time and T_R is the pulse repetition time. Equation (11-29) is derived, under the assumption that the phase coherency of the transverse spin magnetization is completely lost at the time of the next rf pulse application. In the fast SSFP technique the optimal flip angle cannot be defined clearly because the phase coherency is now assumed to be partially preserved at the time when the next rf pulse is applied. The signal amplitudes in fast SSFP imaging are more dependent on the free precession angle which is dependent on field inhomogeneities such as chemical shift, susceptibility, and main field inhomogeneity. The free precession angle θ defined during a pulse repetition interval is given by

$$\theta(r) = \gamma \int_0^{T_R} \mathbf{G}(t) \cdot \mathbf{r} \, dt \tag{11-30}$$

where $\mathbf{r}$ is the spatial coordinate vector, $\mathbf{G}(t)$ is the time-dependent gradient field, γ is the gyromagnetic ratio, and T_R is the repetition time. In the fast SSFP imaging, usually the free precession angle within a voxel follows $2n\pi + \theta$ with sufficiently large n (in practical experiments, n larger than 5 can be easily obtained by lengthening the readout gradient), and it ensures that the average signal intensity of the voxel is independent of the free precession angle. For example, in the pulse sequences shown in Figs. 11-17 and 11-18, the readout gradient is made sufficiently large so that it warrants a uniform distribution of the free precession angle. Assuming that $2n\pi + \theta$ with sufficiently large n is warranted within a voxel, the normalized voxel intensities can be approximated as [24, 25]

$$M^+ = \frac{1}{2\pi} \int_0^{2\pi} \frac{M_0}{D} \left[1 - \exp\left(\frac{-T_R}{T_1} \right) \right] \left[1 - \exp\left(\frac{-T_R}{T_2} \right) \cos\theta \right] \sin\alpha \, d\theta \tag{11-31a}$$

and

$$M^- = \frac{1}{2\pi} \int_0^{2\pi} \frac{M_0}{D} \left[1 - \exp\left(\frac{-T_R}{T_1} \right) \right] \left[\cos\theta - \exp\left(\frac{-T_R}{T_2} \right) \right] \exp\left(\frac{-T_R}{T_2} \right) \sin\alpha \, d\theta \tag{11-31b}$$

where M^+ and M^- represent the normalized voxel intensities of the FID and echo images, respectively, M_0 is the equilibrium spin magnetization, α is the flip angle, θ is the free precession angle, and D is given by

$$D = \left[1 - \exp\left(\frac{-T_R}{T_1} \right) \cos\alpha \right] \left[1 - \exp\left(\frac{-T_R}{T_2} \right) \cos\theta \right]$$
$$- \left[\exp\left(\frac{-T_R}{T_1} \right) - \cos\alpha \right] \left[\exp\left(\frac{-T_R}{T_2} \right) \cos\theta \exp\left(\frac{-T_R}{T_2} \right) \right] \tag{11-32}$$

From Eq. (11-31) optimal flip angles maximizing M^+ and M^- as a function of T_R can be numerically computed. In Fig. 11-20(a) and (b) computed

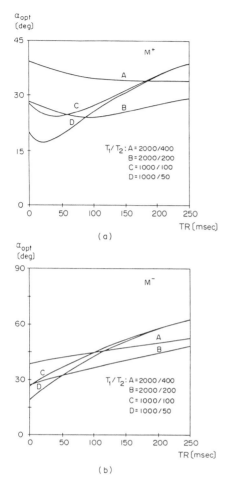

Figure 11-20 Optimal flip angles computed as a function of T_R for both (a) FID (M^+) and (b) echo (M^-) signals in the fast SSFP imaging. Curves A, B, C, and D represent four different T_1/T_2 values of the objects: $A = 200/400$, $B = 2000/200$, $C = 1000/100$, and $D = 1000/50$. (All the units are in milliseconds.)

results of M^+ and M^- for the selected T_1/T_2 values are shown. As seen from the figures, the optimal flip angles for M^+ and M^- as a function of T_R appear relatively constant for most T_1/T_2 values. In Figs. 11-21(a) and (b) normalized intensities of M^+ and M^- computed as a function of the flip angle are shown. In this computation the same T_1/T_2 values as in Fig. 11-20 are used with a T_R/T_E of 40 msec/10 msec. For the M^+ signal the contrast pattern as a function of flip angle appears rather mixed and complex, while in the M^- signal the T_2 contrast seems more pronounced. It is also noticeable that the signal intensities of both M^+ and M^- are maximum at low flip angles and decrease rapidly as the flip angle increases.

Some experimental results of fast SSFP imaging obtained on a 2.0 T superconducting whole-body MRI system are shown in Fig. 11-22. In this sequence both the FID and echo signals are simultaneously acquired,

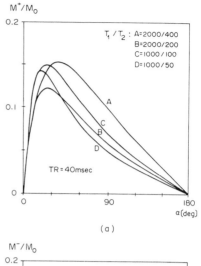

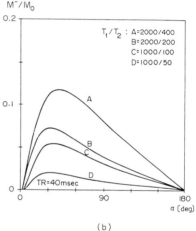

Figure 11-21 Normalized voxel intensities as a function of the flip angle in the images obtained with (a) the FID (M^+) and (b) the echo (M^-) signals in SSFP imaging. Both data sets are obtained under the same conditions as in Fig. 11-20.

and Figs. 11-22(a) and (b) are the images corresponding to the FID (M^+) and echo (M^-) signals, respectively. Both are obtained with a flip angle and T_R/T_E of 30° and 40 msec/11 msec, respectively. In this example with a T_R of 40 msec, the total scan time is only about 10 sec with 256 encoding steps. The flip angle is usually adjusted in reference to the 90° rf pulse with a relatively long repetition time. Data acquisition times for both the FID and echo signals are in the range of 5 msec with a readout gradient strength of 0.5 G/cm. The time interval between the FID and echo signals is approximately 20 msec. If this interval is sufficiently large, interferences between the two signals will be minimal. One drawback of the method is that the images usually suffer from strong susceptibility artifacts, which will be discussed further in Chapter 13 [26, 27].

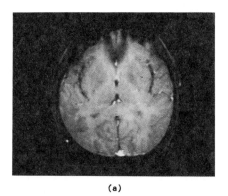

(a)

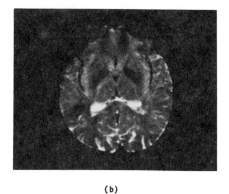

Figure 11-22 Images obtained with a combined pulse sequence for the simultaneous acquisition of the FID (M^+) and echo (M^-) signals in the fast SSFP imaging mode: (a) the FID (M^+) image and (b) the echo (M^-) image. The flip angle and T_R/T_E are 30° and 40 msec/11 msec, respectively.

(b)

Fast SSFP imaging can be differentiated from fast non-SSFP imaging, especially when the spin-spin relaxation time T_2 is comparable to or bigger than the repetition time T_R. Under such a condition, in the former (SSFP), the residual phase coherency of the transverse spin magnetization is sufficiently preserved and utilized for enhancement of the FID (M^+) signal as well as for the generation of the echo (M^-) signal. Because of the revival of the residual phase coherency, a strongly T_2-weighted echo signal is obtained that is usually not available in most of the fast non-SSFP imaging such as the FLASH technique. In the FID image the T_1 contrast is dominant with a mixture of weak T_2 contrast. Contrast in both the FID and echo images can be controlled by adjustments of the flip angles. This fast SSFP imaging of simultaneous data acquisition of FID and echo signals will be an important asset in the areas of fast imaging, where image contrasts are generally poor.

Snapshot FLASH Imaging

Snapshot FLASH imaging is an extension of FLASH imaging to an extremely short repetition time T_R and gradient echo readout time t' [28]. If we assume that any transverse magnetization has been spoiled between two successive rf excitations, the signal $S(t')$ is given by

$$S(t') = \frac{k\rho(x, y)[1 - \exp(-T_R/T_1)]\exp(-t'/T_2)\sin \alpha}{1 - \cos \alpha \exp(-T_R/T_1)} \quad (11\text{-}33)$$

where k denotes a constant given by instrumental conditions and $\rho(x, y)$ is the spin density. In snapshot FLASH (S-FLASH) MRI, the gradient echo time t' and the repetition time T_R are in the range of 1 msec ($t' \ll T_2$) and 3 msec, ($T_R \ll T_1$), respectively, with a flip angle of less than 5° (see Fig. 11-23). Therefore, for most of the biological samples, the ratios t'/T_2 and T_R/T_1 are less than 0.01. In the extreme limit ($\alpha < 5°$, $T_R \ll T_1$, and $t' \ll T_2$), signals will simply become proportional to the spin density $\rho(x, y)$ and the constant k.

For the case of steady state free precession FLASH experiment [33] where transverse magnetization is refocused between the rf pulses, the signal $S(t')$

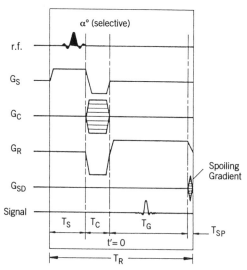

Figure 11-23   The rf pulse and magnetic field gradient timing diagram for snapshot FLASH (S-FLASH) imaging. G_S is the selection gradient, G_C is the phase-encoding gradient, and G_R is the readout gradient for the echo signal, respectively. The gradient G_{SD} serves to spoil the transverse magnetization. This sequence is an extremely fast sequence. For example, T_S, T_C, and t' are in the range of 0.8, 0.4, and 1.6 msec, respectively. The flip angle of the rf pulse is usually less than 5° with a repetition time T_R of less than 3 msec. The total image data acquisition time of the S-FLASH imaging sequence is therefore only on the order of 200 msec for 64 phase-encoding steps.

is given by [35, 36]

$$S(t') = \frac{k\rho(x, y)[1 - \exp(-T_R/T_1)]\exp(-t'/T_2)\sin \alpha}{1 - \exp(-T_R/T_1)\exp(-t'/T_2) - \exp(-T_R/T_1) - \exp(-t'/T_2)\cos \alpha}$$

(11-34)

Again in the case of $T_R \ll T_1$, $t' \ll T_2$, and $\alpha < 5°$, the signal is quite independent of the relaxation times T_1 and T_2, since all the exponential terms and $\cos \alpha$ terms become almost unity, therefore, again signal is dominated only by the spin density $\rho(x, y)$. In both cases it therefore is difficult to observe sufficient image contrast by choosing extremely short values of T_R and t'. However, the magnetic susceptibility artifacts are reduced substantially due to the short gradient duration and are no longer visible, and the effective spin-spin relaxation time T_2^* becomes approximately T_2.

Since it is generally accepted that differences in relaxation times (e.g., T_1 and T_2) are the main factors for the contrast obtained in most of the medical and biological applications of MRI, it appears desirable to incorporate these relaxation-dependent contrasts to this snapshot FLASH imaging, thereby overcoming the contrast limitations inherent to the method [see Eqs. (11-33) and (11-34)]. Hence it is necessary to add the contrast mechanism to S-FLASH, for example, by using another preparation pulse to enhance image contrast. Some of the pulse sequences developed for the contrast enhancement in S-FLASH imaging are discussed next.

Inversion-Recovery Snapshot FLASH Imaging   A pulse sequence of the inversion recovery (IR) coupled to the snapshot FLASH technique is shown in Fig. 11-24. A 180° pulse is added as a preparation pulse for the inversion of the magnetization, and the snapshot FLASH sequence follows with a suitable inversion recovery delay time T_{IR}. During this delay, spoiling gradients are applied to destroy the residual transverse magnetizations resulting from imperfections in the rf pulse. Now the magnetization detected by the S-FLASH sequence depends strongly on the T_1 relaxation, as expected. In all

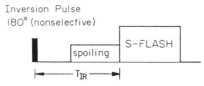

Figure 11-24   A pulse sequence coupled with inversion-recovery (IR) sequence to S-FLASH imaging. The S-FLASH rectangle represents the snapshot FLASH pulse sequence shown in Fig. 11-23. The spoiling gradient is additionally applied to destroy the transverse magnetization developed by rf pulse imperfections. T_{IR} is the inversion-recovery time.

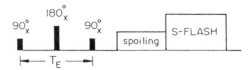

Figure 11-25 Timing diagram of the spin-echo (SE) sequence coupled with S-FLASH imaging. The S-FLASH rectangle represents the snapshot FLASH pulse sequence shown in Fig. 11-23. The spoiling pulse is applied to destroy transverse magnetization developed by rf pulse imperfections. The spin-echo sequence prior to the spoiling is for T_2 labeling.

the inversion-recovery S-FLASH sequences, T_1 contrast is selected by the choice of T_{IR}.

T_2-Weighted Snapshot FLASH Imaging   In Fig. 11-25 a pulse sequence for T_2-weighted snapshot FLASH imaging is shown. Since this is a spin-echo sequence, T_2 contrast can naturally be obtained by suitable adjustment of T_E. In this scheme a set of rf pulses consisting of $90°-180°-90°$ pulses, known as the *driven equilibrium Fourier transform* (DEFT), is added as a preparation pulse. In this way the longitudinal magnetization following the DEFT sequence becomes attenuated by T_2 relaxation during the interval T_E and will be reflected in S-FLASH imaging. The intensity measured by the subsequent S-FLASH experiment therefore heavily depends on the T_2 relaxation. Again a spoiling pulse between the DEFT sequence and the FLASH sequence is added to eliminate the residual magnetization caused by rf pulse imperfections.

Chemical-Shift-Selective (CHESS) Snapshot FLASH Imaging   The pulse sequence for CHESS S-FLASH imaging can be obtained by a straightforward extension of the original CHESS imaging technique [37] and is shown in Fig. 11-26. A frequency-selective 90° pulse, or CHESS pulse, excites or saturates the unwanted spectral region. The FLASH sequence then follows with a spoiling pulse to eliminate the signal from the spectral component(s) that is excited. The imaging sequence will therefore detect those magnetizations unaffected by the CHESS pulse. Detailed descriptions of the CHESS technique have been given elsewhere [37] and are provided in Chapter 13.

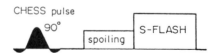

Figure 11-26 The timing diagram for chemical-shift selective (CHESS) snapshot FLASH imaging. The S-FLASH rectangle represents the snapshot FLASH pulse sequence shown in Fig. 11-23. The spoiling pulse is applied to destroy the transverse magnetization caused by the CHESS pulse. One single CHESS rf pulse excites or saturates the unwanted spectral component(s) prior to the S-FLASH experiment.

11-3   NMR MICROSCOPY AND HIGH-RESOLUTION IMAGING

As we have learned, NMR computerized imaging has demonstrated [38–40] resolution capability down to submillimeter and even suggested cellular imaging. NMR imaging has also demonstrated superior performance in diagnostic imaging over many other existing imaging modalities (e.g., X-ray CT). One major advantage of the NMR imaging is the nonionizing nature of the NMR phenomenon whose energy range is only a millionth of an electron volt, in contrast to several kiloelectron volts in the case of electron microscopy. Consequently there is no damage to the cellular objects. Another important characteristic of the NMR is its inherent high-resolution and high-contrast capability, as demonstrated by current medical imaging systems. In this section basic theoretical limits in resolution, voxel size dependent SNR, SNR optimization and some experimental imaging methods will be discussed in context to very high resolution imaging and even microscopy.

11-3-1   Fundamentals of Microscopic and High-Resolution Imaging [41, 42]

Bandwidth-Limited Resolution
Let us consider the basic relationship between desired spatial resolution and bandwidth, which is determined by the gradient amplitude and duration. The basic imaging equation one can start with is given by

$$S(t_x, t_y, t_z, G_x, G_y, G_z) = M_0 \int d^3 \mathbf{r} \rho(\mathbf{r}) \exp\left(i\gamma \mathbf{r} \cdot \int_0^t \mathbf{G}(t)\, dt'\right) A(\cdot) \quad (11\text{-}35)$$

Equation (11-35) can be rewritten as

$$S(\vec{t}, \vec{g}) = M_0 \int\int\int \rho(x, y, z) A(\cdot) \exp\left[i\gamma(xG_x t_x + yG_y t_y + zG_z t_z)\right] dx\, dy\, dz$$

$$(11\text{-}36)$$

where $S(\cdot)$ is the NMR signal, γ is the gyromagnetic ratio, M_0 is the equilibrium magnetization, $\rho(x, y, z)$ is the spatial spin density function including T_1 and T_2 relaxations, G_x, G_y, and G_z are the spatially varying gradients, and $A(\cdot)$ is a signal attenuation factor, which will be discussed in this subsection. As is known from Eq. (11-35), phase encoding can be performed by varying either the gradients G_x, G_y, G_z, or time t_x, t_y, t_z, or both. The resulting phase will then be

$$\phi(\mathbf{r}) = \gamma B_0 t + \gamma \mathbf{r} \cdot \int_0^t \mathbf{G}(t')\, dt' \quad (11\text{-}37)$$

where B_0 is the main static magnetic field and $\gamma B_0 t$ or γB_0 is usually the fixed phase or frequency to be filtered out by quadrature detection.

Now let us first assume that the SNR is sufficiently high and that the detection system is ideal; that is, there is no uncertainty in the measurement. Since NMR imaging is a phase-encoding technique, it is natural to consider the minimal detectable phase difference as a function of the spatial separation between two points (resolution), gradient strength, and the data acquisition period (T_{acq}) for a pair of objects located at $\mathbf{r}_1$ and $\mathbf{r}_2$, where the phases of $\mathbf{r}_1$ and $\mathbf{r}_2$ are given by

$$\phi(\mathbf{r}_1) = \gamma \mathbf{r}_1 \cdot \int_0^{T_{acq}} \mathbf{G}(t')\, dt' \qquad (11\text{-}38)$$

$$\phi(\mathbf{r}_2) = \gamma \mathbf{r}_2 \cdot \int_0^{T_{acq}} \mathbf{G}(t')\, dt' \qquad (11\text{-}39)$$

The phase difference between these two points can be given by

$$\Delta\phi_r = \phi(\mathbf{r}_1) - \phi(\mathbf{r}_2) \qquad (11\text{-}40)$$

Equation (11-40) can also be rewritten as

$$\Delta\phi_r = \gamma(\mathbf{r}_1 - \mathbf{r}_2) \cdot \int_0^{T_{acq}} \mathbf{G}(t')\, dt' = \gamma\, \Delta r G T_{acq} \qquad (11\text{-}41)$$

where a constant amplitude gradient G is assumed. From Eq. (11-41), then the bandwidth-limited intrinsic resolution $(\Delta r)_B$ can be defined as

$$(\Delta r)_B = \Delta\phi_r^{min}/(\gamma G T_{acq}) \qquad (11\text{-}42)$$

where $\Delta\phi_r^{min}$ is the minimal detectable phase. Equation (11-42) is a fundamental relationship representing the intrinsic resolution as a function of the minimal detectable phase and the gradient and time product. The minimal detectable phase $\Delta\phi_r^{min}$ is dependent on the reconstruction algorithm. For example, $\Delta\phi_r^{min} = \pi$ if the Fourier transform technique is used in the reconstruction of a half-echo data set. For a given minimal detectable phase, resolution can be improved by increasing the gradient and time product. Equation (11-42) is shown graphically in Fig. 11-27 for the case of the Fourier transform reconstruction. As implied in Eq. (11-42), while relatively small gradients (0.1–2.0 G/cm) are sufficient for the conventional NMR whole-body imaging, much larger gradients (100–1000 G/cm) will be needed for microscopic resolution imaging.

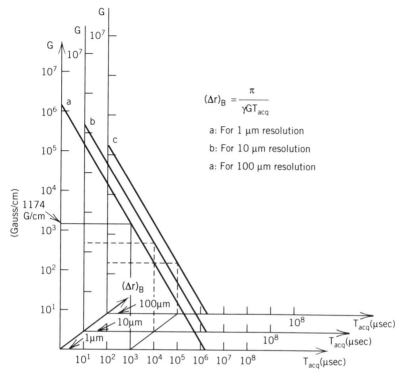

$$(\Delta r)_B = \frac{\pi}{\gamma G T_{acq}}$$

a: For 1 μm resolution

b: For 10 μm resolution

a: For 100 μm resolution

Figure 11-27 A plot of the bandwidth-limited intrinsic resolution $(\Delta r)_B$ in Fourier reconstruction NMR microscopy.

Resolution Limit due to Diffusion

Although it appears that the spatial resolution can be improved by the increase of either gradient G or the acquisition time T_{acq}, other NMR physical parameters such as diffusion will ultimately limit the resolution in very high resolution, such as in microscopy. Here we will consider the effects of diffusion during the data acquisition. Any spatial mapping or coding of a sample in NMR imaging requires the use of magnetic field gradients to map spatial coordinates into the frequency or phase. The Brownian motion of molecules in the material during this coding produces an irrecoverable smearing of the measured point spread function. We will see that this represents an intrinsic resolution limit and that this limit is time dependent such that intrinsic resolution deteriorates as the coding time increases.

The diffusion dependent average square phase fluctuation or "jitter" is given by

$$\left\langle \Delta \phi_D^2 \right\rangle = 2\gamma^2 D \sum_{j=1}^{3} \left[\int_0^{T_{acq}} \left(\int_0^{t'} \mathbf{G}_j(t'') \, dt'' \right)^2 dt' \right] \qquad (11\text{-}43)$$

where D is the diffusion coefficient, T_{acq} is again the data acquisition time during which spin will undergo a diffusion process, and $\mathbf{G}_j$ is the gradient corresponding to the coordinates x, y, and z. In the case that data acquisition follows immediately after a 90° rf pulse, Eq. (11-43) can be written as

$$\langle \Delta\phi_D^2 \rangle = \frac{2}{3}\gamma^2 D G^2 T_{acq}^3 \qquad (11\text{-}44)$$

In deriving Eq. (11-44), only the read gradient G is considered in the diffusion formula, specifically for the acquisition of a half-echo using the diffusion effect reduced gradient pulse sequence. Since the phase fluctuation (rms value) due to the diffusion phenomenon must be smaller than the phase difference due to the spatial differences, the following inequality applies:

$$\Delta\phi_r \geq \sqrt{\langle \phi_D^2 \rangle} \qquad (11\text{-}45)$$

By substituting Eqs. (11-41) and (11-44) into (11-45), we obtain

$$\gamma(\Delta r)GT_{acq} \geq \sqrt{\frac{2}{3}\gamma^2 D G^2 T_{acq}^3}$$

or

$$(\Delta r) \geq (\Delta r)_D \qquad (11\text{-}46)$$

From Eq. (11-46), the diffusion limited resolution can be defined as

$$(\Delta r)_D = \sqrt{\frac{2}{3}DT_{acq}} \qquad (11\text{-}47)$$

Equation (11-47) states that the diffusion associated with image resolution is limited by the diffusion coefficient D and the acquisition time T_{acq}, as plotted in Fig. 11-28. Although this diffusion-limited resolution appears almost negligible in conventional imaging, it could be a significant resolution-limiting factor in microscopic imaging with micron resolution. This diffusion-related resolution limit represents the inherent resolution limit in micron size imaging and should be considered as an intrinsic resolution limit due to the physical parameter. For example, if in a liquid with $D = 10^{-5}$ cm²/sec an acquisition time of 1.5 msec is used, then the diffusion associated resolution limit would be 1.0 μm. This number would increase rapidly if the diffusion coefficient or T_{acq} becomes large. Note that the resolution limit due to bandwidth given in Eq. (11-42) improves the resolution inversely proportional to the acquisition time T_{acq}.

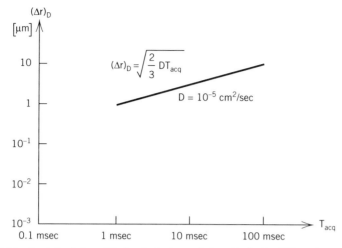

Figure 11-28 A plot of the diffusion-limited resolution $(\Delta r)_D$ in NMR microscopy. The resolution limit is plotted as a function of the acquisition time T_{acq} for a given diffusion coefficient ($D = 10^{-5}$ cm^2/sec).

Resolution Limit due to Signal Decay and Associated Blur

Another interesting effect directly related to the diffusion phenomena is line broadening resulting from the signal amplitude decay during the data acquisition period. This is similar to the Lorentizian broadening due to T_2 decay. The attenuation function $A(t)$ due to the diffusion effect is known as [43]

$$A(t) = A(0)\exp\left\{-\gamma^2 D \int_0^t \left[\int_{t'}^t G(t'') \, dt''\right]^2 dt'\right\} \qquad (11\text{-}48)$$

where $A(0)$ is the initial value. By Fourier transformation of the diffusion affected signal given in Eq. (11-48), the line spread function $P(x)$ can be obtained and is given by

$$P(x) = \frac{1}{A(0)} \int_{-\infty}^{\infty} A(t)\exp(-i2\pi xt) \, dt \qquad (11\text{-}49)$$

where $A(0)$ and $A(t)$ are the same as previously defined in Eq. (11-48).

The line spread given by Eq. (11-49), however, may be restored by an inverse multiplication of the amplitude function of Eq. (11-48) or, similarly, by deconvolution of the blurred image if the diffusion coefficient is known or if the exact amplitude function is given. In this sense the resolution given in Eq. (11-49) (e.g., fwhm of the line spread function) is not an intrinsic resolution compared to the diffusion-limited resolution defined by Eq. (11-46). However, due to difficulties of the restoration process, the line spread function arising from the signal attenuation appears to be a practical limit to the resolution-limiting factor in NMR microscopic imaging.

Application Example of NMR Microscopy

In high-resolution NMR imaging and microscopy, the design of high-field gradients and the development of high-sensitivity rf coils and suitable pulse sequences are major experimental considerations. For the generation of high-gradient fields, a Golay-type gradient coil was developed with cooled water circulation to prevent heat accumulation in case of high-duty cycle gradient applications (short repetition time). The gradient field strengths obtained were about 200 G/cm with pulse rise times of approximately 100 μsec. The rf coil design was based on the solenoidal coil, and the object and coil size were matched to maximize the filling factor.

A number of biological studies, including microscopic studies of cellular objects such as fertilized frog eggs, have been the subject of NMR microscopy. The mechanism by which a fertilized egg becomes a complex organism has been one of the most intriguing and important phenomena in biology. The frog, *Xenopus laevis*, is a convenient and robust model system for this work. The transition from fertilized egg to tadpole takes 7 to 10 days. The egg is relatively large ($\sim$ 1 mm in diameter), and the system does not increase in volume through a significant portion of embryogenesis. Moreover it is a well-studied system, allowing comparison of the NMR microscopy findings with results from other techniques.

Initial experiments have concentrated upon demonstrating the feasibility of using NMR microscopy to obtain *in vivo* images of the frog embryos at a requisite resolution. The fertilized egg or embryo is place in a 2-mm internal diameter NMR tube and surrounded with low-temperature gelling agar. The agar is allowed to gel, thus arresting the sample movement and maintaining a moist environment. The tube is then sealed and placed in the rf coil. As mentioned, the frog embryo is a robust system. Fertilized eggs of embryos continue to develop after this manipulation and with no obvious adverse effects. Figure 11-29 shows an *in vivo* proton NMR microcopy image of *Xenopus laevis* embryos. As seen, distinct morphological structures such as neural tube, somites, and a single layer ectoderm are readily apparent in this image. Pixel resolution is about 12 μm, and slice thickness is about 120 μm in all cases. The signal-to-noise ratio is quite reasonable in these images where the total data acquisition time for a 16-slice volume image was approximately one hour. Calculations show that these experimental conditions will yield a heavily T_1-, T_2-, and diffusion-weighted image. In these untreated embryos local differences in the physical characteristics of the water in the embryos lead to different signal intensities in the images. Thus we are able to identify various morphological features, as is commonly done in clinical NMR imaging.

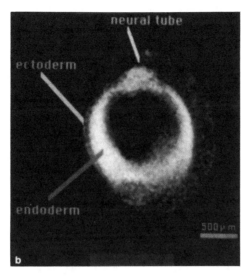

Figure 11-29   The central section of an image of a frog embryo after eight additional hours of development from stage 31. At this time the embryo is in the early stages of neurulation. The ectoderm structure is also seen.

11-3-2   Localized *In vivo* High-Resolution Imaging [44]

Problems and Limitations In vivo High-Resolution Imaging

While microscopic imaging for small objects is progressing well, high-resolution imagings of large objects such as the human body are not readily available, especially *in vivo* high-resolution imaging. For *in vivo* high-resolution NMR imaging using conventional techniques, there are a number of limitations such as the low signal-to-noise ratio and image fold-over due to aliasing and localization. There have been several attempts to localize a small volume and obtain high-resolution images such as the method using a radial coil [45]. Most of the methods, however, were either not readily available or not useful in a clinical setting. This was due to the extensive hardware requirements or other physical limitations.

The basic requirements for the localization technique in high resolution imaging are (1) the size and location of the volume to be localized should be easily adjustable using a simple pulse sequence, (2) the selected region should be uniform and well separated so that the signals from outside the region are well suppressed in comparison to the signal from the selected region, (3) the signal intensity of the selected region should be neither disturbed nor diminished by the localization process, and (4) the pulse sequence should be simple so that other imaging pulse sequences such as the spectroscopic pulse sequences can also be incorporated. Over the past several years a number of localization techniques have been developed, both for the spectroscopic applications and for the localized *in vivo* high-resolution imaging.

Localized In vivo High-Resolution Imaging using Gradient Subencoding

As an alternative to the conventional localization using rf and gradient pulse encoding a gradient subencoding technique can be used, for example, subencoding or weighting in conjunction with the existing phase encoding. Then the rf pulse used is only for slice selection. The principle of localization is based on the convolution operation of the additional subencoding gradients which enable the imaging region to be selected along the phase-encoding direction in the image domain. It is easy to see that the convolution operation of a sinc function in the time domain performed by the subencoding gradient would be equivalent to selecting a rectangular region in the image domain by well-known Fourier convolution theorem. This method requires a large number of subencoding steps. The large number of subencoding steps for localization, however, can be used instead of simple averaging because high-resolution imaging usually requires a large number of averagings. For a 2-D application, localization in the readout direction is subsequently carried out by controlling the bandwidth of the low-pass filter in the receiver channel; thus no complex modification of the pulse sequence is required. Although a high resolution nonaliased image can be obtained by simply oversampling the FID data, it requires much larger data storage and a larger matrix size for the Fourier transform. Usually a subencoding technique is used in combination with a single-cycle SSFP sequence to maximize the signal-to-noise ratio. In the following, a simple analytical description of the method is given.

Let us first consider the well-known basic NMR signal from which an image can be obtained in conventional NMR imaging,

$$S(\omega_x, \omega_y) = \int_x \int_y \rho(x, y) \exp\{i(\omega_x x + \omega_y y)\} \, dx \, dy$$

or
$$= \mathscr{F}_2[\rho(x, y)] \tag{11-50}$$

where

$$\omega_x = \gamma g_x T_x$$
$$\omega_y = \gamma g_y T_y \tag{11-51}$$

Note here that g_x and g_y now represent the variable amplitude of the x and y gradients and T_x and T_y are the corresponding fixed time durations, respectively. In Eq. (11-50), $\mathscr{F}_2[\cdot]$ denotes the 2-D Fourier transform operation. From this basic Fourier transform relation, if a certain one-dimensional weight function $w(x)$ in the phase-encoding direction (x) is multiplied on the density function $\rho(x, y)$ for the purpose of selecting a region of interest in the x direction, Eq. (11-50) can be written as

$$S'(\omega_x, \omega_y) = \mathscr{F}_2[\rho(x, y)w(x)]$$

or

$$= \mathscr{F}_2[\rho(x, y)] * \mathscr{F}_1[w(x)] \qquad (11\text{-}52)$$

where $*$ is the convolution operation. Equation (11-52) is precisely the selection mechanism in NMR imaging using a selection function $w(x)$ in image domain, which is equivalent to the convolution operation in the Fourier domain or, in this case, the time or FID domain. This is equivalent to the localization of the image in the x direction (phase-encoding direction in this example). Equation (11-52) can also be written as

$$S'(\omega_x, \omega_y) = S(\omega_x, \omega_y) * W(\omega_x)$$

or

$$= \int_{\omega_x'} S(\omega_x - \omega_x', \omega_y)W(\omega_x') \, d\omega_x' \qquad (11\text{-}53)$$

where $W(\omega_x) = \mathscr{F}_1[w(x)]$. As mentioned, a sinc shape function $W(\omega_x)$ will result in selection of a region in the x direction (phase-encoding direction) in the image domain. In the numerical operation the right-hand term in Eq. (11-53) represents the summation of the FID signal weighted by $W(\omega_x')$ for a given variable ω_x'. $W(\omega_x')$ is usually in the form of a sinc distribution function, and the variable ω_x' is realized in NMR imaging by introducing the subencoding gradient. The subencoding gradient convolved into the main phase-encoding gradient is illustrated in Fig. 11-30. The total phase-encoding gradient $g_{x,\,total}$ is then the sum of both the main encoding gradient g_x and subencoding gradient g_{xs}:

$$g_{x,\,total} = g_x \pm g_{xs} \qquad (11\text{-}54)$$

The resultant spatial frequency $\omega_{x,\,total}$ is

$$\omega_{x,\,total} = \omega_x \pm \omega_{xs}$$

$$= \gamma g_x T_x \pm \gamma g_{xs} T_{xs} \qquad (11\text{-}55)$$

where T_x and T_{xs} are the time duration of g_x and g_{xs}, respectively. The resultant NMR signal with subencoding gradients can be written as

$$\bar{S}(\omega_x, \omega_y) = \int_x \int_y \rho(x, y)\exp\left[i\gamma\{(\omega_x \pm \omega_{xs})x + \omega_y y\}\right] dx \, dy$$

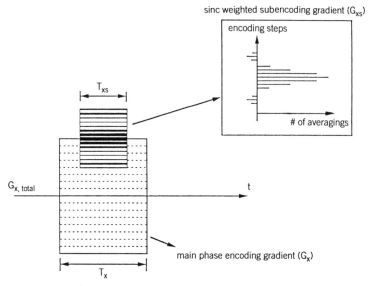

Figure 11-30 The convolution process of the main phase-encoding gradient G_x with the subencoding gradient G_{xs} for localization in the phase-encoding direction (x direction).

or

$$= \int_x \int_y \rho(x, y) \exp\left[i\{\pm\omega_{xs}x\}\right] \exp\left[i\{\omega_x x + \omega_y y\}\right] dx\, dy$$

$$(11\text{-}56)$$

After substituting $\pm\omega_{xs}$ with $-\omega'_x$, Eq. (11-56) can also be written as

$$\bar{S}(\omega_x, \omega_y) = S(\omega_x - \omega'_x, \omega_y) \qquad (11\text{-}57)$$

Taking the summation of Eq. (11-56) or Eq. (11-57) along the subencoding direction after multiplying the weighting function $W(\omega_{xs})$ or $W(\omega'_x)$ will result in a convolution operation in the spatial frequency domain as

$$S(\omega_x, \omega_y)_{\text{sum}} = \int_{-\omega_x}^{\omega_x} S(\omega_x - \omega'_x, \omega_y) W(\omega'_x)\, d\omega'_x$$

or

$$= \bar{S}(\omega_x, \omega_y) * W(\omega_x) \qquad (11\text{-}58)$$

One can easily recognize that Eq. (11-58) is equivalent to Eq. (11-53):

$$S(\omega_x, \omega_y)_{\text{sum}} = S'(\omega_x, \omega_y)$$

or

$$= \int_{-\omega_x}^{\omega_x} S(\omega_x - \omega'_x, \omega_y) W(\omega'_x)\, d\omega'_x \qquad (11\text{-}59)$$

Now by using Eqs. (11-56) and (11-57), Eq. (11-59) can be rewritten as

$$S(\omega_x, \omega_y)_{\text{sum}}$$

$$= \int_{\omega_{xs}} \int_x \int_y \rho(x, y) \exp\{i[(\omega_x \pm \omega_{xs})x + \omega_y y]\}\, dx\, dy\, W(\omega_{xs})\, d\omega_{xs}$$

$$= \int_x \int_y \rho(x, y) \exp\{i(\omega_x x + \omega_y y)\}\, dx\, dy \int_{\omega_{xs}} W(\omega_{xs}) \exp\{i\omega_{xs} x\}\, d\omega_{xs}$$

$$(11\text{-}60)$$

The last integral in Eq. (11-60) represents the Fourier transform of the weighting function $W(\omega_{xs})$ in the subencoding domain, and its Fourier transform $w(x)$ now represents the image domain localization function in the phase-encoding direction (x):

$$S(\omega_x, \omega_y)_{\text{sum}} = \int_x \int_y [\rho(x, y) w(x)] \exp\{i(\omega_x x + \omega_y y)\}\, dx\, dy$$

$$= S'(\omega_x, \omega_y) \qquad (11\text{-}61)$$

where the operation in [ ] represents the localization. Two-dimensional localization is then achieved by adding a low-pass filter $w(y)$ in the readout direction or at the receiver channel:

$$S''(\omega_x, \omega_y) = \int_x \int_y [\rho(x, y) w(x) w(y)] \exp\{i(\omega_x x + \omega_y y)\}\, dx\, dy \quad (11\text{-}62)$$

The weighting function $W(\omega'_x)$ is implemented in NMR imaging by the addition or subtraction of each main encoding gradient and averaged afterward according to the weighting function $W(\omega'_x)$. The NMR signals, which result from all the subencoding gradient steps for each main encoding gradient, are summed up to realize the convolution operation given in Eq. (11-53). The NMR signal corresponding to the negative part of the side lobe of the sinc weighting pulse is reversed in polarity before summation. Finally, by taking the 2-D Fourier transform of the NMR signal $S''(\omega_x, \omega_y)$ in Eq. (11-62), one obtains an image, two-dimensionally localized by the selection function $w(x)$ and $w(y)$. The position of the localized region can also be moved or shifted by multiplying a phase term corresponding to the amount of the position shift x_0. In other words, a new shifted weighting function $W(\omega_x)_{\text{shift}}$ in the image domain can be written as

$$W(\omega_x)_{\text{shift}} = W(\omega_x)\exp(-j\omega_x x_0)$$

or

$$\mathscr{F}[W(\omega_x)_{\text{shift}}] = w(x - x_0) \tag{11-63}$$

The position of the shifted and localized density function $\rho(x, y)$ then becomes $\rho(x, y)w(x - x_0)$. In practice, the complex phase term $\exp(-j\omega_x x_0)$ is multiplied into the NMR signal resulting from each subencoding gradient before taking the average.

Similarly, the localization in the readout direction (y) is performed simply by adjusting the bandwidth of the low-pass filter, which is usually located between the demodulator and the analog-to-digital converter in the receiver system (this low-pass filter is also used to reduce the high-frequency noise and to remove the high-frequency signal components). The relation between the area or width in the y direction (y is the readout direction in this case) and the bandwidth is given by

$$\Delta y = \frac{2\pi \Delta f}{\gamma G_y} \tag{11-64}$$

where Δf is the bandwidth of the low-pass filter. The amplitude of the readout gradient G_y in Eq. (11-64) can be calculated by using other imaging parameters, such as field of view (FOV), the size of the image matrix N, and the duration of the sampling window T_{sw}:

$$G_y = \frac{2\pi N}{\gamma(\text{FOV})T_{sw}} \tag{11-65}$$

Substituting Eq. (11-65) into Eq. (11-64) yields Δy as

$$\Delta y = \frac{\Delta f(\text{FOV})T_{sw}}{N} \tag{11-66}$$

The size of the localization in the readout direction depends therefore on the characteristic of the low-pass filter. The position in the readout direction can also be shifted by changing the carrier frequency of the receiver. The amount of frequency shift Δf_{shift} to be changed for the position shift in the readout

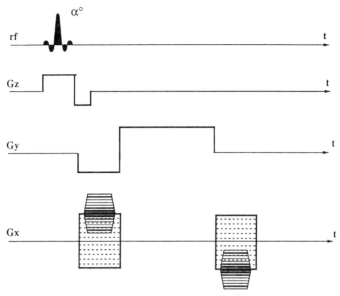

rf

Gz

Gy

Gx

Figure 11-31 Pulse sequence used for the gradient subencoding *in vivo* localized high resolution imaging.

direction can be calculated as

$$\Delta f_{\text{shift}} = \frac{\gamma G_y \, \Delta y_{\text{shift}}}{2\pi} = \frac{N \Delta y_{\text{shift}}}{(\text{FOV}) T_{sw}} \qquad (11\text{-}67)$$

For the experimental test of the subencoding technique, an example of the discrete weighting function is formed by a Gaussian-weighted sinc function, as shown in Fig. 11-30. Usually the total number of averages for this experiment is 100, and the area width selected by the subencoding gradient is set to 5 cm. The number of averages at each subencoding gradient step is therefore governed by the desired selection profile and signal intensity in the real experiment. The low-pass filter used in the receiver side is made with a fourth-order Butterworth filter which possesses maximum flatness in the selected region. The pulse sequence used in the experiment is shown in Fig. 11-31, which is a variation of the SSFP sequence. To reduce the diffusion effect during the application of the readout gradient, a half-echo-like pulse sequence is used. The repetition time and the echo time were 30 msec and 10 msec.

In Fig. 11-32(a) an image of a phantom with normal resolution (~ 1 mm) is shown. The rectangular region inside the image is the region to be seen in high resolution imaging. Figure 11-32(c) shows an image obtained by conven-

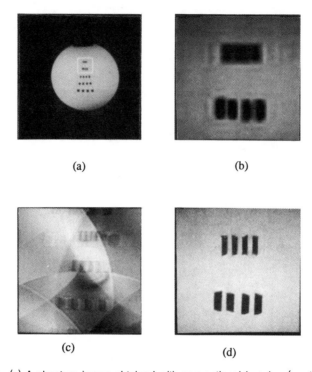

(a)   (b)

(c)   (d)

Figure 11-32 (a) A phantom image obtained with conventional imaging (~ 1-mm resolution). (b) A directly zoomed image of the region marked by a square box in (a). (c) A 10 times expanded (zoomed) image of the same region as in (a) but without the localization technique. The image is degraded by aliasing. (d) A high-resolution image of the same region as in (b) obtained by the localization technique.

tional imaging with normal resolution expansion that is, by increase of gradient strength. In this case, the image is enlarged by simply increasing the gradient; the aliasing effect obscures the image. By using the localization technique, however, we have obtained a clear high-resolution image with an order of magnitude improvement in resolution, as shown in Fig. 11-32(d). This image should be compared with the image shown in Fig. 11-32(b), which is the result of directly zooming the rectangular region of the image shown in Fig. 11-32(a).

REFERENCES

1. E. L. Hahn. *Phys. Rev.* 80:580 (1950).
2. T. C. Farrar and E. D. Becker. *Pulse and Fourier Transform NMR—Introduction to Theory and Methods.* San Diego: Academic Press, 1971.
3. A. Kumar, D. Welti, and R. Ernst. *J. Magn. Reson.* 18:60 (1975).

4. H. W. Park, M. H. Cho, and Z. H. Cho. *Magn. Reson. Med.* 2:534 (1985).

5. H. W. Park, M. H. Cho, and Z. H. Cho. *Magn. Reson. Med.* 3:15 (1956).

6. G. H. Glover and N. J. Pelc. In *Magnetic Resonance Annual 1988*, H. Y. Hressel, ed. New York: Raven Press, 1988, pp. 299–333.

7. W. S. Kim, C. W. Mun, D. J. Kim, and Z. H. Cho. *Magn. Reson. Med.* 13:25–37 (1990).

8. P. Mansfield. *J. Phys. C.* 10:155 (1977).

9. C. B. Ahn, J. H. Kim, and Z. H. Cho. *IEEE Med. Imag.* MI-5:2 (1986).

10. S. Ljunggren. *J. Magn. Reson.* 54:338 (1983).

11. A. Macovski and C. Meyer. *Fifth Annual Meeting of the Society of Magnetic Resonance in Medicine*, WIP, 1986, p. 156.

12. C. Meyer and A. Macovski. *Sixth Annual Meeting of the Society of Magnetic Resonance in Medicine*, 1987, p. 230.

13. A. Haase, J. Frahm, D. Mattaei, W. Hänicke, and K. D. Merboldt. *Book of Abstracts, 4th Annual Meeting of the SMRM*, 1985, p. 980; *J. Magn. Reson.* 67:258 (1986); U.S. Patent No. 4, 707658.

14. J. Frahm, W. Hänicke, and K. D. Merboldt. *J. Magn. Reson.* 72:307 (1987).

15. M. L. Gyngell, N. D. Palmer, and L. M. Eastwood. *Fifth Annual Meeting of the Society of Magnetic Resonance in Medicine*, 1986, p. 666.

16. R. C. Hawkes and S. Patz. *Magn. Reson. Med.* 4:9 (1987).

17. K. Sekihara. *IEEE Trans. Med. Imag.* 6:157 (1987).

18. W. S. Hinshaw, *J. Appl. Physics*, 47:3709 (1976).

19. S. Y. Lee and Z. H. Cho. *Magn. Reson. Med.* 8:142 (1988).

20. R. Graumann, H. Fischer, H. Barfuss, H. Bruder, A. Oppelt, and M. Deimling. *Sixth Annual Meeting of the Society of Magnetic Resonance in Medicine*, 1987, p. 444.

21. T. W. Redpath, R. A. Jones, and J. R. Mallard. *Sixth Annual Meeting of the Society of Magnetic Resonance in Medicine*, 1987, p. 228.

22. T. W. Redpath and R. A. Jones. *Magn. Reson. Med.* 6:224 (1988).

23. H. Bruder, H. Fischer, R. Graumann, and M. Deimling. *Magn. Reson. Med.* 7:35 (1988).

24. D. Shaw. *Fourier Transform NMR Spectroscopy*. New York: Elsevier, 1976.

25. P. Mansfield and P. G. Morris. *NMR Imaging in Biomedicine*. San Diego: Academic Press, 1982.

26. K. M. Ludeke, P. Roschmann, and R. Tischler. *Magn. Reson. Imag.* 3:329 (1985).

27. H. W. Park, Y. M. Ro, and Z. H. Cho. *Phys. Med. Biol.* 33:339 (1988).

28. A. Haase. *Magn. Reson. Med.* 13:77 (1990).

29. R. J. Ordidge, R. Coxon, A. Howsman, B. Chapman, R. Tuner, M. Stehling, and P. Mansfield, *Magn. Reson. Med.* 8:110 (1988).

30. I. L. Pykett and R. R. Rzedaian. *Magn. Reson. Med.* 5:563 (1987).

31. J. Henning, A. Nauerth, and H. Friedburg. *Magn. Reson. Med.* 3:823 (1986).

32. P. Mansfield and B. Chpman. *J. Phys. E.* 19:540 (1986).

33. M. L. Gyngell, N. D. Palmer, and M. Eastwood. *Book of Abstracts, Fifth Annual Meeting of the Society of Magnetic Resonance in Medicine*, 1986, p. 666.

34. J. S. Waugh. *J. Mol. Spectrosc.* 35:298 (1970).

35. P. Mansfield and P. G. Morris. *NMR Imaging in Biomedicine*. San Diego: Academic Press, 1982, pp. 69–83.

36. J. Frahm, W. Hänicke, and K. D. Merboldt. *J. Magn. Reson.* 72:307 (1987).

37. A. Haase, J. Frahm, W. Hänicke, and D. Mattaei. *Phys. Med. Biol.* 30:341 (1982).

38. P. C. Lauterbur. *Nature* 242:190 (1973).

39. Z. H. Cho, H. S. Kim, H. B. Song, and J. Cumming. *Proc. IEEE* 70:1152 (1982).

40. Z. H. Cho. Computerized tomography. In *Encyclopedia of Physical Science and Technology*, vol. 3. San Diego: Academic, 1987, pp. 507–544.

41. Z. H. Cho, C. B. Ahn, S. C. Juh, H. K. Lee, R. E. Jacobs, S. Lee, J. H. Yi, and J. M. Jo. *Med. Phys.* 15:6 (1988).

42. Z. H. Cho, C. B. Ahn, S. C. Juh, J. M. Jo, R. M. Fridenberg, S. E. Fraser, and R. E. Jacobs. *Phil. Trans. R. Soc. Lond.* A, 333:469 (1990).

43. E. O. Stejskal and J. E. Tanner. *J. Chem. Phys.* 42:288 (1965).

44. Z. H. Cho and J. M. Jo. *Med. Phys.* 18(3):350–356 (1991).

45. S. Y. Lee and Z. H. Cho. *Magn. Reson. Med.* 12:56–63 (1989).

12

FLOW AND FLOW-RELATED MAGNETIC RESONANCE IMAGING

The investigation of nuclear magnetic resonance in a flowing liquid has a long history, and its noninvasive nature have made it attractive to many investigators in the field of fluid dynamics as well as medical diagnostic imaging. In particular, the recent advent of MRI has brought about a new dimension in noninvasive clinical diagnoses of many diseases. As stated previously, image contrast with MRI depends on several parameters such as the spin density, the T_1 and T_2 relaxation times, the chemical shift, and the flow. The flow has been of particular interest in MRI because it has significant potential in medical diagnosis and in the investigation of certain patterns of fluid dynamics in body organs [1–3]. The motion of the excited spin produces changes in the amplitude and the phase of the magnetization in NMR. Flow therefore acts like an intrinsic contrast medium in NMR imaging, and this new, noninvasive imaging modality is rapidly gaining clinical acceptance. For example, the high sensitivity of MRI to the motion of the fluid makes it particularly attractive for clinical blood flow measurements. More recently many investigators have made substantial progress in this area, demonstrating that NMR angiography can be accomplished without any contrast enhancing media such as iodine, a toxic contrast agent.

12-1 PRINCIPLES OF BULK FLOW IMAGING

12-1-1 Motion of Spins in a Magnetic Field [2, 5, 7]

As was shown in Chapter 9, the general behavior of the spin magnetizations under the main magnetic field applied in the z direction can be understood by solving the Bloch equation:

$$\frac{\partial \mathbf{M}}{\partial t} = \gamma \mathbf{M} \times \mathbf{H} - \frac{M_x \hat{x}' + M_y \hat{y}'}{T_2} - \frac{(M_z - M_0)\hat{z}'}{T_1} \tag{12-1}$$

where $\hat{x}'$, $\hat{y}'$, and $\hat{z}'$ are the unit vectors in the rotating frame x', y', and z' directions, respectively, t is time, γ is the gyromagnetic ratio, $\mathbf{M}$ is the magnetization vector, $\mathbf{H}$ is the applied magnetic field (including the main magnetic field, the gradient field, and the rf field), and T_1 and T_2 have the usual definitions.

In a rotating frame of reference where the rotating angular frequency is ω, the associated effective magnetic field becomes

$$\mathbf{H}_{\text{eff}} = \mathbf{H} + \frac{\omega}{\gamma} \tag{12-2}$$

In Eq. (12-2), the T_1 and T_2 effects are omitted for simplicity. If ω is equal to the Larmor frequency of the main magnetic field $\mathbf{H}_0$ and if the gradient and rf magnetic fields are applied, Eq. (12-2) can be written as

$$\mathbf{H}_{\text{eff}} = [\mathbf{G} \cdot \mathbf{r}(t)]\hat{z}' + H_{1x'}(t)\hat{x}' + H_{1y'}(t)\hat{y}' \tag{12-3}$$

where $\mathbf{G}$ is the gradient vector, $\mathbf{r}(t)$ is the time-varying position vector of the magnetization, and $H_{1x'}(t)$ and $H_{1y'}(t)$ are the time-varying rf fields applied to the x' and y' coordinate axes, respectively. By solving Eq. (12-1) using the $\mathbf{H}_{\text{eff}}$ given in Eq. (12-3), the complete spin motion during the rf or gradient pulse can be described. In this section we will attempt to solve Eq. (12-1) for a specific case of a selection gradient in conjunction with a spin-echo 180° rf pulse. (See slice selection for flow encoding.)

12-1-2   Spatial and Flow Domain Phase Codings

If one considers a simple case where the time-dependent bipolar gradient pulse $G_x(t)$ is applied after a 90° rf pulse in the positive x direction (neglecting the effects of the relaxation times T_1 and T_2), the resulting phase information of the FID (free induction decay) can be separated into two parts, namely the spatial-position-dependent term Φ_x and the velocity-dependent term Φ_v:

$$\Phi_x = \gamma x \int_0^{2t_p} G_x(t)\, dt = 0$$

and

$$\Phi_v = \gamma v \int_0^{2t_p} G_x(t) t\, dt = \gamma v G_x t_p^2 \tag{12-4}$$

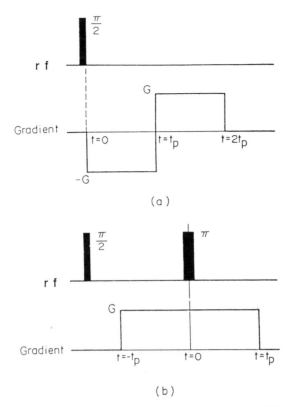

Figure 12-1 Gradient pulse shapes for velocity or flow phase coding: (a) a bipolar gradient in FID detection sequence and (b) an unipolar gradient in spin-echo sequence.

where x, v, and $2t_p$ are the position, flow velocity, and gradient pulse duration, respectively. Using Eq. (12-4), information on the velocity of the moving spins can be inferred by the well-known phase encoding technique [3].

As indicated, Eq. (12-4) leads to $\Phi_x = 0$ but $\Phi_v \neq 0$. Although there are many waveforms that can satisfy these equations, the bipolar gradient waveform shown in Fig. 12-1(a) is a typical waveform that is used for phase coding. The same result can also be obtained by the spin-echo sequence with an unipolar gradient as shown in Fig. 12-1(b) [5].

12-1-3   Phase Encoding for Flow Imaging

As we have learned, a selection gradient with 180° rf pulse in spin echo sequence has exactly the same effect on flow coding as the bipolar gradient in FID detection sequence. It is therefore important to study the flow-coding

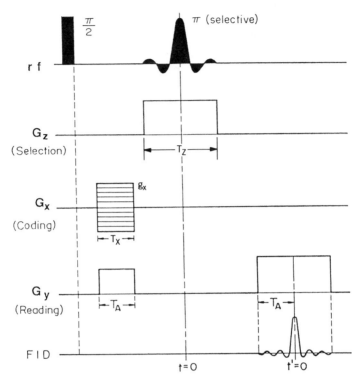

Figure 12-2 A conventional 2-D Fourier imaging pulse sequence with a spin echo where slice selection is achieved by the spin echo using a 180° rf pulse. Note here that the rectangular selection gradient G_z has a similar function as the bipolar pulse shown in Fig. 12-1 (a).

effect of the gradient and rf pulse during the pulse application. In this subsection therefore the slice selection effect in the normal spin-echo imaging sequence (Fig. 12-2) is studied by numerically integrating the Bloch equation to obtain the flow velocity phase relationship [4]. In the present study it is assumed that the flow velocity has only one directional component, namely the z direction or the slice selection direction.

Let us assume that only the z-directional gradient and the time-varying rf pulse are simultaneously applied in the x' direction; then the effective magnetic field in a rotating frame given by Eq. (12-3) becomes

$$\mathbf{H}_{\text{eff}} = G_z(z + v_z t)\hat{z}' + H_{1x'}(t)\hat{x}' \tag{12-5}$$

where z and $H_{1x'}(t)$ are the position of the given magnetization and the intensity of the rf field applied in the x' direction, respectively. By solving the Bloch equation given in Eq. (12-1) using the above effective field $\mathbf{H}_{\text{eff}}$ [Eq.

(12-5)], the behavior of the spins under such a circumstance can be accurately inferred. For the investigation of the spin behavior, let us assume that the initial positions of the spin magnetizations lie somewhere in the transverse plane and that the 180° rf pulse is applied to the x' direction for the selection of the 2-D slice.

It is interesting to note that when we consider the flow of spins in a selected slice, it is necessary to consider 3-D space together with velocity. Flow imaging therefore is 4-D, three dimensions being the spatial coordinates and the other dimension being the velocity coordinate v_z. The NMR signal therefore can be represented in a general equation for different z positions (at $t = 0$) and z-directional velocities as

$$S(t') = \int_{v_z} \int_z \left(\int_y \int_x \rho(x, y, z, v_z) \left\{ \exp[i\gamma G_y y(t' + T_A)] \right. \right.$$

$$\left. \left. \times \mathcal{M}_s(\alpha; z, v_z) \right\} dx\, dy \right) dz\, dv_z \quad (12-6)$$

where $\mathcal{M}_s[\alpha; z, v_z]$ denotes the resulting magnetization affected by the selection operation under a given initial magnetization α ($\alpha = \exp[i\gamma(G_y y T_A + g_x x T_x)]$). Note that the center of the spin-echo signal is defined at $t' = 0$ in Eq. (12-6). Let us consider the resulting magnetization $\mathcal{M}_s(\cdot)$ when the Bloch equation is solved with the two independent initial magnetizations, M'_y and M'_x, which are denoted "1" and "i ($= \sqrt{-1}$)," respectively. The magnetizations resulting from these two initial magnetizations, 1 and i for the given v_z and z, can be represented as

$$\mathcal{M}_s(1; z, v_z) = \mathcal{M}_{SR}^{(1)} + i\mathcal{M}_{SI}^{(1)}$$

and

$$\mathcal{M}_s(i; z, v_z) = \mathcal{M}_{SR}^{(i)} + i\mathcal{M}_{SI}^{(i)} \quad (12-7)$$

where $\mathcal{M}_{SR}^{(1)}$, $\mathcal{M}_{SI}^{(1)}$, $\mathcal{M}_{SR}^{(i)}$, and $\mathcal{M}_{SI}^{(i)}$ are the real and imaginary components of the resulting magnetizations on the transverse plane with the superscripts, 1 and i each denoting the corresponding initial condition. It is worthwhile to remember that $\mathcal{M}_s(\cdot)$ is the resulting magnetization due to the selection operation for a given z, v_z, and $H_{1x}(t)$. Since the Bloch equation is a linear equation, the resulting magnetization from a complex initial magnetization can be represented by the linear combination of $p\mathcal{M}_s(1) + q\mathcal{M}_s(i)$, where p and q are the real and imaginary components of the initial magnetizations, respectively.

After some algebraic operations it can be shown that the terms in the braces $\{\cdot\}$ in Eq. (12-6) can be expressed as

$$(\eta + i\xi)\exp[i\gamma(G_y y t' - g_x x T_x)] \quad (12-8)$$

where η and ξ are given by

$$\eta = \frac{\mathcal{M}_{SR}^{(1)} - \mathcal{M}_{SI}^{(i)}}{2}$$

and

$$\xi = \frac{\mathcal{M}_{SI}^{(1)} + \mathcal{M}_{SR}^{(i)}}{2} \tag{12-9}$$

In both Eqs. (12-8) and (12-9) the phase of the NMR signal is denoted in reference to the spin-echo center. Using Eqs. (12-8) and (12-9), Eq. (12-6) can be written as

$$S(t') = \int_{v_z} \int_z \int_y \int_x \rho(x, y, z, v_z)(\eta + i\xi)\exp\left[i\gamma(G_y yt' - g_x xT_x)\right] dx\, dy\, dz\, dv_z \tag{12-10}$$

Considering a slice of a finite thickness Δz located at $z = z_0$ and assuming that the spin density is uniform along the z direction within the slice thickness, Eq. (12-10) can be further simplified to

$$S_1(t') = \int_{v_z} \int_y \int_x \rho_1(x, y, v_z)\exp\left[i\Phi_{v_z}(x, y)\right]\exp\left[i\gamma(G_y yt' - g_x xT_x)\right] dx\, dy\, dv_z \tag{12-11}$$

where

$$\Phi_{v_z} = \tan^{-1}\left(\frac{\int_{-\Delta z/2}^{\Delta z/2} \xi(v_z, z)\, dz}{\int_{-\Delta z/2}^{\Delta z/2} \eta(v_z, z)\, dz}\right) \tag{12-12}$$

and

$$\rho_1(x, y, v_z) = \int_{-\Delta z/2}^{\Delta z/2} \rho(x, y, z, v_z)\sqrt{\eta^2 + \xi^2}\, dz \tag{12-13}$$

If there is only one velocity component in each spatial location (x, y), then Eq. (12-10) is further reduced to

$$S_2(t') = \int_y \int_x \rho_2(x, y)\exp\left[i\Phi_{v_z}(x, y)\right]\exp\left[i\gamma(G_y yt' - g_x xT_x)\right] dx\, dy \tag{12-14}$$

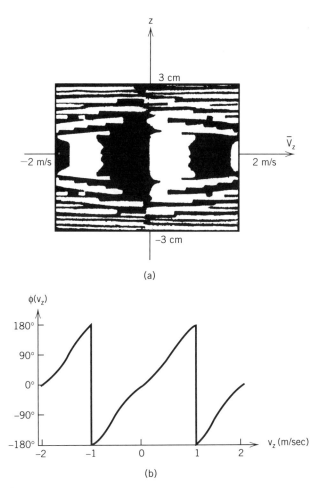

Figure 12-3 Simulation results of the phase-velocity relationship obtained by solving the Bloch equation: (a) the flow-encoded phases [arctan(ξ/η)] as a function of velocity v_z along position z given in Eq. (12-9), and (b) the integrated value of the phases along z direction based on Eq. (12-12).

where $\rho_2(x, y) = \rho_1(x, y, v_z)|_{v_z = \mathrm{const}}$. Figure 12-3(a) and (b) show the phases of $\eta + i\xi$ as a function of v_z at different z positions, and the integrated value of the above phases along z, respectively. This result is obtained by the application of a selective rf pulse, which is of a truncated sinc pulse shape (pulse width: 5 msec, bandwidth: -0.2 G/cm to $+0.2$ G/cm). The region between the two abrupt gray level changes of the integrated phase $\phi(v_z)$ (i.e., from $v_z = -1$ m/sec to $v_z = +1$ m/sec along the v_z axis in the phase map) indicates the useful range (i.e., $-\pi$ to $+\pi$) of the method. The approximate linear velocity phase relationship between -1 m/sec to $+1$ m/sec is the region useful for velocity encoding.

The numerical solution given in Eq. (12-12) (i.e., the calculated velocity encoded phase Φ_{v_z}) agrees well with the result that can be obtained with conventional velocity encoding by a bipolar gradient pulse:

$$\Phi_{v_z} = \left(\frac{\gamma}{4}\right) G_z v_z T_z^2 \tag{12-15}$$

where v_z is the z-directional velocity, T_z is the width of the selection gradient pulse, and Φ_{v_z} now represents the velocity-encoded phase when the selection gradient G_z is applied simultaneously with a 180° rf pulse. In a real imaging situation the magnitude of the selection gradient, G_z, is adjusted so that the encoded phases corresponding to the velocity range to be measured lie between $-180°$ and $180°$. Since this method is easy to incorporate in the spin-echo technique, it can readily be used in many cases of flow imaging.

12-2   FLOW COMPENSATION IN IMAGING

12-2-1   Flow Compensation in the Phase-Encoding Direction (x-Direction)

When the x-direction gradient is used as a phase-encoding gradient in imaging, the velocity phase encoded by the x-gradient can be calculated and is shown in Fig. 12-4. Setting the time origin at the center of the spin echo and assuming that the x-directional velocity v_x is constant, the encoded phase due to the spatial encoding gradient g_x and the bipolar flow phase encoding gradient G_{v_x} can be written as

$$\Phi_x = -\gamma G_x x T_x \tag{12-16a}$$

and

$$
\begin{aligned}
\Phi_{v_x} &= -\tfrac{1}{2}\gamma G_{v_x} v_x \left(t'^2 - T_{v^-}^2\right), & T_{v^-} &< t' < \frac{T_{v^-} + T_{v^+}}{2} \\[4pt]
&= -\tfrac{1}{2}\gamma G_{v_x} v_x \left(t'^2 - \left(\frac{T_{v^-} + T_{v^+}}{2}\right)^2\right), & \frac{T_{v^-} + T_{v^+}}{2} &< t' < T_{v^+} \quad (12\text{-}16b) \\[4pt]
&= -\tfrac{1}{2}\gamma G_x v_x \left(t'^2 - T_a^2\right), & T_a &< t' < T_b
\end{aligned}
$$

The corresponding frequencies ω_x and ω_{v_y} can be represented as

$$\omega_x = \gamma g_x T_x \tag{12-17a}$$

and

$$\omega_{v_x} = \Delta\omega_{v_x, s} + \Delta\omega_{v_x, v} \tag{12-17b}$$

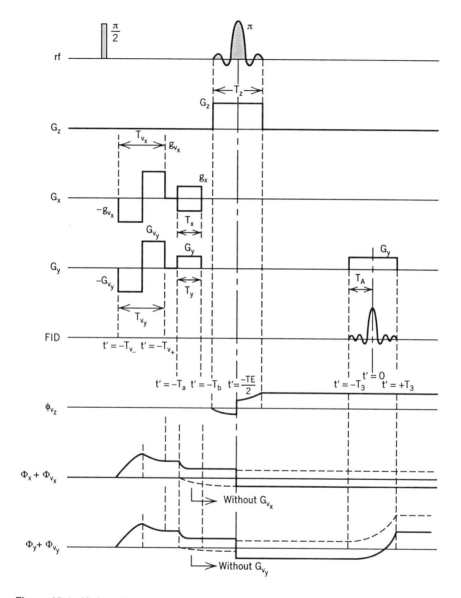

Figure 12-4   Various phases resulting from the application of flow codings and compensating gradients. As shown, while x-directional flow can be fully compensated, y-directional flow is more difficult. In the case of later, phase varies during the signal readout period ($\sim t = \pm T_A$).

where

$$\Delta\omega_{v_x,s} = \frac{\gamma}{2}g_x v_x\left(T_b^2 - T_a^2\right)$$

and

$$\Delta\omega_{v_x,v} = \frac{\gamma}{4}G_{v_x}v_x T_{v_x}^2 \tag{12-18}$$

The time scales T_x and T_{v_x} are the pulse widths of the gradients g_x and G_{v_x}, respectively (see Fig. 12-4). From the preceding equations it can be seen that if x-directional velocity or flow coding is not desired, the x-directional velocity coding Φ_{v_x} can be adjusted so that $\Phi_{v_x} = 0$ during the signal readout period; that is, $-T_3 < t' < +T_3$ by simply controlling G_{v_x} or T_{v_x}. Since the spatial coding gradient g_x varies at each encoding step (see Fig. 12-2), the amplitude of G_{v_x} should vary accordingly in order to make $\Phi_{v_x} = 0$:

$$G_{v_x}T_{v_x}^2 + 2g_x\left(T_b^2 + T_a^2\right) = 0 \tag{12-19}$$

Equation (12-19) shows the relation between the magnitudes and the pulse durations of the spatial and the velocity encoding gradients necessary to compensate for the x-directional flow.

12-2-2 Flow Compensation in the Readout Direction (*y*-Direction)

Let us now consider phase encoding due to the y-gradient G_{v_y} (see Fig. 12-4), which would be needed to compensate for the velocity coding at the center of the FID as well as the phase change due to the flow. If we assume that in Fig. 12-4 the time origin is at the center of the spin echo, the spatially coded and velocity coded phases in the y direction, Φ_y and Φ_{v_y}, are given by

$$\Phi_y = \gamma G_y y t' \tag{12-20a}$$

and

$$\begin{aligned}
\Phi_{v_y} &= -\tfrac{1}{2}\gamma G_{v_y}v_y\left(t'^2 - T_{v-}^2\right), & T_{v-} < t' < \frac{T_{v-} + T_{v+}}{2} \\[2mm]
&= -\tfrac{1}{2}\gamma G_{v_y}v_y\left(t'^2 - \left(\frac{T_{v-} + T_{v+}}{2}\right)^2\right), & \frac{T_{v-} + T_{v+}}{2} < t' < T_{v+} \\[2mm]
&= -\tfrac{1}{2}\gamma G_y v_y\left(t'^2 - T_a^2\right), & T_a < t' < T_b \\[2mm]
&= \frac{\gamma}{2}G_y v_y t'^2, & -T_3 < t' < T_3
\end{aligned} \tag{12-20b}$$

Figure 12-4 shows how Φ_y and Φ_{v_y} change during the readout period. Since we acquire the signal with a finite data readout time $(-T_A$ to $T_A)$, the phase of the signal changes as a function of the time t'. During readout time this varying phase is difficult to compensate, unlike the x component, and poses a problem.

Example: Numerical Integration of the Bloch Equation for Flow Imaging in a Spin-Echo Pulse Sequence

During the z-directional slice selection process using Hahn spin echo, the Bloch equation in the rotating frame can be written as

$$\left(\frac{\partial \mathbf{M}}{\partial t}\right)_{\text{rot}} = \gamma \mathbf{M}(t) \times \mathbf{H}_{\text{eff}}(t) \tag{12-21}$$

where $\mathbf{H}_{\text{eff}}(t)$ is given in Eq. (12-5). As an example, Eq. (12-21) is numerically integrated under the following conditions:

1. G_z: 0.2 G/cm
2. z: $-3.0 \sim +3.0$ cm
3. v_z: $-2.0 \sim +2.0$ m/sec
4. t: $-0.0025 \le t \le +0.0025$ sec
5. $H_{1x}(t)$: $H_{1x}(t) = K \sin (\gamma G_z l t)/t$
6. Initial conditions:

$$\mathbf{M}(t = -0.0025 \text{ sec}) = (0, 1, 0) \text{ or } 1$$

$$\mathbf{M}(t = -0.0025 \text{ sec}) = (1, 0, 0) \text{ or } i \tag{12-22}$$

where the slice thickness l is assumed to be 2 cm and k is the constant required for a 180° flip when $z = 0$ and $v_z = 0$. Here the time axis t is used only in the process of solving the Bloch equation, while t' is used in reference to the spin-echo signal.

By use of the fourth-order Runge-Kutta method [9], one can integrate Eq. (12-21) by following two steps. First, start with t_j, which is defined as

$$t_j = -0.0025 + j \Delta(s) \tag{12-23}$$

where $\Delta(s)$ is the integration time interval in seconds and is set to 0.2 msec. Second, from the initial magnetization $\mathbf{M}(t_0)$ or $\mathbf{M}(-0.0025 \text{ sec})$, calculate $\mathbf{M}(t_2)$, $\mathbf{M}(t_4)$, and so on, by using the equation

$$\mathbf{M}(t_{j+2}) = \mathbf{M}(t_j) + \frac{\Delta}{3}\left[\mathbf{K}_1 + (2 - \sqrt{2})\mathbf{K}_2 + (2 + \sqrt{2})\mathbf{K}_3 + \mathbf{K}_4\right] \tag{12-24}$$

where

$$\mathbf{K}_1 = \gamma \mathbf{M}(t_j) \times \mathbf{H}_{\text{eff}}(t_j)$$

$$\mathbf{K}_2 = \left(\gamma \mathbf{M}(t_j) + \Delta \mathbf{K}_1 \right) \times \mathbf{H}_{\text{eff}}(t_{j+1})$$

$$\mathbf{K}_3 = \left[\gamma \mathbf{M}(t_j) + (-1 + \sqrt{2}) \Delta \mathbf{K}_1 + (2 - \sqrt{2}) \Delta \mathbf{K}_2 \right] \times \mathbf{H}_{\text{eff}}(t_{j+1})$$

$$\mathbf{K}_4 = \left[\gamma \mathbf{M}(t_j) - 2 \Delta \mathbf{K}_2 + (2 + \sqrt{2}) \Delta \mathbf{K}_3 \right] \times \mathbf{H}_{\text{eff}}(t_{j+2}) \qquad (12\text{-}25)$$

where $\Delta = \Delta(s)$. In effect, $\mathbf{K}_1$, $\mathbf{K}_2$, $\mathbf{K}_3$, and $\mathbf{K}_4$ approximate the derivative at each time interval $t_j \leq t \leq t_{j+2}$ at various points [see Eq. (12-21)]. By performing iterative calculations up to $= +0.0025$ sec, the resulting magnetization $\mathbf{M}(t)|_{t=0.0025 \text{ sec}}$ can be obtained.

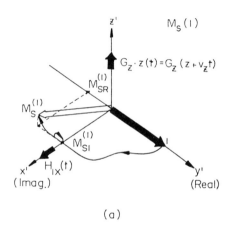

(a)

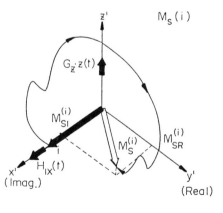

Figure 12-5 The behavior of the magnetizations $\mathcal{M}_s(1)$ and $\mathcal{M}_s(i)$ under the given selection gradient G_z and the 180° rf pulse $H_{1x'}(t)$: (a) $\mathcal{M}_s(1)$ and (b) $\mathcal{M}_s(i)$. The measured time interval is -0.0025 to $+0.0025$ sec.

(b)

Since only transverse components are relevant in NMR imaging, both the initial magnetizations and the resulting magnetizations are represented by complex numbers only in the transverse plane (note that precise 90° rf pulse excitation will result in initial magnetizations only on the transverse components). We denote the resulting complex magnetizations as

$$\mathcal{M}_s(\alpha; z, v_z) = \mathbf{M}_{y'}(t) + i\mathbf{M}_{x'}(t) \tag{12-26}$$

If we designate the initial magnetizations of $(0, 1, 0)$ or $(1, 0, 0)$ as 1 or i in

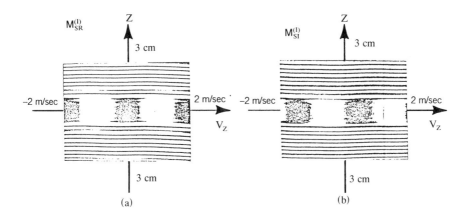

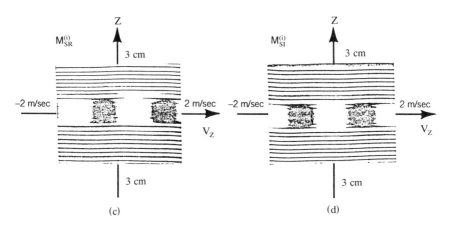

Figure 12-6 Simulated magnetizations resulting from different z and v_z values: (a), (b), (c), and (d) represent $\mathcal{M}_{SR}^{(1)}$, $\mathcal{M}_{SI}^{(1)}$, $\mathcal{M}_{SR}^{(i)}$, and $\mathcal{M}_{SI}^{(i)}$, respectively.

complex form, the resulting magnetizations can be written as (also see the behaviors of the magnetizations with different initial conditions, Fig. 12-5)

$$\mathcal{M}_s(1; z, v_z) = \mathcal{M}_{SR}^{(1)} + i\mathcal{M}_{SI}^{(1)}$$

and

$$\mathcal{M}_s(i; z, v_z) = \mathcal{M}_{SR}^{(i)} + i\mathcal{M}_{SI}^{(i)} \qquad (12\text{-}27)$$

where all the symbols correspond to those in Eq. (12-7). Simulated magnetizations resulting from different z and v_z values are displayed in Fig. 12.6 where (a), (b), (c), and (d) represent $\mathcal{M}_{SR}^{(1)}$, $\mathcal{M}_{SI}^{(1)}$, $\mathcal{M}_{SR}^{(i)}$, $\mathcal{M}_{SI}^{(i)}$, respectively [see Eq. (12-7)].

Since the Bloch equation is a linear equation, for an arbitrary initial magnetization $p + iq$, where p and q are real values, the resulting magnetization $\mathcal{M}_s(p + iq)$ can be written as

$$\mathcal{M}_s(p + iq; z, v_z) = p\mathcal{M}_s(1) + q\mathcal{M}_s(i)$$

$$= p\mathcal{M}_{SR}^{(1)} + q\mathcal{M}_{SR}^{(i)} + i\left(p\mathcal{M}_{SI}^{(1)} + q\mathcal{M}_{SI}^{(i)}\right) \qquad (12\text{-}28)$$

Now using the above results, let us consider the original spin-echo equation. From Eq. (12-6) we have

$$S(t') = \int_{v_z} \int_z \int_x \int_y \rho(x, y, z, v_z)\exp(i\gamma G_y yt')(\cos\theta + i\sin\theta)$$

$$\times \mathcal{M}_s[\cos(\theta + \phi) + i\sin(\theta + \phi; z, v_z)]\, dy\, dx\, dz\, dv_z \qquad (12\text{-}29)$$

where

$$\theta = \gamma G_y yT_A$$

$$\phi = \gamma g_x xT_x$$

$$p = \cos(\theta + \phi)$$

$$q = \sin(\theta + \phi) \qquad (12\text{-}30)$$

In Eq. (12-29) note that the order of the integral operation on x and y is changed in order to show the dephasing effects in the direction of the readout gradient.

By use of Eq. (12-28), Eq. (12-29) can be rewritten as

$$S(t') = \int_{v_z} \int_z \int_x \int_y \rho(x, y, z, v_z) \exp(i\gamma G_y yt')(\cos\theta + i\sin\theta)$$

$$\times \left[\mathcal{M}_s(1)\cos(\theta + \phi) + \mathcal{M}_s(i)\sin(\theta + \phi) \right] dy\, dx\, dz\, dv_z$$

$$= \int_{v_z} \int_z \int_x \int_y \rho(x, y, z, v_z) \exp(i\gamma G_y yt')$$

$$\times \left[\mathcal{M}_s(1; z, v_z)(\cos^2\theta\cos\phi - \cos\theta\sin\theta\sin\phi) \right.$$

$$+ \mathcal{M}_s(i; z, v_z)(\cos^2\theta\sin\phi + \cos\theta\sin\theta\cos\phi)$$

$$+ i\mathcal{M}_s(1; z, v_z)(\cos\theta\sin\theta\cos\phi - \sin^2\theta\sin\phi)$$

$$\left. + i\mathcal{M}_s(i; z, v_z)(\cos\theta\sin\theta\sin\phi + \sin^2\theta\cos\phi) \right] dy\, dx\, dz\, dv_z$$

$$(12\text{-}31)$$

In Eq. (12-31) the real and imaginary axes correspond to the y'- and x'-axes, respectively, for the rotating frame. Note that the center of the spin-echo signal is at $t' = 0$, as shown in Fig. 12-2 or Fig. 12-4. In the process of calculating the terms in the final square brackets, the terms that contain $\cos(2\theta)$ or $\sin(2\theta)$ will vanish when the integration is performed (T_A is assumed large):

$$\int_{-\infty}^{\infty} \rho_y(y)\cos(2\theta)\, dy \to 0$$

or

$$\int_{-\infty}^{\infty} \rho_y(y)\sin(2\theta)\, dy \to 0 \qquad (12\text{-}32)$$

After some algebra and using Eq. (12-27), Eq. (12-31) can be written in a more simplified form as

$$S(t') = \int_{v_z} \int_z \int_x \int_y \rho(x, y, z, v_z)\exp(i\gamma G_y yt')(\eta + i\xi)\exp(-i\phi)\, dy\, dx\, dz\, dv_z$$

$$(12\text{-}33)$$

where

$$\eta = \frac{\mathcal{M}_{SR}^{(1)} - \mathcal{M}_{SI}^{(i)}}{2}$$

and

$$\xi = \frac{\mathcal{M}_{SI}^{(1)} + \mathcal{M}_{SR}^{(i)}}{2} \tag{12-34}$$

From Eq. (12-34) the phase information for a given z and v_z can be derived as

$$\Phi(z, v_z) = \tan^{-1}\left[\frac{\xi(z, v_z)}{\eta(z, v_z)}\right] \tag{12-35}$$

The results of Eq. (12-35) are illustrated in Fig. 12-6.

12-3 MICROSCOPIC FLOW IMAGING: DIFFUSION AND PERFUSION IMAGING

12-3-1 Diffusion (Incoherent Flow) Imaging

The application of nuclear magnetic resonance phenomena to the study of molecular motion (e.g., flow or diffusion depending on the degree of motional coherence involved) has been attempted since the early 1950s [10, 11]. However, most of the studies have been limited to the extraction of diffusion and perfusion parameters from small samples [12, 13]. The developments of recent NMR imaging techniques, however, have made it possible to obtain spatially resolved multidimensional flow images [5, 14]. Some diffusion coefficient images have also been reported recently [15–17].

As in the other NMR imaging techniques, the reconstructed image in diffusion imaging consists of a finite number of resolvable volume elements (voxels) in which all the spins tend to form a detectable signal, as shown in Fig. 12.7. Since the spins always move randomly within a voxel due to thermal agitation, perfect spin rephasing by the spin-echo technique cannot be achieved in an imaging situation where an inhomogeneous magnetic field is always present due to the external gradient fields. As a result the signal from the spins in random motion is attenuated compared to that of the stationary spins. The constant representing the above attenuation process is known as the coefficient of self-diffusion D. The attenuated signal due to diffusion at a given spatial location (x, y) can be expressed as [18]

$$I(x, y) = I_0(x, y)\exp\left[-\gamma^2 D(x, y) \times \sum_{j=1}^{3}\left\{\int_0^{T_E}\left[\int_0^{t'} G_j(t'')\,dt''\right]^2 dt'\right\}\right] \tag{12-36}$$

where $I_0(x, y)$ denotes the intensity in a voxel at (x, y) excluding the effects of diffusion but including T_2 relaxation. In Eq. (12-36), $D(x, y)$ is the

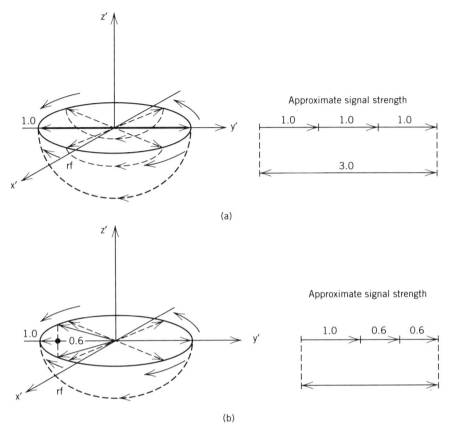

Figure 12-7 Principles of diffusion measurement by the NMR technique. Three spins are given, each having a unit magnitude and experiencing a spatially varying magnetic field. (a) For the stationary spins exact spin rephasing can be achieved after the 180° rf pulse, and the observed signal will be the sum of the vectors (i.e., no attenuation). (b) If the spins are in random Brownian motion with the spatially varying magnetic field, each spin phase introduced during the interval between the 90° and 180° rf pulses will be different, thereby resulting in a smaller signal (i.e., their phases will be different).

diffusion coefficient in a voxel at (x, y); T_E is the echo time, which is defined by the time interval from the 90° rf pulse to the center of spin echo; γ is the gyromagnetic ratio, and G_j is the time-dependent gradient field. As will be shown, the calculation of the diffusion map $D(x, y)$ is possible by taking several data with correspondingly different durations of the gradient field $G_j(t'')$ in the readout direction.

Diffusion Imaging Pulse Sequence

A diffusion imaging technique applicable to the conventional Fourier imaging sequence using spin echo has been proposed by a number of investigators [17,

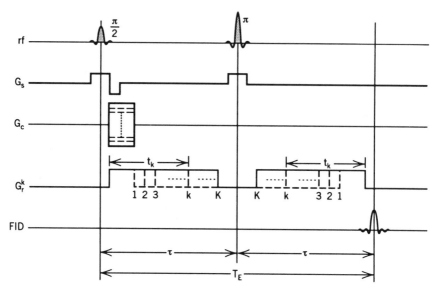

Figure 12-8 The pulse sequence for diffusion imaging by varying the duration of the readout gradient G_r^k.

19] (see Fig. 12-8). The method is based on two different images that have undergone different amounts of diffusion, one image with a small amount of diffusion, thereby, a small signal attenuation, and the other with a much larger amount of diffusion, thereby a large signal attenuation. As will be shown, this can be achieved simply by varying the gradient strength or duration [17, 18].

The simplest way of performing diffusion imaging is the variable length readout gradient method as shown in Fig. 12-8. In this method, a gradient field with a pulse duration t_k, denoted by G_r^k as shown with dotted lines in Fig. 12-8, acts as a diffusion coding gradient. It is assumed that the diffusion coding is predominantly performed by the readout gradient, although the diffusion process is believed to be affected by the other gradients as well, namely phase encoding and selection gradients [16]. Note here that the pulse sequence is so designed that the spin dephasing due to the spin-spin relaxation (T_2) process affects all the images equally, thereby eliminating the necessity of correcting the signal attenuation due to the spin-spin relaxations.

After a set of experiments or imagings is performed, a diffusion map $D(x, y)$ can be extracted by generating a set of spin density images, which is obtained by varying the gradient durations. One can rewrite Eq. (12-36), after taking its logarithm, as

$$\ln\left[\frac{I^k(x, y)}{I_0(x, y)}\right] = -D(x, y)C_k \qquad (12\text{-}37)$$

where I^k is the spin density image obtained with a given gradient duration t_k and C_k is a constant which is given by

$$C_k = -\gamma^2 \sum_{j=1}^{3} \left\{ \int_0^{TE} \left[\int_0^{t'} G_j^k(t'') \, dt'' \right]^2 dt' \right\} \tag{12-38}$$

In principle, $G_j^k(t'')$ in Eq. (12-38) can be set as follows: $G_1^k(t'') = G_s(t'')$, the selection gradient; $G_2^k(t'') = G_c(t'')$, the phase-coding gradient, and $G_3^k(t'') = G_r^k(t'')$, the readout gradient, respectively. Note that in Fig. 12-8, however, only G_r^k is used. Evaluation of Eq. (12-38) for the pulse sequence shown in Fig. 12-8 results in

$$C_k = \gamma^2 t_k^2 G_R^2 \left(T_E - \frac{4t_k}{3} \right) \tag{12-39}$$

where G_R is the amplitude of the readout gradient.

Now using Eq. (12-37), $D(x, y)$ can be calculated directly from the two images obtained with different readout gradient durations, say t_m and t_n:

$$\ln\left[\frac{I^m(x, y)}{I_0(x, y)} \right] - \ln\left[\frac{I^n(x, y)}{I_0(x, y)} \right] = -D(x, y)[C_m - C_n]$$

or

$$D(x, y) = \ln \frac{[I^m(x, y)/I^n(x, y)]}{C_n - C_m}, \qquad m \neq n \tag{12-40}$$

Once the diffusion map $D(x, y)$ is determined, the nondiffused image $I_0(x, y)$ can also be obtained simply by rearranging Eq. (12-37) as

$$I_0(x, y) = I^k(x, y)\exp[D(x, y)C_k], \qquad k = m, n \tag{12-41}$$

More generally, if k differently diffused images are obtained, the extraction of $D(x, y)$ and $I_0(x, y)$ can be achieved by a least squares fit to the experimentally measured data [cf. Eq. (12-37)]. Then the slope and the intersection of the fitted line can be used to compute $D(x, y)$ and $I_0(x, y)$, respectively (see Fig. 12-9).

Data shown in Fig. 12-9 were obtained by a gradient field strength of 2.5 mT/m and a phantom filled with distilled water, acetone, and dimethyl-sulfoxide (DMSO) at room temperature. The echo time T_E was 170 msec with a data acquisition period of 15.4 msec. The average diffusion coefficients of the three materials used in the phantom are listed in Table 12-1 and compared with the previously measured values [13].

For some clinical applications a bulk diffusion coefficient imaging of a human volunteer *in vivo* has also been measured and the results are shown

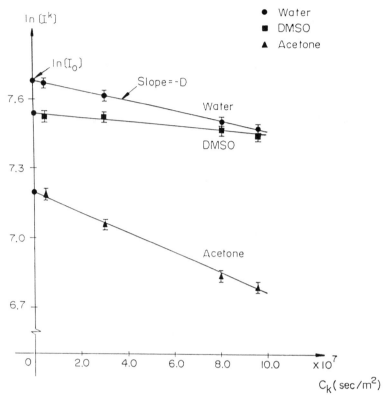

Figure 12-9 The least squares fitting of experimentally measured data. The slope and the intersection of the fitted line with y-axis are used to calculate the diffusion coefficient D and the nondiffused density $\ln I_0$, respectively.

Table 12-1   Mean and standard deviation of diffusion coefficients measured within the region of interest in the diffusion coefficient map of various phantoms

Material	Present Work D (m²/sec)	Previous Work[a] D (m²/sec)
Acetone	$(4.32 \pm 0.26) \times 10^{-9}$	4.47×10^{-9} (at 27.8°C)
DMSO	$(0.84 \pm 0.15) \times 10^{-9}$	
Water	$(2.19 \pm 0.20) \times 10^{-9}$	2.31×10^{-9} (at 28.3°C)

Source: See Fig. 12-9. Also previously measured data are shown for references.
[a] See Cantor and Jonas [13].

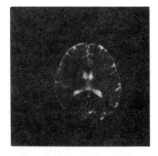

(a)

(b)

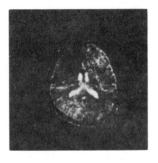

(c)

Figure 12-10 *In vivo* cerebral bulk diffusion coefficient maps of a volunteer obtained by the diffusion imaging technique. In this experiment two different gradient steps were used with an echo time and a repetition time of 140 msec and 2 sec, respectively. A selected data of slice are acquired by varying the gradient pulse length. (a) An *in vivo* diffusion image of a volunteer with $t_1 = 9$ msec. (b) The same image with $t_2 = 60$ msec. (c) The calculated diffusion coefficient maps from the two images. The high-diffusion coefficients of the CSF in the ventricles are noticeable.

in Fig. 12-10. Although the true diffusion coefficients of the *in vivo* human brain and CSF (cerebrospinal fluid) are not accurately known, it is interesting to observe what is believed to be the diffusion coefficients of CSF and other liquids in the brain.

12-3-2 Perfusion (Partially Coherent Flow) Imaging

As has been discussed in the previous section, bulk coherent flow is well known and has been used for various types of flow imaging, for instance, for blood flow in the aorta [2, 4, 20]. The other type of flow, also discussed in the previous section, is the microscopic incoherent flow due to molecular random motion.

One can consider a slightly different form of microscopic flow which is neither an incoherent flow (e.g., diffusion) nor a flow of coherent nature (e.g., bulk flow). Perfusion is an example of such a case [20]. Although it is difficult to quantify the perfusion or random directional quasi-coherent flow micro-scopically, it appears possible to observe the behavior of the aggregated free induction decay signal arising from the microscopic channels or capillaries by employing NMR imaging techniques and to distinguish it from random incoherent flow or diffusion. In practical NMR imaging, diffusion phenomena have been observed by a pulse scheme with varying gradient lengths or amplitudes, as discussed in the previous section. If perfusion is modeled as a capillary flow and if the capillary flow is assumed to be the sum of many distinct coherent flows with randomly oriented directions, it can be refocused by an even echo sequence [21]. Perfusion therefore can be distinguished from diffusion, at least in principle, based on the random directional coherent flow model. Feasibility of capillary flow or perfusion imaging was attempted as a "Gedanken" experiment of perfusion or quasi-coherent random directional flow using a ball ($\sim$ 8 cm in diameter) consisting of a large number of randomly orientated tubes. Using an external water source under variable pressure, it was possible to control the flow velocities in the tubes, thereby controlling the overall capillary flow rate in the ball.

Justification of this "random ball" experiment in an attempt to study perfusion is based on previously known physiological data [22, 23]. The average radius of the capillaries is known to be about 3 μm with an average length of 750 μm. The data also indicates that the mean velocity of flow in the capillaries is about 300 to 500 μm/sec. From the above data, the distance moved during 100 msec (the approximate measuring time in NMR imaging) can be calculated and is found to be about 30 to 50 μm. Since this distance is much smaller than the average capillary length, the flow in the segmented capillaries through that length are almost linear with constant velocities, although the direction of each channel or capillary may be differ-ent. Consideration of the average density of the capillaries ($400-500/\text{mm}^3$) and a typical voxel size in NMR imaging ($1 \times 1 \times 7$ mm) indicates that the number of segmented capillaries in a voxel is over 3000, thus justifying a statistical approach. In the following analysis the segmented capillaries are further assumed to be uniformly distributed in all directions* (see Fig. 12-11). Hence the capillary flow in a voxel is modeled as an aggregate of linear flow elements each flow having a constant velocity within the measurement time ($\sim$ 100 msec). The capillary orientations are assumed to be uniformly dis-tributed. A simple illustration of this capillary flow model is shown in Fig. 12-11.

*This may not be true in some cases.

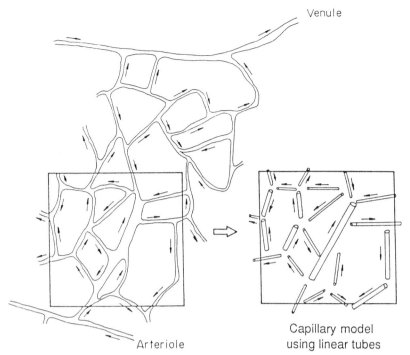

Figure 12-11 Perfusion model as an aggregate of random directional capillary flow. The flow velocity and direction for each small tube are assumed to be constant during the measurement time.

Based on the model developed above, NMR signals from the capillaries or tubes are analyzed. Suppose that a reconstructed image M in an arbitrary voxel is derived using the flow measurement sequence; that is, the external bipolar gradients are applied so that only the phase components of the moving spins are measured, not that of the stationary ones (use of velocity coding gradients). When such a flow measurement sequence is applied, the following analysis can be made: Let k be a tube within a voxel having an orientation in reference to vector $\hat{k}$. If we represent the velocity distribution function in tube k as $f_k(v)$, then the NMR signal from tube k for all the velocity components can be expressed as

$$m_k = m_{0k} \int_0^\infty f_k(v) \exp\left[i\gamma \int_0^t \mathbf{G}(t') \cdot \mathbf{v}t'\, dt'\right] dv$$

$$= m_{0k} \int_0^\infty f_k(v) \exp\left[i\gamma \int_0^t \mathbf{G}(t') \cdot v\hat{k}t'\, dt'\right] dv \qquad (12\text{-}42)$$

where m_{0k} is the equilibrium spin density in the tube at zero velocity, $\mathbf{v}$ is the velocity vector, and the exponential factor $\exp(\cdot)$ is the phase factor for the given tube. In the second part of Eq. (12-42), the velocity vector $\mathbf{v}$ is replaced by the coordinate vector $\hat{k}$ with a scalar velocity magnitude v. If we denote $\boldsymbol{\alpha}$ as a gradient dependent vector which is given by

$$\boldsymbol{\alpha} = \gamma \int_0^t \mathbf{G}(t')t'\,dt' \tag{12-43}$$

where $\mathbf{G}(t')$ is the time varying gradient and if a constant gradient is applied along the x direction with an amplitude $\mathbf{G}_x$ and a duration Δ_x, then at the end of the gradient, $\boldsymbol{\alpha}$ becomes

$$\boldsymbol{\alpha} = -\gamma \mathbf{G}_x \Delta_x^2 \tag{12-44}$$

where we have assumed that the T_1 and T_2 relaxation effects are included in m_{0k}.

Now consider the signals or magnetizations arising from all the flow elements or tubes within a given voxel; then the total signal can be expressed as a summation of m_k for all the tubes in the voxel:

$$
\begin{aligned}
M &= \sum_k m_{0k} \int_0^\infty f_k(v)\exp(iv\boldsymbol{\alpha}\cdot\hat{k})\,dv \\
&= \sum_k m_{0k} \int_0^\infty f_k(v)\exp(iv|\boldsymbol{\alpha}|\cos\theta_k)\,dv
\end{aligned}
\tag{12-45}
$$

where θ_k is the angle between the $\boldsymbol{\alpha}$ and $\hat{k}$ vectors. If we further assume that all the velocity distribution functions are identical [i.e., $f_k(v) = f(v)$], then Eq. (12-45) can also be written as

$$M = M_0 \int f(\theta)\left[\int_0^\infty f(v)\exp(iv|\boldsymbol{\alpha}|\cos\theta)\,dv\right]d\theta \tag{12-46}$$

where M_0 denotes the sum of the equilibrium spin densities for the zero velocity states or the stationary case and $f(\theta)$ is the orientational or angular distribution function for the directions of the tubes. Again it is assumed that the T_1 and T_2 relaxation effects are absorbed in the M_0. Note that in Eq. (12-46), the summation and $f_k(v)$ are now replaced with an integral sign and $f(\theta)$.

By assuming an isotropic distribution of capillaries, the angular distribution function $f(\theta)$ will be a sinusoidal distribution given by

$$f(\theta) = \begin{cases} \dfrac{\sin\theta}{2}, & \text{if } 0 \le \theta \le \pi \\ 0, & \text{otherwise} \end{cases} \tag{12-47}$$

where θ denotes the polar angle in a spherical coordinate system in reference to the directional vector $\boldsymbol{\alpha}$. By substituting Eq. (12-47) into Eq. (12-46) and changing the order of the integration, Eq. (12-46) becomes

$$M = \frac{M_0}{2} \int_0^\infty f(v) \left[\int_0^\pi \sin\theta \exp(iv|\boldsymbol{\alpha}|\cos\theta)\, d\theta \right] dv$$

$$= M_0 \int_0^\infty f(v)\mathrm{sinc}\left(\frac{|\boldsymbol{\alpha}|v}{\pi}\right) dv \qquad (12\text{-}48)$$

where $\mathrm{sinc}(x) = \sin(\pi x)/(\pi x)$. Note that the reconstructed image given by Eq. (12-48) is a real-valued function. This is an interesting and distinct characteristic of aggregated random directional microscopic flow compared to the coherent bulk flow. In the latter the reconstructed image has complex values with phase information, which is related to the flow velocity.

Equation (12-48) can be evaluated for two different types of flow, plug and laminar flow. It can easily be shown that the velocity distribution functions for plug and laminar flow are the delta function and the uniform distribution, respectively. Let us consider these two cases. In the case of plug flow, let v_0 be the velocity of a plug flow that has a velocity distribution function like a delta function, that is, $f(v) = \delta(v - v_0)$. Then Eq. (12-48) becomes

$$M = M_0 \int_0^\infty \delta(v - v_0)\mathrm{sinc}\left(\frac{|\boldsymbol{\alpha}|v}{\pi}\right) dv$$

$$= M_0\, \mathrm{sinc}\left(\frac{|\boldsymbol{\alpha}|v_0}{\pi}\right) \qquad (12\text{-}49)$$

This has an oscillating behavior like a sinc function as shown in Fig. 12-12. In the case of laminar flow with a mean velocity v_0 $(= v_{max}/2)$, the velocity distribution function becomes

$$f(v) = \begin{cases} \dfrac{1}{2v_0}, & \text{if } 0 \le v \le v_0 \\[2mm] 0, & \text{otherwise} \end{cases} \qquad (12\text{-}50)$$

By substituting Eq. (12-50) into Eq. (12-48), one obtains

$$M = \frac{M_0}{(2v_0)} \int_0^{2v_0} \mathrm{sinc}\left(\frac{|\boldsymbol{\alpha}|v}{\pi}\right) dv$$

$$= M_0 \frac{\mathrm{Si}(2|\boldsymbol{\alpha}|v_0)}{2|\boldsymbol{\alpha}|v_0} \qquad (12\text{-}51)$$

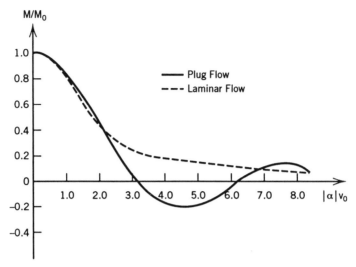

Figure 12-12 Plots of echo signals obtained from randomly oriented directional flow as a function of $|\alpha|v_0$, where $|\alpha|$ is a constant determined by the specific pulse sequence employed and v_0 is the mean velocity of the fluid.

where Si is the sine integral $\text{Si}(x) = \int_0^x \text{sinc}(x'/\pi)\,dx'$. Graphical plots of Eqs. (12-49) and (12-51) as a function of $|\alpha|v_0$ are shown in Fig. 12-12. Note that the aggregated signal or total magnetization for plug flow (delta distribution) takes the form of a damped oscillation, while in the case of laminar flow (uniform velocity distribution), a monotonically decreasing behavior is observed.

As discussed in the previous section, random directional flow in both plug and laminar flow experiences a signal attenuation. Besides this attenuation phenomenon, additional signal attenuations are observed due to diffusion and the T_1 and T_2 relaxation processes. If we assume that the attenuation mechanisms above are independent, the reconstructed image density can be expressed as

$$M = [M_s + M_c A(C)] A(D) A(T_1) A(T_2) \tag{12-52}$$

where M_s is the equilibrium signal intensity of the stationary spin, M_c is the signal intensity of the spins belonging to the capillary flow, $A(C)$ is the attenuation due to the capillary flow as expressed in Eq. (12-48), and $A(D)$, $A(T_1)$, and $A(T_2)$ are the respective attenuation terms due to diffusion and the T_1 and T_2 relaxations. Note that all of these attenuation processes affect only the signal amplitudes, leaving the phases unchanged.

An experimental pulse scheme based on this model is shown in Fig. 12-13. This pulse scheme is composed of two separate measurements each with a

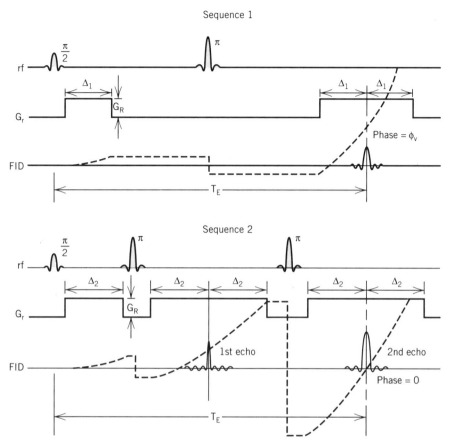

Figure 12-13   A pulse scheme used for the measurement of the capillary density or capillary flow. In sequence 1 the first echo is obtained, while in sequence 2 the second echo is acquired. The latter is believed to be the rephased echo. The phases related to the two sequences are represented by dotted lines.

Fourier spin-echo imaging sequence: one with a single spin echo (sequence 1) and the other with a double spin echo (sequence 2), respectively. In the double-echo sequence, two rf and gradient pulses are adjusted in such a way that the attenuation due to the T_2 decay of the second echo signal is identical to that of the single-echo sequence. The reason for employing such a dual acquisition method is that the amount of attenuation due to capillary flow is different for those two data acquisition sequences; that is, $|\alpha|$ in Eq. (12-48) becomes $\gamma G_R \Delta_1 (T_E - \Delta_1)$ at the center of the echo in sequence 1, while $|\alpha|$ becomes zero at the second echo in sequence 2, thereby making the attenuation due to capillary flow in sequence 2 negligible. This phenomenon is known as "even-echo rephasing"; that is, the phase introduced by the spins moving with a constant velocity with a given directional flow becomes zero at the second spin echo, irrespective of the flow direction and velocity [21]. In sequences 1 and 2 the readout gradient is assumed to be the dominant gradient with a magnitude G_R and duration Δ_1 and Δ_2. The pulse durations will be further adjusted in such a way that the attenuation by diffusion and T_2 relaxation is the same for the two sequences; that is, the attenuation due to the capillary flow is the only difference between the sequence 1 and sequence 2, as discussed earlier.

If we consider the diffusion process alone, the reconstructed images M_1 and M_2 obtained by sequences 1 and 2, respectively, can be written as [11, 22]

$$\frac{M_1}{M_0} = \exp\left[-\gamma^2 G_R^2 D \Delta_1^2 \left(T_E - \frac{4\Delta_1}{3}\right)\right] \quad \text{for sequence 1} \quad (12\text{-}53a)$$

and

$$\frac{M_2}{M_0} = \exp\left[\frac{-\gamma^2 G_R^2 D T_E^3}{48}\right] \quad \text{for sequence 2} \quad (12\text{-}53b)$$

where M_0 is the nondiffused image. In deriving Eq. (12-53b), it is assumed that the readout gradient is applied during the entire period in sequence 2 except the time interval where the slice-selective rf pulse is applied (i.e., $4\Delta_2 \cong T_E$). From Eqs. (12-53a) and (12-53b) the condition for equal attenuation in both sequences is given by

$$\frac{T_E^3}{48} = \Delta_1^2 \left(T_E - \frac{4\Delta_1}{3}\right) \quad (12\text{-}54)$$

The numerical solution of Eq. (12-54) yields $\Delta_1 = 0.163 T_E$. In practice, we choose T_E sufficiently large so that Δ_1 covers a sufficient bandwidth when it is used as a readout gradient in sequence 1.

Finally, if we employ the same repetition time (T_R) for both sequences to ensure identical T_1 dependence for both echo signals, then the reconstructed image intensities [see Eq. (12-52)] for these two sequences become

$$M_1 = [M_s + M_c A(C)] A(D) A(T_1) A(T_2) \quad \text{for sequence 1} \quad (12\text{-}55a)$$

and

$$M_2 = [M_s + M_c] A(D) A(T_1) A(T_2) \quad \text{for sequence 2} \quad (12\text{-}55b)$$

By subtracting M_1 from M_2, the difference image ΔM can be obtained:

$$\Delta M = M_2 - M_1$$
$$= M_c[1 - A(C)]A(D)A(T_1)A(T_2) \qquad (12\text{-}56)$$

Equation (12-56) shows that ΔM is a quantity directly related to the capillary density within a voxel and is independent of the stationary spins. Equation (12-56) can be rewritten using the relationships given in Eqs. (12-48) and (12-53) together with the attenuation formulas for the T_1 and T_2 relaxations:

$$\Delta M(x, y) = M_c(x, y)\left[1 - \int_0^\infty f(v)\operatorname{sinc}\left(\frac{|\alpha|v}{\pi}\right)dv\right] \times \exp\left[\frac{-\gamma^2 G_R^2 D(x, y)T_E^3}{48}\right]$$
$$\times \left[1 - \exp\left(\frac{-T_R}{T_1(x, y)}\right)\right]\exp\left[\frac{-T_E}{T_2(x, y)}\right] \qquad (12\text{-}57)$$

For an experimental demonstration of the method described, the peak amplitudes of the echoes, which amount to the integrated signals over the whole phantom, were measured as a function of the readout gradient field strength using the pulse sequence shown in Fig. 12-13 with a 0.6 T NMR system. The measured amplitudes with sequences 1 and 2 are shown in Fig. 12-14. Note the dependence of $|\alpha| = \gamma G_R \Delta_1(T_E - \Delta_1)$ in sequence 1, while in sequence 2, $|\alpha|$ is equal to zero, making the measurement nearly independent of the readout gradient. As seen in Fig. 12-14, the amplitude of the echo signal decreases rapidly in sequence 1 as the gradient strength increases, while the second echo amplitude in sequence 2 remains nearly constant. The

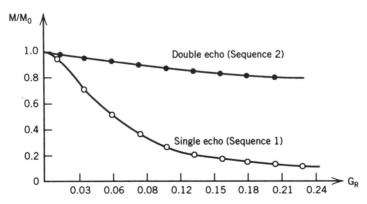

Figure 12-14 Experimentally measured echo amplitudes obtained from the "random ball" experiment. The empty circles denote the measured signals with sequence 1, while the filled circles correspond to sequence 2. These results correspond well to a theoretical calculation based on the laminar flow (solid lines).

slight decrease in the echo amplitude in sequence 2 with increasing gradient strength appears to be due to the diffusion process in which the attenuation is expressed as a function of G_R [Eq. (12-53)]. Some higher-order molecular motion, such as acceleration due to tube bending in the random ball, may also be responsible for the additional attenuations.

Although the medical applications of capillary density or flow rate images are not clearly established or understood, they appear to have significant potential in providing functional images, especially in close correlation with PET (positron emission tomography) where the kinetics of radioactive tracers are measured in conjunction with blood flow or possibly with perfusion [24, 25].

12-4 ANGIOGRAPHY

Flow imaging is one of the promising techniques that is uniquely suited for magnetic resonance imaging, such as identifying and understanding flow and its effects in vascular imaging. Many NMR flow-related imaging techniques have been directed toward the images of blood vessels which may be termed as (nuclear) magnetic resonance angiography (MRA). Inherently the characteristics of the changes in the magnitude and the phase of the magnetization due to the motion of the excited spins within a spatially varying magnetic field provide an inherent contrast between flowing materials and stationary objects [5, 26–32]. Flow therefore acts like an intrinsic contrast medium. NMR images of arteries and veins can be obtained without injecting intravascular contrast agents such as iodine used in X-ray angiography [29]. There is evidence that magnetic resonance angiography may be an alternative to noninvasive vascular imaging which has been the exclusive domain of ultrasound and X-ray angiography [31, 33–36].

12-4-1 Principles and Methods of Angiography

MRA requires that the signal from the static material be reduced or even eliminated in the image, thereby only the signals from the moving or flowing materials such as blood should be present in the image. The principal elements involved in MRA are flow sensitization and the suppression of signals from the stationary material. MRA techniques can be categorized into two broad physically based methods, namely the phase-sensitive method and the in-flow-sensitive method. The former is often called the *phase sensitive or flow velocity sensitive method*, while the latter is called the *in-flow or time-of-flight* (TOF) method.

Phase-Sensitive Method (Flow-Velocity-Sensitive Method)
All phase-sensitive methods of flow measurement or imaging are well known. For the conventional flow measurements, the velocity component

which is in coincident with the magnetic field gradient will induce a phase shift in the transverse spin magnetization [36–38]. Since the velocity-induced phase shift is proportional to the velocity, the variations in the velocity due to the velocity distribution result in dispersion of the phase shifts. The dispersion of phase shifts can result in unequal signal attenuation or loss. Although this signal loss due to the loss of phase coherency can be prevented by employing flow compensation using such techniques as the bipolar gradient as discussed in the previous section, it is nevertheless incompatible with our main goal of phase-sensitive flow measurement.

Although the phase sensitive method has good sensitivity, it has limitations. The first limitation is its sensitivity to the pulsatile and nonuniform flow. Although the sensitivity to the pulsatile flow can be overcome by cardiac gating to ensure that the blood velocity is consistent for each acquired echo or by averaging many echoes over the cardiac cycle to obtain an average flow, this process still poses a problem. A second limitation is the sensitivity to instrumental imperfections such as eddy currents induced in the metallic bore of the magnet by gradient pulses. Inadequate suppression of these eddy currents results in failure in improper subtraction of the stationary tissue signal. A third limitation is that the method is also sensitive to motion occurring anywhere within the imaging volume [35, 39].

In-flow-Sensitive Method (Time-of-Flight (TOF) Method)

The principles of the in-flow technique are simple; when a slice or line (projection of slice) is repeatedly pulsed, static samples will be saturated while, on the other hand, fresh blood or materials newly injected into the slice will give rise to large signals. In the in-flow method therefore one can simply measure the signal intensity either in one dimension (projection of a slice) or two dimensions (2-D planar scanning). This TOF method is less sensitive to the errors that result from pulsatile flow, rf inhomogeneities, eddy currents, and so on, due to the fact that TOF procedures use only longitudinal magnetization; thus it is insensitive to flow-induced phase shifts in transverse magnetization [34, 35, 40]. Using the recently developed gradient echo sequences of various types, NMR angiography with one-dimensional line scannings or two-dimensional slice scannings can be performed without a presaturation pulse. In this in-flow NMR angiography, the presaturation technique and the selection of a thin contiguous two-dimensional slice and data acquisition make it possible to distinguish between arterial and venous vessels [21, 41] and even possible to distinguish between arteries and veins simultaneously [41]. Since these techniques do not require subtraction of one image from the other to eliminate the image of the stationary object, overall data acquisition time is reduced by half and is less vulnerable to misregistration artifacts [40] due to the eddy current effect. In-flow techniques also have some limitations, since they are essentially qualitative data or images rather than quantitative and the signal intensity is not sensitive to the flow velocity; in other words, they are more or less constant as long as the flow is over a

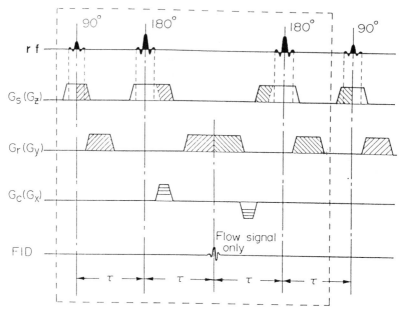

Figure 12-15   The pulse sequence used for the static sample signal suppression. This pulse sequence is sometimes referred to as the "composite" pulse sequence.

certain critical velocity. The latter, however, appears advantageous in some cases.

Because the signal from the blood vessel represents only a small percentage of the total signal from the slice or volume, all the MRA methods require suppression of the static background signals. An example of a static sample signal suppression technique using a composite pulse sequence is shown in Fig. 12-15. The result of this type of static sample suppression technique has a suppression ratio of better than $10^4:1$ over the static sample. Another static signal or image suppression technique applicable to both line scan and planar scan imaging is the large flip angle (90°) SSFP sequence, as will be detailed later (see the pulse sequence shown in Fig. 12-16).

12-4-2   Angiography Techniques

As discussed in the previous section, currently two types of MR angiography techniques are most widely used, namely the phase-sensitive method [36, 37, 39, 42, 43] and the in-flow or time-of-flight method [33, 41, 44]. The former uses bipolar gradient pulses for the flow coding, while the latter uses the saturation effect of the spins in the static samples. In the phase-sensitive method the subtraction of two images, each produced with different velocity phase codings, was used. This method, however, is sensitive to eddy currents

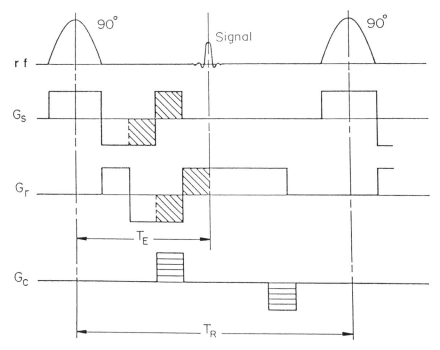

Figure 12-16   The pulse sequence used for 3-D volume MR angiography by scanning of the 2-D planar images. G_s, G_r, and G_c are the selection, readout, and coding gradients, respectively. This sequence is repeated $N_c \times N_s$ (N_c: encoding steps for a slice image; N_s: number of slices in 3-D volume) times to complete the 3-D volume angiogram. Each 2-D image obtained by using this sequence is accumulated until the desired 3-D volume image is obtained. Note that the additional bipolar pulses shown are the flow compensation gradients [41].

and other motion-dependent image misregistrations [36, 42, 43]. The in-flow method, on the other hand, utilizes the contrast that results from the fresh in-flow spins, which are not saturated [33, 44, 45], thereby giving a large signal compared with the signal obtained from the static samples. Conventional projection techniques, however, require extremely high suppression of the static sample signal [45], as mentioned. If the in-flow technique is applied to 2-D planar imaging, the contrast ratio requirement can be relaxed somewhat.

Three-Dimensional MR Angiography with Two-Dimensional Planar Image Scanning

A method of forming 3-D MR volume angiograms using 2-D planar image scanning with a fast gradient echo or steady state free precession (SSFP) pulse sequence with a large flip angle (90°) has been proposed [41]. Since, for example, each slice or planar image formation requires, 128 or more encodings, the static samples in the selected slice will be saturated immediately after the application of the series of rf pulses, especially when the flip angle is large (90°). This sequence therefore provides a highly suppressed static sample signal (reduced to about 5% of the flow signal). Each selected slice image obtained with this 2-D sequence can thus be stacked to form a 3-D volume image. In this approach a planar image is obtained using the SSFP gradient echo sequence, and the image data of each slice are obtained in a short time (~ 8 sec). A total of 64 to 128 slice images are usually obtained and stacked to form a volume image. This method offers 3-D volume images of arbitrary size and field of view. It is found that the method is quite insensitive to the velocity variations of the spin flow as long as the flow velocities are higher than a certain critical velocity (e.g., about 3 cm/sec in the experiment). This method is also basically a nonsubtraction technique and therefore is free from misregistration artifacts.

When images are obtained by the fast imaging sequence where the repetition time (T_R) is on the order of 10 msec with a small flip angle, flow signals tend to show a small signal enhancement. The optimal flip angles for this kind of imaging technique are usually much less than 90°. However, when a large flip angle such as 90° is used in conjunction with the SSFP sequence, it is found that the flow-related signal enhancement is significant compared with the static background signal simply due to the fact that the static samples are largely saturated. Although the suppression ratio is not as high as for the other methods such as the composite pulse sequence [45], a 90° flip angle SSFP can be utilized for 3-D MR angiography in conjunction with the 2-D planar scanning method described above. In addition, if the slice thickness is thin, the contrast will be independent of the in-flow rate of the spins because in-flow spins will effectively replace the entire volume of the blood vessel, thereby enhancing the flow signal contrast over the background.

The pulse sequence used for angiography (i.e., the planar 2-D scan 3-D volume angiogram) is shown in Fig. 12-16. The shaded regions are the flow-phase-compensated gradient pulses used for the removal of the artifacts in the readout and selection directions. This imaging technique is basically the same as the line scan angiography technique [44] except that each line is now replaced with a 2-D image, thereby forming a 3-D volume image rather than the 2-D projection image. After the completion of each slice data acquisition with N_c-encoding steps, the next adjacent slice is imaged like the line scan angiography. In actual imaging, before the start of each slice imaging, several presaturation rf pulses are added to saturate the static samples in the newly selected slice. In this imaging scheme the slice thickness (Δz) therefore defines the resolution in the selection (z) direction. Because of the velocity saturation effect the proposed method has a relatively uniform sensitivity to the flow over a wide velocity range.

The amount of background signal usually observed in this method is in the range of 5% of the in-flow spin signal. This is usually considered poor in

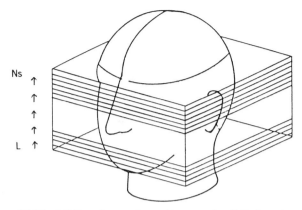

Figure 12-17 A 3-D angiogram formed by scanning 2-D planar images.

projection angiography (they require on the order of 10^{-4}–10^{-5}). It is sufficient, however, when the final image is of the 3-D form, which will further be enhanced by the maximum pixel ray tracing algorithm. The field of view in the z direction is equal to the number of 2-D imaging slices (N_s) multiplied by the slice thickness, Δz. The total imaging time T is therefore proportional to the volume of interest:

$$T = N_s\big[(N_c \times T_R) + T_D\big]$$

$$\simeq N_s\big[(N_c \times T_R)\big], \qquad T_D \ll N_c \times T_R \qquad (12\text{-}58)$$

where N_C, T_R, and T_D are the number of encoding steps in the phase encoding direction, the repetition time, and the preshot or preparation time, respectively. Figure 12-17, gives an illustrative example of 3-D volume angiography formed by planar 2-D scan.

A slice image experimentally obtained from a 3-D angiogram of a volunteer's head using the 2-D planar imaging pulse sequence is shown in Fig. 12-18(a). Figure 12-18(b) shows the summed or projected image of 64 slices similar to the one in Fig. 12-18(a). The velocity-compensated gradient pulse is used in both the selection and the readout directions. The single main lobe sinc pulse was used as an excitation rf pulse to decrease the echo time (T_E) since a short echo time is important for the reduction of the higher-order motion effect. A thin slice selection is also an important factor for sensitivity improvement of low-velocity flow and for the improvement of the resolution in the selection direction. In the above experiment, a thickness $\Delta z = 1.2$ mm was chosen by using a 1.33-G/cm gradient field and a 0.16-G bandwidth rf field, while the readout and phase encoding directional resolutions in the experiment were 0.86 and 1.1 mm, respectively. The field of view in the x and y directions was 220 mm. Two hundred encoding steps, N_c, were used in the

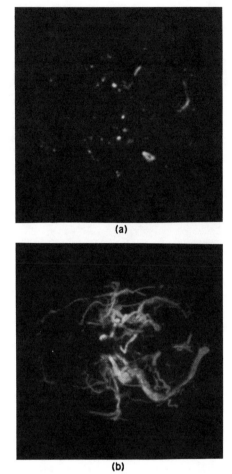

Figure 12-18 (a) An axial slice image obtained with a 90° flip-angle SSFP pulse sequence. (b) A projection image obtained by summation of 64 slice images like (a).

phase encoding direction for each slice imaging. The imaging time for each slice was 8.8 sec, including the time for 20 preshot pulses where each preshot pulse period was 40 msec. The total imaging time for the 100 slices was therefore 14.67 min. Figure 12-19(a), (b), and (c) show the three sagittal view images at three different view angles obtained after the 3-D volume image was reconstructed.

Simultaneous Three-dimensional Angiography of Arteries and Veins (SAAV) [41]

Since the 2-D planar scan 3-D angiography imaging sequence utilizes the fresh in-flow spin signal, it is easy to separate the direction of flow by using some form of directional saturation. There are currently several methods to

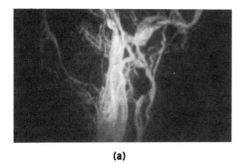

(a)

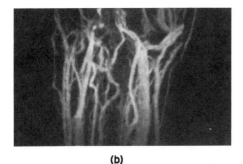

(b)

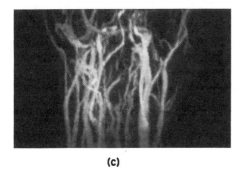

(c)

Figure 12-19 Sagittal view images at three different view angles obtained after the 3-D volume image is reconstructed by 2-D planar scanning.

separate the arteries and veins by means of taking two or three imaging sequences with different saturations or inversion techniques [46–48].

It is also possible to generate images of arteries and veins simultaneously by a single acquisition of data. This is achieved by selecting a thick saturation region and folding this region by two imaging slices, namely an imaging slice for the arteries and one for the veins. In each sequence a middle saturation region is excited first before the excitation of the arteries and veins. This is then followed by time-multiplexed dual-slice imaging. The pulse-timing diagram of this SAAV sequence is shown in Fig. 12-20. In this sequence the

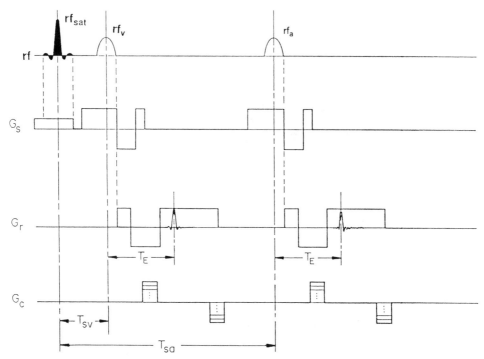

Figure 12-20 The sequence shown in Fig. 12-16 is extended for the SAAV angiogram. In this scheme the rf_{sat} pulse is added before the excitation rf pulses for the vein and artery, which are noted as rf_v and rf_a, respectively.

minimum T_R is somewhat longer than the normal 2-D planar imaging sequence, the total imaging time, however, does not increase more than 20%.

As shown in Fig. 12-20, three rf pulses are used to excite a thick volume and two slices in sequence: rf_{sat}, rf_v, and rf_a, represent the rf pulses for saturation, and venous and arterial excitations, respectively. Figure 12-21 illustrates how artery and vein imagings are separately obtained in one scan. First, an rf_{sat} pulse is applied at $t = 0$ to saturate the in-flow signals from both the artery and vein to the region, a slab shown in Fig. 12-21 (a). After the application of the second rf pulse rf_v at $t = T_{sv}$ in Fig. 12-21 (b), fresh spins, which are continuously injected into the venous imaging slice, will produce signals while the spins in the arterial vessels that originated from the saturated region and are injected into the imaging slice will not produce observable signals. By the third rf pulse rf_a at $t = T_{sa}$ in Fig. 12-21 (c), the spins in the venous blood injected into the arterial imaging slice (lower slice) are saturated while spins in the arterial blood in the slice are fresh, thereby giving signals only from the artery. If the velocities of the blood in the arteries and veins are too high, there could be a certain confusion between the arterial and venous bloods. The optimal saturated slice thickness (W_s)

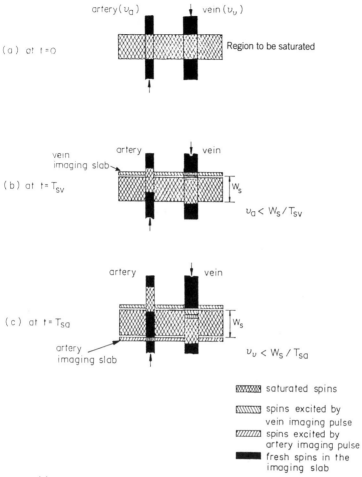

Figure 12-21 (a) The rf_{sat} pulse is applied at $t = 0$ on the thick slab to saturate all the in-flow signals both from the artery and vein. (b) By applying rf_v at $t = T_{sv}$, only the fresh spins from the vein are injected into the imaging slice, thereby giving venous signals only, while the spins in the arterial vessels that originated from the saturated region will not produce observable signals. (c) By the third rf pulse rf_a an arterial imaging slice at the lower side of the saturated slab is selected. The spins injected into the imaging slice from the vein are then saturated while spins in the arterial blood in the slice are fresh, thereby producing signals that are from the artery.

therefore has to be chosen accordingly. If the time intervals between rf_{sat} and rf_v and between rf_{sat} and rf_a are denoted as T_{sv} and T_{sa}, respectively, the unwanted vessel signals can be eliminated by satisfying the following relations:

$$v_a \leq \frac{W_s}{T_{sv}}$$

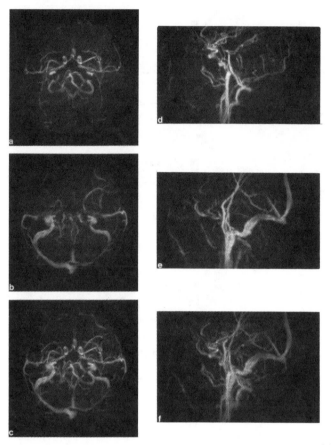

Figure 12-22 An axial view of angiograms obtained by the SAAV technique. (a), (b), and (c) are the artery, vein, and combined angiogram of (a) and (b), respectively. (d), (e), and (f) are the same 3-D images seen by lateral views (i.e., the artery, vein, and their combined angiograms, respectively).

and

$$v_v \leq \frac{W_s}{T_{sa}} \tag{12-59}$$

where v_a and v_v are the blood velocities in the arteries and veins while W_s is the thickness of the saturation region or the slab.

In Fig. 12-22 the experimental results from the simultaneous 3-D angiography of an artery and vein using the SAAV imaging sequence are shown. Figures 12-22(a), (b), and (c) show the projected axial view angiograms corresponding to the artery, the vein, and combined image of the artery and vein, respectively. Corresponding lateral view images of the artery, the vein, and the combined image of artery and vein are shown in (d), (e), and (f), respectively.

REFERENCES

1. J. R. Singer. *J. Phys. E: Sci. Instrum.* 11:281 (1978).
2. P. R. Moran. *Magn. Reson. Imag.* 1:197 (1982).
3. P. R. Moran, R. A. Moran, and N. Korstaedt. *Radiology.* 154:433 (1985).
4. A. Constantinesco, J. J. Malet, A. Bonmartin, C. Lallot, and A. Briguet. *Magn. Reson. Imag.* 2:335 (1984).
5. Z. H. Cho, C. H. Oh, Y. S. Kim, C. W. Mun, O. Nalcioglu, S. J. Lee, and M. K. Chung. *J. Appl. Phys.* 60:1256 (1986).
6. C. H. Oh, H. S. Kim, W. W. Park, W. S. Kim, S. W. Lee, and Z. H. Cho. *IEEE Trans. Nucl. Sci.* NS-20:1899 (1983).
7. Z. H. Cho, H. S. Kim, H. B. Song, and J. Cumming. *Proc. IEEE* 70:1152 (1982).
8. P. Van Dijk. *J. Comput. Assist. Tomogr.* 8:429 (1984).
9. B. Carnahan, H. A. Luther, and J. O. Wikes. *Applied Numerical Methods.* New York: Wiley, 1969, p. 361.
10. E. L. Hahn. *Phys. Rev.* 80:580 (1950).
11. H. Y. Carr and E. M. Purcell. *Phys. Rev.* 94:630 (1954).
12. E. O. Stejskal and J. E. Tanner. *J. Chem. Phys.* 42:288 (1965).
13. D. M. Cantor and J. Jonas. *J. Magn. Reson.* 28:157 (1977).
14. C. H. Oh and Z. H. Cho. *Phys. Med. Biol.* 31:1237 (1986).
15. D. G. Taylor and M. C. Bushell. *Phys. Med. Biol.* 30:345 (1985).
16. G. E. Taylor and M. E. Moseley, and R. L. Ehman. *Biomedical Magnetic Resonance*, T. L. James and A. R. Margulis, eds. San Francisco: Radiology Research and Education Foundation, 1984, p. 63.
17. D. L. Bihan, E. Breton, and A. Syrota. In *Abstracts of Society of Magnetic Resonance in Medicine*, 1985, p. 1238.
18. R. F. Karlicek, Jr. and I. J. Lowe. *J. Magn. Reson.* 37:75 (1980).
19. C. B. Ahn, S. Y. Lee, O. Nalcioglu, and Z. H. Cho. *Med. Phys.* 13:789 (1986).
20. F. Ståhlberg, A. Ericsson, T. Greitz, B. Nordell, B. Persson, and G. Sperber. In *Abstracts of Society of Magnetic Resonance in Medicine*, 1985, p. 611.
21. V. Waluch and W. G. Bradley. *J. Comput. Assist. Tomogr.* 8:594 (1984).
22. C. A. Keele, E. Neil, and N. Joels. *Applied Physiology*, 13th ed. Oxford: Oxford University Press, 1982, p. 81.
23. B. Folkow and E. Neil. *Circulation.* Oxford: Oxford University Press, 1971, p. 97.
24. M. E. Phelps, E. J. Hoffman, N. A. Mullani, and M. M. Ter-Pogossian. *J. Nucl. Med.* 16:210 (1976).
25. T. F. Budinger, S. E. Derenzo, R. H. Huseman, and J. L. Cahoon. *Proc. Soc. Photo-Opt. Instrum. Eng.* 372:3 (1982).
26. Z. H. Cho, C. H. Oh, C. W. Mun, and Y. S. Kim. *Magn. Reson. Med.* 3:857–862 (1986).

27. D. G. Norris. In *Abstracts of Society of Magnetic Resonace in Medicine*, 1985, pp. 593–594.

28. G. L. Nayler, D. N. Firmin, and D. B. Longmore. *J. Comput. Assist. Tomogr.* 10:715 (1986).

29. D. G. Nishimura, A. Macovski, and J. M. Pauly. *IEEE Trans. Med. Imag.* MI-5 (1986).

30. S. J. Lee, M. K. Chung, C. W. Mun, and Z. H. Cho. *Experiments in Fluids* 5:273 (1987).

31. R. J. Alfidi, T. J. Masaryk, E. M. Haake, G. W. Lenz, J. S. Ross, M. T. Modic, A. D. Nelson, J. P. LiPuma, and A. M. Cohen. *AJR* 149:1097 (1984).

32. Y. S. Kim, C. W. Mun, K. J. Jung, and Z. H. Cho. *Magn. Reson. Med.* 4:289 (1987).

33. J. Henning, M. Mueri, H. Friedburg, and P. Brunner. *J. Comput. Assist. Tomogr.* 11:872 (1987).

34. C. L. Dumoulin, H. E. Cline, S. P. Souza, W. A. Wagle, and M. F. Walker. *Magn. Reson. Med.* 11:35 (1989).

35. P. J. Keller, B. P. Drayer, E. K. Fram, K. D. Williams, C. L. Dumoulin, P. Souza. *Radiology* 173:527 (1989).

36. L. Axel and D. Morton. *J. Comput. Assist. Tomogr.* 11:31 (1987).

37. G. A. Laub and W. A. Kaiser. *J. Comput. Assist. Tomogr.* 12:377 (1988).

38. J. N. Lee, S. J. Riederer, and N. J. Pelc. *Magn. Reson. Med.* 12:1 (1989).

39. C. L. Dumoulin, S. P. Souza, M. F. Walker, and W. A. Wagle. *Magn. Reson. Med.* 9:139 (1989).

40. G. T. Gullberg, F. W. Wehrli, A. Shimakawa, and M. A. Simons. *Radiology* 165:241 (1987).

41. J. H. Kim and Z. H. Cho. *Magn. Reson. Med.* 14:554–561 (1990).

42. C. L. Dumoulin and H. R. Hart. *Radiology* 161:717 (1986).

43. C. L. Dumoulin, S. P. Souza, and H. R. Hart. *Magn. Reson. Med.* 5:238 (1987).

44. J. Frahm, K. D. Merboldt, W. Hänicke, M. L. Gyngell, and H. Bruhn. *Magn. Reson. Med.* 7:79 (1988).

45. Z. H. Cho, J. H. Kim, and K. D. Lee. *J. Magn. Reson.* 87:447 (1990).

46. E. M. Haacke and G. W. Lenz. *AJR* 148:1251, June (1987).

47. D. G. Nishimura, A. Macovski, J. M. Pauly, and S. M. Conolly. *Magn. Reson. Med.* 4:193 (1987).

48. J. Frahm, A. Haasse, and D. Matthaei. *Magn. Reson. Med.* 3:321 (1986).

13

CHEMICAL-SHIFT AND SPECTROSCOPIC IMAGING

13-1 CHEMICAL-SHIFT IMAGING [1 – 12]

In NMR the Larmor frequency is uniquely defined for a nucleus if a uniform field strength B_0 is given. However, the magnetic field may not be constant for all nuclei. The magnetic field in the vicinity of a nucleus is often affected by the local conditions. The local magnetic field B_{loc} experienced by a nucleus in a constant external magnetic field B_0 is given by

$$B_{loc} = (1 - \sigma) B_0 \qquad (13\text{-}1)$$

where σ is the screening (or shielding) constant which is mainly influenced by the diamagnetic, paramagnetic, and interatomic current effects:

$$\sigma = \sigma_{dia} + \sigma_{para} + \sigma' \qquad (13\text{-}2)$$

where σ_{dia}, σ_{para}, and σ' are the screening constants due to the diamagnetic, paramagnetic, and interatomic current effects, respectively.

Then the Larmor frequencies for two different nuclei of the same species are given by

$$v_k = \gamma(1 - \sigma_k) B_0$$

$$v_{ref} = \gamma(1 - \sigma_{ref}) B_0 \qquad (13\text{-}3)$$

where γ is the gyromagnetic ratio and the subscripts "k" and "ref" indicate the sample and the reference materials, respectively. The chemical shift is given by the difference of these two equations:

$$\omega_k \equiv v_k - v_{ref} = \gamma(\sigma_{ref} - \sigma_k)B_0 \qquad (13\text{-}4)$$

The first point to note is that the chemical shift ω_k is field dependent. To eliminate the field dependency of ω_k, a relative chemical shift δ_k is defined as

$$\delta_k = \frac{v_k - v_{ref}}{v_{ref}} \times 10^6 = \frac{\sigma_{ref} - \sigma_k}{1 - \sigma_{ref}} \times 10^6 \text{ ppm} \qquad (13\text{-}5)$$

In proton NMR spectroscopy, tetramethylsilane (TMS) is usually used as a reference material. A positive value of δ_k means that the nuclei of the sample resonate at a higher frequency than the reference material. In a high magnetic field the spectrum of a particular substance may split into several peaks due to the chemical shift, and the frequency difference between the peaks becomes larger with increasing magnetic field strength B_0. High-resolution NMR spectra therefore can be obtained with high magnetic field which is usually obtained by a superconducting magnet.

Although chemical shift plays a key role in NMR spectroscopy, chemical shift is often the main source of artifacts in NMR imaging, especially with a high-field superconducting magnet. The patterns of the artifacts are characterized in accordance with the imaging methods. Here the chemical-shift artifacts are analyzed for conventional two-dimensional Fourier imaging with spin-echo sequence.

Let us assume that an NMR signal is obtained with a conventional Fourier imaging pulse sequence as shown in Fig. 13-1 and is given by

$$S(\omega_x, \omega_y) = \int \int \int \rho(x, y; \omega_k) \exp\left\{-i\left[\left(\frac{\omega_k}{\gamma G_y} + y\right)\omega_y + x\omega_x\right]\right\} dx\, dy\, d\omega_k$$

$$(13\text{-}6)$$

where $\omega_x = \gamma G_x t_x$ and $\omega_y = \gamma G_y t_y$. In Eq. (13-6), ω_k is $\gamma \delta_k B_0 \times 10^{-6}$ (rad/sec) and $\rho(x, y; \omega_k)$ is the spatial spin density distribution at (x, y) with the chemical shift ω_k. The readout gradient time variable t_y is measured with respect to the time of the spin-echo formation. The spin-spin and spin-lattice relaxation terms are neglected for simplicity in this equation. As usual the spin density distribution can be calculated by the inverse Fourier transform of the NMR signal:

$$\tilde{\rho}(x, y) = \int \int S(\omega_x, \omega_y) \exp\left[i(\omega_x x + \omega_y y)\right] d\omega_x\, d\omega_y \qquad (13\text{-}7)$$

Now $\tilde{\rho}(x, y)$ is the reconstructed spin density distribution with chemical shift.

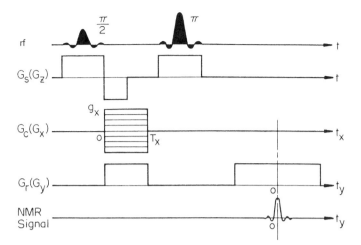

Figure 13-1 The basic form of the pulse sequence for 2-D Fourier spin echo technique widely used in NMR imaging. Here the amplitude variation scheme is used for phase encoding G_x, while the amplitudes of the slice selection and the readout gradients are constant.

Assuming a point source located at the origin with a single chemical-shift component with frequency $\hat{\omega}_k$, the spin density $\rho(0, 0; \hat{\omega}_k)$ can be written as

$$\rho(0, 0; \hat{\omega}_k) = \rho(x, y; \omega_k)\, \delta(x)\, \delta(y)\, \delta(\omega_k - \hat{\omega}_k) \qquad (13\text{-}8)$$

where $\delta(\cdot)$ is the Dirac delta function. From Eqs. (13-6), (13-7), and (13-8) the reconstructed spin density image $\rho(x', y')$ can also be expressed as

$$\rho(x', y') = \rho(x, y; \hat{\omega}_k)\, \delta\!\left(y - \frac{\hat{\omega}_k}{\gamma G_y}\right)\delta(x) \qquad (13\text{-}9)$$

where the y direction is assumed to be the readout gradient direction. When $\hat{\omega}_k = 0$, one obtains the reconstructed spin density distribution of the reference substance,

$$\rho(x', y') = \rho(x, y; 0)\, \delta(x)\, \delta(y)$$
$$= \rho(0, 0) \qquad (13\text{-}10)$$

From Eqs. (13-9) and (13-10) we observe that for the reference material (i.e., the material with no chemical shift) the computed spin density of a point source at the origin is also a point source at the origin. However, when $\hat{\omega}_k \neq 0$, namely when the material has a chemical shift as indicated in Eq. (13-9), the point at the origin is shifted by a distance $\hat{\omega}_k/(\gamma G_y)$ along the readout gradient direction (y direction in this case) resulting in a chemical-shift-dependent image misregistration or degradation.

13-1-1   Chemical-Shift-Imaging Methods

As mentioned earlier, there are several chemical shift imaging techniques that are in practical use. These techniques can be classified into three categories: the chemical-shift-selective technique, four-dimensional Fourier imaging, and echo time encoded spectroscopic imaging.

Chemical-Shift-Selective (CHESS) Imaging [13, 14]

When only a single spectral peak is of interest such as for water or fat selective proton chemical shift imaging, the best-known technique is the chemical-shift-selective (CHESS) technique. This technique uses an imaging method similar to the conventional method together with the selective excitation of the spectral peak of interest. Among the several CHESS techniques, the selective rf pulse technique and the gradient reversal technique are the two most often used methods.

Selective rf Pulse Technique for CHESS [13, 14]   Most of the CHESS techniques employ a narrow band, selective rf pulse without a selection gradient to excite a single spectral peak. Figure 13-2 shows several variations of the CHESS rf pulse technique. In the pulse sequence of Fig. 13-2(a), the spatially selective 90° rf pulse of the conventional imaging sequence is replaced with a CHESS 90° rf pulse without a selection gradient. Note here that the method applies to single-slice imaging only since the whole volume is excited by the CHESS 90° rf pulse without any gradients. All the other CHESS techniques shown in Fig. 13-2 have the same property of single-slice chemical shift imaging. The pulse sequence of Fig. 13-2(b) takes advantage of the Fourier transform relationship between the time domain rf pulse waveform and the frequency domain selection profile; namely the selection profile of the square-shaped 180° rf pulse is approximately sinc shaped, having several zero crossings at the side lobes. For example, when only two spectral peaks are of interest, the sinc shape in the frequency domain, resulting from the square 180° rf pulse, would select the spectral peak of interest that lies in the center of the main lobe, while the other spectral peak to be eliminated lies in the zero crossing point of the selection profile so that it would not be selected. Then this 180° rf pulsing generates an echo signal of the spectral peak of interest only. As described above, the pulse sequences shown in Figs. 13-2(a) and (b) are both applicable for the imaging of a selected spectral peak only.

On the other hand, instead of selective excitation, one can also selectively excite and suppress the spectral peak. The CHESS techniques of Figs. 13-2(c) and (d) are suitable sequences for such a purpose. When one spectral peak is too strong compared with the other spectral peaks, the dominant

Chemical Shift Selective (CHESS) Techniques

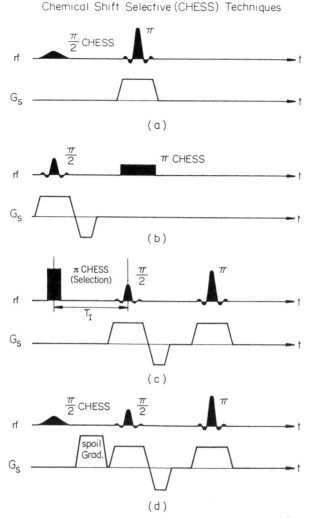

Figure 13-2 Various pulse sequences for the CHESS technique: (a) the 90° ($\pi/2$) chemical-shift-selective excitation technique, (b) the 180° (π) selective excitation technique, (c) the 180° (π) selective inversion technique which selectively suppresses the unwanted spectral peak by inversion, and (d) the 90° ($\pi/2$) selective saturation technique.

peak should be suppressed to improve the dynamic range. In NMR spectroscopy therefore the water peak, for example, is often suppressed by a suppression technique similar to the CHESS method. In Fig. 13-2(c) a 180° spectral selective inversion pulse is applied, and the spin-echo sequence follows at the time of the zero crossing of the T_1 value of the spectral peak of interest. In other words, if the spin-lattice relaxation time of the spectral (dominant) peak to be suppressed is T_1, a suitable selection of the inversion time, T_I, would give a zero NMR signal:

$$S(t) = M_0 \left[1 - 2 \exp \left(- \frac{T_I}{T_1} \right) \right] = 0 \qquad (13\text{-}11)$$

This technique, however, may not be useful when the dominant spectral peak has multiple T_1-values.

Finally, Fig. 13-2(d) shows a selective saturation technique. In this method the 90° CHESS rf pulse is applied to selectively excite the spectral peak and subsequently saturates the peak by using a spoiling gradient. Since the saturated spectral peak has no net magnetization, a NMR signal will not be generated when the conventional spin-echo imaging sequence is applied.

One of the main drawbacks of these four pulse sequences is the lack of multislice imaging capability due to the inherent limitation of the method; that is, the method requires, in one way or another, excitation or saturation of the entire volume. In the following discussion we will introduce a gradient reversal CHESS technique with which multislice imaging can be performed.

Gradient Reversal Technique for CHESS [15]

Spectral Selective Imaging   The chemical-shift effect usually appears as positional shifts in both the readout and the selection gradient directions in the conventional two-dimensional Fourier imaging. By use of the spectroscopic imaging technique, the position shift in the readout gradient direction can be corrected. The chemical-shift effect in the direction of selection gradient is, however, different and requires the following considerations. Let the amplitude of the selection gradient and the frequency bandwidth of the rf pulse be G_s gauss/cm and F_B Hz, respectively (see the pulse sequence of Fig. 13-3); the selected slice thickness is then determined by those two parameters and is given by

$$L_s = \frac{2\pi F_B}{\gamma G_s} \text{ cm} \qquad (13\text{-}12)$$

If the object is, however, off-resonance with a frequency F_{off} Hz, the selected slice is shifted by an amount L_c cm, as given by (see Fig. 13-4)

$$L_c = \frac{2\pi F_{\text{off}}}{\gamma G_s} \text{ cm} \qquad (13\text{-}13)$$

Figure 13-4 shows the relationships between the rf bandwidth and the off-resonance frequency together with the region that will be selected in conventional spin-echo Fourier imaging. Since most of the proton chemical shift imaging in the human body has two spectral peaks, namely water and

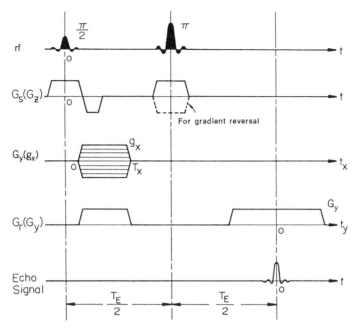

Figure 13-3 The pulse sequences for conventional 2-D Fourier imaging (the solid line) and for the gradient reversal technique (dotted lines in G_S during the 180° rf pulse represent the additional gradient pulse needed for the technique). Note that the only difference is the additional sequence with the gradient reversal at the 180° rf pulse.

lipid protons, one of the peaks can be set at on-resonance, whereas the other can be set at off-resonance. In this case the selected regions of these two peaks are separated by L_c cm provided that the resonance frequency difference between the two peaks is F_{off} Hz. As will be discussed in the next section, this slice-selective property can be utilized for the selection of a particular spectral peak of interest.

Let us assume that only two spectral peaks are involved; then the first 90° rf with gradient will select the spectral peak of interest, and the following 180° rf will again select the same slice (see Fig. 13-3 with solid lines). This situation is illustrated in Fig. 13-4. However, if a gradient-reversed pulse sequence (gradient with dotted lines) is applied, the combined situation appears as illustrated in Fig. 13-5. As seen in the figure, the region of peak A selected by the 90° rf pulse does not overlap with that of the 180° rf pulse. That is, the spectral peak A selected by the first 90° rf pulse is unable to produce echo signals by 180° rf pulse. On the other hand, the spectral peak B, which is on-resonance, would select the same region by both the 90° and the 180° rf pulses, thereby producing an echo signal. For gradient reversal CHESS imaging the desired peak should therefore be set at on-resonance (e.g., B), while the other unwanted peak can be placed at off-resonance with

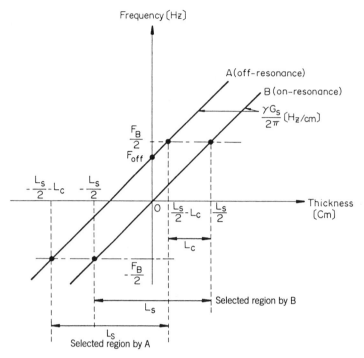

Figure 13-4 The region selected by the rf pulse and the selection gradient in conventional Fourier imaging. Substance B is on-resonance, whereas that of A is off-resonance with an offset frequency F_{off} (Hz). The region selected by A is shifted from that of B by an amount L_C (cm). Note, however, that the slice thickness is not changed and remained same.

a frequency bandwidth set by

$$F_B < \frac{\gamma B_0 \delta_k \times 10^{-6}}{\pi} \text{ Hz} \tag{13-14}$$

The selected region B then appears as shown in Fig. 13-15 (thick line). Some experimental results obtained with a high-field (2.0 T) superconducting NMR imager are shown in Fig. 13-6. Figures 13-6(a) and (b) show the chemical-shift separated images of water and fat in the human knee obtained by the gradient reversal CHESS sequence with an rf pulse frequency bandwidth of 500 Hz.

Slice Selection Error Correction [16, 17] The slice selection error due to the chemical shift can also be corrected by use of a gradient reversal technique similar to the gradient reversal CHESS imaging sequence discussed above. In this case both the A and the B peaks are now set at two different off-resonance conditions (i.e., $+F_{off}$ and $-F_{off}$) as shown in Fig. 13-7. When

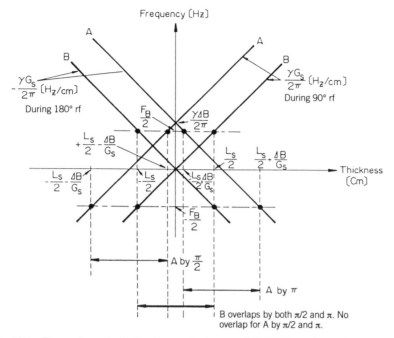

Figure 13-5   The region selected by the gradient reversal CHESS imaging technique shown in Fig. 13-3. The substance *B* is at on-resonance, while that of *A* is at off-resonance with an offset frequency of $\gamma \Delta B/2\pi$ (Hz), consequently only substance *B* will be selected.

the chemical-shift difference between the water and the lipid protons is δ_k ppm and the two peaks are both set at two different off-resonances (i.e., one at upward off-resonance $+F_{\text{off}}$ Hz and the other at downward off-resonance $-F_{\text{off}}$ Hz) it is easy to show that the selected slice would overlap only at the center with a thickness L_s, which is related to F_{off} and the bandwidth F_B by

$$F_B = \frac{\gamma G_s L_s}{2\pi} + 2F_{\text{off}} \qquad (13\text{-}15)$$

where

$$F_{\text{off}} = \frac{\gamma B_0}{2\pi} \frac{\delta_k}{2} \times 10^{-6} \text{ Hz} \qquad (13\text{-}16)$$

The important advantage of this technique when applied to CHESS imaging is that there is no need for additional rf pulses for the chemical-shift selection of water or fat imaging, it requires only a single experiment. In addition this technique also provides a selection capability for both water and lipid protons in the same slice, regardless of the chemical shift.

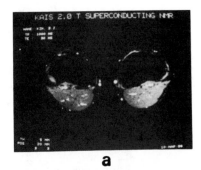

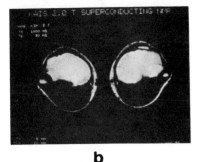

Figure 13-6 The *in vivo* human chemical-shift images obtained by the gradient reversal CHESS technique: (a) and (b) are the chemical-shift-separated images obtained experimentally that correspond to water and lipid protons, respectively.

Four-dimensional Fourier Imaging [18]

Four-dimensional Fourier NMR imaging was first proposed by Maudsley et al., and it offered new possibilities of doing spatially resolved high-resolution spectroscopy. This four-dimensional NMR technique is a variation of the three-dimensional Fourier imaging technique with an added spectral dimension. This new spectral dimension represents the chemical shift information. Figure 13-8 shows the pulse sequence for four-dimensional Fourier NMR imaging. Note the total absence of a readout gradient in any direction except the three-dimensional coding gradients G_x, G_y, and G_z. Collected data is then transformed into the spatial domain by a four-dimensional Fourier transform to generate the NMR spectra as well as the 3-D image; in other words, the NMR spectrum at each voxel in the spatially resolved 3-D volume image. The measured NMR signal is then given by

$$S(\omega_x, \omega_y, \omega_z, t_x)$$

$$= \int_{\omega_k} \int_z \int_y \int_x \rho(x, y, z, \omega_k) \exp\left[-i(x\omega_x + y\omega_y + z\omega_z + \omega_k t_k)\right] dx\, dy\, dz\, d\omega_k$$

$$(13\text{-}17)$$

where $\omega_x = \gamma g_x T_x$, $\omega_y = \gamma g_y T_y$, $\omega_z = \gamma g_z T_z$, and g_x, g_y, and g_z are the amplitude variables of the x, y, and z gradients, respectively. A three-dimen-

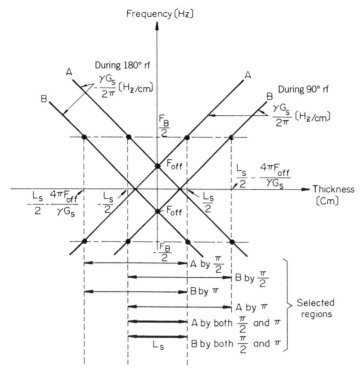

Figure 13-7 A variation of the gradient reversal technique shown in Fig. 13-5. In this case the selected region will overlap for both A and B in the region from $-L_S/2$ to $+L_S/2$ thereby select a slice with L_S thickness.

sionally resolved volume spectral image naturally can be reduced to a two-dimensional slice spectral image by simply converting any one of the three coding gradients into the selection gradient. Full four-dimensional Fourier imaging, however, requires an imaging time of $N_x N_y N_z T_R$ sec for spectrally resolved three-dimensional volume imaging. Here N_x, N_y, N_z, and T_R are the number of encodings of the x, y, and z gradients and the repetition time, respectively. N_x, N_y, and N_z then will represent the number of image pixels in the spatial domains x, y, and z, respectively. As seen, even for the case of two-dimensional slice selected spectroscopic imaging, quite a large number of coding steps will be required, and they are often too long for human *in vivo* imaging. The advantage of this four-dimensional NMR technique however, is that the spectral resolution is independent of the number of encoding steps, thereby always very high resolution spectra are obtained. Four-dimensional NMR is therefore ideally suited for high resolution spectroscopic imaging with limited resolution in the spatial domain.

For example, phosphorus, ^{31}P, would be an ideal candidate for four-dimensional NMR or three-dimensional NMR with selected-volume or se-

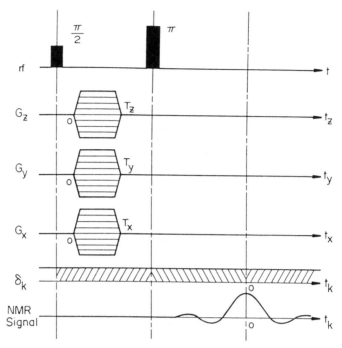

Figure 13-8 Pulse sequence of the 4-D Fourier NMR for spectroscopic imaging. This scheme is ideally suited for high spectral resolution imaging rather than high spatial resolution imaging due to the requirement of large number of encoding steps, i.e., large imaging time.

lected-slice imaging having relatively poor spatial resolution. High-resolution *in vivo* spectroscopic imaging of ^{31}P has been successfully performed with the four-dimensional Fourier NMR imaging technique [18].

Echo Time Encoded Spectroscopic Imaging [19, 20]

As discussed in the previous sections, in an attempt to resolve the spectrum at each pixel in the reconstructed image plane, both Dixon's method and four-dimensional NMR are limited either in the spectral resolution or spatial resolution. For example, in Dixon's method [13] the spectral resolution is limited, while in three-dimensional NMR spectroscopic imaging with a selected-slice, long imaging time is the practical limitation. The above two techniques are therefore often found to be difficult to use for high-resolution human *in vivo* spectroscopic imaging. These difficulties, however, can be overcome by the use of echo time encoded spectroscopic imaging [20]. In this scheme the spectral resolution can be arbitrarily adjusted without being limited by the spatial resolution, thereby allowing us to choose either a high spectral resolution image or a high spatial resolution image, depending on the need. These parameters can be separately controlled by optimum selection of the number of echo time encoding steps or spatial resolution encoding steps.

In Fig. 13-9 the pulse sequence for the echo time encoded (ETE) spectroscopic imaging based on the Fourier imaging technique is shown. Initially this imaging method was used for chemical shift artifact correction in proton imaging in a high magnetic field [19]. The basic difference of the present method compared with conventional single-slice Fourier imaging is that the time position of the 180° rf pulse and the corresponding selection gradient (z-gradient) are shifted a given number of steps depending on the desired spectral resolution. For instance, the higher the required spectral resolution is, the larger the number of encoding steps should be. If there are only two peaks—such as water and lipid protons or lipid and lactate protons in the proton spectroscopic imaging—it is acceptable to take only two encoding steps, which are enough to resolve the two peaks in the spectral domain (i.e., equal to Dixon's method). It is, however, often necessary to take spectral resolution higher than simply two points, even though there are only two spectral components, such as water and lipid protons. This is mainly due to the fact that the spectrum of each pixel is affected by a number of other factors, including the magnetic susceptibility, the static field inhomogeneity, and chemical shift.

The following is the basic principle of ETE spectroscopic imaging with which arbitrarily selected spectral and spatial resolutions can be obtained within a given imaging time. Let us consider the single-slice spectroscopic imaging pulse sequence shown in Fig. 13-9. In this scheme the measured NMR signal can be expressed as

$$S(\omega_x, \omega_y; t_k)$$

$$= \int_{\omega_k} \int_y \int_x \rho(x, y; \omega_k) \exp\left[-i\left\{\omega_x x + \omega_y\left(y + \frac{\omega_k}{\gamma G_y}\right) + \omega_k t_k\right\}\right] dx\, dy\, d\omega_k$$

$$(13\text{-}18)$$

where $\rho(x, y; \omega_k)$ is the two-dimensional spatial spin density distribution at (x, y) with the chemical shift ω_k, $\omega_x = \gamma g_x T_x$, $\omega_y = \gamma G_y t_y$, and the other parameters (g_x, G_y, T_x, t_y, and t_k) are the parameters given in Fig. 13-9. In this equation the spin-lattice (T_1) and spin-spin (T_2) relaxation effects are omitted for simplicity (the effects will be the same as those for conventional Fourier NMR imaging). From the principles of discrete signal processing, spectral resolution is defined as

$$\text{Spectral resolution} = \frac{1}{W(t_k)}$$

$$= \frac{1}{N_k \, \Delta t_k} \qquad (13\text{-}19)$$

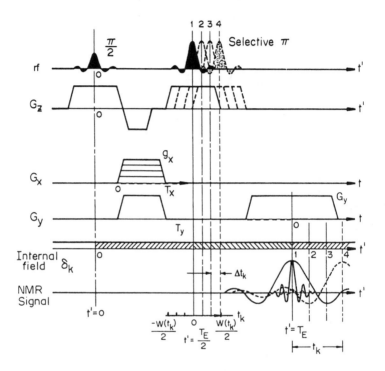

Figure 13-9 Pulse sequence of the echo time encoded spectroscopic imaging. Note the position of the 180° rf pulses and the corresponding z-gradient pulses (selection gradient) are synchronously shifted. The resultant echo signal is now weighted by the spectral coding according to the 180° rf pulse time position. The internal field consists of the chemical shift, the field inhomogeneity, the magnetic susceptibility, and so on. In this example, four signals are illustrated: The narrow echo signal shown in pulse 1 is the echo signal with the readout gradient G_y, while the broad signal is the one without the readout gradient. It can be interpreted that pulse 1 corresponds to the case where both the rf echo and the gradient echo coincide, thereby weighting the gradient echo peak to a maximum; while the others (2, 3, and 4) are the cases where the rf echoes do not coincide with the gradient echo.

where $W(t_k)$ is the total time window of the echo time encoding, N_k is the number of encoding steps for the spectral resolution, and Δt_k is the time interval of the rf encoding step. The encoding time range is therefore given by

$$-\tfrac{1}{2}W(t_k) \le t_k \le \tfrac{1}{2}W(t_k) \tag{13-20}$$

The advantages of the echo time encoding method are the flexible imaging time due to the adjustable number of encoding steps; that is, only a small number of encoding steps will be required, if the high spectral resolution is not the prerequisite. For example, in high-resolution proton spectroscopic imaging, a high spatial resolution image with a modest spectral resolution within a reasonable imaging time is usually needed. In this case the echo time encoding scheme is ideally suited for such a purpose, since this scheme allows us to trade off the spatial resolution with the spectral resolution, and vice versa.

Let us now consider an actual implementation of the echo time encoded technique. The following two procedures are usually used:

1. *Preprocessing method*: Each echo signal is multiplied by $\exp(-i\omega_k t_y)$ before the Fourier transform to compensate for the phase shift due to chemical shift, and then the three-dimensional inverse Fourier transform is performed to obtain the final spectrally resolved image data:

$$\mathscr{F}_3^{-1}\!\left[S(\omega_x, \omega_y; t_k)\exp(-i\omega_k t_y); \omega_x \to x, \omega_y \to y, t_k \to \omega_k\right] = \tilde{\rho}(x, y, \omega_k) \tag{13-21}$$

where $\mathscr{F}_3^{-1}[\cdot]$ is a three-dimensional inverse Fourier transform operator. As shown in Eq. (13-21), the spectroscopic image is obtained by using the three-dimensional Fourier transform of the echo signal compensated by $\exp(-i\omega_k t_y)$. The compensation applied by $\exp(-i\omega_k t_y)$ corrects the geometric shift due to the chemical shift.

2. *Postprocessing method*: As an alternative to the first method where the correction is applied before the Fourier transform, a postprocessing can also be applied. This postprocessing method is often preferred from the computational viewpoint simply because it offers spectral image by a direct three-dimensional Fourier transform of the echo signal. The result is a spatially resolved 2-D spectra however, with a geometrical shift:

$$\tilde{\rho}(x, y; \omega_k) = \mathscr{F}_3\!\left[S(\omega_x, \omega_y; t_k); \omega_x \to x, \omega_y \to y, t_k \to \omega_k\right]$$

$$= \rho\!\left(x, y - \frac{\omega_k}{\gamma G_y}; \omega_k\right) \tag{13-22}$$

Note that the spectral image obtained in Eq. (13-22) is nothing more than an image shifted in the y direction (i.e., the readout gradient direction) by a fixed value of $\omega_k/(\gamma G_y)$, which can easily be corrected after the spectral image is reconstructed. The final corrected image would then appear as

$$\rho(x, y; \omega_k) = \tilde{\rho}\left(x, y + \frac{\omega_k}{\gamma G_y}; \omega_k\right) \qquad (13\text{-}23)$$

The resultant equations given in Eqs. (13-21) and (13-23) will provide a spectrally resolved two-dimensional image or a spectral shift (artifact) corrected two-dimensional image. The latter is simply obtained by the summation of the spectrally resolved images. In other words, the corrected image $\rho(x, y)$ is given by

$$\rho(x, y) = \int \rho(x, y; \omega_k)\, d\omega_k \qquad (13\text{-}24)$$

For example, at a field strength of 2.0 T where the Larmor frequency of a proton is 85.15 MHz, the spectral difference between water and lipid

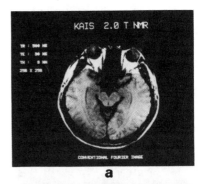

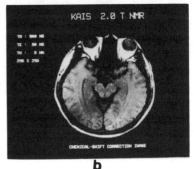

Figure 13-10 Images obtained with and without the spectral shift artifact correction. (a) is the image obtained by the conventional Fourier imaging. Observe the large spaces between the eyeballs and retrobulbar fat tissue around the optic nerves due to the chemical shift in the vertical direction (the vertical direction is the y or readout gradient direction). (b) is the corrected image of (a) using the echo time encoded spectroscopic imaging technique. The repetition time and echo time were $T_R = 500$ msec and $T_E = 30$ msec, respectively.

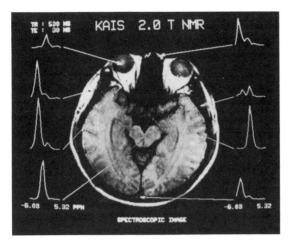

Figure 13-11 A spectrally resolved proton NMR image of a human head obtained by the echo time encoded spectroscopic imaging. A few representative pixel points are shown with their corresponding spectra.

protons appears to be approximately 300 Hz which is about 3.5 ppm. To resolve 300 Hz with reasonable accuracy, a 0.96 msec encoding time interval with 16 encoding steps [i.e., $W(t_k) = 0.96 \times 16$ msec or 65 Hz $= 1/W(t_k)$] was used, and the data (echo signal) were then sampled by a 30-μsec interval. The number of encoding steps for the x-gradient amplitude was selected as 256 so that 256×256 pixels were obtained for each spectral value. With the above conditions, a spectral resolution of 65 Hz $[= 1/(W(t_k)]$ was obtained with a spatial resolution of 1.0 mm (where the frequency difference between adjacent pixels was also set to approximately 65 Hz in the x and y directions). This 65 Hz is about 0.76 ppm at 85.15 MHz, and should be larger than the field inhomogeneity within the imaging volume of interest.

Figure 13-10(a) shows a head of a human volunteer, with the spectral shift artifact mainly due to the chemical shift (see the shifted fat around the optic nerves), while Fig. 13-10(b) shows the artifact-corrected image of (a) using the above-discussed echo time encoded spectroscopic imaging method [see Eq. (13-24)]. In Fig. 13-11 a spectrally resolved image (also an artifact-corrected image) with a few selected spectra corresponding to those indicated pixels is shown.

With the echo time encoded spectroscopic imaging sequence, it is possible to obtain high resolution *in vivo* spectroscopic images of humans within reasonable imaging times. The imaging time can further be reduced by use of the gradient echo technique. In addition the method offers a simple way to correct the spectral shift artifact in high-field proton NMR imaging.

13-1-2 Field Inhomogeneity, Chemical Shift, and Susceptibility

Field Inhomogeneity Effects in NMR Imaging [21–23]

Static field inhomogeneity is an important factor determining the image quality in NMR imaging and is generally kept as low as possible. For instance, a 2.0-T superconducting magnet system for whole body NMR imaging has a field inhomogeneity of about 5 ppm over a 30 cm DSV (diameter of spherical volume) with an active shim set. Although this 5-ppm field inhomogeneity is not the critical factor for conventional NMR imaging, it would seriously affect chemical shift-related imaging, since the chemical shifts involved in medical applications are also within a few ppm. To obtain a chemical shift image with high spectral resolution, the field inhomogeneity should be kept well below the desired spectral resolution, or otherwise some form of correction scheme should be applied.

For the conventional imaging, there has been much work recently toward obtaining undistorted NMR images in the presence of a field inhomogeneity. Most of these techniques utilize the a priori information on the field map in the spatial domain, and the inhomogeneity term is then corrected by using this information. The field homogeneity map can usually be obtained from the phase information of the image reconstructed using the echo time encoding technique. For example, an NMR signal which is measured with the echo time encoded pulse sequence (Fig. 13-12) can be given as

$$S(\omega_x, \omega_y)_{\Delta_t}$$

$$= \int\int \rho(x, y) \exp\left[-i\left(x\omega_x + y\omega_y + \gamma E(x, y)\, \Delta_t + \frac{E(x, y)}{G_y}\omega_y\right)\right] dx\, dy$$

$$(13\text{-}25)$$

where $\omega_x = \gamma g_x T_x$, $\omega_y = \gamma G_y t_y$, $E(x, y)$ is the field inhomogeneity term [the field difference from B_0 at each point (x, y)], and $2\Delta_t$ is the time interval between the rf echo center and the gradient echo center. By using the coordinate transform given by

$$\hat{x} = x$$

$$\hat{y} = y + \frac{E(x, y)}{G_y} \qquad (13\text{-}26)$$

and by substituting Eq. (13-26) into Eq. (13-25), the measured NMR signal can be simplified to

$$S(\omega_x, \omega_y)_{\Delta_t} = \int\int f(\hat{x}, \hat{y}) \exp\left[-i(\omega_x \hat{x} + \omega_y \hat{y})\right] \exp\left(-i\gamma \hat{E}(\hat{x}, \hat{y})\, \Delta_t\right) d\hat{x}\, d\hat{y}$$

$$(13\text{-}27)$$

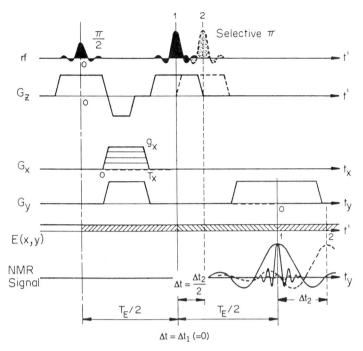

Figure 13-12   The pulse sequence designed for the measurement of the field inhomogeneity map. This sequence is close to the pulse sequence used for the conventional Fourier imaging except for the echo time delay of Δ_{t_2}. The echo time delay encodes the field inhomogeneity $E(x,y)$ in terms of the phase. Usually two echo time delays are used, Δ_{t_1} and Δ_{t_2} [see Eq. (13-25)].

where $\hat{E}(\hat{x}, \hat{y})$ is the field inhomogeneity in the distorted domain, which is assumed to be $\hat{E}(\hat{x}, \hat{y}) = E(x, y)$, and $f(\hat{x}, \hat{y})$ is

$$f(\hat{x}, \hat{y}) = \rho(x, y) |J(x, y)|^{-1} \tag{13-28}$$

In Eq. (13-28), $J(x, y)$ is the Jacobian resulting from the coordinate transformation:

$$J(x, y) = \begin{vmatrix} \dfrac{\partial \hat{x}}{\partial x} & \dfrac{\partial \hat{x}}{\partial y} \\[2ex] \dfrac{\partial \hat{y}}{\partial x} & \dfrac{\partial \hat{y}}{\partial y} \end{vmatrix}$$

$$= 1 + \frac{1}{G_y} \frac{\partial E(x, y)}{\partial y} \tag{13-29}$$

The reconstructed image $\tilde{\rho}(\hat{x}, \hat{y})_{\Delta_t}$ can be obtained from $S(\omega_x, \omega_y)_{\Delta_t}$ through 2-D Fourier transform,

$$\tilde{\rho}(\hat{x}, \hat{y})_{\Delta_t} = \int\int S(\omega_x, \omega_y)_{\Delta_t} \exp\big(i\big(\omega_x\hat{x} + \omega_y\hat{y}\big)\big) d\omega_x \, d\omega_y$$

$$= \rho(x, y)|J(x, y)|^{-1} \exp\big[-i\gamma\hat{E}(\hat{x}, \hat{y}) \Delta_t\big] \qquad (13\text{-}30)$$

By using a nonzero value of Δ_t in Eq. (13-30) and taking the argument of $\tilde{\rho}(\hat{x}, \hat{y})_{\Delta_t}$, an inhomogeneity map of $\hat{E}(\hat{x}, \hat{y})$ can be obtained:

$$\hat{E}(\hat{x}, \hat{y}) \equiv E(x, y) = -\frac{1}{\gamma\Delta_t} \big[\arg\big(\tilde{\rho}(\hat{x}, \hat{y})_{\Delta_t}\big) + 2\pi k\big] \qquad (13\text{-}31)$$

where k is an integer necessary to account for the slowly varying function $\hat{E}(\hat{x}, \hat{y})$, since the argument is defined from $-\pi$ to π.

From the inhomogeneity term obtained from Eq. (13-31) the geometrical shift $E(x, y)/G_y$ in the readout gradient direction can be estimated and corrected:

$$\hat{y} = y + \frac{\hat{E}(\hat{x}, \hat{y})}{G_y} \qquad (13\text{-}32)$$

The original y therefore can be obtained by

$$y = \hat{y} - \frac{\hat{E}(\hat{x}, \hat{y})}{G_y} \qquad (13\text{-}33)$$

Note that the x-directional shift is assumed to be negligible [i.e., $\hat{x} = x$; see Eq. (13-26)]. From the measured or estimated inhomogeneity $\hat{E}(\hat{x}, \hat{y})$ in Eq. (13-31), the geometrical shift-corrected image $\rho(x, y)_{\Delta_t}$ can be obtained and is given by [from Eq. (13-30)]

$$\rho(x, y)_{\Delta_t} = \tilde{\rho}(\hat{x}, \hat{y})_{\Delta_t}|J(x, y)|$$

$$\equiv \rho(x, y)\exp\big[-i\gamma E(x, y) \Delta_t\big] \qquad (13\text{-}34a)$$

In Eq. (13-34a), $\hat{E}(\hat{x}, \hat{y})_{\Delta_t} = E(x, y) \Delta_t$ is assumed. From Eq. (13-34) the true image $\rho(x, y)$ can finally be obtained as

$$\rho(x, y) \equiv \rho(x, y)_{\Delta_t} \exp\big[i\gamma E(x, y) \Delta_t\big] \qquad (13\text{-}34b)$$

Correction of Field Inhomogeneity Effects in Chemical-Shift Imaging [24, 25]

In vivo proton spectroscopic imaging in humans usually involves only two spectral peaks: water and lipid (fat) protons. A simpler inhomogeneity correction technique can be found. Let us divide the spin-density function $\rho(x, y)$ in Eq. (13-25) into $\rho_w(x, y)$ and $\rho_f(x, y)$ representing the water and fat density functions, respectively. Equation (13-25) then can be rewritten as

$$S(\omega_x, \omega_y)_{\Delta_t} = \int\int \left\{ \rho_w(x, y) + \rho_f(x, y) \exp\left[-i\left(\omega_k \Delta_t + \omega_k \frac{\omega_y}{\gamma G_y} \right) \right] \right\}$$

$$\times \exp\left[-i\left(x\omega_x + y\omega_y + \gamma E_h(x, y) \Delta_t + \frac{E_h(x, y)}{G_y} \omega_y \right) \right] dx\, dy$$

$$(13\text{-}35)$$

Here we have assumed that the water is at on-resonance while the fat is at off-resonance with $\omega_k = \gamma \delta_k B_0 \times 10^{-6}$, and that $E_h(x, y)$ is the field inhomogeneity excluding the chemical shift. By Fourier transform the reconstructed image becomes

$$\tilde{\rho}(\hat{x}, \hat{y})_{\Delta_t} = \left[\rho_W(x, y) + \rho_f\left(x, y - \frac{\omega_k}{\gamma G_y} \right) \exp(-\omega_k \Delta_t) \right]$$

$$\times |J(x, y)|^{-1} \exp\left[-i\gamma E_h(x, y) \Delta_t \right] \qquad (13\text{-}36)$$

To obtain the water or the fat density function in a separate form using Eq. (13-36), two encoding times Δ_{t1} and Δ_{t2} are required:

$$\Delta_{t1} = 0$$

$$\Delta_{t2} = \frac{\pi}{\gamma \delta_k B_0 \times 10^{-6}} = \frac{\pi}{\omega_k} \qquad (13\text{-}37)$$

When the above conditions are applied to Eq. (13-36), the reconstructed images become

$$\tilde{\rho}(\hat{x}, \hat{y})_{\Delta_{t1}} = \left[\rho_w(x, y) + \rho_f\left(x, y - \frac{\omega_k}{\gamma G_y} \right) \right] |J(x, y)|^{-1}$$

$$\tilde{\rho}(\hat{x}, \hat{y})_{\Delta_{t2}} = \left[\rho_w(x, y) - \rho_f\left(x, y - \frac{\omega_k}{\gamma G_y} \right) \right] |J(x, y)|^{-1} \exp(-i\gamma E_h(x, y) \Delta_{t2})$$

$$(13\text{-}38)$$

Since the spin density functions and the Jacobian are real, the phase term $\exp(-i\gamma E_h(x, y) \Delta_{t2})$ can be estimated from Eq. (13-38). Using the phase information and addition and subtraction of Eq. (13-38), the reconstructed water and fat density functions (still geometrically distorted) can be obtained and are given by

$$\tilde{\rho}_W(\hat{x}, \hat{y}) = \frac{1}{2}\left[\tilde{\rho}(\hat{x}, \hat{y})_{\Delta_{t1}} + \tilde{\rho}(\hat{x}, \hat{y})_{\Delta_{t2}} \exp(i\gamma E_h(x, y)\Delta_{t2}\right]$$

$$= \rho_W(x, y)|J(x, y)|^{-1}$$

$$\tilde{\rho}_f\left(\hat{x}, \hat{y} - \frac{\omega_k}{\gamma G_y}\right) = \frac{1}{2}\left[\tilde{\rho}(\hat{x}, \hat{y})_{\Delta_{t1}} - \tilde{\rho}(\hat{x}, \hat{y})_{\Delta_{t2}} \exp(i\gamma E_h(x, y)\Delta_{t2}\right]$$

$$= \rho_f\left(x, y - \frac{\omega_k}{\gamma G_y}\right)|J(x, y)|^{-1} \quad (13\text{-}39)$$

Since the field inhomogeneity term $E_h(x, y)$ or the phase term $\gamma E_h(x, y)\Delta_{t2}$ are already known, the geometrical-shift corrected images of $\rho_w(x, y)$ and $\rho_f(x, y)$ can be obtained by use of the field inhomogeneity correction

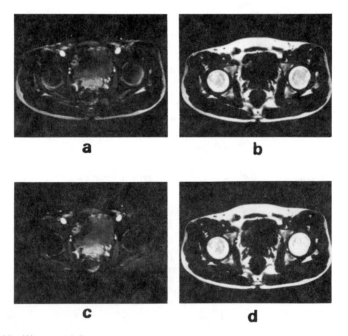

Figure 13-13 Water and fat separated images under a large field inhomogeneity and inhomogeneity corrected chemical shift images obtained by using the correction method shown in Fig. 13-12. (a) and (b) are the water and fat images without the field inhomogeneity correction, whereas (c) and (d) are the field inhomogeneity corrected images of (a) and (b), respectively [see Eq. (13-39)].

algorithm given in the previous section. Figures 13-13(a) and (b) are the water and fat images without the field inhomogeneity correction, whereas Figs. 13-13(c) and (d) are the field-inhomogeneity-corrected water and fat images using Eq. (13-39) and the geometrical shift correction algorithm given in the previous section. Note in the latter that there is a clear separation of water and fat as well as a uniform correction despite the large field inhomogeneity (field inhomogeneity of 10 ppm is assumed in the image volume).

Magnetic Susceptibility Effects on NMR Imaging [25, 26, 27]

Another important inhomogeneity component is, as mentioned earlier, susceptibility, since in NMR the object to be imaged consists of both paramagnetic and diamagnetic substances where the paramagnetic material appears as a positive susceptibility while the diamagnetic material appears as a negative susceptibility. Examples of paramagnetic substances are potassium, oxygen, tungsten, and the rare earth elements. Diamagnetic substances are the ones that will slightly decrease a magnetic field inside the sample, such as the inert gases, copper, bismuth, sodium chloride, and sulfur. Even if neither paramagnetic nor diamagnetic substances are added to water, such as air often causes a susceptibility effect in NMR imaging. The susceptibility of air appears positive compared with that of the water, as will be demonstrated shortly.

Magnetic susceptibility [26], similar to the chemical shift and the main magnetic field inhomogeneity, distorts the image geometrically as well as the intensities. Again, similar to the chemical shift artifact, the amount of image distortion due to the susceptibility is proportional to the main magnetic field strength and inversely proportional to the gradient strength.

Even though the effects of the magnetic susceptibility, the chemical shift, and the main field inhomogeneity are similar, there are some characteristic differences between them. The main magnetic field inhomogeneity is usually less than a few parts per million in the imaging region, and its field variation is a slowly varying function of space therefore the field is nearly uniform within an image pixel. In chemical shift imaging on the other hand two peaks (water and fat) are usually of interest with a known quantity. It can, therefore, usually be corrected. Lastly the susceptibility is somewhat different from the other two. It is rapidly varying in space, and its field variation is much larger than both the main magnetic field and chemical shift dependent field variations per unit distance. Often the field variation due to the susceptibility is so large that it is appreciable even within a pixel (e.g., susceptibility effects at air-water boundary). This unique characteristic of the susceptibility can be exploited to extract or separate out the susceptibility effect alone from the other inhomogeneity effects as discussed in the following.

In conventional Fourier NMR imaging with echo time variation in the presence of magnetic field inhomogeneities, the NMR signal to be obtained is written as Eq. (13-27). Further, if one is interested in the separation of the chemical shift from the total field inhomogeneities, Eq. (13-27) may be rewritten as

$$S(\omega_x, \omega_y)_{\Delta_t} = \int \int f(\hat{x}, \hat{y}) \exp\left\{-i\gamma\left[\hat{h}_c(\hat{x}, \hat{y}) + \hat{h}_s(\hat{x}, \hat{y}) + \hat{h}_0(\hat{x}, \hat{y})\right]\Delta_t\right\}$$

$$\times \exp\left[-i\left(\omega_x\hat{x} + \omega_y\hat{y}\right)\right] dx\, dy \qquad (13\text{-}40)$$

Equation (13-40) is obtained by use of the fact that total field inhomogeneity $\hat{E}(\hat{x}, \hat{y})$ can now be broken into $\hat{h}_c(\hat{x}, \hat{y})$, $\hat{h}_s(\hat{x}, \hat{y})$, and $\hat{h}_0(\hat{x}, \hat{y})$ which are the chemical shift, the magnetic susceptibility and the main field inhomogeneity, respectively. Since $\hat{h}_c(\hat{x}, \hat{y})$ is usually known for the case of two spectral peaks such as water and fat in proton NMR, the phase term $\gamma\hat{h}_c(\hat{x}, \hat{y})\Delta_t$ due to the chemical shift can be made either 0 or a multiple of 2π, thereby the chemical shift term $(\exp[-i\gamma\hat{h}_c(\hat{x}, \hat{y})\Delta_t])$ can be made unity. In this case $\hat{h}_c(\hat{x}, \hat{y})$ can be defined as

$$\hat{h}_c(\hat{x}, \hat{y}) = \begin{bmatrix} 0, & \cdot & \text{for water} \\ \delta_k B_0 \times 10^{-6} & \text{for fat} \end{bmatrix} \qquad (13\text{-}41)$$

where δ_k is the chemical shift in ppm between water and fat (i.e., about 3.5 ppm). When the chemical shift-dependent phase term is made either 0 or a multiple of 2π, Eq. (13-40) can be reduced to

$$S(\omega_x, \omega_y)_{\Delta_{t1,2}} = \int \int f(\hat{x}, \hat{y}) \exp\left\{-i\gamma\left[\hat{h}_s(\hat{x}, \hat{y}) + \hat{h}_0(\hat{x}, \hat{y})\right]\Delta_{t1,2}\right\}$$

$$\times \exp\left[-i\left(\omega_x\hat{x} + \omega_y\hat{y}\right)\right] d\hat{x}\, d\hat{y} \qquad (13\text{-}42)$$

where Δ_{t1} and Δ_{t2} are the two chemical-shift-synchronized echo time shifts that satisfy the following conditions:

$$\gamma\delta_k B_0 \times 10^{-6}\Delta_{t1} = 0 \quad \text{or} \quad 2\pi$$

$$\gamma\delta_k B_0 \times 10^{-6}\Delta_{t2} = n2\pi \quad \text{for } n \geq 2 \qquad (13\text{-}43)$$

Now, the remaining phase terms are the ones due to the susceptibility and the main magnetic inhomogeneity. Under this condition reconstruction of the spin density (image) function $\tilde{\rho}(\hat{x}, \hat{y})$ can be obtained by the inverse Fourier transform of Eq. (13-42):

$$\tilde{\rho}(\hat{x}, \hat{y})_{\Delta_{t1,2}} = \int \int S(\omega_x, \omega_y)_{\Delta_{t1,2}} \exp\left[i\left(\omega_x\hat{x} + \omega_y\hat{y}\right)\right] d\omega_x\, d\omega_y$$

$$= f(\hat{x}, \hat{y}) \exp\left[-i\hat{\phi}(\hat{x}, \hat{y})\right]_{\Delta_{t1,2}} \qquad (13\text{-}44)$$

where $\hat{\phi}(\hat{x}, \hat{y})_{\Delta_{t1,2}} = \gamma[\hat{h}_s(\hat{x}, \hat{y}) + \hat{h}_0(\hat{x}, \hat{y})]\Delta_{t1,2}$.

Let us now consider the characteristics of Eq. (13-44), especially within a pixel when two echo time shifts are used. Since the image is reconstructed in the discrete domain, the image function has the physical pixel size Δ_S. When the discrete image function $\tilde{\rho}_D(i, j)$ of a pixel at the point (i, j) has a center position $(\hat{x}_i, \hat{y}_j)$, it can be approximated as

$$\tilde{\rho}_D(i, j) \, \Delta_{t1,2} = \int_{\hat{y}_j - \Delta s/2}^{\hat{y}_j + \Delta s/2} \int_{\hat{x}_i - \Delta s/2}^{\hat{x}_i + \Delta s/2} \tilde{\rho}(\hat{x}, \hat{y}) \, \Delta_{t1,2} \, d\hat{x} \, d\hat{y} \qquad (13\text{-}45)$$

By taking the magnitude of Eq. (13-45), the following relationship can be established at each pixel:

$$\left| \tilde{\rho}_D(i, j) \right|_{\Delta_{t1}} \geq \left| \tilde{\rho}_D(i, j) \right|_{\Delta_{t2}} \quad \text{for } \Delta_{t1} \leq \Delta_{t2} \qquad (13\text{-}46)$$

Equation (13-46) is a unique property of the susceptibility effect.

Let us now discuss how the differences in the main field inhomogeneity and the magnetic susceptibility will affect Eq. (13-46). Since the main magnetic field is slowly varying and the total inhomogeneity is only a few parts per million in the entire imaging region, the phase variation within a pixel is therefore negligible. The two values in Eq. (13-46) are then nearly identical. These two values, however, will be different if the field inhomogeneity within a pixel is appreciable. Since the main magnetic field inhomogeneity is slowly varying, Eq. (13-46) is strictly valid only for the case where the magnetic susceptibility is present, and it suggests that there will be severe signal attenuation due to the susceptibility effect or signal weighting which is proportional to Δ_t, especially when the phase variation is large within a pixel.

From Eq. (13-46) the magnetic susceptibility can be related with the amplitude of the reconstructed image as

$$\frac{\left| \tilde{\rho}_D(i, j) \right|_{\Delta_{t1}} - \left| \tilde{\rho}_D(i, j) \right|_{\Delta_{t2}}}{\left| \tilde{\rho}_D(i, j) \right|_{\Delta_{t1}}} \propto (\Delta_{t1} - \Delta_{t2}) \nabla \hat{\phi}(\hat{x}_i, \hat{y}_j) \qquad (13\text{-}47)$$

where $\nabla \hat{\phi}(\hat{x}_i, \hat{y}_j)$ is the phase gradient within a pixel, which is given by

$$\nabla \hat{\phi}(\hat{x}_i, \hat{y}_j) = \frac{\partial \hat{\phi}(\hat{x}, \hat{y})}{\partial x} + \frac{\partial \hat{\phi}(\hat{x}, \hat{y})}{\partial y} \Bigg|_{\substack{\hat{x} \leftarrow \hat{x}_i \\ \hat{y} \leftarrow \hat{y}_j}} \qquad (13\text{-}48)$$

Equation (13-47) should also satisfy the following relation

$$(\Delta_{t2} - \Delta_{t1}) \nabla \hat{\phi}(\hat{x}_i, \hat{y}_j) \leq \frac{1}{2\Delta_S} \qquad (13\text{-}49)$$

where Δ_S is the size of the pixel in the reconstructed image.

Since the reconstructed image $\bar{\rho}(\hat{x}, \hat{y})$ in Eq. (13-44) still represents a geometrically distorted image due to the inhomogeneity $E(x, y)$, further correction of the geometrical distortion is needed. For this distortion correction the field inhomogeneity correction algorithm described in the previous section can be used [23, 24]. If this correction method is applied to the image function $\bar{\rho}(\hat{x}, \hat{y})_{\Delta_{t1,2}}$ given in Eq. (13-44), the geometrically corrected image $\rho(x, y)$ will be obtained. The geometrically corrected susceptibility effect or map can then finally be obtained from the corrected images; that is, $\tilde{\rho}_D(i, j)_{\Delta_{t1}}$ and $\tilde{\rho}_D(i, j)_{\Delta_{t2}}$.

Experimental results are obtained using the method discussed above. The field strength of the magnet was 2.0 T. As described, at each view or encoding step, two echo time encoding steps were taken, $\Delta_{t1} = 4$ msec and $\Delta_{t2} = 20$ msec. Δ_{t1} was made relatively short to simulate $\Delta_t \cong 0$ for minimal phase and therefore small signal attenuation, but Δ_{t1} was also adjusted for the chemical shift cancellation by setting $\Delta_{t1} = 2\pi/(\gamma\delta_k B_0 \times 10^{-6})$; that is, $\Delta_{t1} = 4$ msec. Subsequently $\Delta_{t2} = 20$ msec was used for large susceptibility weighting so that $\tilde{\rho}_D(i, j)_{\Delta_{t2}}$ experiences maximum attentuation. Simultaneously it is designed so that it satisfies the condition for the chemical shift cancellation; that is, Δ_{t2} is set to form a multiple of 2π (10π in this case).

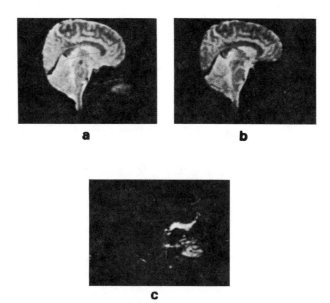

Figure 13-14 Susceptibility maps or images of a human head obtained with the echo time weighted technique. (a) and (b) correspond to $\Delta_{t_1} = 4$ and $\Delta_{t_2} = 20$ msec, respectively. The latter, (b), shows the strong susceptibility effect at the nasal cavity. The repetition time and the echo time were 3000 and 60 msec, respectively. (c) is the susceptibility map or image obtained by the relation given in Eq. (13-47).

A human head image demonstrates the possible applications of the technique to the many clinical cases. In Figs. 13-14(a) and (b) are shown two images obtained with the echo time weighted sequence shown in Fig. 13-12 with two different echo time weightings: $\Delta_{t1} = 4$ msec and $\Delta_{t2} = 20$ msec. In both images, the repetition time T_R and echo time T_E were set to 3000 msec and 60 msec, respectively. Figure 13-14(c) shows the map of the susceptibility effects obtained by the relation given by Eq. (13-47). As shown in the figure the most interesting examples are found in head images where nasal cavities and other air-tissue boundaries exhibit strong susceptibility effects.

With the magnetic susceptibility imaging technique the susceptibility effect can be singled out and imaged. Since this technique effectively generates susceptibility weighted images, it allows one to single out the susceptibility effect amongst other inhomogeneity effects such as the chemical shifts and static inhomogeneity.

Correction and Enhancement of Susceptibility Effect in Gradient Echo Imaging [28, 29]

Susceptibility Artifact Correction Method [28] Since the introduction of the gradient echo technique, it has become possible to obtain many fast MR images using techniques such as the SSFP, FLASH, and GRASS. In clinical practice these techniques are often difficult to use because of severe inhomogeneity artifacts due to the susceptibility. Consequently the use of these gradient echo techniques has been limited. While inhomogeneities due to the chemical shifts or static fields can be corrected, the correction of the susceptibility effects arising from the air-tissue interface has been particularly difficult, for example, around the nasal cavity in the human head. This is mainly due to the fact that gradient echo imaging is particularly sensitive to the local field inhomogeneity, such as the inhomogeneities induced by susceptibility. In other words, the precession frequencies of the spins within a voxel become sufficiently different from one another due to the local field inhomogeneity. Consequently the magnetization of the dephased spins in a voxel mutually cancel each other thereby the sum signal from the voxel also becomes small. Correction of these highly localized field inhomogeneities due to the susceptibility has been especially difficult because of the relatively sudden changes or highly localized field gradient. The susceptibility artifacts are especially pronounced when the thickness of the slice selection is large. Greater thickness means larger phase-spreads along the slice selection direction. We now turn the discussion to the characteristics of the inhomogeneity due to the susceptibility, resulting phase dispersions along the direction of the slice selection, and a possible correction scheme that could restore the signal strength.

The selected-slice thickness in most MR imaging techniques tends to be larger than the resolution in the transverse plane. Therefore this thickness-related inhomogeneity in gradient echo techniques tends to disperse the spin phase during the echo time and results in dispersion of the spin phases within

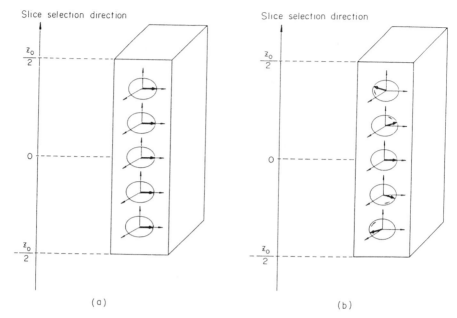

Figure 13-15   The simplified illustrations of the spin phase distributions in a voxel after 90° rf excitation: (a) When the fields are homogeneous, all the spins remain in the same phase after spin-echo rephasing; (b) when the fields are not homogeneous, all the spins are dephased even after the spin-echo rephasing.

the voxel. This situation is illustrated in Fig. 13-15. Here we have assumed that the signal loss resulting from the susceptibility in a voxel is mainly due to the finite thickness of the image plane. The spins excited by the rf pulse with a slice selection gradient are flipped onto the transverse plane and are dephased due to the field inhomogeneity, as shown in Figs. 13-15(a) and (b). Figure 13-15(a) illustrates an ideal case with no field inhomogeneity along the slice selection direction, while (b) illustrates the case with a strong field inhomogeneity along the slice selection direction. If in the case of no field inhomogeneity, a perfect linear gradient and an ideal sinc rf selection pulse will provide well-rephased spins at the time of the echo position; consequently a large signal will result due to the increased vector sum of the spins. On the other hand, when the field is nonlinear and inhomogeneous, rephased spins will not result in a coherent vector sum, as shown in Fig. 13-15(b).

Let us consider more specific cases, as shown in Figs. 13-16(a) and (b). In the case of an ideal homogeneous field as shown in Fig. 13-16(a), complete spin rephasing will result. If a field inhomogeneity due to the susceptibility is introduced, a strong localized gradient field will develop within the voxel, as shown in Fig. 13-16(b), with the resulting phase distribution appearing in the upper right-hand corner of the figure. The resulting vector sum will produce a much weaker signal.

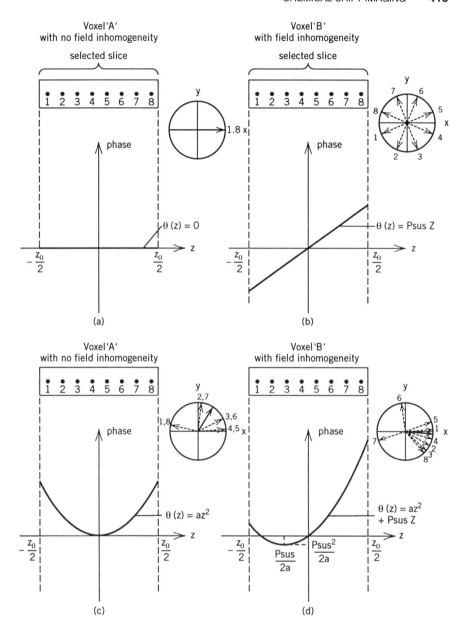

Figure 13-16 (a) The phase distribution of the spins in a voxel when the field is homogeneous or constant within the voxel. We observe maximum signal strength (coherency) in this case. (b) An example of phase distribution of spins in a voxel when a strong localized field gradient exists (e.g., susceptibility). In this case the spins become incoherent, and the signal is reduced substantially. (c) The phase distribution of the spins in a voxel when a quadratic phase rf pulse is added onto a voxel with a homogeneous field. In this case the signal strength is reduced but not as much as in the case of (b). (d) The combined phase distribution of the spins in a voxel when a quadratic phase rf pulse is superimposed onto a voxel which has a strong build in localized linear field gradient due to e.g., susceptibility. Note in the latter the substantially enhanced spin coherency and therefore the signal strength.

The total signal obtainable in NMR is given by

$$S = \sqrt{R^2 + I^2} \tag{13-50}$$

where S represents the detected signal and R and I are the real and imaginary components of magnetization in a voxel, respectively. Because phase dispersion is due to field inhomogeneity, both the real and imaginary components represent the sum of the transverse magnetization components in the voxel:

$$R = \int_{\text{voxel}} M \cos \theta(v) \, dv$$

$$= \int_x \int_y \int_z M \cos \theta(x, y, z) \, dx \, dy \, dz \tag{13-51}$$

and

$$I = \int_{\text{voxel}} M \sin \theta(v) \, dv$$

$$= \int_x \int_y \int_z M \sin \theta(x, y, z) \, dx \, dy \, dz \tag{13-52}$$

where v is a volume representing $v = v(x, y, z)$, M is the magnetization, and $\theta(x, y, z)$ is the phase distribution of spins in three dimensions. To simplify the analysis, we have also assumed that the resolutions in the transverse plane (x, y) are negligible compared with the slice thickness (z) and that the slice has been selected from $-z_0/2$ to $z_0/2$ in the z direction so that the slice thickness equals z_0. With the above assumptions, R and I in Eqs. (13-51) and (13-52) can be rewritten as

$$R = \int_z M \cos \theta(z; x, y) \, dz$$

$$= \int_{-z_0/2}^{z_0/2} M \cos \theta(z) \, dz \tag{13-53}$$

and

$$I = \int_z M \sin \theta(z; x, y) \, dz$$

$$= \int_{-z_0/2}^{z_0/2} M \sin \theta(z) \, dz \tag{13-54}$$

where $\theta(z; x, y)$ or $\theta(z)$ is the phase along the z or slice-thickness direction. One can also assume that the value of $\theta(z)$ is linearly proportional to the position along the slice thickness, as implied in Fig. 13-16(b), such that $\theta(z) = P_{\text{sus}} z$. This assumption is valid since the field inhomogeneity due to the susceptibility is usually highly localized; therefore quite steep gradients are common, as shown in Fig. 13-16(b). One can define P_{sus} as a phase gradient arising from the susceptibility, and it is given by

$$P_{\text{sus}} = \gamma T_E G_{\text{sus}} \qquad (13\text{-}55)$$

where γ is the gyromagnetic ratio, T_E is the echo time, and G_{sus} is the field gradient created by the susceptibility effect. The signal S in Eq. (13-50) then can be rewritten as

$$S = \left\{ \left[\int_{-z_0/2}^{z_0/2} M \cos(P_{\text{sus}} z)\, dz \right]^2 + \left[\int_{-z_0/2}^{z_0/2} M \sin(P_{\text{sus}} z)\, dz \right]^2 \right\}^{1/2} \qquad (13\text{-}56)$$

Note here that the second bracket corresponding to the imaginary part will become zero in normal cases, since $M \sin(P_{\text{sus}} z)$ is an odd function. The first bracket, however, will lead to the well-known $\mathrm{sinc}(\cdot)$ function:

$$S = M z_0 \left| \mathrm{sinc}\left(\frac{P_{\text{sus}}}{2\pi} z_0 \right) \right| \qquad (13\text{-}57)$$

The implications of Eq. (13-57) will be discussed in the following.

Let us now consider two different field inhomogeneities within a given voxel: one that has a constant or homogeneous field like voxel A, and another that has a linear gradient field with a phase distribution $\theta(z) = P_{\text{sus}} z$ like voxel B, as shown in Figs. 13-16(a) and (b). The latter could be the case where the local field inhomogeneity is induced by the susceptibility.

Signal loss due to the susceptibility or the phase gradient created by the susceptibility can be minimized by using a suitably tailored rf pulse. The rf pulse in the conventional imaging generally has a constant phase distribution; the spin phases within the selected slice (voxel) are constant in the direction of the slice selection. If the rf pulse is suitably tailored such that it has a quadratic phase $[\theta_p(z) = \alpha z^2]$ distribution along the slice selection direction as shown in Fig. 13-16(c), it can be used to compensate the phase gradient developed within the slice due to the susceptibility. In other words, by superimposing the phase-compensating rf pulse on the field inhomogeneity (created because of the susceptibility), it is possible to create a new combined distribution that has minimal total phase dispersion. An example of the superimposition of the quadratic phase on a linear field inhomogeneity is illustrated in Fig. 13-16(d), and it is given by

$$\theta(z) = P_{\text{sus}} z + \theta_p(z)$$

$$= P_{\text{sus}} z + \alpha z^2 \qquad (13\text{-}58)$$

where αz^2 denotes the quadratic phase distribution of the rf pulse with a coefficient α chosen as the design parameter of the rf pulse. Figure 13-16(c) shows a sample case where a quadratic phase rf pulse is applied to voxel A where the field is homogeneous. Figure 13-16(d) represents the phase distribution of the spins when the same rf pulse is applied to voxel B where a linear field gradient is developed due to the susceptibility. When the quadratic phase generated by the rf pulse is superimposed on the local inhomogeneity (linear phase $P_{sus}z$), the acquired real and imaginary parts of the signal can be written as

$$R = \int_{-z_0/2}^{z_0/2} M \cos\left(\alpha z^2 + P_{sus} z\right) dz \tag{13-59}$$

and

$$I = \int_{-z_0/2}^{z_0/2} M \sin\left(\alpha z^2 + P_{sus} z\right) dz \tag{13-60}$$

Then Eq. (13-56) would be

$$S = \left\{ \left[\int_{-z_0/2}^{z_0/2} M \cos\left(\alpha z^2 + P_{sus} z\right) dz \right]^2 + \left[\int_{-z_0/2}^{z_0/2} M \sin\left(\alpha z^2 + P_{sus} z\right) dz \right]^2 \right\}^{1/2} \tag{13-61}$$

Note here that the imaginary part [Eq. (13-60)] is no longer zero. Two cases, namely, a homogeneous field and an inhomogeneous field, which are given by Eqs. (13-57) and (13-61) are calculated numerically as a function of the phase gradient (P_{sus}), and the results are shown in Figs. 13-17(a) and (b). Figure 13-17(a) represents the signal intensity obtainable with a conventional slice selection rf pulse as a function of the linear phase gradient strength (P_{sus}) in a voxel where P_{sus} or the inhomogeneity is created by the susceptibility, namely when the field inhomogeneity is the same as that in Fig. 13-16(b). In this case the signal intensity is severely reduced as the strength of the field inhomogeneity increases. When the quadratic phase rf pulse is applied, however, the total phase distribution in the voxel is modified, as seen in Fig. 13-16(d), and the signal is significantly enhanced, as seen in Fig. 13-17(b).

Equations (13-57) and (13-61), together with Figs. 13-17(a) and (b), clearly indicate that a quadratic phase rf pulse can be used to enhance the signal intensity provided that the field gradient due to susceptibility follows a linear field gradient pattern. Moreover the large uniform region of the signal graph in Fig. 13-17(b) indicates that the signal strength is kept at the same level as in the case of no field inhomogeneity up to a quite strong field gradient or phase gradient (i.e., up to $2\pi/z_0$).

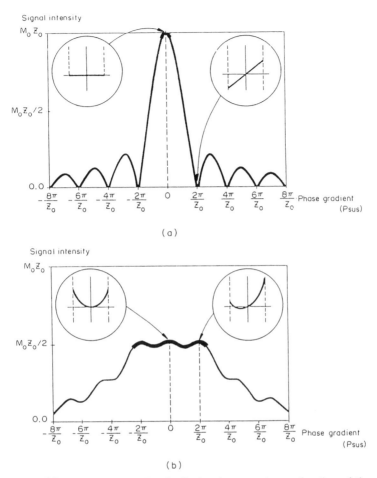

Figure 13-17 (a) The signal intensity distribution in a voxel as a function of the phase gradient or strength of the field inhomogeneity [see Fig. 13-16(b)].(b) Same as (a) but with the superposition of a quadratic phase rf pulse on the field inhomogeneity shown in Fig. 13-16(b). As seen, the signal intensity as a function of the strength of the field inhomogeneity (susceptibility) improved substantially in comparison with (a). Note, however, that the peak signal strength is now reduced to a half of that of the homogeneous field case.

Based on the theoretical discussions above, experiments were performed with a 2.0 T NMR system using the gradient echo sequence. The rf pulse designed for the quadratic phase distribution in the selected slice is shown in Fig. 13-18(c) and its actual magnitude (selection profile) and phase distributions within the selected slice are shown in Fig. 13-18(d). This result was obtained by numerical computation of the Bloch equation. To compare this result with that of the conventional rf pulse, the same numerical calculation

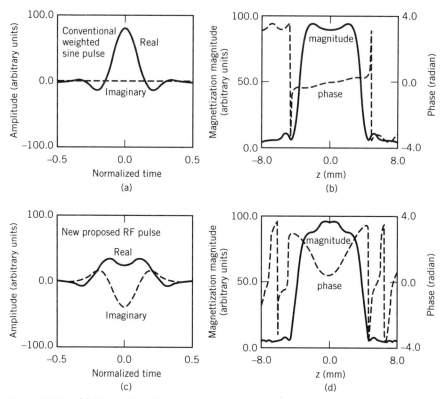

Figure 13-18 (a) The real and imaginary parts of the conventional rf pulse that will select a rectangular slice. (b) The magnitude and phase distribution obtained with the conventional rf pulse shown in (a). Note the nearly constant phase variation within the selected slice. (c) A tailored rf pulse designed to provide a quadratic phase distribution in the selected slice. (d) Result of a numerical calculation of the magnitude and phase distribution in the selected slice obtained by using the quadratic rf pulse shown in (c). As seen, the phase distribution follows a quadratic pattern within the selected slice.

was performed for the conventional rf pulse (Fig. 13-18(a)) and the results are shown in Fig. 13-18(b) for comparison.

To demonstrate the reduction of the susceptibility artifacts, a human head imaging near the nasal cavities was performed with and without a quadratic phase rf pulse. In the experiment, the repetition time was 500 msec with an echo time of 15 msec and a slice thickness of 1 cm. The image shown in Fig. 13-19(a) was obtained using the conventional rf pulse (without a quadratic phase) for the area around the nasal cavities. As is seen, a strong susceptibility artifact appears near the nasal cavities. Figure 13-19(b) is the image obtained by applying the quadratic phase rf pulse we have discussed. In this latter image the susceptibility artifact is significantly reduced and all the tissues previously lost due to the susceptibility-dependent signal voids near

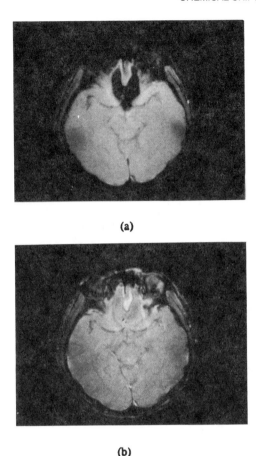

(a)

(b)

Figure 13-19 (a) A human head image obtained with the conventional gradient echo technique. Note the signal voids around the nasal cavities. (b) The same image as (a) obtained with the quadratic phase rf pulse. Note the complete recovery of the signals near the nasal cavities.

the nasal cavities (the dark area) are now recovered. In conclusion, the quadratic phase rf pulse technique is found to be a useful method for the compensation of the strong local inhomogeneity effects due to, for example, susceptibility.

Susceptibility Effect Enhancement [29]

Further extension of the above susceptibility artifact correction technique using tailored rf pulse, a susceptibility effect enhancement technique using yet another kind of tailored rf pulse has been developed and applied for angiographic and functional imaging applications. For example blood containing deoxyhemoglobin is more paramagnetic than surrounding tissue and thereby produces susceptibility effect at blood-tissue interfaces. In this case, by use of a tailored rf pulse which suppress the signal from the normal tissues but enhances the signal from the regions with susceptibility, that is the blood-tissue interfaces. Details of the technique and applications are discussed by Cho and co-workers [29]. Susceptibility effect and blood deoxygenation, that is, the production of oxygen extracted or depleted blood, deoxyhemoglobin, which strongly exhibits the susceptibility effect are utilized actively in the various functional studies where blood flow and oxygenated blood provide information on regional cerebral blood flow (rCBF) and regional cerebral blood volume [30, 31].

A Generalized Field Inhomogeneity Correction Technique [32]

In the previous discussion we considered various inhomogeneity effects such as the chemical shift, magnetic susceptibility, and static field inhomogeneity in proton NMR imaging and their correction and utilization techniques. Now we will present a generalized inhomogeneity correction scheme known as the "view angle tilting technique." It includes the correction of the static field inhomogeneities, such as the effects of chemical shift, susceptibility, and the main magnetic field inhomogeneity. Let us assume the total sum of the inhomogeneity to be $E(x, y, z)$, or simply $E(x, y)$, for a given slice. For the slice selection process, the NMR signal can be written as

$$S(t_x, g_y) = \int_y \int_x \int_{z_1}^{z_2} \rho(x, y, z) \exp\left[-i\gamma E(x, y) t_x\right]$$

$$\times \exp\left[-i\gamma (xG_x t_x + yg_y T_y)\right] dz\, dx\, dy$$

or

$$= \int_y \int_x \int_{-(L_s/2) + L_c(x, y)}^{(L_s/2) + L_c(x, y)} \rho(x, y, z)$$

$$\times \exp\left\{-i\gamma\left[\left(\frac{x + E(x, y)}{G_x}\right)G_x t_x + yg_y T_y\right]\right\} dz\, dx\, dy \quad (13\text{-}62)$$

where γ is the gyromagnetic ratio, $\rho(x, y, z)$ is the spin density function, G_x and g_y are the readout and coding gradient strengths, L_s is the slice thickness determined by the radio frequency (rf) bandwidth F_B and the selection gradient field strength G_s, L_c is the position variation due to the inhomogeneity, and z_1 and z_2 are the lower and upper limits of the region selected by selective rf pulse, respectively:

$$L_s = \frac{2\pi F_B}{\gamma G_s} \text{ cm}$$

$$L_c(x, y) = -\frac{E(x, y)}{G_s} \text{ cm}$$

$$z_1 = -\frac{L_s}{2} + L_c(x, y)$$

$$z_2 = \frac{L_s}{2} + L_c(x, y) \tag{13-63}$$

As noted earlier, if we apply (along the slice selection direction) a compensation gradient of the same magnitude (in amplitude) as the selection gradient simultaneously with the readout gradient (see the broken line in Fig. 13-20), Eq. (13-62) can be written as

$$S(t_x, g_y) = \int_y \int_x \int_{-(L_s/2)+L_c(x, y)}^{(L_s/2)+L_c(x, y)} \rho(x, y, z) \exp(-i\gamma z G_z t_z)$$

$$\times \exp\left\{-i\gamma\left[\left(\frac{x + E(x, y)}{G_x}\right)G_x t_x + y g_y T_y\right]\right\} dz\, dx\, dy \tag{13-64}$$

By a change of variable, $z = \hat{z} - E(x, y)/G_s$, and by assuming that $t_z = t_x$ and that $G_z = G_s$, Eq. (13-64) becomes

$$S(t_x, g_y) = \int_y \int_x \int_{\hat{z}_1}^{\hat{z}_2} \rho\left[x, y, \hat{z} - \frac{E(x, y)}{G_S}\right] \exp\left\{-i\gamma\left[\hat{z} - \frac{E(x, y)}{G_S}\right]G_s t_x\right\}$$

$$\times \exp\left\{-i\gamma\left[\left(x + \frac{E(x, y)}{G_S}\right)G_x t_x + y g_y T_y\right]\right\}|J|\, d\hat{z}\, dx\, dy \tag{13-65}$$

where $\hat{z}_1$ and $\hat{z}_2$ now represent $-L_s/2$ and $L_s/2$, respectively, and J is the Jacobian which is unity in this case:

$$J(x, y) = \frac{\partial z}{\partial \hat{z}} = \frac{1}{\partial \hat{z}/\partial z} = 1 \tag{13-66}$$

Equation (13-65) can be further simplified by eliminating the inhomogeneity

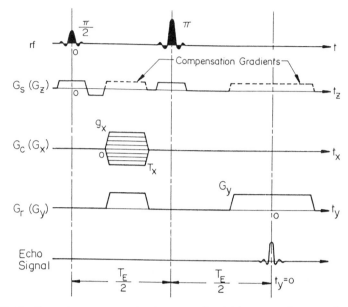

Figure 13-20 The pulse sequence for the generalized inhomogeneity correction scheme. This sequence is based on the conventional spin-echo sequence (solid line) with the addition of the compensation gradient (view angle tilting) G_S as shown (broken line). The strength of a compensation gradient G_S should be identical to the selection gradient and be applied simultaneously with the readout gradient G_y. For this case the view angle tilting appears as $\theta = \tan^{-1} G_S/G_y$.

terms related to t_x:

$$
S(t_x, g_y) = \int_y \int_x \int_{-L_s/2}^{L_s/2} \rho\left[x, y, \hat{z} - \frac{E(x,y)}{G_s}\right]
$$

$$
\times \exp(-i\gamma \hat{z} G_s t_x)\exp\left[-i\gamma(xG_x t_x + yg_y T_y)\right] d\hat{z}\, dx\, dy \quad (13\text{-}67)
$$

For simplicity, let us assume that the spin density function $\rho(x, y, z)$ is constant with respect to the z direction within the selected slice whose thickness is L_s. With this assumption the spin density function $\rho(x, y, \hat{z} - [E(x, y)/G_s]$ of Eq. (13-67) can be replaced with $\rho(x, y, \hat{z}_0 - [E(x, y)/G_s])$, where $\hat{z}_0$ is a constant value of $\hat{z}$. Thus Eq. (13-67) can be written as

$$
S(t_x, g_y) = \int_{-L_s/2}^{L_s/2} \exp(-i\gamma \hat{z} G_s t_x)\, d\hat{z} \int_y \int_x \rho\left[x, y, \hat{z}_0 - \frac{E(x,y)}{G_S}\right]
$$

$$
\times \exp\left[-i\gamma(xG_x t_x + yg_y T_y)\right] dx\, dy
$$

or

$$= \left[L_s \, \text{sinc}\left(\gamma G_s \frac{L_s}{2} t_x \right) \right] \int_y \int_x \rho \left[x, y, \hat{z}_0 - \frac{E(x,y)}{G_s} \right]$$

$$\times \exp\left[-i\gamma \left(x G_x t_x + y g_y T_y \right) \right] \, dx \, dy \qquad (13\text{-}68)$$

The reconstructed image function $\tilde{\rho}(x, y)$ can be obtained by a 2-D Fourier transform of Eq. (13-68):

$$\tilde{\rho}(x, y) = \int_y \int_x S(t_x, g_y) \exp\left[i(\omega_x x + \omega_y y) \right] \, d\omega_x \, d\omega_y$$

$$= \left\{ \int_y \int_x \left[L_s \, \text{sinc}\left(\gamma G_s \frac{L_s}{2} t_x \right) \right] \exp\left[i(\omega_x x + \omega_y y) \right] \, d\omega_x \, d\omega_y \right\}$$

$$* \rho \left[x, y, \hat{z}_0 - \frac{E(x,y)}{G_s} \right]$$

$$= \frac{2}{\gamma G_x} \prod \left[\frac{x}{2\pi F_B / \gamma G_x} \right] * \rho \left[x, y, \hat{z}_0 - \frac{E(x,y)}{G_s} \right] \qquad (13\text{-}69)$$

where $*$ is the convolution operator and $\prod$ is a rectangular function defined by

$$\prod(x) = \begin{cases} 1, & -\tfrac{1}{2} \le x \le \tfrac{1}{2} \\ 0, & \text{otherwise} \end{cases} \qquad (13\text{-}70)$$

Equation (13-69) shows that the image function $\rho(x, y, \hat{z}_0 - [E(x, y)/G_s])$ is now convolved (blurred) with a rectangular function $\prod[x/(2\pi F_B/\gamma G_x)]$. In practice, however, $\prod[\cdot]$ is made relatively narrow, therefore the resulting image-blur is usually negligible:

$$\tilde{\rho}(x, y) \cong \rho \left[x, y, \hat{z}_0 - \frac{E(x,y)}{G_s} \right] \qquad (13\text{-}71)$$

By applying a compensation gradient simultaneously with the readout gradient, the view angle is tilted by $\theta = \tan^{-1}(G_z/G_x)$. Therefore the view angle will decrease by increasing G_x or by decreasing G_z. It should also be mentioned that the optimal condition $G_z = G_s$ is independent of the inhomogeneity term $E(x, y)$, so that the total inhomogeneity artifacts, including the chemical shift and the susceptibility, are simultaneously corrected.

Figure 13-21 gives a step-by-step illustration of the chemical shift correction process. First, the chemical shift in the z direction is shown in Fig. 13-21(a), and then the combined shifts in both the selection (z) and readout (x) gradient directions are illustrated in Fig. 13-21(b). In Fig. 13-21(c) the projection image with an artifact is shown. Finally, Fig.

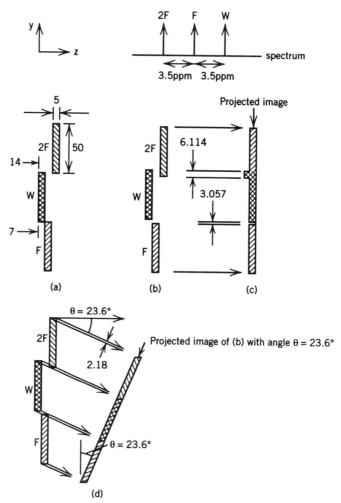

Figure 13-21   A simplified step-by-step diagram of the generalized inhomogeneity correction method. (a) shows the chemical shift in the z direction only. (b) shows the chemical shifts in both the z and y directions (i.e., a combined z- and y-directional shift) (c) is the resultant image that will be obtained by the conventional technique. In (c) note the overlap of the 2F and water. Finally, (d) shows the view angle tilted image of the two combined shifts with an angle θ. The projected image with an angle θ would produce a corrected image.

13-21(d) represents the eventual tilting of the view, thereby eliminating the inhomogeneity effects. Here $\bar{\rho}(x, y)$ represents the inhomogeneity corrected image with small blurring due to the view angle tilting, as illustrated in Fig. 13-21(c).

To demonstrate the correction ability of the view angle tilting method for the chemical shift and susceptibility dependent geometrical distortions, we have devised a phantom that has both the chemical shift and susceptibility effects. For all of the images shown, the vertical direction is the direction of the readout gradient and the field of view is 256 mm. All the experiments were carried out with a 2.0-T whole-body superconducting NMR system. Figure 13-22(a) shows the phantom with which both the chemical shift and

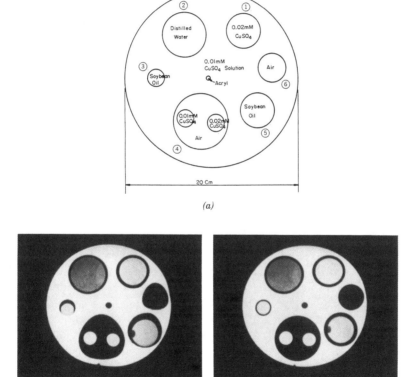

Figure 13-22 Experimental results of the chemical-shift and susceptibility effect imaging of a complex phantom that consists of water, fat (soybean oil), and air: (a) is the phantom, and (b) and (c) are the images obtained by using the pulse sequence shown in Fig. 13-20 with and without view angle tilting, respectively. The field strength used for the compensation gradient was 0.1 G/cm with a y-directional readout gradient strength of 0.458 G/cm which eventually resulted in a tilting angle of 12.3°.

susceptibility (air-water boundary) dependent geometrical shift effects can be measured and corrected. This phantom consists of a column of distilled water with a relatively long T_1 value compared with ordinary water, three columns of 0.02 or 0.01 mM CuSO$_4$ solutions with short T_1's, two columns of air representing a negative susceptibility compared to the background, two soybean oil columns for fat substitution, and an acryl (which does not generate a signal). In Figs. 13-22(b) and (c) experimentally obtained images of the phantom are shown. Figure 30-22(b) is an image obtained using a normal spin-echo sequence with $T_R = 500$ msec and $T_E = 30$ msec. In this image clear chemical shift effects are visible; that is, the two fat columns (circles) are shifted downward while the other water columns (circles) remained still. The two air circles are now clearly distorted by the susceptibility effect. Figure 13-22(c) gives the corrected image of the same phantom using the proposed view angle tilting technique. This perfectly corrected image of the complex phantom contains chemical shift, susceptibility, and other field homogeneity effects. The compensation gradient and the readout gradient employed and the subsequent view tilting angle are 0.1 G/cm, 0.458 G/cm, and 12.3°, respectively, with the same T_R and T_E as given in Fig. 13-22(b).

In summary, the view angle tilting technique appears to be a generalized field inhomogeneity correction technique with which both the chemical shift and the susceptibility can be corrected simultaneously by a single sequence. This technique utilizes an additional selection gradient G_z of the same magnitude as the selection gradient in simultaneity with the readout gradient, thereby producing a tilted viewing angle which in turn automatically corrects the field inhomogeneity dependent geometrical shifts. One disadvantage of the method is that the method tends to blur if the slice becomes thick.

13-2 SPECTROSCOPY AND SPECTROSCOPIC IMAGING

Nuclear magnetic resonance spectroscopy is a unique tool in obtaining quantitative information regarding biochemical parameters noninvasively. For example, phosphorus-31 (^{31}P) spectroscopy provides information such as the cellular energy state and intracellular pH, as well as phospholipid metabolism, whereas water-suppressed proton spectroscopy can quantify the concentrations of various intermediary metabolites including amino acids and lactate. Most of the spectroscopy techniques critically depend upon the quality of the spectral resolution that can be obtained. Good resolution can be achieved by optimizing the magnetic field homogeneity over the sample volume under investigation. One way to achieve good homogeneity is by limiting the volume of interest by some form of volume selection mechanism. Along this line a number of volume selection methods have been developed. Among them are rotating-frame zeugmatography [33–34], DRESS [35], SPARS [36, 37], STEAM [38, 39], and other localization techniques using high-order gradient fields and multidimensional localization [40–61]. In this section SPARS, STEAM, and other methods using high-order radial gradient coils and spiral scanning techniques will be detailed [36, 38, 46, 54, 56, 61].

13-2-1 Localization Techniques and Methods

3-D Volume Localization Using SPARS for Spectroscopy

Spatially resolved spectroscopy (SPARS) [43] has been developed and used for NMR spectroscopy to obtain NMR spectra from a well-defined volume of interest. By combining a set of selective radio frequency pulses with pulsed gradients, one can select a volume and thereby suppress MR signals from outside of the sample volume of interest. This method is the modified volume selective excitation (VSE) sequence originally proposed by Aue et al. [41, 42].

The SPARS sequence is flexible; therefore it can easily be combined with different pulse sequences such as the water suppression pulse sequence, which we will discuss later. By suppressing water or fat, the dynamic range of the ADC (analog-to-digital converter) can be greatly enhanced allowing even small metabolites such as lactate to be observed.

The basic pulse sequence for SPARS, shown in Fig. 13-23, consists of a sequence of three rf pulses with pulsed gradients. The sample is first excited by a 90° nonselective rf pulse, followed (after a short delay) by a 180° nonselective refocusing pulse. These two pulses will then saturate the entire volume. An additional selective 90° rf pulse, which follows the two preceding

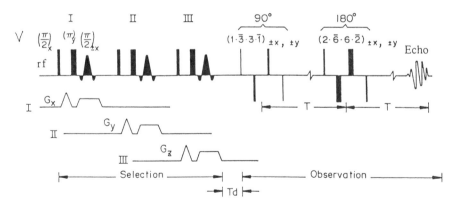

Figure 13-23 The spatially resolved spectroscopy (SPARS) with volume selection sequence, combined with the $1\bar{3}\bar{3}1 - 2\bar{6}\bar{6}2$ sequence for water signal suppressed proton spectroscopy. First, the basic selection sequence is repeated for the x, y, and z directions. After the completion of the selection sequence, an observation sequence is followed with a pulse sequence such as the water suppressed 90° $- \tau -$ 180° spin-echo pulse sequence. Different observation sequences may be applied after the selection sequence instead of the $1\bar{3}\bar{3}1 - 2\bar{6}\bar{6}2$ sequence.

Table 13-1   Selection (x, y, z) phase-cycling scheme

	$[x]$	$[y]$	$[z]$
1	x	x	x
2	$-x$	x	x
3	x	$-x$	x
4	x	x	$-x$
5	$-x$	$-x$	x
6	$-x$	x	$-x$
7	x	$-x$	$-x$
8	$-x$	$-x$	$-x$

Note: Combinations $= 2^3$.

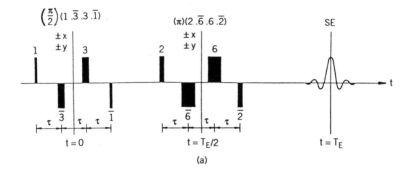

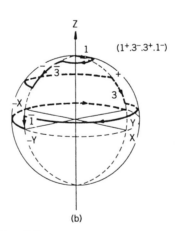

Figure 13-24 (a) The $1\bar{3}3\bar{1} - 2\bar{6}6\bar{2}$ spectral suppression spin-echo pulse sequence. (b) The magnetization trajectory for the sequence $1\bar{3}3\bar{1}$ at an offset frequency of 1 KHz ($\sim 1/2\tau$). The time interval τ between the pulses within a 90° or 180° rf pulse group provides rotation of the spin magnetization 180° around the z-axis in the xy-plane by its natural precession during the τ interval. $\pm x$ and $\pm y$ are the phase alternations used for the exorcycle phase cyclings (2^4 combinations).

rf pulses, in the presence of a selection gradient will complete the selection of a slice in any one gradient direction. An appropriate correction gradient (spoiling gradient) is included between the first 90° pulse and the second 180° pulse for an optimal spin echo sequence (see the triangular pulse preceding the selection gradient in Fig. 13-23). The net result of the three consecutive pulse sequences, each one for selecting a predetermined slice in the x, y, and the z direction, assures the preservation of the longitudinal magnetization in the selected volume within the object. On the other hand, outside the selected volume the magnetizations remain saturated or dephased in the transversal plane. Following these volume selection sequences, a signal from this volume may be obtained by applying an observation pulse sequence. As previously described [43], imperfections in the volume selection resulting from rf inhomogeneities or off-resonance effects can be corrected by introducing a suitable phase-cycling scheme. This is done by alternating the phases of the selective reset pulses and later changing the polarity of the corresponding signal. By combining all phase alternations for the three selective pulses, a total of eight different sets are obtained (see Table 13-1).

After a volume is selected, the SPARS sequence can be combined with a spin-echo spectral suppression pulse sequence, such as the water suppression sequence. For example, a spectral suppression pulse such as the $1\bar{3}3\bar{1}$ pulse can be used to suppress the water signal in high resolution NMR spectroscopy [44]. The $1\bar{3}3\bar{1}$ pulse is a tailored rf pulse that enables us to selectively excite a spectral region of interest but exclude a specific resonance frequency or spectrum to be rejected, such as water. The $1\bar{3}3\bar{1}$ pulse can be used with the SPARS sequence and can even be extended to the spin-echo technique using an additional 180° equivalent $2\bar{6}6\bar{2}$ pulse. In Fig. 13-24 the $1\bar{3}3\bar{1}$ pulse and the $2\bar{6}6\bar{2}$ pulse are depicted together with a phase diagram corresponding to the 90° flip by the $1\bar{3}3\bar{1}$ pulse [see (b)]. By combining the volume selective sequences and spectral selective $1\bar{3}3\bar{1}$ and $2\bar{6}6\bar{2}$ pulses, the following combinations of pulse sequences are possible:

$$[X]-[Y]-[Z]-\text{Td}-90°-T-180°-T-\text{Acq.} \qquad \text{(Sequence 1)}$$

$$[X]-[Y]-[Z]-\text{Td}-1\bar{3}3\bar{1}-T-180°-T-\text{Acq.} \qquad \text{(Sequence 2)}$$

$$[X]-[Y]-[Z]-\text{Td}-1\bar{3}3\bar{1}-T-2\bar{6}6\bar{2}-T-\text{Acq.} \qquad \text{(Sequence 3)}$$

where the notation $[X]-[Y]-[Z]$ denotes the SPARS volume selection sequence. Td is the eddy current delay period, and T is the spin-echo delay time.

In most of the spin-echo experiments, the SPARS phase cycling (2^3 combinations) is combined with exorcycle phase cyclings (2^4 combinations) shown in Figs. 13-24(a) and (b), leading to a total of 128 cyclings (see Tables 13-1 and 13-2), thereby eliminating the possible accumulation of phase errors likely to arise due to the multiple flips and spin echoes involved in the sequence.

Table 13-2 Exorcycle phase cycling and the relative phases of the rf pulses and the receiver

rf Phase		Receiver Phase
First 90° Pulse	Second 180° Pulse	
$+x\,(x^+, x^-, x^+, x^-)$	$+x\,(x^+, x^-, x^+, x^-)$	$+$
$+x$	$-x\,(x^-, x^+, x^-, x^+)$	$+$
$+x$	$+y\,(y^+, y^-, y^+, y^-)$	$-$
$+x$	$-y\,(y^+, y^-, y^+, y^-)$	$-$
$-x\,(x^-, x^+, x^-, x^+)$	$+x$	$+$
$-x$	$-x$	$+$
$-x$	$+y$	$-$
$-x$	$-y$	$-$
$+y\,(y^+, y^-, y^+, y^-)$	$+x$	$-$
$+y$	$-x$	$-$
$+y$	$+y$	$+$
$+y$	$-y$	$+$
$-y\,(y^-, y^+, y^-, y^+)$	$+x$	$-$
$-y$	$-x$	$-$
$-y$	$+y$	$+$
$-y$	$-y$	$+$

Note: Combinations $= 2^4$. Examples of $+x$ and $-x$ (same for y) are

$$+x = (x^+, x^-, x^+, x^-), \quad -x = (x^-, x^+, x^-, x^+)$$
$$+y = (y^+, y^-, y^+, y^-), \quad -y = (y^-, y^+, y^-, y^+)$$

where superscripts $+$ and $-$ denote spin flip directions corresponding to clockwise and anticlockwise directions, respectively.

3-D Volume Localization Using STEAM for Spectroscopy

Similar to the previous volume selection technique a new technique known as stimulated echo acquisition mode (STEAM) is being developed. This method uses the properties of the stimulated echo (STE) for the selection of a volume [45]. To spatially select a volume of interest within a three-dimensional object, it is generally required that at least three selective rf pulses be applied in the presence of orthogonal magnetic field gradients. This condition is met by the stimulated echo sequence [see Chapter 9 for STE].

For localized spectroscopy, the stimulated echo sequence used for volume selection is shown in Fig. 13-25. In this case volume selection is achieved by using three rf pulses with the corresponding selection gradients. A stimulated echo then arises from the spins in the small region (cube) overlapped by the three orthogonally selected slices. A problem with this sequence is the unwanted signal from the entire slice selected by the last (third) pulse; it is usually much larger than the stimulated echo signal arising from the small volume selected from the overlap of the three orthogonal slices. To discriminate against this large unwanted signal and to maximize the small stimulated

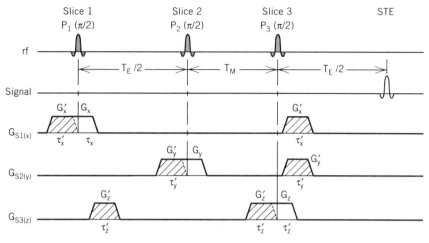

G_x', G_y', G_z': STE refocusing but FID Dephasing

Figure 13-25 The rf and slice selection gradient pulses for the volume selective STEAM spectroscopy pulse sequence. G_x', G_y', and G_z' are the STE rephasing gradients.

echo signal arising from the selected cube, a series of rephasing and dephasing gradients are used in conjunction with the selective pulses. For example, dephasing due to the G_x and G_y gradients at the P_1 and P_2 rf pulses are rephased by G_x' and G_y' at the end of P_3. The reason for this delay is to dephase the z-slice signal arising from the P_3 rf pulse. The last G_z gradient pulse, however, is handled differently because of the space selection. In this case the rephasing gradient G_z' is inserted between the P_1 and P_2 pulse, thereby refocusing the stimulated echo but not the FID. Each pulse sequence then will result in a spectrum of the selected volume.

Naturally other pulse sequences, such as the water or fat suppression pulse sequences, can be added to this STEAM sequence for high-resolution proton spectroscopy. It is worth noting, however, that the signal obtained by the STEAM spectroscopy sequence is only half of that obtainable from the conventional spin echo. The sequence shown in Fig. 13-25, however, offers an elegant means to determine the local T_1 and T_2 relaxation times. This can be accomplished simply by varying the length of the corresponding intervals T_M or T_E in a series of experiments without additional pulses. Metabolic proton spectroscopy, however, requires the suppression of the water signal and possibly lipid proton signals as well. In this case one may attempt to exploit the inherent suppression capabilities of the sequence, that is independent adjustments of T_1 (lipid resonances) or T_2 (water resonance) weightings.

It should be noted that there are two extensions of the STEAM sequence with which the efficiency of the spectroscopic examinations can be improved. The first extension of the method is the one-dimensional multipoint version of the sequence shown in Fig. 13-25. It is obtained by extending a 1-D point scan by applying a series of third pulses, each with a suitable center frequency shift (at the expense of slightly increased T_M values). In this case P_1 and P_2 are applied once, and a series of P_3's will follow. Further extension of the method produces 2-D multislicing, thereby extending the region in the form of a two-dimensional array. In this latter case P_2 will vary and select the slice along the y direction.

2-D Localization Using a Radial Gradient Coil [46]

A volume selection can also be accomplished by using a fourth coil, a radial gradient coil in conjunction with the conventional x, y, and z coil set for localization and for localized high-resolution NMR imaging and spectroscopy [46]. The principle of the method is the use of a radial gradient in conjunction with a selective rf pulse. To selectively excite the spins inside a cylindrical volume located along the z-axis ($r = 0$, $\phi = 0$) in cylindrical coordinates (see Fig. 13-26), the radial magnetic field gradient required is $B_z(r, \phi, z) = G_r r$, where B_z is the z-component of the magnetic field, G_r is the radial gradient strength, and the main magnetic field is assumed to be along the z direction. A first-order approximation of such a magnetic field can be achieved by a circular loop coil as shown in Fig. 13-26(a). The configuration of the circular loop coil placed coaxially with the z-axis, along with the main magnetic field B_z therefore can be considered as an additional gradient field which is superimposed on to the main magnetic field B_0. The magnetic field represented by $G_r r$ is a radially increasing field toward the periphery [see Fig. 13-27(a)], and a rapidly diverging field from the center ($z = 0$) toward both ends of the z-axis, as shown in Fig. 13-27(b). By applying a selective rf pulse in the presence of a radial gradient field, a desired cylindrical volume centered around the z-axis can be selected. The diameter of the selected cylindrical volume, L_2, will then be determined by the adjustment of the gradient strength and the bandwidth of the selective rf pulse; that is, $L_2 = \text{BW}/\gamma G_r$, where γ is the gyromagnetic ratio and BW is the rf bandwidth.

Since the circular loop coil produces an axially symmetrical magnetic field, the magnetic field along the radial direction (x or y direction) is also symmetric and increases while the field along the z direction decreases from the maximum field at $z = 0$. The excited or selected regions or volumes in the x or y and the z directions obtained using a radial gradient coil are shown in Fig. 13-28. In this example, a selective rf pulse consisting of a Gaussian weighted sinc pulse with eight zero crossings $u(t) = [\sin(8\pi t/t_p)/8\pi t/t_p]\exp(-4t^2/t_p^2)$ is used, where t_p is the rf pulse width. In practice, however, the circular loop coil produces a radial gradient field with an offset field ΔB_z at the center. It therefore requires compensation of this offset field or adjustment of the center frequency of the selective rf pulse. This has been achieved by offsetting the field at the center by using a Helmholtz coil pair so that the Larmour frequency at the center matches that

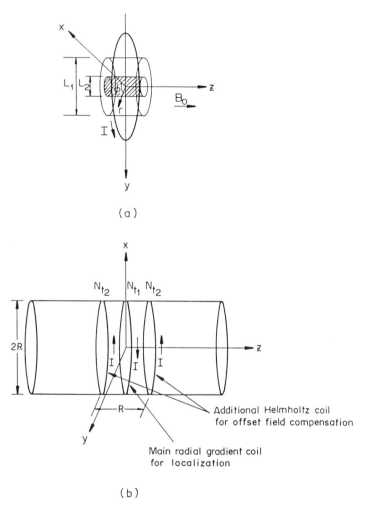

Figure 13-26 (a) A radial gradient coil and an example of a small selected volume with a diameter L_2 using the radial gradient field. The radial gradient field is generated by a circular loop coil of radius R placed at the center ($z = 0$). B_0 is the uniform main magnetic field. (b) A complete radial gradient coil set, which consists of a main circular loop radial gradient coil and a serially coupled Helmholtz coil for the compensation of the offset field. N_{t_1} and N_{t_2} are the numbers of turns of the main circular loop radial gradient coil and the Helmholtz coil for the compensation, respectively.

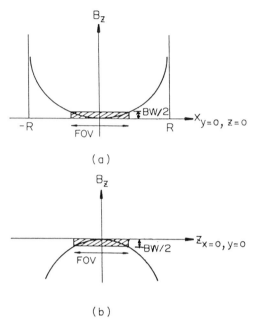

Figure 13-27 Cut views of the z-directional magnetic fields along (a) the x-axis or radial direction and (b) the z-axis at the center i.e., $x = 0, y = 0$.

of the rf center frequency [see the Helmholtz coil pair used for this purpose shown in Fig. 13-26(b)]. The Helmholtz pair connected in series with the main circular loop is designed so that it generates a field opposite to that of the circular loop coil, thereby canceling the offset field produced by the main loop coil. Figures 13-28(a) and (b) show a quasi-cylindrical volume selected by using the radial coil and the spin-echo sequence with a suitable z-gradient and selective 180° rf pulse.

2-D Localization Using Spiral Scan
Recently a new class of rf pulses with which two-dimensional spatial localization can be achieved was introduced [47–50]. These pulse sequences consist of an rf excitation applied in the presence of a net magnetic field gradient that effectively reorients the spins in two dimensions [51–53]. Pauly and coworkers have used a k-space approach with small tip-angle excitation pulses for the localization of a two-dimensional space [54, 55]. These pulses produce an excited 2-D space after Fourier transform of the resulting NMR signal. The selected 2-D space can be considered as the result of a weighted trajectory in k-space such as a spiral. The accompanying rf waveform, normalized by the k-space velocity then becomes the weighting function for the k-space trajectory. This method has been used to produce a cylindrical volume excitation with a Gaussian profile [54].

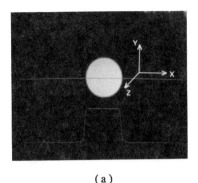

(a)

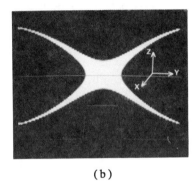

(b)

Figure 13-28 Cut views of the selected volume at (a) $z = 0$ and (b) $x = 0$. Selection profiles corresponding to the center lines of each view are also shown.

Let us consider a set of pulses that will for example, produce radially symmetric excitation profiles by the Hankel transform relation. A useful Hankel transform pair for the selection of a disklike 2-D space can be obtained by the Fourier transform relation:

$$\text{Circ}\left(\frac{\mathbf{r}}{2\mathbf{r}_0} \right) \overset{\mathscr{F}}{\leftrightarrow} \mathbf{r}_0 J_1(k \mathbf{r}_0)$$

Straightforward application of these techniques leads to a number of two-dimensional excitation profiles that have potential usefulness in NMR imaging and spectroscopy, including circles, squares, and annuli. For example, to obtain a spiral trajectory in **k**-space, x- and y-directional **k**-space functions can be defined as

$$k_x(t) = \kappa\left(1 - \frac{t}{T} \right)\cos(\omega t)$$

$$k_y(t) = \kappa\left(1 - \frac{t}{T} \right)\sin(\omega t) \qquad (13\text{-}72)$$

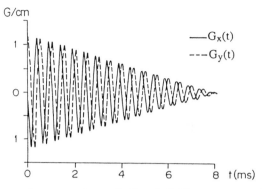

Figure 13-29 The gradient wave forms $G_x(t)$ and $G_y(t)$ necessary to form a converging spiral trajectory in **k**-space.

The corresponding waveforms for $G_x(t)$ and $G_y(t)$ are given by

$$G_x(t) = \frac{1}{\gamma} \frac{dk_x(t)}{dt}$$

$$G_y(t) = \frac{1}{\gamma} \frac{dk_y(t)}{dt} \tag{13-73}$$

An example of the gradient waveforms, $G_x(t)$ and $G_y(t)$, for the values $\omega = 2\pi n/T$, $n = 16$, and $0 \le t \le T$ are plotted in Fig. 13-29. If the rf excitation is of the form $B_1 \equiv B_{1x} + iB_{1y}$, the rf waveform necessary to excite a desired 2-D profile $P(\mathbf{r})$ can be made by weighting the **k**-space trajectory as [54]

$$B_1(t) = |\mathbf{G}(t)| W[\mathbf{k}(t)] \tag{13-74}$$

where $W[\mathbf{k}(t)]$ and $|\mathbf{G}(t)|$ are given by

$$W[\mathbf{k}(t)] = \int_{-\infty}^{\infty} \int_{-\infty}^{\infty} P(\mathbf{r}) e^{i\mathbf{k}(t)\cdot\mathbf{r}} \, dx \, dy \tag{13-75}$$

$$|\mathbf{G}(t)| = \frac{\kappa}{\gamma T} \sqrt{\left[2\pi n\left(1 - \frac{t}{T}\right)\right]^2 + 1} \tag{13-76}$$

κ is a constant related to the strength of the gradient field and $P(\mathbf{r})$ is the desired 2-D spatial domain function. Note that $|\mathbf{G}(t)|$ is also given by

$$|\mathbf{G}(t)| = \sqrt{G_x^2(t) + G_y^2(t)} \tag{13-77}$$

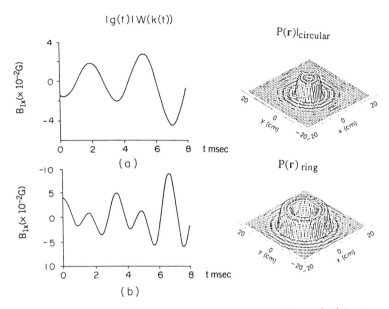

Figure 13-30 The profiles (right) and corresponding B_1 pulse shapes (left) for two radially symmetric magnetizations or excitations. These magnetizations contain only the real part, M_x. The gradients used were the two oscillating gradients shown in Fig. 13-29. The tip angle used was 90° for both pulses.

To obtain a weighting function which would result in a circularly symmetric distribution, Eq. (13-75) can be converted to **k**-space by using the Hankel transform of the desired circular function $P(\mathbf{r})$ as

$$W[k(t)] = 2\pi \int_0^\infty P(r) r J_0[k(t)r]\, dr \qquad (13\text{-}78)$$

It is interesting to note that $W[\mathbf{k}(t)]$ is equal to $B_1(t)/|\gamma \mathbf{G}(t)|$ and is a moving sampling of a time-independent weight function $W(k)$. In general, for a nonsymmetric profile Eq. (13-75) is solved numerically. The rf excitation is complex, requiring both real and imaginary channels. The magnetization profiles obtained by this method will correspond closely to those desired provided that the **k**-space has been adequately sampled by the gradient wave forms, that is, when the **k**-space have been filled sufficiently well covered by a spiral scan.

Figure 13-30 shows two circularly symmetric 2-D magnetization or excitation profiles [$P(\mathbf{r})$ at the right] and the corresponding rf pulses (B_{1x} at the left). The oscillating gradient waveforms of Fig. 13-29 were used and the rf waveforms were determined from Eq. (13-74). The profiles were produced by numerically solving the Bloch equations, neglecting relaxations. As will be described, the pulses illustrated here have potential applications in NMR imaging and spectroscopy.

3-D Volume Localization Using Spiral Scan with a Radial Gradient Coil for Spectroscopy [56]

A localized 3-D volume imaging technique using a radial gradient coil [46] has been developed using the conventional spin-echo sequence. As we have learned from the preceding discussion, 3-D localization can also be obtained by using oscillating gradients and a suitable rf pulse [54, 57]. In general, most of the volume selection techniques with gradient fields suffer from excessive T_1 and T_2 decays. For instance, the localization method using the spiral scan technique requires an additional 180° rf pulse for the final volume selection and will therefore suffer T_2 decay. Here we introduce the spiral scan method which uses a single rf pulse in combination with a radial gradient coil for the localization of a volume. Since, in this technique, the volume selection time is relatively short, the resulting signal is free from T_1 or T_2 relaxation. To obtain a well-defined volume for localization, we depend on the Bessel function of the first kind to shape the rf pulse and the interlacing technique for k-space scanning.

Based on the k-space analysis of small flip-angle excitation, the resulting transverse magnetization $M_{xy}(\mathbf{r}, T)$ is given by [54, 57]

$$M_{xy}(\mathbf{r}, T) = i\gamma M_0(\mathbf{r}) \int_{\mathbf{k}} p(\mathbf{k}) \, e^{i\mathbf{r}\cdot\mathbf{k}} \, d\mathbf{k} \tag{13-79}$$

where

$$p(\mathbf{k}) = \int_0^T \frac{B_1(t)}{|\dot{\mathbf{k}}(t)|} \left\{ {}^3\delta(\mathbf{k}(t) - \mathbf{k})|\dot{\mathbf{k}}(t)| \right\} dt \tag{13-80}$$

As has been discussed earlier, $\mathbf{k}(t)$ is the time varying k-space trajectory formed by two oscillating gradients, in this case $G_z(t)$ and $G_r(t)$. In Eq. (13-80), T is the duration of the rf pulse, ${}^3\delta(\cdot)$ is the 3-D Dirac delta function, $\dot{\mathbf{k}}(t) = d\mathbf{k}(t)/dt$, and $\mathbf{k}(t)$ is the well-known k-space trajectory derived from the relations given in Eqs. (13-72) and (13-73):

$$\mathbf{k}(t) = -\gamma \int_t^T \mathbf{G}(t') \, dt' \tag{13-81}$$

Note here that $|\mathbf{G}(t)| = \sqrt{G_z^2(t) + G_r^2(t)}$. In Eq. (13-80), $p(\mathbf{k})$ is considered to be the weighted k-space trajectory, and $\dot{\mathbf{k}}(t)$ as the velocity in the k-space scanning. In other words, through the simultaneous application of $B_1(t)$ and the two oscillating gradients, namely G_z and G_r, one can obtain a spiral trajectory in the 3-D k-domain. Note that in Eq. (13-80) the selected volume is the Fourier transform of the 3-D k-space trajectory weighted by the velocity-compensated rf pulse.

Compared with the conventional 2-D slice selection, volume selection requires the coverage of the 3-D k-domain by a large number of spiral turns

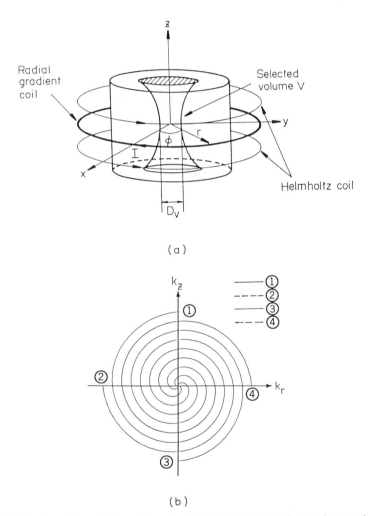

(a)

(b)

Figure 13-31   A radial gradient coil based volume selection technique using a spiral scan and an rf pulse. In this scheme the oscillating gradients in the z and radial directions form a localized volume at the center. (a) Radial gradient coil and expected cylindrical volume to be selected. (b) k-space trajectories for the two-turn spiral scans with four interlacings ($N = 2$, $L = 4$).

in order to provide the Nyquist sampled trajectory [54, 57, 58]. The method also requires a relatively large oscillating gradient at the initial phase; it requires a large peak gradient G_{max} to circumvent the distortion that arises from the chemical shift during volume selection. This is due to the reduction of the effective gradient strength G_{eff} of the oscillating gradient. This can be remedied by the interlacing technique, since G_{max} and G_{eff} are related to the number of spiral turns N as [58]

$$G_{eff} = \frac{G_{max}}{2\pi N} \tag{13-82}$$

From Eq. (13-82) one can see that a large number of spiral turns N would reduce the effective gradient strength for a given maximum gradient strength.

By using combined oscillating radial- and z-gradient fields (instead of the conventional 3-D volume selection technique in which x-, y-, and z-gradient fields are applied in series with multiple rf pulses) a 3-D volume selection can be achieved instantly with one rf excitation and a relatively small effective gradient strength [56]. Then, the spiral $\mathbf{k}$-space trajectory can be decomposed into $k_r(t)$ and $k_z(t)$ as given by

$$k_r(t) = -\gamma \int_t^T G_r(t') \, dt' = K_{max}\left(1 - \frac{t}{T}\right)\cos\left(\frac{2\pi Nt}{T}\right)$$

$$k_z(t) = -\gamma \int_t^T G_z(t') \, dt' = K_{max}\left(1 - \frac{t}{T}\right)\sin\left(\frac{2\pi Nt}{T}\right) \tag{13-83}$$

where K_{max} is the maximum spatial frequency in $\mathbf{k}$-space. It should be noted that the oscillating gradients in Eq. (13-83) provide an inherently refocused excitation [54, 57].

To increase the effective gradient G_{eff} for a given maximum required gradient G_{max}, N should be reduced and interlacing should be introduced [59, 60]. A fine sampling interval or the filling of the $\mathbf{k}$-space finely to provide the Nyquist sampling rate is realized by interlacing the several spiral loci based on small flip-angle excitation. As shown in Fig. 13-31 (b), two spiral turns with four interlacing loci yield the same performance as eight spiral turns without interlacing. Then the effective gradient G_{eff} can be increased in proportion to the number of interlacings under the same imaging conditions.

By simple modification of Eq. (13-83), $\mathbf{k}$-space loci using the interlacing technique can be realized:

$$k_{rl}(t) = -\gamma \int_t^T G_{rl}(t') \, dt' = K_{max}\left(1 - \frac{t}{T}\right)\cos\left(\frac{2\pi N't}{T} + \frac{2\pi l}{L}\right)$$

$$k_{zl}(t) = -\gamma \int_t^T G_{zl}(t') \, dt' = K_{max}\left(1 - \frac{t}{T}\right)\sin\left(\frac{2\pi N't}{T} + \frac{2\pi l}{L}\right)$$

$$\text{for } l = 1, 2, \ldots, L; \; N' = \frac{N}{L} \tag{13-84}$$

where the combination of $k_{rl}(t)$ and $k_{zl}(t)$ represents the lth locus in **k**-space, L is the number of interlacings, and $G_{rl}(t)$ and $G_{zl}(t)$ are the corresponding radial and z-directional oscillating gradients:

$$G_{rl}(t) = \frac{1}{\gamma} \frac{dk_{rl}(t)}{dt}$$

$$= -G_{\max}\left\{\left(1 - \frac{t}{T}\right)(2\pi N')\sin\left(\frac{2\pi N't}{T} + \frac{2\pi l}{L}\right) + \cos\left(\frac{2\pi N't}{T} + \frac{2\pi l}{L}\right)\right\}$$

$$G_{zl}(t) = \frac{1}{\gamma} \frac{dk_{zl}(t)}{dt}$$

$$= +G_{\max}\left\{\left(1 - \frac{t}{T}\right)(2\pi N')\cos\left(\frac{2\pi N't}{T} + \frac{2\pi l}{L}\right) + \sin\left(\frac{2\pi N't}{T} + \frac{2\pi l}{L}\right)\right\}$$

$$(13\text{-}85)$$

and $G_{\max} = K_{\max}/\gamma T$. In the interlacing technique a complete data set from the selected volume can be obtained after L interlaced scannings with a repetition time of T_R. This increases the overall data acquisition time, but it also increases the SNR proportionately. It should be noted that this method requires only one rf pulse with a short duration in each scan so that the effect of T_2 decay can be reduced (see Fig. 13-32).

Now the exciting rf pulse waveform should produce a properly weighted **k**-space trajectory as given in Eq. (13-80). If one uses a 2-D Bessel function of

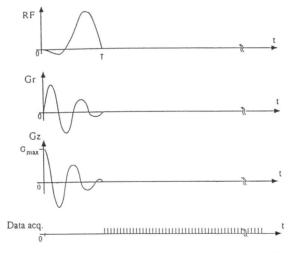

Figure 13-32 A radial gradient coil based volume selective spectroscopic pulse sequence using spiral scan oscillating gradients and an rf pulse. In this sequence G_r and G_z will form the spiral scan in the k-domain, while the rf pulse weight the spiral trajectory up to time T. Note here that G_r is already in two dimensions. Therefore the resultant trajectory formed together with the oscillating gradient G_z will be three-dimensional in the k-domain.

the first kind of order one for the volume selection, the rf pulse is given by [see Eqs. (13-74), (13-75), and (13-76)]

$$B_1(t) = \frac{J_1(\alpha|\mathbf{k}(t)|)}{|\mathbf{k}(t)|} \left(\frac{K_{max}}{T}\right) \sqrt{1 + (2\pi N')^2 \left(1 - \frac{t}{T}\right)^2} \quad (13\text{-}86)$$

where α is a coefficient proportional to the size of the selected volume. It is noted that the rf pulse waveform is common to all the loci. By simultaneously applying an rf pulse $B_1(t)$ and two oscillating gradients, namely $G_{rl}(t)$ and $G_{zl}(t)$, in each interlaced scan, one can localize a 3-D volume at the center of the object. The pulse sequence of the radial gradient coil based volume selective spectroscopy using oscillating gradients is shown in Fig. 13-32.

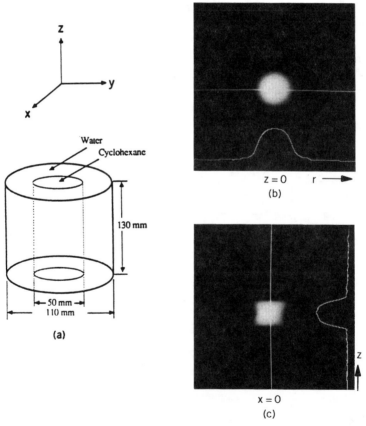

Figure 13-33 An example of the radial coil based volume selection using the spiral scans: (a) a phantom consisting of cyclohexane (fat) and water, (b) an axial view of the selected volume (cyclohexane) at $z = 0$, (c) a sagittal view (image at z-y-plane) of the selected volume at $x = 0$.

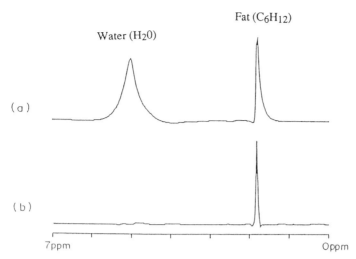

Figure 13-34 Proton spectra obtained from the phantom shown in Fig. 13-33 (a) using the radial gradient coil based spiral scan technique: (a) a spectrum obtained from the whole phantom without volume selection and (b) a spectrum obtained from the localized volume at the center (C_6H_{12}). The pulse sequence shown in Fig. 13-32 was used for both experiments.

In the experiment the Gaussian-weighted Bessel function of the first kind of order one is used for the rf pulse waveform to select a volume of 2.0 cm in diameter. The rf pulse duration used was 2 msec. In this case the effective gradient amplitude G_{eff} was chosen to be 0.13 $G/$cm for both G_r and G_z, which is considered to be strong enough to eliminate the selection blur due to the chemical shift in proton spectroscopy. Figures 13-33(b) and (c) show the selection profiles obtained along the r ($z = 0$ plane) and z ($x = 0$ plane) directions using a 90° flip angle and interlaced scannings with two spiral turns. The spectra obtained from the phantom shown in Fig. 13-33(a), which contains both water and cyclohexane, are shown in Fig. 13-34. The spectrum obtained from the whole phantom is shown in Fig. 13-34(a), while the spectrum of the localized volume obtained by the radial gradient coil based spiral scan technique is shown in Fig. 13-34(b). As seen in these figures the spectrum obtained by the radial gradient coil based spiral scan technique shows a clean and narrow peak of fat (cyclohexane) alone, suggesting that the selection technique works as expected.

3-D Volume Localization Using Projective Scan with a Radial Gradient Coil for Spectroscopy [61]

Another volume localization technique based on the radial gradient coil is the projective scan technique which uses the projection-like scan method shown in Fig. 13-35. Since the effective gradient strength in the spiral scan is inversely proportional to the number of spiral turns, it is important to reduce

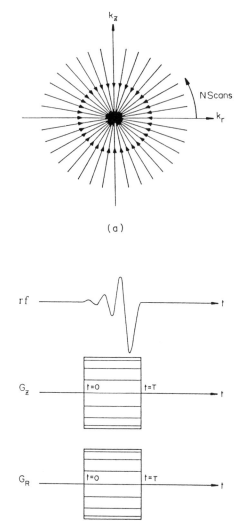

Figure 13-35 The k-space trajectory and the pulse sequence of a projective scan using a radial gradient coil: (a) the k-space trajectory and (b) the pulse sequence. This is similar to the projection reconstruction technique except for the rf pulse, which is now tailored by a Bessel function.

the number of spiral turns. An extreme case of this situation is the use of two constant (flat) gradient pulses, instead of two oscillating gradients, in combination with an rf pulse. k-space trajectories of this projective scan volume selection technique then look like the one shown in Fig. 13-35(a). Since this is virtually the same as the projection scan, the pulse sequence would be the one shown in Fig. 13-35(b). Volume selection is completed after N scans [59]. One could consider this projective scan method as a variant of the spiral scan technique with a very large number of interlacings (L interlacings).

From Eq. (13-84), by assuming that L is large and N is small, the gradient pulses for the projective scan can be obtained as

$$G_{rl}(t) = -G_{max} \cos\left(\frac{2\pi l}{L}\right) \quad \text{for } 0 \le t \le T \tag{13-87a}$$

$$G_{zl}(t) = G_{max} \sin\left(\frac{2\pi l}{L}\right) \quad \text{for } 0 \le t \le T; l = 1, 2, \dots, L \tag{13-87b}$$

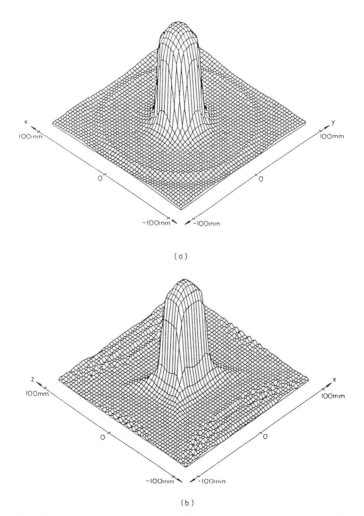

(a)

(b)

Figure 13-36 Computer simulation results of the central region obtained by the projective scan method: (a) the axial view and (b) the coronal view. The selected volume has a cylindrical shape.

The resulting **k**-space trajectory then becomes

$$K_{rl}(t) = K \cos\left(\frac{2\pi l}{L}\right)(T - t) \quad \text{for } 0 \le t \le T \tag{13-88a}$$

$$K_{zl}(t) = K \sin\left(\frac{2\pi l}{L}\right)(T - t) \quad \text{for } 0 \le t \le T; l = 1, 2, \ldots, L \tag{13-88b}$$

where the constant K is equal to $-\gamma G_{\max}/T$. Since the rf pulse shape is the same for all the projective loci, the same $B_1(t)$ can be used throughout the projective scans. The rf pulse shape can be obtained from Eq. (13-74) as

$$B_1(t) = J_1(\alpha|\mathbf{k}(t)|)|\dot{\mathbf{k}}(t)| \tag{13-89}$$

Some computer simulations of the volume selection were performed. In the simulations the T_1 effects were neglected, and the rf pulse given in Eq. (13-89) with a 90° flip angle and a T of 2 msec was used. The radial gradient field, close to the practical field used in the whole-body system, was generated by a radial coil with a diameter of 40 cm. The maximum radial- and z-gradient field strengths were $G_r = 0.17$ G/cm^2 and $G_z = 0.5$ G/cm, respectively. Seventy-four projective scannings were used to minimize the signal contamination from outside the volume of interest (VOI). The size of the selected cylindrical volume was 4.5 cm (diameter) × 3.5 cm (height). Figure 13-36 shows the computer simulated results of the selected areas in axial and coronal views.

13-2-2 Applications of the Localization Techniques to the Area of Spectroscopy

Proton Spectroscopy [39 – 45]
Proton magnetic resonance (MR) spectroscopy is an important tool for the study of *in vivo* metabolisms in animal and human. Several important metabolites, such as aminobutyric acid (GABA) and lactate, have been identified in the MR spectra obtained from living rats and rabbits. The effect of physiologic perturbations, such as hypoxia or hypoglycemia, in relation to the concentrations of these metabolites have been studied. The concentration of lactate is an important indicator of pathologic condition, and the animal studies have demonstrated that it can be measured with MR spectroscopy. MR signals of other metabolites may also have diagnostic significance. For example, the concentration of *N*-acetyl aspartate differs for normal brain tissue and for tumors; thus measurements of the compound may help characterize tumors. Hydrogen MR spectroscopic measurements of low molecular weight metabolites in the human brain may also be of value in evaluating patients.

However, the techniques used in in situ measurements of metabolites with MR spectroscopy in animals must be modified to be useful for the *in vivo* human measurements. Many of the animal studies were performed with narrow-bore magnets, which have a magnetic field strength several times higher than that of the whole-body magnets available today for human studies. Because spectral resolution is proportional to field strength, it is more difficult to resolve resonances at the lower-field strengths available with whole-body magnets. The problem of resolving resonances at low-field strengths is further complicated by the relatively low signal intensity of those metabolites. In addition the high-intensity signals from water and lipids severely interfere with the observation of the weak signals from low molecular weight metabolites such as lactates. For example, the tissue-water signal is typically four orders of magnitude more intense than that of the metabolites. Because of these limitations it is generally difficult to observe the weak signals from metabolites in the presence of the intense water signal. As discussed previously, proton spectroscopy therefore requires some form of water signal suppression technique to overcome the large dynamic range problem. Several such techniques have been used in analytical NMR spectrometers and have been successful [38, 65]. Further suppression of other signals such as the one from fat is also important. In some *in vivo* studies of humans such as brain studies, it is often easier to observe signals from metabolites because brain tissues contain little fat.

Animal studies are usually performed with surface coils and with the overlying tissues removed to ensure that only signals from the organ of interest are detected. This procedure is particularly important for observing metabolites with MR because the intense signals from fat, which is often present in the overlying tissue, can obscure the signals from the metabolites in the organ of interest. However, for studies on human subjects, techniques that suppress the unwanted signals from the overlying tissue must be used. Since, in spectroscopic study, a specific region is evaluated rather than whole organs or regions, the region where the spectrum is to be obtained must be well defined. This region preferably should be selected on the basis of an image.

Phosphorus Spectroscopy [61, 63]

Phosphorus spectroscopy plays a central role in NMR spectroscopy especially in *in vivo* human studies. *In vivo* phosphorus spectroscopy has been performed using one of the localization methods discussed in the previous sections, namely projective scanning with a radial gradient coil, and the volume selection technique shown in Fig. 13-35. Figures 13-37(a) and (c) show the proton images in the coronal view obtained by the conventional spin-echo sequence where each VOI is identified by the rectangular box. The projected coronal images of the two selected volumes of approximately 4.5 cm (diameter) $\times$ 3.5 cm (height) at the center and slightly off-center in the brain are shown in Figs. 13-37(b) and (d), respectively. The corresponding

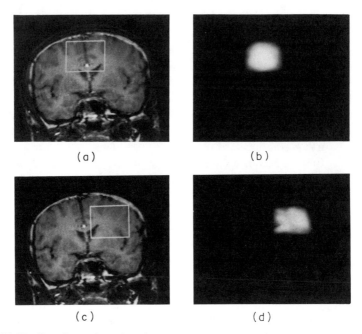

Figure 13-37 Experimental results of the volume localization *in vivo* spectroscopy of the human brain obtained by the projective scan method using a radial gradient coil. (a) and (c) are the proton images of the coronal view obtained by the conventional spin-echo sequence. The rectangular boxes indicated in the images are the volumes to be selected. (b) and (d) are the corresponding volumes indicated in (a) and (c) selected by the projective scan method.

spectra obtained from these two volumes are shown in Figs. 13-38(a) and (b).

In phosphorus spectroscopy, measurements of the T_1 and T_2 relaxation times of the metabolites are often important and can be made by using the STEAM technique. The evaluated T_1 and T_2 relaxation times of phosphorus metabolites in the adult human brain are summarized in Table 13-3. The T_1 relaxation times were calculated for four different repetition times, while the T_2 values were obtained by using five different echo times [63].

Measurements of the T_2 relaxation times of homonuclear spin-spin coupled resonances are affected by J modulation. In STEAM sequences a first nulling of the signal amplitudes of a doublet occurs at $T_E = 1/J$ (i.e., about 60 msec for the ATP phosphates). To minimize the influence of J modulation, the T_2 relaxation times of ATP were evaluated from spectra recorded at echo times of $T_E < 20$ msec. When compared to human skeletal muscle, brain ATP T_2 values show no significant differences, whereas T_2 relaxation times of phosphor creatine (PCr) are considerably longer in muscle [64].

Relative metabolite concentrations can also be calculated by measuring the areas or spectral peaks and correcting the values by means of the

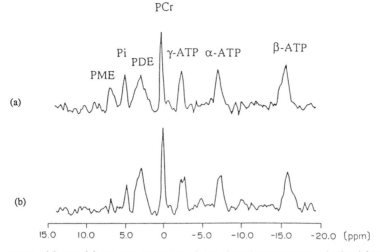

Figure 13-38 (a) and (b) are the examples of the phosphorus spectra obtained from the selected volumes shown in Figs. 13-37 (b) and (d), respectively. Sixty-four projective scans were performed with a T_R of 3 sec. In each scan 8192 sampling points were obtained, each with a sampling time of 20 μsec. The size of the selected volume was 4.5 cm (diameter) $\times$ 3.5 cm (height), and the total measurement time was 30 min.

Table 13-3 T_1 and T_2 relaxation times in localized phosphorus NMR spectra of the adult human brain in vivo obtained by STEAM (2.0 T)

Compound	δ (ppm)	T_1 (sec)	T_2 (msec)
PME	6.75	—	—
Pi	4.83	2.5	80
PDE	2.90	—	—
PCr	0	3.0	150
γ-ATP	-2.57	0.7	30
α-ATP	-7.62	0.7	30
β-ATP	-16.3	1.0	20

measured T_1 and T_2 relaxation times. The values are normalized with respect to PCr. When PCr is taken as an internal reference with an absolute concentration of about 5.0 mM, the numbers may be read as absolute concentrations in millimolar. The absolute concentrations of phosphate metabolites in normal human brain reported in recent studies range from 1.0 to 2.6 mM for Pi, 2.7 to 4.3 mM for PCr, 2.1 to 5.7 mM for α-ATP, and 1.8 to 3.5 mM for β-ATP and γ-APT, respectively.

REFERENCES

1. A. Abragam. *The Principles of Nuclear Magnetism*. Oxford: Oxford University Press, 1961.
2. D. Shaw. *Fourier Transform NMR Spectroscopy*. Amsterdam: Elsevier Scientific, 1976.
3. H. Gunther. *NMR Spectroscopy—An Introduction*. New York: Wiley, 1980.
4. P. C. Lauterbur. *Nature* 242:190 (1973).
5. R. Damadian. *Science* 171:1151 (1971).
6. T. C. Farrar and E. D. Becker. *Pulse and Fourier Transform NMR—Introduction to Theory and Methods*. San Diego: Academic Press, 1971.
7. P. Mansfield and P. G. Morris. *NMR Imaging in Biomedicine*. San Diego: Academic Press, 1982.
8. Z. H. Cho (ed.). Development of methods and algorithms for Fourier transform nuclear magnetic resonance tomographic imaging. KAIS ISS Lab. Report No. 2, Seoul, Korea, 1980.
9. Z. H. Cho, H. S. Kim, H. B. Song, and J. Cumming. *Proc. IEEE* 70:1152 (1982).
10. W. S. Hinshaw and A. H. Lent. *Proc. IEEE* 71:338 (1983).
11. A. Haase, J. Frahm, W. Hänicke, and D. Matthaei. *Phys. Med. Biol.* 30:341 (1985).
12. B. R. Rosen, V. J. Wedeen, and T. J. Brady. *J. Comput. Assist. Tomogr.* 8:813 (1984).
13. W. T. Dixon. *Radiology* 153:189 (1984).
14. R. E. Sepponen, J. T. Sipponen, and J. I. Tamttu. *J. Comput. Assist. Tomogr.* 8:585 (1984).
15. H. W. Park, D. J. Kim, and Z. H. Cho. *Magn. Reson. Med.* 4:526 (1987).
16. Z. H. Cho and H. W. Park. *Advances in Magnetic Resonance Imaging* 1:1–48 (1989).
17. H. W. Park and Z. H. Cho. *Magn. Reson. Med.* 3:448 (1986).
18. A. A. Maudsley, S. K. Hilal, W. H. Perman, and H. E. Simon. *J. Magn. Reson.* 51:147 (1983).
19. Z. H. Cho, H. W. Park, J. B. Ra, S. W. Lee, and S. K. Hilal. *Proc. of Third Annual Meeting of Society of Magnetic Resonance in Medicine* (Abstract), 1984, p. 155.
20. Z. H. Cho, O. Nalcioglu, H. W. Park, J. B. Ra, and S. K. Hilal. *Magn. Reson. Med.* 2:253 (1985).
21. M. L. Bernardo, Jr., P. C. Lauterbur, and L. K. Hedges. *J. Magn. Reson.* 61:168 (1985).
22. K. Sekihara, M. Kuroda, and H. Kohno. *Phys. Med. Biol.* 29:15 (1984).
23. E. Feig, F. Greenhleaf, and M. Perlin. *Phys. Med. Biol.* 31:1091 (1986).
24. Y. S. Kim, C. W. Mun, and Z. H. Cho. *Magn. Reson. Med.* 4:452 (1986).
25. A. A. Maudsley and S. K. Hilal. *Magn. Reson. Med.* 2:218 (1985).
26. K. M. Ludeke, P. Roschmann, and R. Tischler. *Magn. Reson. Imag.* 3:329 (1985).
27. H. W. Park, Y. M. Ro, and Z. H. Cho. *Phys. Med. Biol.* 33:339 (1987).

28. Z. H. Cho and Y. R. Ro. *Magn. Reson. Med.* 23:193–200 (1992).

29. Z. H. Cho, Y. M. Ro, and T. H. Lim. *Magn. Reson. Med.* 28:25–38 (1992).

30. J. W. Belliveau, D. N. Kennedy, R. C. McKinstry. et al. *Science* 254:716 (1991).

31. S. Ogawa and T. Lee. *Magn. Reson. Med.* 16:68 (1990).

32. Z. H. Cho, D. J. Kim, and Y. K. Kim. *Med. Phys.* 15:7 (1987).

33. P. Styles, C. A. Scott, and G. K. Radda. *Magn. Reson. Med.* 2:402 (1985).

34. M. Garwood, T. Schliech, G. B. Matson, and G. Acosta. *J. Magn. Reson.* 60:268 (1984).

35. P. A. Bottomley, T. H. Foster, and R. D. Darrow. *J. Magn. Reson.* 59:338 (1984).

36. P. R. Luyten, A. J. H. Marien, B. Sijtsma, and J. A. D. Hollander. *J. Magn. Reson.* 9:79 (1989).

37. P. R. Luyten and A. J. H. Hollander. *Radiology* 161:795 (1986).

38. J. Frahm, H. Bruhn, M. L. Gyngell, K. D. Merboldt, W. Hänicke and R. Sauter. *Magn. Reson. Med.* 9:79 (1989).

39. J. Frahm, H. Bruhn, M. L. Gyngell, K. D. Merboldt, W. Hänicke and R. Sauter. *Magn. Reson. Med.* 11:47 (1989).

40. P. R. Luyten, A. J. H. Marien, B. Sijtsma, and J. A. D. Hollander. *J. Magn. Reson.* 67:148 (1986).

41. W. P. Aue, S. Mueller, T. A. Cross, and J. Seelig. *J. Magn. Reson.* 56:350 (1984).

42. S. Mueller, W. P. Aue, and J. Seelig. *J. Magn. Reson.* 63:530 (1985).

43. P. R. Luyten and J. A. D. Hollander. *Proc. SMRM* 2:1021 (1985).

44. P. J. Hore. *J. Magn. Reson.* 55:283 (1983).

45. J. Frahm, K. D. Merboldt, and W. Hänicke. *J. Magn. Reson.* 72:502 (1987).

46. S. Y. Lee and Z. H. Cho. *Magn. Reson. Med.* 12:56 (1989).

47. C. J. Hardy and H. E. Cline. *J. Magn. Reson.* 82:647 (1989).

48. P. A. Bottomley and C. J. Hardy. *J. Appl. Phys.* 62:4284 (1987).

49. P. A. Bottomley and C. J. Hardy. *J. Magn. Reson.* 74:550 (1987).

50. C. J. Hardy, P. A. Bottomley, and P. B. Roemer. *J. Appl. Phys.* 63:4741 (1988).

51. C. J. Hardy, P. A. Bottomley, M. O'Donnel, and P. B. Roemer. *J. Magn. Reson.* 77:223 (1988).

52. S. Kirkpatrick, C. D. Gelatt, and M. P. Vecchi. *Science* 220:671 (1983).

53. N. Metropolis, A. W. Rosenbluth, A. H. Teller, and E. Teller. *J. Chem. Phy.* 21:1987 (1953).

54. J. Pauly, D. Nishimura, and A. Macovski. *J. Magn. Reson.* 81:43 (1989).

55. J. Pauly, D. Nishimura, and A. Macovski. *Proc. SMRM* 7:654 (1988).

56. J. B. Ra, C. Y. Rim, and Z. H. Cho. *Magn. Reson. Med.* 17:423 (1991).

57. C. J. Hardy and H. E. Cline. *J. Magn. Reson.* 82:647 (1989).

58. C. B. Ahn, J. H. Kim, and Z. H. Cho. *IEEE Tran. Med. Imag.* 5:1 (1986).

59. C. Y. Rim, J. B. Ra, and Z. H. Cho. *Proc. SMRM* 8:30 (1989).

60. C. J. Hardy and H. E. Cline. *Proc. SMRM* 8:26 (1989).

61. C. Y. Rim, J. B. Ra, and Z. H. Cho. *Magn. Reson. Med.* (forthcoming).

62. M. Gyngell, J. Frahm, K. D. Merbolt, W. Hänicke, and H. Bruhn. *J. Magn. Reson.* 77:596 (1988).

63. K. D. Merboldt, D. Chien, W. Hänicke, M. L. Gyngell, and H. Bruhn. *J. Magn. Reson.* 89:343 (1990).

64. C. Thomsen, K. Z. Jesen, and O. Henriksen. *Magn. Reson. Imag.* 7:557 (1989).

65. J. Frahm, H. Bruhn, M. L. Gyngell, K. D. Merboldt, W. Hänicke, and R. Sauter. *Magn. Reson. Med.* 8:49 (1988).

IV

ULTRASOUND AND ULTRASONIC IMAGING

14

ULTRASOUND PHYSICS

Acoustics is an old science which, surprising to many, continues to evolve and innovate. For example, the theories of nonlinear phenomena, solitons, and chaos all had their early origins in acoustics. Today various aspects of acoustics find application in almost every field of science, engineering, and human endeavor, ranging from the design of concert halls to medical ultrasonics. It is this latter topic that concerns us here, the propagation of acoustical waves in the low MHz frequency range and their interaction with tissue. The objective of medical ultrasound is to use our knowledge of acoustics and the propagation/interaction process to produce acoustical images of tissue and to extract additional information from the image or interaction process that may prove to be clinically relevant. This chapter is designed to provide the reader with a sufficient understanding of the *physics* of ultrasound so that he or she can fully understand present imaging systems, appreciate ongoing research efforts, and become a productive member of the research and engineering community developing new medical ultrasound methods and techniques. The reader will note that in this text somewhat more time is devoted to ultrasound physics than to, say, the physics of ionizing and other nonionizing radiations. This emphasis is the result of the fact that electromagnetism, atomic, and nuclear physics are well covered in most university curricula, whereas acoustics is not. It is rare for a student of either physics or engineering at either the graduate or undergraduate level to have a comprehensive course in acoustics. In most cases wave propagation and mechanical radiation are covered as a small and simplified part of freshman physics. Although our coverage of the topic will overcome these deficiencies, it is clearly unrealistic in the space available to provide a complete and rigorous treatment of all the topics of acoustics relevant to medical ultrasonics. The interested reader is therefore referred to the references given at the end of this chapter and in particular to section 14.7 which reviews the acoustical literature as it relates to medical ultrasonics.

14-1   SIMPLE WAVE PROPAGATION AND NONLINEAR ACOUSTICS

In this section we derive the basic equations that describe the propagation of sound in a homogeneous and nondissipative medium, and then develop and define appropriate parameters that aid in describing the propagation process. Although our initial results (subsection 14-1-1) are in a linearized form, we later show (subsection 14-1-4) that this general wave equation is in fact nonlinear and discuss the implications of this result for medical applications. The basic formalism developed here will be added to and expanded in future sections of this chapter to include propagation in fluids, solids, and tissue.

14-1-1   The Linear Wave Equation for Propagation in a Nondissipative Medium

Here we derive from first principles a set of equations which will describe the propagation of the simplest of sound waves (a plane wave) in the simplest medium we can imagine (a homogeneous and nondissipative fluid). The effects of absorption and attenuation as well as the effects of more complex wave fronts will be added later. The reader might well ask why we should begin with such a simple situation and not go directly to the arrangement of our primary interest, the propagation of an ultrasonic pulse in real tissue, which is inhomogeneous and absorptive, and, on occasion, nonisotropic. There are at least two reasons for this seemingly pedantic approach. First, we believe that it is pedagogically correct to begin with the simplest situation, adding layers of complexity as required. With the basic foundations well understood, new situations can be addressed as needed. Second, there are many practical situations in medical ultrasound where even the simplest model will provide new insights as well as an appropriate computational framework. For any given problem in medical ultrasound (or in medical imaging) the successful student should be able to select an appropriate model of sufficient complexity to address the questions at hand but not overly complex so as to be overly cumbersome. With these comments, let us proceed with the promised derivation.

Once again let us assume a medium that is homogeneous, continuous, of infinite extent, and nondissipative (i.e., no energy is lost or dissipated as the sound wave propagates). Although these assumptions may seem over idealized, in reality this is a reasonable first-order model for most materials, including tissue. The effects of absorption and/or scattering are simply added to the model as required. To our knowledge there are only two general cases where these restrictions on the medium do not lead to a reasonable model: rarefied gases and solids in which the wavelength of the sound wave is on the order of or smaller than the interatomic distances.

Let us further assume that a sound wave propagates in this medium along a broad front and that the nodes of compression and rarefaction by which the sound wave propagates are all of equal magnitude and are all parallel. Given these assumptions, we can establish a rectangular coordinate system $[x, y, z]$ in the medium such that the wave propagates in the x direction only and that all motions along x are independent of both the y and z coordinates. This description of propagation is better known as a *plane wave*.

As the wave propagates, the particles of the medium will be displaced from some equilibrium position. Here we have required that this displacement be in the same direction as the wave propagates; this defines a *longitudinal plane wave*. *Transverse waves* or waves that propagate perpendicular to the direction of propagation can also be generated. Perhaps the best example of a transverse wave is electromagnetic radiation. Transverse acoustical waves or shear waves can also be generated but not in a fluid. In fact one definition of a fluid is a material that will not support a shear stress. Although ultrasonic shear waves have been used to study bone, such waves will not propagate in fluids or soft tissue.

Given a longitudinal plane wave propagating in the x direction in our homogeneous, nondissipative fluid, let us examine what happens when this wave impinges upon a small fluid element defined by the boundaries x and $x + dx$, as shown in Fig. 14-1. The wave propagating from left to right will produce a displacement ξ at the first boundary and a displacement of $(\xi + d\xi)$ at the second. Note that by permitting the displacements to be

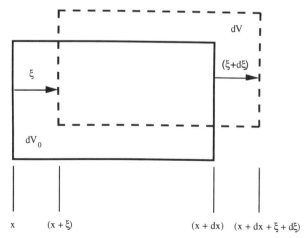

Figure 14-1   A small volume element of fluid dV_0, defined by the boundaries x and $x + dx$ is deformed by an incident plane wave (propagating from left to right) into a new volume element dV defined by $x + \xi$ and $x + dx + \xi + d\xi$, where ξ is the displacement.

different at the two boundaries, we have allowed the fluid to be compressible. The volume of the fluid element before (dV_0) and after (dV) which the sound wave passes through is then given by

$$dV_0 = dx\,dy\,dz \tag{14-1}$$

and

$$dV = (dx + d\xi)\,dy\,dz \tag{14-2}$$

respectively. Note that no change occurs in either the y or z directions, since the front of the plane wave only changes along x.

Let ρ_0 be the density of fluid element dV_0 and ρ the density of the element dV. Since the mass of the fluid element must remain constant (i.e., mass is conserved as the sound wave propagates), then

$$\rho_0\,dV_0 = \rho\,dV \tag{14-3}$$

Substituting Eqs. (14-1) and (14-2) into (14-3) gives

$$\rho = \rho_0\left(\frac{dx}{dx + d\xi}\right)$$

or

$$\rho = \frac{\rho_0}{1 + \partial\xi/\partial x} \tag{14-4}$$

Let us return again to Fig. 14-1 and consider the net force F (to the right) which the sound wave places on the fluid element dV_0. From the definition of force we may write

$$F = \text{net pressure} \times \text{cross-sectional area}$$

If p is the pressure, then

$$F = \left[p - \left(p + \frac{\partial p}{\partial x}\,dx\right)\right]dy\,dz$$

or

$$F = -\left(\frac{\partial p}{\partial x}\right)dx\,dy\,dz \tag{14-5}$$

Using Newton's law of motion, we can write an alternate expression for the force on the fluid element dV_0. Thus

$$F = \text{mass of } dV_0 \times \text{acceleration of } dV_0$$

or

$$F = (\rho_0 \, dx \, dy \, dz) \frac{\partial^2 \xi}{\partial t^2} \tag{14-6}$$

Equating Eqs. (14-5) and (14-6), we have

$$-\frac{\partial p}{\partial x} = \rho_0 \frac{\partial^2 \xi}{\partial t^2} = \rho_0 \frac{\partial u}{\partial t} \tag{14-7}$$

where u, the particle velocity, is defined as

$$u = \frac{\partial \xi}{\partial t}$$

This result is easily generalized to three dimensions, so we can write

$$-\nabla p = \rho_0 \frac{\partial u}{\partial t} \tag{14-8}$$

This is an important equation of motion which is sometimes known as the *linear inviscid force equation*. Later (in Section 14-1-4) we will see that Eq. (14-8) is simply a reduction of Euler's equation for the case of an ideal fluid, without viscosity. Note that since ∇p in Eq. (14-8) points in the direction of increasing pressure, the acceleration must be in the direction of decreasing pressure.

In our calculations leading to Eqs. (14-4) and (14-8), and using Fig. 14-1, we began with an element of fluid dV_0 that was subjected to the forces of a propagating sound wave. Now let us replace this fluid element with a rigid frame of the same dimensions and calculate the rate of mass influx through this box, as shown in Fig. 14-2. The rate of mass influx through the left-hand side of the box is clearly

$$\text{density} \times \text{particle velocity} \times \text{cross-sectional area}$$

or

$$\rho u \, dy \, dz \tag{14-9}$$

Similarly the rate of mass outflow on the right-hand side of the box is

$$[\rho u + d(\rho u)] \, dy \, dz$$

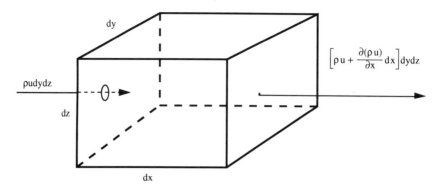

Figure 14-2 Rate of mass influx through a fixed volume element $dx\,dy\,dz$.

or

$$\left[\rho u + \frac{\partial(\rho u)}{\partial x}\,dx\right] dy\,dz \qquad (14\text{-}10)$$

Subtracting Eq. (14-10) from Eq. (14-9) gives the rate of net mass influx, from left to right, through the fixed element. The result is

$$-\frac{\partial(\rho u)}{\partial x}\,dV_0 \qquad (14\text{-}11)$$

Clearly the rate of net mass influx through the volume element is also the rate of increase of mass in the element, or

$$\frac{\partial\rho}{\partial t}\,dV_0 \qquad (14\text{-}12)$$

Equating these last two expressions gives

$$-\frac{\partial\rho}{\partial t} = \frac{\partial(\rho u)}{\partial x} \qquad (14\text{-}13)$$

This result is also easily generalized to three dimensions, giving

$$-\frac{\partial\rho}{\partial t} = \nabla(\rho u) \qquad (14\text{-}14)$$

which is the well-known equation of continuity. Note that this is a nonlinear equation. We can obtain a linearized form of the continuity equation by writing Eq. (14-14) in a somewhat different form and explicitly ignoring all terms of second order or higher. To accomplish this, it will first be convenient if we define the condensation s as

$$s \equiv \frac{\rho - \rho_0}{\rho_0} \tag{14-15}$$

Substituting Eq. (14-4) into (14-15) gives

$$s = \frac{-\partial \xi / \partial x}{1 + \partial \xi / \partial x}$$

which, to first order, is

$$s \approx -\frac{\partial \xi}{\partial x} \tag{14-16}$$

Substituting Eq. (14-16) back into (14-4) gives, to the first order,

$$\rho \approx \rho_0(1 + s) \tag{14-17}$$

Substituting Eq. (14-17) into the equation of continuity, Eq. (14-13), gives

$$-\frac{\partial \rho}{\partial t} = -\rho_0 \frac{\partial s}{\partial t} = \rho_0 \frac{\partial u}{\partial x} + \rho_0 s \frac{\partial u}{\partial x} + u \rho_0 \frac{\partial s}{\partial x}$$

The last two terms can be ignored because they both contain products of differentials and will be second order or higher in magnitude. Thus the last equation becomes

$$-\frac{\partial s}{\partial t} = \frac{\partial u}{\partial x} \tag{14-18}$$

which is the linearized version of the equation of continuity.

Next let us assume that the pressure is a function of the density, or

$$p = p(\rho) \tag{14-19}$$

which thermodynamically is the classical model of a compressible fluid at constant entropy. Writing Eq. (14-19) as a series expansion gives

$$p = \left(\frac{\partial p}{\partial \rho}\right)(\rho - \rho_0) + \cdots \tag{14-20}$$

Substituting Eq. (14-15) into (14-20) and ignoring higher-order terms gives

$$p \approx \rho_0 \left(\frac{\partial p}{\partial \rho}\right) s \tag{14-21}$$

Now let us return to Eq. (14-7) and differentiate with respect to x. The result is

$$-\frac{\partial^2 p}{\partial x^2} = \rho_0 \frac{\partial}{\partial x}\left(\frac{\partial u}{\partial t}\right) \tag{14-22}$$

Returning to Eq. (14-18), let us differentiate with respect to t:

$$-\frac{\partial^2 s}{\partial t^2} = \frac{\partial}{\partial t}\left(\frac{\partial u}{\partial x}\right) \tag{14-23}$$

Combining these last two equations, we have

$$\frac{\partial^2 p}{\partial x^2} = \rho_0 \frac{\partial^2 s}{\partial t^2} \tag{14-24}$$

Substituting Eq. (14-21) into (14-24) gives

$$\frac{\partial^2 p}{\partial x^2} = \frac{1}{(\partial p/\partial \rho)}\frac{\partial^2 p}{\partial t^2} \tag{14-25}$$

Finally, let us consider the term $(\partial p/\partial \rho)$. A simple review of units will show that this term has units of (velocity)^2. Thermodynamic considerations far more involved than we can discuss here show that

$$\left(\frac{\partial p}{\partial \rho}\right) = c^2 \tag{14-26}$$

where c is the speed of sound. Substituting Eq. (14-26) into (14-25) gives our final result:

$$\frac{\partial^2 p}{\partial x^2} = \frac{1}{c^2}\frac{\partial^2 p}{\partial t^2} \tag{14-27a}$$

This is the basic wave equation that describes the propagation of a plane wave in a homogeneous, nondissipative fluid. The result is clearly generalizable to three dimensions:

$$\nabla^2 p = \frac{1}{c^2}\frac{\partial^2 p}{\partial t^2} \tag{14-27b}$$

Note that this simple wave equation is based on a linearization of the equation of continuity and a first-order expansion of the pressure in terms of density. Retaining these higher-order terms leads to a more general nonlinear equation, as we will show in Subsection (14-1-4).

14-1-2 Acoustical Parameters and Plane Wave Propagation

Thus far we have used the conservation of mass, Newton's law of motion, a linearized form of the equation of continuity, and the assumption that the pressure can be written as a series expansion of the density to derive the basic wave equation, Eqs. (14-27). These two equations are fundamental to linear acoustics and to much of medical ultrasound. As derived here, Eqs. (14-27) describe the propagation of a plane wave in a homogeneous, nondissipative fluid. Proceeding with our development of linear acoustics we now define some additional parameters that will also be useful to our study of medical ultrasonics.

In electrodynamics the potential plays an important role in the theoretical development of the field. Similarly in acoustics it is useful to define a *velocity potential* ϕ such that its gradient is equal to the particle velocity:

$$\frac{\partial \phi}{\partial x} = u = \frac{\partial \xi}{\partial t} \tag{14-28a}$$

or

$$\nabla \phi = u \tag{14-28b}$$

To develop a useful equation using the velocity potential, let us return to Eq. (14-7), the equation of motion. Substituting Eq. (14-28a) into (14-7) and integrating with respect to x gives

$$-p = \rho_0 \frac{\partial \phi}{\partial t} + f(t) + C$$

where f is an arbitrary function of time and C is a constant, both determined by the physics of the initial conditions. Since this equation must be valid even when there is no sound wave propagating (i.e., when $\partial \phi / \partial t = 0$), it follows that $f(t) = 0$ and $C = -p_0$, where p_0 is some equilibrium pressure. Thus

$$p - p_0 = -\rho_0 \frac{\partial \phi}{\partial t}$$

Since the excess pressure $(p - p_0)$ is really the parameter of interest, for notational convenience we define $p \equiv (p - p_0)$ and write

$$p = -\rho_0 \frac{\partial \phi}{\partial t} \tag{14-29}$$

which is the desired result.

In the previous section we defined the *condensation s* as

$$s \equiv \frac{\rho - \rho_0}{\rho_0}$$

and showed that to first order

$$s \approx \frac{\partial \xi}{\partial x}$$

This parameter will also prove to be useful in our development.

Next we turn to considerations of energy using, once again, the small volume element, dV_0 shown in Fig. 14-1. The kinetic energy dE_k associated with the volume element is clearly

$$dE_k = \tfrac{1}{2}\rho_0 u^2 \, dV_0 \qquad (14\text{-}30)$$

where the mass of the element $\rho_0 \, dV_0$ is expressed in terms of the density and volume of the undisturbed fluid. Note that the kinetic energy of the fluid element is essentially a function of the particle velocity u.

The potential energy dE_p associated with the volume element is, by definition,

$$dE_p = -\int_{dV_0}^{dV} p \, dV \qquad (14\text{-}31)$$

where the negative sign means that the potential energy will increase as work is done on the element by the action of a positive acoustic pressure.

Using Eqs. (14-3), (14-15), (14-17), and (14-21), it can be shown that Eq. (14-31) reduces to

$$dE_p = \tfrac{1}{2}\rho_0 c^2 s^2 \, dV_0 \qquad (14\text{-}32a)$$

or

$$dE_p = \frac{p^2}{2\rho_0 c^2} \, dV_0 \qquad (14\text{-}32b)$$

The total acoustical energy dE of the volume element is then given by

$$dE = \tfrac{1}{2}\rho_0(u^2 + c^2 s^2) \, dV_0 \qquad (14\text{-}33a)$$

or

$$dE = \tfrac{1}{2}\rho_0\left(u^2 + \frac{p^2}{\rho_0^2 c^2}\right) dV_0 \qquad (14\text{-}33b)$$

It is convenient to define the *instantaneous energy density* ε_i as

$$\varepsilon_i = \frac{dE}{dV_0} \qquad (14\text{-}34)$$

The *mean energy density* ε is then the time average of ε_i, or

$$\varepsilon \equiv \frac{1}{t} \int_0^t \varepsilon_i \, dt \tag{14-35}$$

Although most of the measuring devices in acoustics are pressure sensitive rather than intensity or energy sensitive, it is still useful to consider the *acoustical intensity I*, which is defined as the average rate of energy flow through a unit area normal to the direction of propagation. Thus

$$I = c\varepsilon \tag{14-36}$$

Electrical analogs have historically played a significant role in acoustics, especially in transducer design. The simplest such analog associates voltage with pressure and current with particle velocity. Thus the acoustical equivalent of Ohm's law becomes

$$Z = \frac{p}{u} \tag{14-37}$$

where Z is the *specific acoustical impedance*.

From the parameters defined above we now turn to an example to compute their values for the specific case of a plane harmonic wave. Suppose that the particle velocity is given by

$$u = u_0 e^{-i(kx - \omega t)} \tag{14-38}$$

which is a plane harmonic wave propagating from left to right where u_0 is a real constant, k is the wave number, and ω is the angular frequency. We leave as an exercise to the reader the calculation of the displacement ξ, the velocity potential ϕ, the condensation s, the pressure p, the instantaneous energy density ε_i, the mean energy density ε, the intensity I, and the specific acoustical impedance Z. The results are as follows:

$$u = u_0 e^{-i(kx - \omega t)}$$
$$\xi = -iu/\omega$$
$$\phi = iu/k$$
$$s = u/c$$
$$p = \rho_0 cu$$
$$\varepsilon_i = \rho_0 u^2$$
$$\varepsilon = \tfrac{1}{2}\rho_0 u_0^2$$
$$I = \tfrac{1}{2}\rho_0 cu_0^2$$
$$Z = \rho_0 c$$

In the case of a plane wave note that the specific acoustic impedance reduces to the product of the density and the speed of sound. This product is known as the *characteristic impedance*.

14-1-3   Spherical and Cylindrical Waves

In Section 14-1-1 we derived the basic wave equation for a plane wave in terms of the pressure p (see Eq. 14-27). Similar equations can be obtained in terms of other acoustical parameters such as the displacement ξ and the velocity potential ϕ. Of particular interest is the formulation

$$\frac{\partial^2 \phi}{\partial x^2} = \frac{1}{c^2} \frac{\partial^2 \phi}{\partial t^2} \tag{14-39}$$

whose derivation we leave as an exercise for the reader. Note that the general solution for this equation can be written as

$$\phi = f(t \pm x/c) \tag{14-40}$$

where f is a general function; the minus sign represents a wave propagating from left to right, and the plus sign represents a wave propagating from right to left. A harmonic wave such as

$$\phi = \phi_0 e^{\pm i(kx - \omega t)} \tag{14-41}$$

represents a special example of f where the sign $\pm$ has the same meaning as in the general solution.

Although a plane wave analysis will serve as a useful tool for ultrasonics, other waveform geometries are also important. In particular, it will be useful to consider waves with spherical symmetry (e.g., from a point source) and waves with cylindrical symmetry (e.g., from a line source). To obtain such formalisms, we simply apply the appropriate coordinate transformation to our original wave equation. We will find it convenient to begin with Eq. (14-39), a wave equation for ϕ in rectangular cartesian coordinates. Transforming this equation into spherical coordinates [1] we have

$$\frac{1}{r} \frac{\partial^2 (r\phi)}{\partial r^2} = \frac{1}{c^2} \frac{\partial^2 \phi}{\partial t^2} \tag{14-42}$$

where r is the radius vector from the focal point to the edge of the spherical wave front. The general solution to the equation has the form

$$\phi = \frac{1}{r} f(t \pm r/c) \tag{14-43}$$

where f is a general function; the minus sign represents a divergent spherical wave, and the plus sign represents a converging spherical wave.

In a similar fashion we can obtain a formalism with cylindrical symmetry. Thus, transforming Eq. (14-39) from rectangular coordinates into cylindrical coordinates [1] gives

$$\frac{1}{r}\frac{\partial}{\partial r}\left(r\frac{\partial\phi}{\partial r}\right) = \frac{1}{c^2}\frac{\partial^2\phi}{\partial t^2} \tag{14-44}$$

where r is the radius vector from a line to the edge of the cylindrical wavefront centered on the line. The general solution to this equation has the form

$$\phi = \frac{1}{\sqrt{r}}f(t \pm r/c) \tag{14-45}$$

where f is a general function; the minus sign represents a divergent cylindrical wave, and the plus sign represents a convergent cylindrical wave. The reader is encouraged to verify that the general solutions given above [Eqs. (14-43) and (14-45)] do indeed satisfy their respective wave equations.

Harmonic solutions to the wave equation are useful for many applications in medical ultrasonics. Such solutions can take the following forms:

$$\phi = \phi_0 e^{-i(kx-\omega t)} \tag{14-46}$$

represents a plane wave propagating from left to right along the x-axis,

$$\phi = \phi_0\left(\frac{1}{r}\right)e^{-i(kr-\omega t)} \tag{14-47}$$

represents a spherical wave diverging from the origin at $r = 0$, and

$$\phi = \phi_0\left(\frac{1}{\sqrt{r}}\right)e^{-i(kr-\omega t)} \tag{14-48}$$

represents a cylindrical wave diverging from a line located at $r = 0$. These three wave types are shown schematically in Fig. 14-3.

In Section 14-1-2 we calculated a number of acoustical parameters for a plane wave defined in terms of the particle velocity. We encourage the reader to repeat such a calculation using the three wave forms given above in terms of the velocity potential. The results are shown in Table 14-1. Note that many of these quantities are complex so that some care must be exercised in relating them to actual physical measurements. For example, note that the specific acoustical impedance for the spherical wave is complex, which indicates that the pressure and particle velocity are not in phase. It is

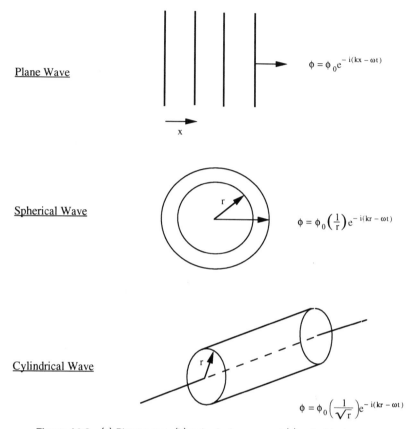

Plane Wave

$$\phi = \phi_0 e^{-i(kx - \omega t)}$$

Spherical Wave

$$\phi = \phi_0 \left(\frac{1}{r}\right) e^{-i(kr - \omega t)}$$

Cylindrical Wave

$$\phi = \phi_0 \left(\frac{1}{\sqrt{r}}\right) e^{-i(kr - \omega t)}$$

Figure 14-3   (a) Plane wave, (b) spherical wave, and (c) cylindrical wave.

instructive to examine this quantity in the limiting case of high frequency or large distance from the source; that is, where $kr \gg 1$. Rewriting this quantity, we have

$$Z = \frac{i\omega\rho_0 r}{1 + ikr} = \frac{i\rho_0 \omega r}{1 + k^2 r^2} + \frac{\rho_0 \omega kr^2}{1 + k^2 r^2}$$

Taking the limit as $kr \to \infty$ gives

$$Z \to 0 + \frac{\rho_0 \omega}{k} = \rho_0 c$$

Thus, as expected, the specific acoustical impedance associated with a spherical wave becomes, at large distances, equivalent to a plane wave, since the wave front of a spherical source appears planar at such distances.

Table 14-1 Acoustical parameters for plane, spherical, and cylindrical wave fronts

Parameter / General Expression for:	Harmonic Plane Wave (Propagating Left to Right)	Divergent Harmonic Spherical Wave	Divergent Harmonic Cylindrical Wave
Velocity potential, ϕ	$\phi = \phi_0 e^{-i(kx-\omega t)}$	$\phi = \phi_0\left(\dfrac{1}{r}\right) e^{-i(kr-\omega t)}$	$\phi = \phi_0\left(\dfrac{1}{\sqrt{r}}\right) e^{-i(kr-\omega t)}$
Particle velocity, u $(u = \nabla\phi)$	$u = \dfrac{\partial\phi}{\partial x} = -ik\phi$	$u = \dfrac{\partial\phi}{\partial r} = -\left(\dfrac{1}{r} + ik\right)\phi$	$u = \dfrac{\partial\phi}{\partial r} = -\left(\dfrac{1}{2r} + ik\right)\phi$
Condensation, s $\left(s = \dfrac{\rho - \rho_0}{\rho_0} = -\dfrac{1}{c^2}\dfrac{\partial\phi}{\partial t} = -\nabla\xi\right)$	$s \approx -\dfrac{\partial\xi}{\partial x}$ $s = -\dfrac{i\omega\phi}{c^2} = -\dfrac{ik\phi}{c}$	$s = -\dfrac{i\omega\phi}{c^2} = -\dfrac{ik\phi}{c}$	$s = -\dfrac{i\omega\phi}{c^2} = -\dfrac{ik\phi}{c}$
Pressure, p $(p = -\rho_0\dot{\phi})$	$p = -i\rho_0\omega\phi$ $p = \rho_0 cu$	$p = -i\rho_0\omega\phi$	$p = -i\rho_0\omega\phi$
Specific acoustical impedance, z $\left(z = \dfrac{p}{u}\right)$	$z = \rho_0 c$	$z = \dfrac{i\omega\rho_0 r}{1 + ikr}$	$z = \dfrac{i\omega\rho_0 r}{(1/2) + ikr}$

14-1-4 General Wave Equation for Propagation in a Nondissipative Medium: Implications of Nonlinear Acoustics and Propagation of Waves of Finite Amplitudes

The formalism developed, primarily in Section 14-1-1, to describe the propagation of a sound wave in a homogeneous and nondissipative medium relied on two major approximations: the linearization of the equation of continuity [see Eqs. (14-14) and (14-18)] and the retention of only first-order terms in the expression for the condensation [see Eq. (14-16)]. Here we show that if these approximations are not made, a wave equation can still be obtained, but the equation is fundamentally nonlinear. We also show the physical meaning of such nonlinearities and indicate the implications for medical ultrasonics.

Let us begin by returning to Eq. (14-4):

$$\rho = \frac{\rho_0}{1 + \partial\xi/\partial x}$$

which the reader will recall was obtained directly from the conservation of mass. Differentiating with respect to x, we have

$$\frac{\partial\rho}{\partial x} = \frac{-\rho_0}{(1 + \partial\xi/\partial x)^2} \frac{\partial^2\xi}{\partial x^2} \tag{14-49}$$

Next we note that the equation of motion Eq. (14-7) can be written as

$$-\frac{\partial p}{\partial x} = -\left(\frac{\partial p}{\partial \rho}\right)\left(\frac{\partial \rho}{\partial x}\right) = \rho_0\frac{\partial^2\xi}{\partial t^2}$$

or

$$\frac{\partial\rho}{\partial x} = -\frac{\rho_0}{\partial p/\partial \rho}\frac{\partial^2\xi}{\partial t^2} \tag{14-50}$$

Equating Eqs. (14-49) and (14-50) gives

$$\frac{\partial^2\xi}{\partial t^2} = \frac{\partial p/\partial \rho}{(1 + \partial\xi/\partial x)^2}\frac{\partial^2\xi}{\partial x^2} \tag{14-51a}$$

or, making the identification from thermodynamics that $c^2 \equiv \partial p/\partial \rho$, see Eq. (14-26), we have

$$\frac{\partial^2\xi}{\partial t^2} = \frac{c^2}{(1 + \partial\xi/\partial x)^2}\frac{\partial^2\xi}{\partial x^2} \tag{14-51b}$$

which is clearly a nonlinear wave equation for the displacement ξ. What is remarkable and what makes this result so fundamental is the fact that this equation is a direct consequence of the conservation of mass and Newton's law of motion, both of which are fundamentally linear relationships. Further insights are gained if we consider specific relationships between the pressure and density as well as take advantage of the equation of continuity, which itself is nonlinear.

Suppose that our homogeneous medium were an ideal gas. Then from thermodynamics

$$p = p_0 \left(\frac{\rho}{\rho_0} \right)^\gamma \tag{14-52}$$

where γ is the ratio of specific heats. Differentiating with respect to density gives

$$\left(\frac{\partial p}{\partial \rho} \right) \equiv c^2 = \frac{\gamma p_0}{\rho_0} \left(\frac{\rho}{\rho_0} \right)^{\gamma - 1}$$

$$= \frac{\gamma p_0}{\rho_0} \left(\frac{1}{1 + \partial \xi / \partial x} \right)^{\gamma - 1} \tag{14-53}$$

where we have also used Eq. (14-4). Substituting Eq. (14-53) into Eq. (14-51b), we have

$$\frac{\partial^2 \xi}{\partial t^2} = \frac{\gamma c_0^2}{(1 + \partial \xi / \partial x)^{\gamma + 1}} \frac{\partial^2 \xi}{\partial x^2} \tag{14-54}$$

where $c_0^2 = (p_0 / \rho_0)$.

Next let us suppose that our homogeneous medium is governed by a somewhat more general thermodynamic relationship than that for an ideal gas. Specifically let us assume that

$$p = p(\rho, S)$$

where S is the entropy. Expanding this expression gives

$$p = p_0 + \left(\frac{\partial p}{\partial \rho} \right)_{S, \rho = \rho_0} \times (\rho - \rho_0) + \frac{1}{2} \left(\frac{\partial^2 p}{\partial \rho^2} \right)_{S, \rho = \rho_0} \times (\rho - \rho_0)^2 + \cdots \tag{14-55}$$

Let us now define two coefficients A and B such that Eq. (14-55) can be rewritten as

$$p - p_0 = A\left(\frac{\rho - \rho_0}{\rho_0}\right) + \frac{B}{2}\left(\frac{\rho - \rho_0}{\rho_0}\right)^2 \tag{14-56}$$

where we have retained only terms to the second order. The ratio B/A, known as the *parameter of nonlinearity*, is one of the most important parameters in nonlinear acoustics whose significance will soon become apparent.

Returning now to the case of the ideal gas, let us rewrite Eq. (14-52) as follows:

$$p = p_0(\rho/\rho_0)^\gamma = p_0\left(1 + \frac{\rho - \rho_0}{\rho_0}\right)^\gamma$$

or

$$p = p_0 + \gamma p_0\left(\frac{\rho - \rho_0}{\rho_0}\right) + \frac{\gamma(\gamma - 1)p_0}{2}\left(\frac{\rho - \rho_0}{\rho_0}\right)^2 + \cdots \tag{14-57}$$

Comparing Eqs. (14-56) and (14-57), we can make the following identification:

$$\frac{B}{A} \equiv \gamma - 1 \tag{14-58}$$

Substituting this result into Eq. (14-54) gives

$$\frac{\partial^2 \xi}{\partial t^2} = \frac{c_0^2}{(1 + \partial\xi/\partial x)^{B/A+2}} \frac{\partial^2 \xi}{\partial x^2} \tag{14-59}$$

which is the general wave equation for the propagation of sound in a homogeneous, nondissipative fluid. A similar derivation, which we leave as an exercise for the reader, leads to an equation in terms of the pressure p. Thus

$$\frac{\partial^2 p}{\partial t^2} = \frac{c_0^2}{(1 + \partial\xi/\partial x)^{B/A+2}} \frac{\partial^2 p}{\partial x^2} \tag{14-60}$$

and we see that the wave equation for the simplest physical situation imaginable—a plane wave propagating in a homogeneous, nondissipative medium—is fundamentally nonlinear. We will discuss the meaning and implications of this result later; for now let us consider in more detail the parameter of nonlinearity.

From the definition of the coefficients A and B we see, by comparing Eqs. (14-56) and (14-55), that

$$\frac{B}{A} = \frac{\rho_0}{c_0^2}\left(\frac{\partial^2 p}{\partial \rho^2}\right)_{S,\,\rho=\rho_0} \tag{14-61}$$

Applying a series of thermodynamic transformations, which are much too involved to detail here, one can show that [2, 3]

$$\frac{B}{A} = 2\rho_0 c_0 \left(\frac{\partial c}{\partial p}\right)_{T,\,\rho_0} + \frac{2\beta T c_0}{c_p}\left(\frac{\partial c}{\partial T}\right)_{p,\,\rho_0} \tag{14-62}$$

where $\beta = (1/V)(\partial V/\partial T)_p$ and c_p is the specific heat at constant pressure. Note that all of the parameters in this equation can be obtained experimentally and that together they provide a unique representation of material properties. Thus the parameter of nonlinearity is a fundamental acoustical property of materials. As we will see in later sections, B/A is now playing an increasingly important role in the quantitative characterization of tissue.

Next we return to the wave equation for pressure, Eq. (14-60) and explore the physical meaning of this nonlinear equation. Note that this equation would be linear if it were not for the term

$$\left(1 + \frac{\partial \xi}{\partial x}\right)^{B/A+2}$$

which divides into the square of the sound speed. Note further that the nonlinear term depends primarily upon the gradient of the displacement. Thus the larger the displacement, the greater is the nonlinear effect. Since the term

$$\frac{c_0^2}{\left(1 + \partial \xi/\partial x\right)^{B/A+2}}$$

represents an effective sound speed squared, the propagation velocity of the sound wave will become amplitude dependent. Clearly, if the displacement is small (i.e., of *infinitesimal* amplitude), the gradient of the displacement is very, very small, the nonlinear term is equal to unity, and the sound speed is a constant c_0. In this case Eq. (14-60) reduces to an ordinary linear wave equation. On the other hand, if the displacement is large (i.e., of *finite* amplitude), the gradient of the displacement is no longer small, the nonlinear term is no longer unity, and the sound speed becomes amplitude dependent. Thus a sound wave of finite amplitude will propagate such that the higher amplitude portions of the wave front will travel at a higher propagation

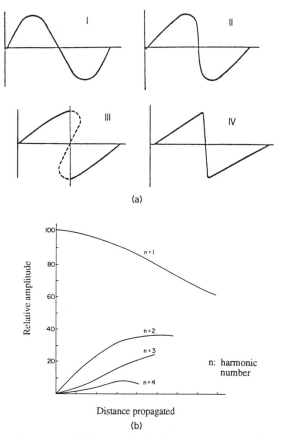

Figure 14-4 (a) A sine wave of finite amplitude distorts as it propagates because higher amplitude portions of the wave travel at higher speeds than do lower amplitude portions. The sine wave is fully distorted into a shock wave after traveling a distance l = the discontinuity distance. (b) As the sine wave distorts, the relative amplitude of the fundamental frequency declines and the harmonics increase in amplitude.

velocity than those portions of the wave front with lower amplitude. This is illustrated in Fig. 14-4(a) where we begin with a sine wave of finite amplitude and show how it becomes distorted as it propagates. The distance over which a sine wave must travel until it is fully distorted into a shock wave is known as the *discontinuity distance l*, which can be shown [2, 3] to assume the following analytical form:

$$l = \frac{c_0^2}{(B/2A + 1)\omega u_0}$$

$$= \left[\left(\frac{B}{2A} + 1 \right) Mk \right]^{-1}$$

where the wave number $k = \omega/c_0$ and $M \equiv u_0/c_0$ is the acoustic mach number. Note that the discontinuity distance depends on the properties of the material $(B/A, c_0)$ as well as the properties of the wave (ω, u_0). Note that as the wave propagates the relative amplitude of the fundamental frequency declines, being replaced by harmonics of ever increasing amplitude. This process is illustrated in Fig. 14-4(b).

After the above discussion the reader will be surprised to learn that to date nonlinear acoustics has not played a major role in medical ultrasonics. Why then should we bother with this topic? There are several reasons. First, it is extremely important for the student to realize that the basic equations of acoustics as well as the basic acoustical processes are fundamentally nonlinear. Any attempt to use the greatly simplified linear forms of acoustics must be thoroughly justified. Such justifications cannot be made without a full understanding of both linear and nonlinear acoustics and the approximations and conditions that lead from one to the other.

Second, although most ultrasound imaging devices operate within a range of parameters for which linear acoustics provides an adequate description, some instruments, particularly those designed for Doppler or color flow imaging, operate on the border line between linear and nonlinear acoustics. Since there are examples where conventional equipment has produced non-linear effects, the student should be prepared to recognize such effects should they occur and apply the appropriate analysis if required.

Third, many therapeutic ultrasound devices operate in the nonlinear regime. Such devices range from low-frequency continuous-wave instruments designed for internal heating for cancer treatment to high-frequency pulsed instruments designed to break down kidney stones (lythotripsy). To fully understand these techniques requires an understanding of nonlinear acoustics.

Finally, the study of the biological effects of ultrasound involves many phenomena that can only be explained in terms of nonlinear acoustics. This includes such things as cavitation, acoustic streaming, and radiation pressure. Readers interested in these important topics will have to consult the more than adequate literature currently available [2, 3, 4]. Further guidelines may be found in Section 14-7.

14-2 REFLECTION AND TRANSMISSION OF PLANE WAVES

The reflection and transmission of plane waves across planar boundaries is a classical acoustics problem whose solution is well known and well documented in the literature [5]. It also provides the basis and formalism for much of the modeling in medical ultrasonics even for situations of far greater complexity. Here we develop in some detail the classical boundary value problem associated with the propagation of a plane wave across a planar boundary. In contrast to other treatments in the literature, we make a clear distinction between alternate formalisms in terms of pressure or in terms of intensity. Since most of our measuring devices in acoustics are pressure sensitive rather than intensity or energy sensitive, it is important to clearly understand the differences between the two formalisms and to realize that the results of one is simply not the square of the results of the other. Having detailed the boundary value problem for the simplest case, the reader should be well prepared to apply a similar analysis to more complicated situations.

14-2-1 Propagation across a Planar Boundary

The reflection (and transmission) of a plane acoustical wave from (and across) a planar boundary has served as a starting point for much of the theoretical developments in acoustics for over 100 years. This problem provides us with the acoustical analog to Snell's law in optics and gives us simple results that can be universally applied with surprisingly good effect to situations far beyond their range of applicability.

In the simplest formulation of the problem, a plane acoustical wave propagating in a homogeneous medium of uniform density ρ_1 and of constant velocity (or sound speed) c_1 is normally incident on a plane boundary separating the first medium from a second homogeneous medium of different acoustical properties represented by ρ_2 and c_2. Solving the simple boundary value problem, which requires that the pressure as well as the particle velocity be equal across the boundary, we find that the wave can be both reflected and transmitted at the boundary and that this reflection/transmission process is dependent upon the acoustical properties (in this case ρ and c) of the two media. Most, if not all, of the theoretical foundations of acoustics are extensions or extrapolations from this simple problem. These extensions include such problems as propagation through multiple boundaries, multiple reflections, propagation at nonnormal angles, and the reflection of nonplane waves from complex geometries. Although the mathematics associated with these problems can be complex, the basic physics is the same and is quite simple. Thus a propagating acoustical wave is reflected if and only if it encounters a change in impedance (or a change in density and/or velocity). These same physical principles serve as a basis for all scattering theory in acoustics. Thus scattering, even from tissue (as we will see in Section 14.6), is a result of changes in impedance or fluctuations in density and sound speed. Since the speed of sound can (as we will see later) be related to the elasticity or the compressibility, most descriptions of scattering are in terms of fluctuations in density and compressibility.

Let us now consider in more detail the propagation of a plane wave across a planar discontinuity in impedance, as shown in Fig. 14.5. Here a plane harmonic wave p_i is propagating (from left to right) in a homogeneous medium defined by its density ρ_1 and its sound speed c_1. We assume that no energy loss occurs during the propagation process; thus the absorption coefficient is zero everywhere. No scattering occurs since the medium is homogeneous. This propagating or incident pressure wave may therefore be

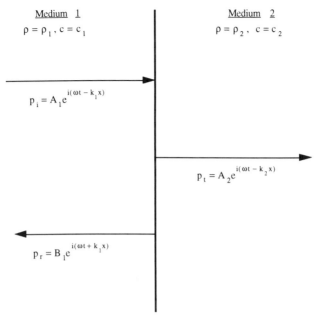

Figure 14-5   The reflection and transmission of a plane wave at a planar boundary.

represented as

$$p_i = A_1 e^{i(\omega t - k_1 x)} \tag{14-63}$$

where A_1 is a constant equal to the amplitude of the wave, t is the time, x is the spatial location, ω is the angular frequency, and k_1 is the wave number (in medium #1). Recall that $k_1 = \omega / c_1$.

Let us assume that p_i is normally incident on a plane parallel boundary that separates the first homogeneous medium from a second homogeneous medium with different acoustical properties. We assume that the second medium is defined by its density ρ_2 and by its sound speed c_2. Our intuition suggests that a portion of the wave will be transmitted across the boundary and that a portion will be reflected. This suggestion is confirmed and quantified by solving the appropriate boundary value problem related to the propagation process. Before undertaking this task, first note that the reflected wave may be described by

$$p_r = B_1 e^{i(\omega t + k_1 x)} \tag{14-64}$$

where B_1 is a constant giving the amplitude of the wave and $+k_1$ denotes propagation from right to left, but in the opposite direction from $-k_1$ in

Eq. (14-63). Similarly the transmitted wave is described by

$$p_t = A_2 e^{i(\omega t - k_2 x)} \tag{14-65}$$

where A_2 is a constant equal to the amplitude of p_t and k_2 is the wave number of the wave in the second medium. This situation is described schematically in Fig. 14-5.

Note that the pressure reflection coefficient r, defined as the ratio of the reflected wave to the incident wave at the boundary, is given by

$$r \equiv \left(\frac{p_r}{p_i} \right) \bigg|_{x=0} = \frac{B_1}{A_1} \tag{14-66}$$

Similarly the pressure transmission coefficient τ, defined as the ratio of the transmitted wave to the incident wave, is given by

$$\tau \equiv \left(\frac{p_t}{p_i} \right) \bigg|_{x=0} = \frac{A_2}{A_1} \tag{14-67}$$

Our goal is to solve explicitly for r and τ. We accomplish this by applying boundary conditions based on fundamental conservation principles. Specifically the application of two boundary conditions yields two equations relating p_i, p_r, and p_t. The simultaneous solution of the two equations allows us to eliminate one constant from the set (A_1, B_1, A_2) and therefore to solve for either r or τ, as shown in Eqs. (14-66) and (14-67).

As the first boundary condition we require that the pressures must be equal at the boundary (which we conveniently position at $x = 0$). That is, conservation of energy requires that the total pressure to the left of the boundary must equal the total pressure to the right of the boundary:

$$p_i|_{x=0} + p_r|_{x=0} = p_t|_{x=0} \tag{14-68}$$

Substituting Eqs. (14-63), (14-64), and (14-65) into Eq. (14-68) gives

$$A_1 + B_1 = A_2 \tag{14-69}$$

which is the final result from the first boundary condition.

As the second boundary condition we require that the particle velocities normal to the interface be equal at the boundary. Thus, if u represents the particle velocity, we require that

$$u_i|_{x=0} + u_r|_{x=0} = u_t|_{x=0} \tag{14-70}$$

Before we can evaluate this boundary condition we must first develop a general expression for the particle velocity. The reader will recall the analysis leading to Eq. (14-7) which is a restatement of Newton's law as it applies to the propagation of a sound wave. Integrating Eq. (14-7) gives

$$u = -\left(\frac{1}{\rho}\right)\int\left(\frac{\partial p}{\partial x}\right)dt \qquad (14\text{-}71)$$

Now, if p is harmonic (as well as plane), then the spatial and temporal dependences can be separated such that

$$p(x, t) \equiv p(x)e^{i\omega t} \qquad (14\text{-}72)$$

Substituting Eq. (14-72) into Eq. (14-71) gives

$$u = -\frac{1}{i\omega\rho}\left[\frac{\partial p(x)}{\partial x}\right]e^{i\omega t}$$

which, using Eq. (14-72) again becomes

$$u = -\frac{1}{i\omega\rho}\frac{\partial p(x, t)}{\partial x} \qquad (14\text{-}73)$$

which is the general expression for the particle velocity that we have sought. Successive substitutions of Eqs. (14-63), (14-64), and (14-65) into Eq. (14-73) gives the particle velocity of the incident wave

$$u_i = -\frac{1}{i\omega\rho_1}\left(\frac{\partial p_i}{\partial x}\right) = \frac{A_1}{\rho_1 c_1}e^{i(\omega t - k_1 x)} \qquad (14\text{-}74)$$

the particle velocity of the reflected wave

$$u_r = -\frac{1}{i\omega\rho_1}\left(\frac{\partial p_r}{\partial x}\right) = \frac{-B_1}{\rho_1 c_1}e^{i(\omega t + k_1 x)} \qquad (14\text{-}75)$$

and the particle velocity of the transmitted wave

$$u_t = -\frac{1}{i\omega\rho_2}\left(\frac{\partial p_t}{\partial x}\right) = \frac{A_2}{\rho_2 c_2}e^{i(\omega t - k_2 x)} \qquad (14\text{-}76)$$

Substituting these last three equations into Eq. (14.70) gives, at $x = 0$,

$$\frac{A_1}{\rho_1 c_1} - \frac{B_1}{\rho_1 c_1} = \frac{A_2}{\rho_2 c_2} \qquad (14\text{-}77)$$

which is the final result from the second boundary condition.

Substituting Eq. (14-69) into Eq. (14-77), we can eliminate the constant A_2. Thus

$$\frac{A_1}{\rho_1 c_1} - \frac{B_1}{\rho_1 c_1} = \frac{A_1}{\rho_2 c_2} + \frac{B_1}{\rho_2 c_2}$$

or

$$A_1\left(\frac{1}{\rho_1 c_1} - \frac{1}{\rho_2 c_2}\right) = B_1\left(\frac{1}{\rho_1 c_1} + \frac{1}{\rho_2 c_2}\right) \qquad (14\text{-}78)$$

Substituting Eq. (14-78) into our definition of the pressure reflection coefficient, Eq. (14-66), we have, after collecting terms,

$$r = \frac{B_1}{A_1} = \frac{\rho_2 c_2 - \rho_1 c_1}{\rho_2 c_2 + \rho_1 c_1} \qquad (14\text{-}79)$$

which is the well-known expression for the reflection of a plane wave from a planar boundary.

We follow a similar process to calculate the pressure transmission coefficient. Thus we substitute Eq. (14-69) into Eq. (14-77) once again, but this time eliminating the constant B_1 rather than A_2. The result is

$$\frac{A_1}{\rho_1 c_1} - \frac{A_2 - A_1}{\rho_1 c_1} = \frac{A_2}{\rho_2 c_2}$$

or

$$A_1\left(\frac{2}{\rho_1 c_1}\right) = A_2\left(\frac{1}{\rho_1 c_1} + \frac{1}{\rho_2 c_2}\right) \qquad (14\text{-}80)$$

Substituting Eq. (14-80) into our definition of the pressure transmission coefficient, Eq. (14-67), we have, after collecting terms,

$$\tau = \frac{A_2}{A_1} = \frac{2\rho_2 c_2}{\rho_1 c_1 + \rho_2 c_2} \qquad (14\text{-}81)$$

which is the expression we have sought describing the transmission of a plane wave across a planar boundary.

It will be useful to consider the expression

$$1 + r$$

Substituting our expression for the pressure reflection coefficient, Eq. (14-79), into this last equation and collecting terms, we can show that

$$1 + r = \tau \tag{14-82}$$

At first glance Eq. (14-82) appears to violate basic conservation principles. Recall, however, that this expression deals with pressure rather than energy or intensity, so its form is perfectly appropriate. The (perhaps) more familiar relationship between the intensity (or energy) reflection and transmission coefficients can be derived in a similar fashion to the above analysis by merely substituting the correct expression for intensity for that of pressure.

For our purposes here it is easier to calculate the intensity directly (and from that the energy reflection and transmission coefficients) rather than repeat the earlier boundary value problem. Recall from Section 14-1-2 that the intensity of a plane wave is given by

$$I = \tfrac{1}{2}\rho c u^2 \tag{14-83}$$

Successive substitutions of Eqs. (14-74), (14-75), and (14-76) into Eq. (14-83) gives

$$I_i = \frac{A_1^2}{2\rho_1 c_1}$$

$$I_r = \frac{B_1^2}{2\rho_1 c_1}$$

$$I_t = \frac{A_2^2}{2\rho_2 c_2} \tag{14-84}$$

Defining the energy (or intensity) reflection coefficient R as

$$R \equiv \frac{I_r}{I_i} \tag{14-85}$$

we have with Eqs. (14-84) and (14-79)

$$R = \frac{B_1^2}{A_1^2} = r^2 \tag{14-86}$$

Defining the energy (or intensity) transmission coefficient T as

$$T \equiv \frac{I_t}{I_i} \tag{14-87}$$

we have with Eqs. (14-84) and (14-81)

$$T = \left(\frac{A_2^2}{A_1^2} \right) \left(\frac{\rho_1 c_1}{\rho_2 c_2} \right) = \tau^2 \left(\frac{\rho_1 c_1}{\rho_2 c_2} \right) \tag{14-88}$$

Combining Eqs. (14-86) and (14-88), we have

$$R + T = 1 \tag{14-89}$$

which is the familiar relationship between reflection and transmission that is a direct result of the conservation of energy.

It is perhaps useful to summarize our findings here for the propagation of a plane wave across a planar boundary. In terms of the characteristic impedance $Z = \rho c$, we can write

$$r \equiv \frac{p_r}{p_i} = \frac{Z_2 - Z_1}{Z_1 + Z_2}$$

$$\tau = \frac{p_t}{p_i} = \frac{2Z_2}{Z_1 + Z_2}$$

$$1 + r = \tau$$

$$R = \frac{I_r}{I_i} = \left(\frac{Z_2 - Z_1}{Z_1 + Z_2} \right)^2 = r^2$$

$$T = \frac{I_t}{I_i} = \frac{4Z_1 Z_2}{(Z_1 + Z_2)^2} = \tau^2 \left(\frac{Z_1}{Z_2} \right)$$

$$R + T = 1 \tag{14-90}$$

14-2-2   Propagation through a Layer

It will prove useful to consider the propagation of a plane wave through a planar layer. Suppose that the two homogeneous half-planes of Fig. 14-5 are separated by a layer of thickness l. Our task is to calculate the transmission coefficient for a plane wave that travels through the layer. The situation is shown schematically in Fig. 14-6 and is known as the three-layer problem. Although the algebraic details are too involved to give here, the transmission coefficient can easily be found following the analysis of Section 14-2-1. Since it is instructive to examine the results for a specific special case, we simply write down the energy (or intensity) transmission coefficient from medium 1 into medium 3 (i.e., across the boundary). The result is

$$T_{13} \equiv \frac{I_{t3}}{I_{i1}} = \frac{A_3^2/2Z_2}{A_1^2/2Z_1} \tag{14-91}$$

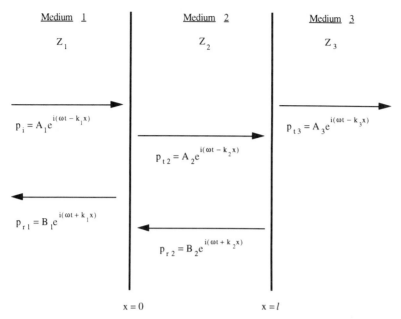

Figure 14-6   Propagation through a layer. Under certain conditions 100% of the energy can be transmitted from medium 1 into medium 3.

which, after application of the boundary conditions at $x = 0$ and at $x = l$, becomes

$$T_{13} = \frac{4}{2 + [(Z_3/Z_1) + (Z_1/Z_3)]\cos^2 k_2 l + [(Z_2^2/Z_1 Z_3) + (Z_1 Z_3/Z_2^2)]\sin^2 k_2 l} \tag{14-92}$$

The reader can easily show that

$$T_{13} \equiv 1 \tag{14-93}$$

if

$$l = \frac{(2n - 1)\lambda_2}{4} \tag{14-94}$$

where n is an integer, $n \geq 1$, and if

$$Z_2 = \sqrt{Z_1 Z_3} \tag{14-95}$$

Thus 100% of the energy in medium 1 can be transmitted across the layer into medium 3 provided that the layer is a quarter wavelength thick, or a

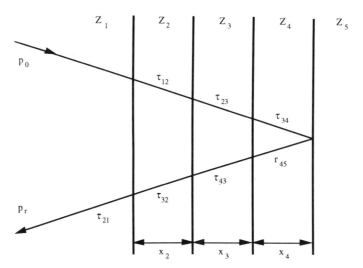

Figure 14-7   Notation for tracing an ultrasonic wave through several layers.

$(2n - 1)$ multiple, and provided that the impedance of the layer is equal to the geometric mean of the adjacent impedances. This result is the basis for the so-called quarter-wavelength matching layer used with medical ultrasonic transducers. Such analysis provides a means for maximizing the amount of energy transferred from the transducer (medium 1) into the human body (medium 3).

14-2-3   Propagation through Multiple Layers

The propagation of ultrasound in tissue is inherently a problem of propagation through multiple layers. For many situations, and certainly for order-of-magnitude estimates, tissue can be modeled as a series of parallel layers. In these cases the formalism of the previous two sections provides a means for making such calculations. As a practical matter it is certainly not necessary to re-solve the boundary value problem each time. In fact the use of simple notation, as illustrated in Fig. 14-7 allows us to trace an ultrasound pulse through a series of layers and return. Here the notation is key. Note that the pressure reflection coefficient for the reflection from the jth layer of a wave propagating in the ith layer is

$$r_{ij} = \frac{Z_j - Z_i}{Z_i + Z_j} \qquad (14\text{-}96)$$

Similarly

$$\tau_{ij} = \frac{2Z_j}{Z_i + Z_j} \tag{14-97}$$

Using this notation, we can easily calculate the amplitude of the pressure wave p_r that has propagated through the layers, as indicated in Fig. 14-7, and returned to medium 1. By inspection the result is

$$p_r = p_0 \tau_{12} \tau_{23} \tau_{34} r_{45} \tau_{43} \tau_{32} \tau_{21} \tag{14-98a}$$

Recalling that $1 + r = \tau$ and that

$$\tau_{ij} = 1 + r_{ij}$$
$$\tau_{ji} = 1 + r_{ji} = 1 - r_{ij}$$

Eq. (14-98a) can be further simplified to

$$p_r = p_0 \left(1 - r_{12}^2\right)\left(1 - r_{23}^2\right)\left(1 - r_{34}^2\right) r_{45} \tag{14-98b}$$

The effects of absorption can easily be included in this formalism. If α_i is the absorption coefficient associated with the ith layer whose thickness is given by x_i, then the term

$$\exp\left[-2(\alpha_2 x_2 + \alpha_3 x_3 + \alpha_4 x_4)\right] \tag{14-99}$$

when multiplied by the right-hand side of Eq. (14-98b) includes the effects of absorption.

14-3 RADIATION AND RECEPTION

Thus far in our discussion of ultrasound physics we have limited ourselves to the propagation of sound. Now we turn our attention to the radiation and reception of sound. We will show how even a complex radiator can be described in terms of a collection of simple sources and how the radiation from simple sources can be derived from first principles. Finally, we introduce reciprocity techniques as a means for both calibration and measurement. Our goal is not to provide a description of a particular transducer but rather to develop the framework within which all sources and receivers may be described.

14-3-1 Simple Sources

Assuming that even the most complex acoustical source can be modeled as a collection of simple sources (i.e., a distribution of monopole and/or dipole sources), we seek to obtain an analytical expression that describes the

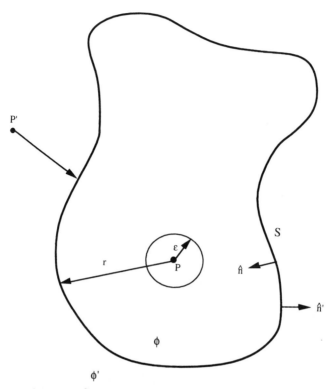

Figure 14-8   Surface S within which the functions ϕ and Ψ are defined.

radiation field produced by appropriate distributions of simple sources. Let us begin with an integral identity known as Green's theorem. If ϕ and Ψ are continuous and have continuous first derivatives in a region bounded by the closed surface S and the volume V, then

$$\int_V (\phi \nabla^2 \Psi - \Psi \nabla^2 \phi)\, dV = \int_S \left(\phi \frac{\partial \Psi}{\partial \hat{n}} - \Psi \frac{\partial \phi}{\partial \hat{n}} \right) dS \qquad (14\text{-}100)$$

which is a statement of Green's theorem. Here $\hat{n}$ is a unit normal vector pointing inward as shown in Fig. 14-8. As a further restriction on ϕ and Ψ, let us assume that both satisfy the ordinary wave equation [e.g., Eq. (14-27b)] and have a harmonic time dependence (i.e., $e^{i\omega t}$). Under such conditions

$$\nabla^2 \phi = -\left(\frac{\omega^2}{c^2} \right) \phi$$

$$\nabla^2 \Psi = -\left(\frac{\omega^2}{c^2} \right) \Psi$$

Substituting this result into Eq. (14-100), we find that the volume integral on the left-hand side of the equation is identically zero,

$$\int_S \left(\phi \frac{\partial \Psi}{\partial \hat{n}} - \Psi \frac{\partial \phi}{\partial \hat{n}} \right) dS = 0 \qquad (14\text{-}101)$$

if ϕ and Ψ are solutions to the wave equation. Let us further assume that Ψ has a particularly simple form, namely that it represents a spherical wave solution to the wave equation.

$$\Psi = \frac{e^{-ikr}}{r}$$

Clearly Ψ is not defined at the point of origin P. To get around this singularity, we construct a small sphere of radius ε around point P, integrate along S as well as the surface of radius ε, and finally take the limit as $\varepsilon \to 0$. Substituting this form for Ψ into Eq. (14-101) and integrating along S as well as the sphere of radius ε gives

$$\int_S \phi \frac{\partial}{\partial \hat{n}} \left(\frac{e^{-ikr}}{r} \right) dS - \int_S \left(\frac{e^{-ikr}}{r} \right) \frac{\partial \phi}{\partial \hat{n}} \, dS$$

$$+ \phi_p \frac{\partial}{\partial \hat{n}} \left(\frac{e^{-ik\varepsilon}}{\varepsilon} \right) 4\pi\varepsilon^2 - \left(\frac{e^{ik\varepsilon}}{\varepsilon} \right) \left(\frac{\partial \phi}{\partial \hat{n}} \right)_p 4\pi\varepsilon^2 = 0 \quad (14\text{-}102)$$

where the integral over the sphere of radius ε is replaced by the integrand. Evaluating the last two terms of this equation and taking the limit as $\varepsilon \to 0$ gives

$$-4\pi\phi_p$$

where $(\partial\varepsilon / \partial\hat{n}) = 1$ and ϕ_p is the value of ϕ at point P. Thus Eq. (14-102) becomes

$$\phi_p = \frac{-1}{4\pi} \int_S \frac{e^{-ikr}}{r} \frac{\partial \phi}{\partial \hat{n}} \, dS + \frac{1}{4\pi} \int_S \phi \frac{\partial}{\partial \hat{n}} \left(\frac{e^{-ikr}}{r} \right) dS \qquad (14\text{-}103)$$

Let us now suppose that the point of origin is outside the surface S at P'. Repeating the above derivation, we obtain the same result with the following modifications:

$$\phi_{p'} \equiv 0$$
$$\phi \text{ (within } S) \to \phi'(\text{outside } S)$$
$$\hat{n} \to \hat{n}'$$

as shown in Fig. 14-8. Thus, for points outside the surface S, Eq. (14-103) becomes

$$0 = \frac{-1}{4\pi} \int_S \frac{e^{-ikr}}{r} \left(\frac{\partial \phi'}{\partial \hat{n}'} \right) dS + \frac{1}{4\pi} \int_S \phi' \frac{\partial}{\partial \hat{n}'} \left(\frac{e^{-ikr}}{r} \right) dS \quad (14\text{-}104)$$

Adding together Eqs. (14-103) and (14-104) and using the fact that $(\partial/\partial \hat{n}') = -(\partial/\partial \hat{n})$, we have for all space

$$\phi_p = \frac{-1}{4\pi} \int_S \frac{e^{-ikr}}{r} \left(\frac{\partial \phi}{\partial \hat{n}} - \frac{\partial \phi'}{\partial \hat{n}} \right) dS + \frac{1}{4\pi} \int_S (\phi - \phi') \frac{\partial}{\partial \hat{n}} \left(\frac{e^{-ikr}}{r} \right) dS$$

$$(14\text{-}105)$$

Since S can be any surface, let us take it to be a plane perpendicular to the z-axis of some rectangular coordinate system and therefore parallel to or coincident with the $x - y$ plane. Now we have a choice of two boundary conditions: At the boundary either the functions ϕ and ϕ' are equal or their normal derivatives are equal. Choosing the first of these boundary conditions, we have

$$\phi(x, y, -z) = \phi'(x, y, z)$$

which means that

$$\frac{\partial \phi}{\partial \hat{n}} = -\frac{\partial \phi'}{\partial \hat{n}}$$

Substituting this result into Eq. (14-105) gives

$$\phi_p = \frac{-1}{4\pi} \int_S \left(\frac{e^{-ikr}}{r} \right) \left(2 \frac{\partial \phi}{\partial \hat{n}} \right) dS \quad (14\text{-}106)$$

This is the diffraction integral first used by Lord Rayleigh to represent the radiation field associated with a distribution of point sources on a surface. Note that the term

$$\frac{e^{-ikr}}{r}$$

represents the radiation from a point source (which generates a spherical wavelet). If this term is multiplied by the density of such point sources on a surface and the product integrated over the surface the result is simply the value of some wave parameter at any point P in space. This is an extremely important result for it allows us, with some knowledge of the acoustical source, to compute the effects of that radiation at any point in space. For example, suppose that S is the surface of an ultrasonic transducer that we model as a collection of point sources on the surface. If ϕ is the velocity potential, which can be defined and measured at the surface of the transducer, then $2(\partial\phi/\partial\hat{n})$ represents the density of point sources that produces the radiation field, and ϕ_p gives us the value of the velocity potential at the field point P. In the section that follows we use the formalism of Eq. (14-106) to describe the radiation of a plane piston source, which is perhaps the best model for current medical ultrasound transducers.

For completeness let us return to Eq. (14-105) and apply the second possible boundary condition. In this case

$$\frac{\partial\phi(x, y, -z)}{\partial\hat{n}} = -\frac{\partial\phi'(x, y, z)}{\partial\hat{n}}$$

which means that

$$\phi = -\phi'$$

at the boundary. Substituting this result into Eq. (14-105) gives

$$\phi_p = \frac{1}{4\pi}\int_S 2\phi \frac{\partial}{\partial\hat{n}}\left(\frac{e^{-ikr}}{r}\right) dS \qquad (14\text{-}107)$$

Note that the term

$$\frac{\partial}{\partial\hat{n}}\left(\frac{e^{-ikr}}{r}\right)$$

represents the normal derivative to the planar surface S of a spherical source at the surface. This is of course just a dipole source. Thus Eq. (14-107) describes the radiation of a collection of dipole sources distributed with a density 2ϕ on the surface S. This result is clearly important for the calculation of more complex radiation fields.

14-3-2   The Plane-Piston Source

The basic and most fundamental model for all ultrasonic transducers is the plane piston source, that is, a disk of a radius a that moves back and forth like a piston along its major axis to generate a sound wave. Although many transducers today have different geometries and are even formed into arrays, the same basic analysis used for the piston source serves as the basis for all transducer modeling. Since the analysis for even a simplified model of the plane piston source is rather involved, we can only outline a calculation here and urge the interested reader to complete the analysis and consult the extensive literature for more realistic situations.

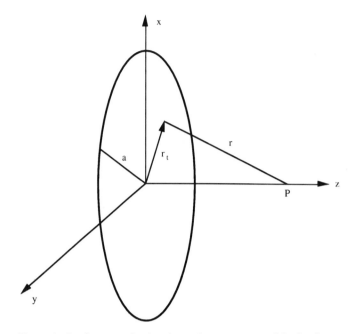

Figure 14-9   Geometry for the plane-piston source, a disk of radius a.

We begin by returning to Eq. (14-106), which we apply to the circular disk of Fig. 14-9. Let P be a point along the z-axis and ϕ the velocity potential. Let the disk of radius a be contained in the $x - y$ plane and centered on the z-axis. We assume that the vibrating disk is fully clamped at its boundaries (clearly a condition that cannot be realized in practice) and moves as if it were mounted in an infinitely rigid wall or baffle. The boundary conditions are then given by

$$u = \begin{cases} \dfrac{\partial \phi}{\partial \hat{n}} = u_0 e^{i\omega t}, & r_t \le a \\ 0, & r_t > a \end{cases}$$

Substituting this result into Eq. (14-106), we have

$$\phi_p = -\frac{u_0 e^{i\omega t}}{2\pi} \int_0^a \frac{e^{-ikr}}{r} 2\pi r_t \, dr_t$$

which reduces to

$$\phi_p = -\frac{iu_0 e^{i\omega t}}{k} [e^{-ikr_a} - e^{-ikz}]$$

where $r_a^2 = z^2 + a^2$. Using the expression

$$p = -\rho_0 \dot{\phi}$$

to calculate the pressure and the expression

$$I = \frac{\left\langle [\mathrm{Re}(p)]^2 \right\rangle_{\mathrm{ave}}}{\rho_0 c}$$

to calculate the intensity, we have finally the approximate result for the on-axis intensity:

$$I \approx 2\rho_0 c u_0^2 \sin^2 \left[\left(\frac{\pi}{2} \right) \left(\frac{a^2/\lambda}{z} \right) \right] \qquad (14\text{-}108)$$

A graph of this result is shown in Fig. 14-10. Note that the axial intensity goes through a number of oscillations for axial positions smaller than a^2/λ. For positions greater than this last maximum the intensity slowly declines (actually the result of beam spreading). The so-called focal zone for the plane piston source located at $z = a^2/\lambda$ represents a transition between the near field (Fresnel zone) and the far field (Fraunhofer zone). A more complete analysis of the plane-piston source shows that the pressure profile in the near field is quite complex while the pressure in the far field is uniform, spreading slowly with increasing distance. Similar beam structures are seen even with transducer arrays.

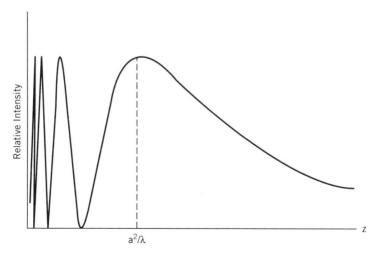

Figure 14-10 The on-axis intensity for a plane-piston source.

14-3-3 Reciprocity and Transducer Measurement

Generally the absolute measurement of the pressure of an acoustical wave, it turns out, is an exceedingly difficult task. Thus most of our measurements of pressure or intensity are relative ones (hence the decibel scale). However, given one transducer that has been subjected to absolute calibration, other transducers can be calibrated from this one using the principle of reciprocity. Given two transducers that are uncalibrated but are known to be identical, then reciprocity once again permits an absolute calibration. Even more impressive, the concept of self-reciprocity allows us to calibrate a single transducer from a set of simple physical measurements. Thus the concept of reciprocity is essential to any transducer measurement and is important to almost every aspect of ultrasonic imaging.

To develop the formalism of acoustical reciprocity, we return once again to Green's theorem, Eq. (14-100), which reduces to Eq. (14-101) provided that both ϕ and Ψ satisfy the wave equation. Let us make the following identifications in Eq. (14-101):

$\phi = p_1 =$ pressure produced by transducer #1
$\Psi = p_2 =$ pressure produced by transducer #2

Then, given that $p = i\omega\rho_0\phi$ with $u = \nabla\phi$, we have

$$\int_S (p_1 \times u_2 - p_2 \times u_1) \cdot \hat{n}\, dS \qquad (14\text{-}109)$$

Let us assume that both sources are spherical and of radius a and that they are small with respect to a wavelength. The pressure is then uniform over the source and can be removed from the integrand. In addition the integral can be replaced by the area of the source. Thus Eq. (14-109) becomes

$$p_1 \times 4\pi a^2 u_{2_0} = p_2 \times 4\pi a^2 u_{1_0} \qquad (14\text{-}110)$$

Defining the source strength Q as the product of the area of the source with the amplitude of the particle velocity, we have

$$Q_1 \equiv 4\pi a^2 u_{1_0}$$

and Eq. (14-110) becomes

$$\frac{Q_1}{p_1} = \frac{Q_2}{p_2} \qquad (14\text{-}111)$$

The ratio of the source strength to the pressure is a constant J_s and is known as the (spherical) wave reciprocity parameter. Using earlier expressions for both Q and p, we can now write

$$\frac{Q}{p} = \frac{4\pi a^2 u_0}{\rho_0 c u_0 a^2 k/r} = \frac{4\pi r}{\rho_0 c k} = \frac{2\lambda r}{\rho_0 c} \equiv J_s \tag{14-112}$$

To understand how this parameter can be used for transducer calibration, let us first look at the reciprocity arrangements common for electroacoustics. Two electrical circuits are reciprocal if the ratio of voltage e to current i is constant:

$$\frac{e_1}{i_1} = \frac{e_2}{i_2} \tag{14-113}$$

Since the acoustical analog of voltage is pressure (or force F) and the acoustical analog of current is particle velocity, we can rewrite Eq. (14-113) in its electroacoustical form as

$$\frac{e}{u} = \frac{F}{i} \tag{14-114}$$

Using Eq. (14-112), the pressure p_s produced by a spherical source is

$$p_s = \frac{\rho_0 c Q}{2\lambda r} = \frac{A \rho_0 c u}{2\lambda r} \tag{14-115}$$

where A is the surface area of the source.

If the same transducer is used as a microphone (i.e., as receiver or hydrophone), then the incident pressure wave p_i produces a force

$$F = p_i A \tag{14-116}$$

Combining the last three equations, the electroacoustical reciprocity relation becomes

$$\frac{e}{p_i A} = \frac{p_s}{i} \left(\frac{2\lambda r}{A \rho_0 c} \right) \tag{14-117}$$

Defining the receiving (or microphone) response M as

$$M \equiv \frac{e}{p_i} \tag{14-118a}$$

and the transmitting (or source) response S as

$$S \equiv \frac{p_s}{i} \tag{14-118b}$$

Eq. (14-117) becomes

$$\frac{M}{S} = \frac{2\lambda_r}{\rho_0 c} = J_s \tag{14-119}$$

where we have compared the results with Eq. (14-112). Thus the (spherical) wave reciprocity parameter not only can be expressed in terms of the physical parameters of the medium but also is equal to the ratio of the receiving and transmitting responses of the transducer.

Similar expressions can be derived for transducers (and waves) of different geometries. Here we merely state the results

$$J_p = \frac{2A(\lambda r)^0}{\rho c} = \frac{2A}{\rho c} \qquad \text{(plane-wave reciprocity parameter)}$$

$$J_c = \frac{2L(\lambda r)^{1/2}}{\rho c} \qquad \text{(cylindrical-wave reciprocity parameter)}$$

$$J_s = \frac{2(\lambda r)}{\rho c} \qquad \text{(spherical-wave reciprocity parameter)} \tag{14-120}$$

Here A is the area of the plane-wave transducer and L is the length of the line source that would produce cylindrical waves.

The application of this formalism to transducer calibration should be evident. Given two identical transducers and a particular physical arrangement the applicable reciprocity parameter is calculated. Using one of the transducers as a source and the other as a receiver, measurements of input voltage and output current are made. Reversing the transducers, similar measurements are made. Incorporating these experimental measurements into Eqs. (14-118) and (14-119), we have a set of equations from which we can determine the pressure. This in turn gives us values for M and S, which completes the calibration. A single transducer can also be calibrated using an appropriate experimental arrangement. We leave the specifications of such self-reciprocity procedures as an interesting exercise for the reader.

14-3-4   Intensity of Pulsed Fields

Finally, in this section dealing with the formalism of acoustical measurement we should at least mention the problem associated with the definition of intensity when applied to pulsed fields. For a continuous acoustical wave the definition of intensity is clear and straightforward [e.g., Eq. (14-36)]. However, this definition becomes ambiguous when applied to pulses of acoustical energy. With pulsed fields there are in fact four different ways in which the intensity can be defined. They are

I_{SATA}: spatial average, temporal average intensity

I_{SATP}: spatial average, temporal peak intensity

I_{SPTP}: spatial peak, temporal peak intensity

I_{SPTA}: spatial peak, temporal average intensity

The name associated with each of these intensities are suggestive of the associated measurement procedure. For example, for I(SPTA), which is particularly relevant for biomedical applications, the peak spatial intensity of the pulse is determined and then averaged over time, taking into account the pulse duration and repetition rate.

14-4   PROPAGATION IN FLUIDS

Thus far our discussion of ultrasound physics has assumed that the medium in which the acoustical wave is propagating is an ideal fluid; homogeneous, loss-less, and only able to support longitudinal waves. Although real fluids can be homogeneous and, for the most part, do not support a shear stress, they are seldom loss-less. Here we examine the acoustical properties of "real" fluids and review two models that taken together can largely explain their behavior.

14-4-1   Viscosity and Propagation in Classical Fluids

When an ultrasonic wave propagates in a real fluid some of the energy associated with the wave is absorbed or transformed into other forms of energy. This loss of energy by frictional forces was first described by Sir George Stokes in 1845 who analyzed the effects of viscosity on the propagation of sound in a gas. Gustav Kirchhoff in 1868 extended the work of Stokes to include the effects of heat conduction. Taken together their work forms the basis for what has become known as the classical theory of absorption. A wave equation can be formulated that includes the effects of viscosity and heat conduction. Such a formulation now known as the Navier-Stokes equation [6] draws from classical mechanics as well as thermodynamics and describes a process that is reversible, adiabatic, and isentropic. A plane-wave solution to this equation (which time constraints do not allow us to derive) could be of the form

$$p = p_0 e^{-i(kx - \omega t)} e^{-\alpha x} \qquad (14\text{-}121)$$

where α is the absorption coefficient. Substituting this expression for pressure into the wave equation and solving for α gives

$$\alpha_{\text{class}} = \frac{\omega^2}{\rho_0 c^3}\left[\frac{4\eta_s}{3} + \frac{(\gamma - 1)\chi}{C_p}\right]\tag{14-122}$$

where α_{class} specifically denotes absorption due to viscosity and heat conduction, η_s is the coefficient of shear viscosity, γ is the ratio of specific heats, C_p is the heat capacity at constant pressure, and χ is the thermal conductivity. The important result here is that the classical theory of absorption yields an absorption coefficient that is proportional to the square of the frequency. Thus

$$\alpha_{\text{class}} \sim \omega^2$$

or

$$\frac{\alpha_{\text{class}}}{\omega^2} = \text{constant}$$

Although the classical theory of absorption can describe, at least qualitatively, the loss mechanism in a number of real fluids, it is clear from experimental studies that other effects are also involved. For example, although the absorption of sound in pure water is proportional to the square of the frequency, the magnitude of the absorption, as predicted by Eq. (14-122), is several orders of magnitude too low. The excess absorption, it turns out, is due to ionic disassociations that occur in water and can be described in terms of various relaxation effects as detailed next.

14-4-2 Relaxation Processes

In addition to the frictional forces associated with viscosity and heat conduction, which result in the so-called classical mechanisms of absorption, there exist other mechanisms that contribute to the absorption of sound in fluids. Extensive experimental studies conducted over many years have identified a variety of processes that remove energy from the interrogating sound wave and return it at an appreciably later time in the wave cycle. Such processes are most easily described in terms of a relaxation phenomenon and an associated relaxation time as shown in Fig. 14-11. For example, the translational motion of the sound wave could have an effect on the vibrational or rotational structure of the fluid such that at certain frequencies structural rearrangements could occur fueled by the energy of the sound wave and cause an effective increase in absorption, as shown in Fig. 14-11. Such

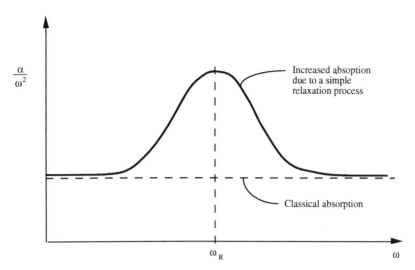

Figure 14-11   Increased absorption due to a single relaxation peak at ω_R. The relaxation time is $\tau = 1/\omega_R$.

processes are no longer isentropic, although they may be adiabatic. A full analysis requires irreversible thermodynamics.

As the structural complexity of a fluid increases, the number of relaxation processes required to describe the absorption of sound also increases. The absorption coefficient α_R for a collection of relaxation processes is most conveniently written as the following sum:

$$\alpha_R = \omega^2 \sum_{i=1}^{n} \frac{A_i}{1 + \left(\omega/\omega_{R_i}\right)^2} \qquad (14\text{-}123)$$

where A_i is a descriptive constant or function associated with the ith process. The total absorption coefficient α is then given by the sum of Eqs. (14-122) and (14-123), or

$$\alpha = \alpha_{\text{class}} + \alpha_R \qquad (14\text{-}124)$$

In general, relaxation processes not only raise the magnitude of the absorption over its "classical" value but also change the frequency dependence. As the number of relaxation processes increases, the absorption coefficient goes from $\alpha \sim \omega^2$ to $\alpha \sim \omega$. In fact it can be shown that as the number of processes becomes infinite [$n \to \infty$ in Eq. (14-123)], the frequency dependence of α goes to unity. This analysis is in keeping with experiment:

Complex solutions of macromolecules (as well as tissue) have absorption coefficients that have a near-unity dependence on frequency.

14-4-3   Propagation in Real Fluids and Tissue

Equation (14-124), which represents the sum of so-called classical absorption and absorption due to a variety of relaxation processes, provides an appropriate formalism to describe the absorption of sound in "real" fluids and gives considerable insight to the propagating of sound in tissue. Given a detailed knowledge of the structure of a fluid, this equation can be used, with appropriate physical modeling, to compute the absorption of sound as a function of frequency. Such calculations are, almost without exception, in good agreement with experiment. The inverse problem, determining the structure of the fluid from a knowledge of the absorption coefficient, is much more difficult, and in most cases not unique, but under certain conditions and restrictions it can provide a powerful investigative tool. As we will see later, similar conclusions apply to tissue. In the remaining paragraphs of this section we briefly detail the acoustical properties of a number of selected fluids in the context of our model represented by Eq. (14-124). We begin with water and continue with solutions of ever increasing complexity.

Although pure water would seem to be the most simple of fluids, the ionic disassociation that occurs greatly enhances the magnitude of the absorption (described by a broad relaxation process) while keeping the frequency dependence the same as that for classical absorption. Seawater exhibits additional excess absorption that can be explained by two chemical relaxation mechanisms: one below 1 kHz due to a small amount of boric acid and a second below 500 kHz due to magnesium sulfate.

The absorption of sound in simple electrolyte solutions (e.g., sodium sulfate, formic acid, acetic acid, copper acetate, and ammonia) is well described by a single relaxation process (plus classical absorption). Since the ionic structure imposes a denser local order, an increase in concentration increases the sound speed and broadens the relaxation curve. A number of nonelectrolyte solutions are also characterized by a single relaxation process. These include water solutions of acetone, methanol, and ethanol.

Amino acids, the basic building blocks of proteins, are relatively simple organic molecules consisting of at least one amino group and one carboxyl group connected by a wide variety of other organic groups [see Fig. 14-12(a)]. In water, amino acids can exist in a number of forms depending on the pH and the ionic strength of the solution. At low pH the carboxyl groups are un-ionized, while the amino groups are ionized. The situation is reversed at high pH. At intermediate pH the amino acid can take on dipole or multipole forms, as shown in Fig. 14-12(b) for glycine, a particular amino acid. Sound propagation in solutions of amino acids depends very strongly on the structure assumed by the molecule and therefore is determined to a great extent by the environment (concentration, pH, etc.). Surprisingly a single relaxation

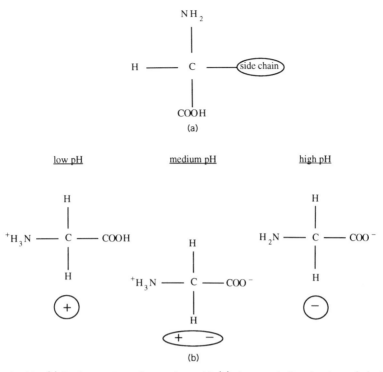

Figure 14-12 (a) Basic structure of an amino acid; (b) changes in the structure of glycine as a function of pH.

process is sufficient to describe the absorption of sound in amino acid solutions, at least in the 1- to 100-MHz frequency range. However, the details of the relaxation peak are easily altered by environmental factors, as might be expected.

Peptides are strings or chains of identical amino acids, each one connected to its immediate neighbor by a peptide bond. Polypeptides are just peptides with a large number (≥ 100) of amino acid residues. Large polypeptides may have rather complex structures consisting of (1) a primary structure consisting of a chain or backbone sequence of amino acids, (2) a secondary structure produced by intrachain bonding and interactions with the surrounding medium (e.g., water), and (3) a tertiary structure produced by 3-D orientation.

The absorption of sound in the simplest of peptides can be described by a single relaxation process, which is clearly a function of such parameters as temperature, concentration, and pH. The more complex polypeptides require a series of relaxation processes to affect an appropriate description. For example, many polypeptides have a secondary structure that is helical in form and is maintained by weak hydrogen and hydrophobic interactions. An ultrasonic wave, given the right conditions, can disrupt these weak bonds leading to a perfectly normal random coil configuration. The energy required to produce this change in structure comes from the ultrasound and represents an additional component to the total absorption coefficient.

Proteins are large biopolymers whose repeating subunits are the amino acids. They range in molecular weights from 5000 to 10^6. Proteins are generally linear in form but may have helical secondary structure based on hydrogen bonding as well as intrachain and interchain higher-order structuring formed by covalent sulfur bridges.

It is constructive if we examine in more detail the structure of one particular protein. Our choice is hemoglobin, an important globular protein with a molecular weight of 68,000. With only minor differences this protein is present in all mammals as well as in many lower species. Its prime function is the transport of oxygen from the lungs to the tissue and to carry away carbon dioxide. Hemoglobin consists of four polypeptide chains: two identical α-chains and two identical β-chains. Each of the four chains contains about 140 amino acid residues that interlink and adhere together to form a characteristic globular aggregate. Within the molecule there are four levels of structural hierarchy:

1. Primary: the backbone amino acid sequences.
2. Secondary: the helical sequences of the chain.
3. Tertiary: the folding and interdigitating of the helical bonds in space.
4. Quaternary: the bonding between the four chains.

Clearly this is much more complex than polypeptides. As expected, the absorption of sound in hemoglobin is characterized by a broad spectrum of relaxation frequencies. Given the complexity of the interactions and structures, attempts to predict the absorption from the structure have been quite successful, at least in a number of specific situations.

The propagation of sound in cells and cell suspensions is qualitatively similar to that involving proteins. Clearly a broad spectrum of relaxation frequencies is involved. However, the level of complexity is so much greater that most attempts to predict the absorption from the structure have not been successful. More fundamentally, our knowledge of the interaction of ultrasound with the cell is at best sketchy. Certainly the intrusion of ultrasound into a complex and dynamic system such as the cell can be expected to give rise to interactions of varying degrees of importance and possibly to changes of biological significance. Some cells (e.g., nerve and muscle) should experience high stresses at lower intensities because fatigue mechanisms are likely to occur. The sensitivities of different cell components to different parameters of the ultrasonic beam has yet to be fully explored. Apparently there is considerable variability in the relative fragility of chromosomes, nuclei, and cell membranes. In short, the propagation of ultrasound in cells is still far from understood. The mechanisms have yet to be fully quantified, and their dependence on such factors as temperature, pH, aggregation of cells, and parameters of the ultrasound beam have yet to be explored.

Finally, we turn to the propagation of sound in tissue. Surprisingly the greater complexities lead to phenomenalogical descriptions of considerable simplicity. For example, the spectrum of relaxation frequencies that describes the absorption of sound in hemoglobin leads to a plot of α versus ω that is quite complex. Soft tissue, on the other hand, with an even larger number of relaxation frequencies has a relationship between absorption and frequency that is almost linear and that is near constant in slope over the range of diagnostic frequencies. Although a detailed understanding may not be at hand, relatively simple relationships seem to exist between the acoustical properties of tissue and tissue type/tissue state. To zeroth order soft tissue might be viewed as a homogeneous media characterized by absorption and sound speed. A first-order description of tissue would have to include scattering and the basic inhomogeneous nature of tissue which in fact makes imaging possible. As we will see in Section 14.6, when we discuss scattering in some detail, tissue can perhaps best be modeled as a lossy medium with velocity and impedance inhomogeneities.

14-5 PROPAGATION IN SOLIDS

So far our development of ultrasound physics has assumed that the medium in which the sound wave is propagating is fluid or fluidlike and therefore only able to support longitudinal waves. The propagation of sound in solids is quite different because solids (by their definition) can support a shear stress. Thus both transverse (or shear) and longitudinal waves can be propagated in a solid. In general, for any given direction of propagation in a solid, three different modes with mutually orthogonal displacements are possible: one longitudinal wave and two transverse waves. Although the details of the propagation process are complex, they clearly depend on the structure of the solid.

Since soft tissue will generally not support a shear stress and is better modeled as a fluid rather than a solid, why then should we be concerned with sound propagation in solids? There are four reasons. First, some soft tissues apparently do support shear wave propagation, at least over a limited range. Second, bone and some cartilage are in fact solids. Third, mode conversion, the apparent attenuation that occurs at a fluid/solid interface when the energy associated with one mode of propagation is transformed into a second, can play an important role in describing the propagation of sound in tissue. And fourth, ultrasonic transducers can only fully be described by using the theory of elasticity.

In this section we briefly outline the formalism necessary to describe the propagation of sound in solids, oriented toward medical ultrasound applications. For a more complete treatment the reader is referred to the extensive literature available [7, 8, 9].

14-5-1 A Generalized Description of Stress and Strain

Suppose two points in a solid are separated by the distance dl. Given the coordinate system (x_1, x_2, x_3), this distance can be represented by

$$(dl)^2 = (dx_1)^2 + (dx_2)^2 + (dx_3)^2 \tag{14-125}$$

An acoustical wave propagating in the solid will produce a deformation that will alter the relative positions of the two points in question. Thus after deformation the separation between the two points will be given by

$$(dl')^2 = (dx_1')^2 + (dx_2')^2 + (dx_3')^2 \tag{14-126}$$

where the deformation is described by

$$\xi_i = x_i' - x_i, \qquad i = 1, 2, 3 \tag{14-127}$$

Since $dx_i' = d\xi_i + dx_i$, Eq. (14-126) becomes

$$(dl')^2 = \sum_{i=1}^{3} \left(d\xi_i^2 + dx_i^2 + 2d\xi_i \, dx_i \right)$$

or

$$(dl')^2 = d\xi_i \, d\xi_i + dx_i \, dx_i + 2d\xi_i \, dx_i \tag{14-128}$$

where we have used the Einstein summation convention. That is, a product of two or more terms with repeated indices represents a summation on those indices. Thus

$$a_i b_i \equiv a_1 b_1 + a_2 b_2 + a_3 b_3$$

It will prove convenient to use this notation for the remaining portions of this section. Since

$$d\xi_i = \frac{\partial \xi_i}{\partial x_k} dx_k$$

Eq. (14-128) becomes

$$(dl')^2 = (dl)^2 + \frac{\partial \xi_j}{\partial x_i} dx_i \frac{\partial \xi_j}{\partial x_k} dx_k + 2\frac{\partial \xi_i}{\partial x_k} dx_i \, dx_k \tag{14-129}$$

Let us now make the following definition:

$$u_{ik} \equiv \frac{1}{2}\left(\frac{\partial \xi_i}{\partial x_k} + \frac{\partial \xi_k}{\partial x_i} + \frac{\partial \xi_j}{\partial x_i}\frac{\partial \xi_j}{\partial x_k} \right) \tag{14-130}$$

We term u_{ik} the *strain tensor*. A further simplification results if we assume that the strain is small enough to only produce small deformations. Then the second-order term can be ignored, and we are left with

$$u_{ik} = \frac{1}{2}\left(\frac{\partial \xi_i}{\partial x_k} + \frac{\partial \xi_k}{\partial x_i} \right) \tag{14-131}$$

Such a definition is in keeping with our conceptual notions of strain. For example, we say that a structure is strained when the relative positions of the points in the structure are altered. In one dimension we define strain as

$$u = \frac{\text{increase in length}}{\text{original length}} = \frac{\Delta l}{l}$$

We will see that our definition of the strain tensor is consistent with this simple example. Combining Eqs. (14-129) and (14-130), we have

$$(dl')^2 = (dl)^2 + 2u_{ik}\, dx_i\, dx_k \tag{14-132}$$

Stress is defined as the force applied to a structure per unit area. The stresses on a solid are most conveniently expressed as a tensor because given the interconnecting structures of a solid, a force applied in one direction can result in net forces in other directions. Thus we define the stress tensor symbolically as

$$T_{ij}$$

By convention, we regard this as describing a force applied along the ith direction producing a stress in the solid along the jth direction. Thus T_{11}, T_{22}, and T_{33} represent tensile stresses, while all other T_{ij}'s $(i \neq j)$ represent shear stresses.

From the simple one-dimensional Hook's law we know that stress is proportional to strain. That is, the force applied to a body must be related in some way to the deformations that the force produces. Extending this concept to the stress and strain tensors, we can write

$$T_{ij} = C_{ijkl} u_{kl} \tag{14-133}$$

Here T_{ij} is the stress tensor, u_{kl} is the strain tensor [see Eq. (14-131)], and C_{ijkl} is the elastic modulus.

Since C_{ijkl} is a fourth-rank tensor, it has 81 components. For computational purposes it is clearly important to reduce this number. Basic symmetries in T_{ij} and u_{kl} lead to the following equalities:

$$C_{ijkl} = C_{jikl} = C_{ijlk} = C_{klij}$$

which reduces the number of independent elastic constants from 81 to 21. Further reductions can occur given structural symmetries in the solid. For example, solids with a cubic crystal system, such as sodium cloride and aluminum, only have three independent elastic constants. A hexagonal system, such as PZT, cadmium, and magnesium, has five while a trigonal system, such as quartz, has six or seven depending on the cut. An isotropic solid has only two independent moduli.

For many applications it is convenient to reformulate Eq. (14-133) into what is commonly called *reduced notation*. Thus we transform the second-order tensors in three dimensions (T_{ij}, u_{ij}) into first-order tensors (or vectors) of six dimensions. First, it will be useful if we rewrite the strain tensor using the following notation: Using Eq. (14-131), let

$$\varepsilon_{ik} \equiv u_{ik} = \frac{\partial \xi_i}{\partial x_k} \qquad \text{if } i = k$$

and

$$\varepsilon_{ik} = 2u_{ik} = \frac{\partial \xi_i}{\partial x_k} + \frac{\partial \xi_k}{\partial x_i} \qquad \text{if } i \neq k \qquad (14\text{-}134)$$

Then Eq. (14-133) becomes

$$T_{ij} = C_{ijkl}\varepsilon_{kl} \qquad (14\text{-}135)$$

Going to reduced notation, we define a pair of indices (with each element running 1 to 3) by a single index (running from 1 to 6) such that

$$(11) \rightarrow 1 \qquad (23) \rightarrow 4$$
$$(22) \rightarrow 2 \qquad (13) \rightarrow 5$$
$$(33) \rightarrow 3 \qquad (12) \rightarrow 6$$

Then Eq. (14-135) and the general stress/strain relation becomes

$$T_i = C_{ij}\varepsilon_j \qquad (14\text{-}136)$$

where the indices now run from 1 to 6. Note that using reduced notation automatically reduces the number of components of the elastic modulus from 81 to 36. Further reductions depend on symmetry. For example, the symmetries in a cubic crystal result in a C_{ij} matrix of only three independent components. The elastic modulus tensor for a cubic crystal is in fact given by

$$C_{ik} = \begin{pmatrix} C_{11} & C_{12} & C_{12} & 0 & 0 & 0 \\ C_{12} & C_{11} & C_{12} & 0 & 0 & 0 \\ C_{12} & C_{12} & C_{11} & 0 & 0 & 0 \\ 0 & 0 & 0 & C_{44} & 0 & 0 \\ 0 & 0 & 0 & 0 & C_{44} & 0 \\ 0 & 0 & 0 & 0 & 0 & C_{44} \end{pmatrix} \qquad (14\text{-}137)$$

If the solid is also isotropic

$$C_{44} = \tfrac{1}{2}(C_{11} - C_{12}) \qquad (14\text{-}138)$$

and we are left with two independent elastic constants.

There are a number of additional terms widely used in the literature for discussions of elasticity. It will prove helpful for the reader if we define several of these here in the context of the proceeding formalism.

First, the elastic constants of an isotropic solid are often defined in terms of what are called the *Lame constants*: λ and μ. In the context of Eq. (14-137) we have

$$C_{11} \equiv \lambda + 2\mu$$
$$C_{12} \equiv \lambda$$
$$C_{44} \equiv \mu$$

Note that this set of relationships satisfies Eq. (14-138).

Second, Young's modulus Y_0 is defined as

$$Y_0 \equiv \frac{\text{extensional stress}}{\text{extensional strain}}$$

Hook's law is sometimes shown graphically as a plot of stress versus strain. On such a graph Y_0 is just the slope of the curve.

In a solid suppose that we have tension along the x-axis with $T_1 = T_2 = 0$. Then

$$Y_0 = \frac{T_3}{\varepsilon_3} = \frac{\mu(3\lambda + 2\mu)}{(\lambda + \mu)}$$

in terms of the Lame constants.

Third, Poisson's ratio $\mathscr{P}$ is defined as

$$\mathscr{P} \equiv \frac{\text{longitudinal extensional displacement}}{\text{displacement perpendicular to the axis}}$$

For an isotropic solid

$$\mathscr{P} = -\frac{\varepsilon_1}{\varepsilon_3} = \frac{\lambda}{2(\lambda + \mu)}$$

Fourth, the bulk modulus B is defined as

$$B \equiv \frac{-\text{hydrostatic pressure}}{\text{relative change in volume}} = \frac{-p_0}{V}$$

For an isotropic solid note that

$$-p_0 = T_1 = T_2 = T_3$$

and

$$\Delta V = \varepsilon_1 + \varepsilon_2 + \varepsilon_3$$

so that

$$B = \lambda + \frac{2\mu}{3}$$

Finally, the shear modulus G is

$$G = \frac{\text{shear stress}}{\text{shear strain}}$$

which for an isotropic solid becomes

$$G = \mu$$

14-5-2 Propagation of Elastic Waves

Here we use the formalism developed in subsection 14-5-1 to obtain the equations of motion that will describe the propagation of sound in solids. We seek an expression analogous to Eq. (14-7), or

$$-\frac{\partial p}{\partial x} = \rho_0 \frac{\partial^2 \xi}{\partial t^2}$$

Since the components of the stress tensor are pressure, we can immediately write

$$\frac{\partial T_{ij}}{\partial x_j} = \rho_0 \frac{\partial^2 \xi_i}{\partial t^2} \tag{14-139}$$

where the summation convention is still in effect. Substituting Eqs. (14-133) and (14-131) into (14-139) yields

$$\rho_0 \frac{\partial^2 \xi_i}{\partial t^2} = \frac{1}{2} C_{ijkl} \frac{\partial}{\partial x_j} \left(\frac{\partial \xi_k}{\partial x_l} + \frac{\partial \xi_l}{\partial x_k} \right)$$

which, using the symmetry properties of C_{ijkl}, becomes

$$\rho_0 \frac{\partial^2 \xi_i}{\partial t^2} = C_{ijkl} \frac{\partial^2 \xi_j}{\partial x_k \partial x_l} \tag{14-140}$$

Suppose that a plane harmonic wave of frequency ω and wave vector k is propagating in the solid. The displacement is given by

$$\xi_i = \xi_{0i} \exp\left[-i(\mathbf{k} \cdot \mathbf{r} - \omega t)\right] = \xi_{0i} \exp\left[-i(k_m \cdot r_m - \omega t)\right] \tag{14-141}$$

Substituting this into Eq. (14-140) gives

$$\rho_0 \omega^2 \xi_{0i} = C_{ijmn} k_j k_m \xi_{0n} \tag{14-142}$$

Using the notation

$$\delta_{ik} = \begin{cases} 1, & i = k \\ 0, & i \neq k \end{cases}$$

Eq. (14-142) becomes

$$(M_{im})(\xi_{0m}) = 0 \tag{14-143a}$$

where

$$M_{im} = C_{ijmn} k_j k_n - \delta_{im} \omega^2 \rho_0 \tag{14-143b}$$

These equations are satisfied provided that

$$|M_{im}| \equiv 0 \tag{14-143c}$$

This is clearly a cubic equation in ω^2, whose three roots represent three different waves propagating with mutually orthogonal displacements. Here it is instructive to consider a specific example. Using reduced notation and with $k_3 = k$ and $k_1 = k_2 = 0$, Eq. (14-143c) becomes

$$\begin{vmatrix} C_{55}k^2 - \omega^2\rho_0 & C_{45}k^2 & C_{35}k^2 \\ C_{45}k^2 & C_{44}k^2 - \omega^2\rho_0 & C_{34}k^2 \\ C_{35}k^2 & C_{34}k^2 & C_{33}k^2 - \omega^2\rho_0 \end{vmatrix} = 0$$

For an isotropic crystal this reduces to

$$\begin{vmatrix} C_{44}k^2 - \omega^2\rho_0 & 0 & 0 \\ 0 & C_{44}k^2 - \omega^2\rho_0 & 0 \\ 0 & 0 & C_{11}k^2 - \omega^2\rho_0 \end{vmatrix} = 0$$

whose solutions are one longitudinal wave propagating with velocity

$$c_{\text{long}} = \frac{\omega}{k} = \sqrt{\frac{C_{11}}{\rho_0}}$$

and two shear (transverse) waves propagating with velocity

$$c_{\text{trans}} = \frac{\omega}{k} = \sqrt{\frac{C_{44}}{\rho_0}}$$

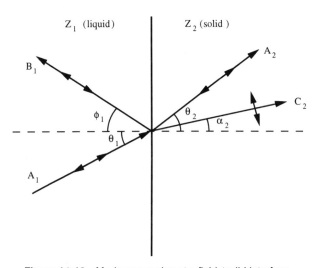

Figure 14-13 Mode conversion at a fluid/solid interface.

One of the more interesting applications dealing with the propagation of waves in a medium that will support a shear stress in the problem of mode conversion. We leave as an exercise for the reader to complete the analysis for the problem outlined in Fig. 14-13. Here a plane wave of amplitude A_1 propagating in a fluid of impedance Z_1 is incident with angle θ_1 to a solid structure of impedance $Z_2 > Z_1$. Some of the energy will be reflected (wave B_1) and some will propagate into the solid. Note that mode conversion creates two waves in the solid, one longitudinal (A_2) and one transverse (C_2).

14-6 PROPAGATION IN TISSUE

Our development of ultrasound physics has proceeded quite purposefully from the simple to the more complex. We began with the propagation of sound in a homogeneous loss-less medium, then a homogeneous lossy medium, and next a homogeneous medium that could support shear. Here we add a final level of complexity: the propagation of sound in inhomogeneous media. This added formalism will provide the appropriate framework for describing the propagation of sound in tissue.

14-6-1 Sources of Scattering: Propagation of Sound in an Inhomogeneous Medium

As we have seen earlier, an acoustical wave propagating in a homogeneous medium can be altered if it encounters a change in acoustical properties. If the change is abrupt and is of a size much greater than the wavelength of the interrogating wave, then the process is described in terms of reflection. Diffraction and refraction, in analogy with optics, can also be described with the same formalism.

The acoustical wave can also be altered by the nature of the medium and the propagation process. Frictional forces as well as certain relaxation phenomena can produce frequency-dependent losses, which we have termed *absorption*. Scattering is yet another mechanism that not only alters the sound beam but also produces an apparent loss of energy. We define scattering as the reflection from structures that are on the order of or smaller than a wavelength. The analytical description of scattering can be quite complex in contrast to the description of reflection. However, understanding this process is essential to a description of medical ultrasonics since ultrasound images are essentially mappings of the scattering process.

Scattering redirects a portion of the interrogating beam in all directions. The backscattered wave form serves as the basis for all current ultrasound imaging systems. The remaining scattered signal is not utilized and represents an apparent loss in energy of the incident beam. This loss of energy due to scattering is added to the loss caused by absorption to give a total energy loss associated with the propagating wave. This total loss (by all mechanisms) is termed *attentuation*. Clearly

$$\text{Attenuation (total loss)} = \text{scattering} + \text{absorption}$$

Experimentally it is very difficult, especially *in vivo*, to separate out the effects of scattering from those of absorption. Thus most measurements deal with attenuation.

What are the mechanisms that produce scattering? What causes scattering in tissue? It turns out these questions were actually answered by Lord Rayleigh some 100 years ago in his studies of London fog. Lord Rayleigh was interested in the mechanisms by which foghorn sounds were seemingly redirected by the fog, providing mariners with misinformation. He concluded that the foghorn signals were scattered by the fog and that fluctuations in density and compressibility provided the mechanism. It is precisely the same mechanism that produces scattering in tissue and that serves as the basis for medical ultrasonic imaging.

Clearly an ultrasonic pulse propagating in a uniform homogeneous medium experiences no reflection or scattering. Thus any mechanisms that describe scattering must involve some local or small change in the acoustical properties. From our analysis of the reflection process (Section 14-2) it should be evident that changes in density as well as changes in sound velocity (or elasticity or compressibility) could produce scattering. Simple physical arguments as well as a derivation from first principles will support this hypothesis, as we will soon see.

Consider a homogeneous medium in which is embedded a small inclusion that has a different density from the surrounding material. An acoustical wave incident on the density inclusion will exert a force on the inclusion, causing it to move in the direction of sound propagation (we assume that the inclusion is incompressible). Once the acoustical wave has passed, the inclusion will oscillate back and forth around its equilibrium position because of the pressure rarefaction that follows the acoustical wave and because energy absorbed by the inclusion from the sound wave must be dissipated. The back-and-forth motion of the density inclusion acts like a dipole source.

Next consider the same homogeneous medium in which this time is embedded a small inclusion that has a different compressibility from the surrounding material. An acoustical wave incident on this inclusion will exert a force that will compress it. Once the acoustical wave has passed, the inclusion will oscillate back and forth as above, but unlike the density inclusion this inclusion in compressibility will oscillate in all directions. Thus the inclusion in compressibility acts like a monopole source.

Therefore, whether from fog or tissue, scattering is the result of fluctuations in density and compressibility. Changes in density act like a dipole source, whereas changes in compressibility act like a monopole source. The scattering process acts as if the scatterers extracted a small amount of energy from the incident beam, redistributed the energy among a large collection of dipole and monopole sources, and then reradiated the energy by these same sources.

This rather intuitive description of scattering can be placed on solid mathematical footing and can even be derived from first principles, as we will now see. Following a derivation similar to that used in Section 14-1 for the plane-wave equation, let us begin with Newton's law, which, in its acoustical analogue, can be written as

$$\frac{\partial p}{\partial x} = -\rho(x)\frac{\partial u}{\partial t} \qquad (14\text{-}144\text{a})$$

as derived in Eq. (14-7). Differentiating and substituting the original equation into the results gives

$$\frac{\partial^2 p}{\partial x^2} = \frac{1}{\rho}\left(\frac{\partial \rho}{\partial x}\right)\left(\frac{\partial p}{\partial x}\right) - \rho\frac{\partial^2 u}{\partial x\,\partial t} \qquad (14\text{-}144\text{b})$$

Next we write down for later use the linearized form of the continuity equation in accordance with Eq. (14-18).

$$\frac{\partial \rho}{\partial t} = -\rho_0\frac{\partial u}{\partial x} \qquad (14\text{-}145)$$

where we have ignored second-order and higher terms.

Third, let us assume, as we did in Eq. (14-19), that the pressure is a function of density:

$$p = p(\rho)$$

which essentially means that we are dealing with an adiabatic process. Taking the time derivative we have

$$\frac{\partial p}{\partial t} = \frac{\partial p}{\partial \rho}\frac{\partial \rho}{\partial t} = \frac{1}{\rho_0\kappa}\frac{\partial \rho}{\partial t} \qquad (14\text{-}146)$$

where κ is the compressibility and is defined as

$$\kappa(x) \equiv \frac{1}{\rho_0}\left(\frac{\partial \rho}{\partial p}\right)_{\Delta S = 0} \qquad (14\text{-}147)$$

Next substitute Eq. (14-145) into Eq. (14-146) and the result into (14-144b). This yields

$$\frac{\partial^2 p}{\partial x^2} - \rho\kappa\frac{\partial^2 p}{\partial t^2} = \left(\frac{1}{\rho}\right)\left(\frac{\partial \rho}{\partial x}\right)\left(\frac{\partial p}{\partial x}\right) \qquad (14\text{-}148)$$

Now let us define $\gamma(x)$ as a fluctuation in compressibility and $\mu(x)$ as a fluctuation in density such that

$$\kappa = \kappa_0(1 + \gamma(x)) \tag{14-149a}$$

$$\rho = \frac{\rho_0}{1 - \mu(x)} \tag{14-149b}$$

Substituting Eq. (14-149) into (14-148) gives

$$\frac{\partial^2 p}{\partial x^2} - \frac{1}{c_0^2}\frac{\partial^2 p}{\partial t^2} = \frac{\gamma(x)}{c_0^2}\frac{\partial^2 p}{\partial t^2} + \frac{\partial}{\partial x}\left(\mu(x)\frac{\partial p}{\partial x}\right) \tag{14-150a}$$

where $c_0^2 \equiv 1/\kappa_0\rho_0$ and c_0 is the mean sound speed in the medium. Equation (14-150a) is an inhomogeneous wave equation in which the left-hand side is just the ordinary homogeneous wave equation while the right-hand side contains the scattering terms. This equation derived from first principles and an assumed adiabatic process clearly describes scattering from fluctuations in density and compressibility. It is instructive to examine each of the scattering terms. The first term on the right-hand side of Eq. (14-150a) describes a fluctuation in compressibility that has isotropic emission and an intensity that is dependent on the acceleration of the source boundaries by the acoustical pressure as determined by the second time derivative. Thus the fluctuation in compressibility acts like a monopole source.

The second term on the right has a nonisotropic directivity pattern (because of the first gradient) and a strength that depends on the differential force on the inclusion. The result is equivalent to an oscillating particle along the x-axis in a stationary medium. Thus the fluctuation in density acts like a dipole source. Our formal analysis has led to a description of scattering that is identical to our intuitive modeling.

Equation (14-150a) can easily be transformed into a 3-D format:

$$\nabla^2 p(r,t) - \frac{1}{c_0^2}\ddot{p}(r,t) = \frac{\gamma(r)}{c_0^2}\ddot{p}(r,t) + \nabla \cdot (\mu\nabla p) \tag{14-150b}$$

or

$$\nabla^2 p(r,t) - \frac{1}{c_0^2}\frac{\partial^2 p(r,t)}{\partial t^2} = \frac{1}{c_0^2}\frac{\partial^2 p(r,t)}{\partial t^2}\left[\frac{\kappa(r) - \kappa_0}{\kappa_0}\right]$$
$$+ \nabla\left\{\left[\frac{\rho(r) - \rho_0}{\rho(r)}\right]\nabla p(r,t)\right\} \tag{14-150c}$$

Equations (14-150) describe the propagation of an acoustical wave in a nonabsorbing, inhomogeneous medium in which scattering is produced by static fluctuations in density and compressibility. This fundamental result from classical acoustics will serve as the basis for our description of the scattering of sound from tissue. Note that nonlinear and shear wave propagation effects are not included, nor are they needed in most cases. More important, absorption effects have also been omitted; however, in many cases they can be included on an ad hoc basis as a multiplicative factor to the loss-less solution. When absorption cannot be so treated, then recourse must be made to wave equations of far greater complexity than Eqs. (14-150).

14-6-2 Scattering of Sound from Tissue

Here we seek a general solution to Eqs. (14-150) that will serve as a model for the description of the scattering of sound from tissue. We then examine the implications such a solution has for medical imaging.

In practice, obtaining a solution to Eq. (14-150c) requires that we make further assumptions and approximations. Let us therefore consider the following situation which is consistent with an appropriate model for medical ultrasonic imaging. Assume that at time $t = 0$ a plane-wave piston source transducer emits a pulse of ultrasonic energy that travels through a homogeneous, loss-less medium of sound velocity c_0. At some later time $t = t_R \sim R/c_0$, the pulse encounters a region of volume V located at some large distance R from the transducer, which contains static fluctuations in density ρ and compressibility κ. Let us place the origin of the coordinate system that describes Eq. (14-150c) within the volume V such that the far-field condition $R \gg r$ holds for all position vectors r within volume V. In addition, we assume that the scattering within the region V is weak. Formally this means that multiple scattering can be neglected. Weak scattering is assured provided that

$$|\rho(r) - \rho_0| \equiv |\rho_1(r)| \ll \rho_0$$

and

$$|\kappa(r) - \kappa_0| \equiv |\kappa_1(r)| \ll \kappa_0$$

Weak scattering also implies that the field p_0 *inside* the scattering region is, to a first approximation, a solution of the *homogeneous* wave equation:

$$\nabla^2 p_0(r, t) - \frac{1}{c_0^2} \frac{\partial^2 p_0(r, t)}{\partial t^2} = 0 \tag{14-151}$$

Since in medical ultrasound the structure of the interrogating pulse is well known, it is convenient to assume the following form for p_0:

$$p_0(r, t) = A(R + z - c_0 t) B(x, y) \tag{14-152}$$

where $r = (x, y, z)$, A is the axial pulse, and B is the beam profile. Note that p_0 represents a pulse traveling in the $+z$ direction, has substantial nonzero values only when the argument of A is near zero, and is present within the scattering volume for times

$$t = \frac{R + z}{c_0} \approx \frac{R}{c_0}$$

The alert reader will have noted that Eq. (14-152) is not an exact solution to Eq. (14-151). Although an exact solution can be forced through, further (and unrealistic) restrictions on the beam profile are required. We choose to retain the original solution which is physically correct although mathematically, at least in the context of the homogeneous wave equation, somewhat inexact.

Assuming that Eq. (14-152) represents a solution to the homogeneous wave equation, a solution to the inhomogeneous equation [Eq. (14-150c)] can be obtained via Green's function methods. Since the details for obtaining this solution are lengthy but are also straightforward and well documented in the literature [10, 11], we simply state the result here. Thus, given the above conditions, the solution to Eq. (14-150c) for the backscattered wave p_s reaching the transducer at $r = R$ is

$$p_s(R, t) = \frac{1}{4\pi R} \int A(2R + 2z - c_0 t) H(z) \, dz \qquad (14\text{-}153a)$$

where

$$H(z) \equiv \frac{1}{4} \frac{\partial^2}{\partial z^2} \int \left[\frac{\rho_1(x, y, z)}{\rho_0} - \frac{\kappa_1(x, y, z)}{\kappa_0} \right] B(x, y) \, dx \, dy$$

$$(14\text{-}153b)$$

Note that p_s is a convolution integral in which the axial wave form of the interrogating pulse A is convolved with the function H which is essentially the impulse response of the system. Note that H only depends on the physical properties of the tissue averaged over the beam profile cross section of the pulse. Thus both our physical modeling and the solution to the wave equation are consistent with a linear systems model of the reflection process. Such a model would view the interrogating pulse A as an input to the system, the backscattered signal p_s as the output of the system, and the impulse response H as the characterizing system parameter. Then, if reflection is a linear process,

$$p_s = A * H$$

or the backscattered signal is equal to the convolution of A with H.

Further examination of Eq. (14-153b) shows that

$$\left[\frac{\rho_1}{\rho_0} - \frac{\kappa_1}{\kappa_0}\right]$$

is just the characteristic impedance $Z(x, y, z)$. Then

$$\int\left[\frac{\rho_1}{\rho_0} - \frac{\kappa_1}{\kappa_0}\right]B(x, y)\, dx\, dy$$

is just the cross-sectional beam profile averaged impedance, which we define as the effective impedance

$$Z_{\mathrm{eff}}(z)$$

Then Eq. (14-153b) becomes

$$H(z) = \frac{1}{4}\frac{d^2}{dz^2}\left[Z_{\mathrm{eff}}(z)\right] \qquad (14\text{-}153\text{c})$$

From the structure of Eqs. (14-153) it is clear that the backscattered signal is produced by fluctuations in impedance. This is consistent with our earlier intuitive model of scattering as fluctuations in density and compressibility. The monopole and dipole sources add up in such a way that the backscattered signal can be identified with fluctuations in impedance. Forward scattering (in the direction of pulse propagation) can then be described in terms of velocity fluctuations. Because of multipath propagation and variation of acoustical properties over the pulse's cross section, different parts of the pulse may arrive at slightly different times. Since dipole radiation associated with changes in density does not contribute to orthogonal (or 90°) scattering, such signals are a result of fluctuations in compressibility alone.

For purposes of ultrasonic imaging we can then view tissue as a lossy medium with inhomogeneities in density and compressibility (or velocity and impedance). The absorption of sound is a result of frictional forces as well as a spectrum of relaxation effects. Scattering, which produces the signals used in all ultrasonic imaging systems, is a result of the tissue inhomogeneities. The backscattered signal, utilized in all conventional imaging systems and the basis for most proposed imaging techniques, is a result of fluctuations in impedance. The formalism developed here to model tissue and to describe the propagation of sound in tissue will be utilized in the next chapter to discuss ultrasonic imaging.

A further note is in order concerning the solution of the inhomogeneous wave equation, Eq. (14-150c). The solution we have outlined departs somewhat from the so-called Born approximation because of the way in which we have specified the pressure field within the scattering volume [Eq. (14-152)].

Other solutions, which are more general and less restrictive, can be obtained for the same equation still in the context of the first Born, or even the first Rytov approximation. Such solutions [12, 13], still obtained via Green's function techniques, are mathematically quite complex and add little to either our physical understanding or our ability to develop better imaging algorithms. If the physical constraints of the scattering process are such that higher-order Born terms must be included, then the Lippman-Schwinger formalism [14] offers a more appropriate approach. This makes the problem equivalent to the solution of a Fredholm integral equation. The resulting complications can be largely circumvented via the use of propagator/reflector operators as detailed in Chapter 15.

14-7 ULTRASOUND PHYSICS AND THE ACOUSTICS LITERATURE

For general reading on acoustics, the following are recommended:

1. L. E. Kinsler, A. R. Frey, A. B. Coppens, and J. V. Sanders, *Fundamentals of Acoustics*, *Third Edition*, Wiley (1982).
2. Allan Pierce, *Acoustics*, Acoustical Society of America (1989).
3. E. Skudrzyk, *The Foundations of Acoustics*, Springer (1971).
4. P. M. Morse and U. Ingard, *Theoretical Acoustics*, McGraw-Hill (1968).
5. Robert T. Beyer, *Nonlinear Acoustics*, Department of the Navy/Academic Press (1974).
6. V. A. Shutilov (M. E. Alferieff, trans.), *Fundamental Physics of Ultrasonics*, Gordon and Breach (1988).
7. A. P. Dowling and J. E. Ffowcs-Williams, *Sound and Sources of Sound*, Horwood (1983).

For books dealing primarily with ultrasonics and ultrasound measurements, the following are recommended:

1. Gordon Kino, *Acoustic Waves: Devices, Imaging, and Analog Signal Processing*, Prentice Hall (1987).
2. Lawrence C. Lynnworth, *Ultrasound Measurements for Process Control*, Academic Press (1989).
3. R. T. Beyer and S. V. Letcher, *Physical Ultrasonics*, Academic Press (1969).

For books dealing at least in part with medical ultrasonics, the following are recommended:

1. C. R. Hill (ed.), *Physical Principles of Medical Ultrasonics*, Horwood/Wiley (1986).
2. Steve Webb (ed.), *The Physics of Medical Imaging*, Adam Hilger (1988).

3. Francis A. Duck, *Physical Properties of Tissue*, Academic Press (1990).
4. Albert Macovski, *Medical Imaging Systems*, Prentice Hall (1983).

For books dealing strictly with the *clinical* aspects of medical ultrasonics, the following are recommended:

1. C. M. Rumack, S. R. Wilson, and J. W. Charboneau, *Diagnostic Ultrasound*, vols. 1, 2, Mosby/Year Book (1991).
2. W. Swobodnik, M. Herraman, J. E. Altwein, and R. F. Basting, *Atlas of Ultrasound Anatomy*, Thieme (1991).
3. D. Sarti, *Diagnostic Ultrasound: Text and Cases*, 2nd ed., Year Book (1987).

Medical Ultrasonics is a very interdisciplinary field, so the research ranging from theoretical to clinical is reported in a wide range of journals. The following are recommended for further reading:

1. *Ultrasound in Medicine and Biology*
2. *Journal of the Acoustical Society of America*
3. *IEEE Transactions on Ultrasonics, Ferroelectrics and Frequency Control*
4. *Ultrasonic Imaging*
5. *IEEE Transactions on Biomedical Engineering*
6. *Journal of Ultrasound in Medicine*
7. *IEEE Transactions on Medical Imaging*

REFERENCES

1. G. Arfken. *Mathematical Methods for Physicists*, 3d ed. San Diego: Academic Press, 1985.
2. R. T. Beyer and Stephen V. Letcher. *Physical Ultrasonics*. San Diego: Academic Press, 1969.
3. R. T. Beyer. *Nonlinear Acoustics*. San Diego: Academic Press/U.S. Department of the Navy, 1974.
4. C. R. Hill (ed.). *Physical Principles of Medical Ultrasonics*. Chichester, England: Ellis Horwood Limited, 1986.
5. L. E. Kinsler, A. R. Frey, A. B. Coppens, and J. V. Sanders. *Fundamentals of Acoustics*. 3d ed. New York: Wiley, 1982.
6. P. M. Morse and U. Ingard. *Theoretical Acoustics*. New York: McGraw-Hill, 1968.
7. L. D. Landau and E. M. Lifshitz. *Theory of Elasticity*. J. B. Sykes and W. H. Reid, transl. Oxford: Pergamon, 1959.
8. H. Schlichting. *Boundary—Layer Theory*, 6th ed., J. Kestin, transl., McGraw-Hill, 1968.

9. L. S. Sokolnikoff. *Mathematical Theory of Elasticity*, 2d ed., New York: McGraw-Hill, 1956.

10. J. C. Gore and S. Leeman. Ultrasonic backscattering from human tissue: A realistic model. *Phys. Med. Biol.* 22:317–326 (1977).

11. R. J. Dickinson. Reflection and scattering. In *Physical Principles of Medical Ultrasonics*, C. R. Hill, ed., Chichester, England: Ellis Horwood Limited, 1986, pp. 225–260.

12. G. F. Roach. *Green's Functions*. 2d ed. Cambridge: Cambridge University Press, 1982.

13. J. M. Blackledge, M. A. Fiddy, S. Leeman, and L. Zapalowski. Three-dimensional imaging of soft tissue with dispersive attenuation. In *Acoustical Imaging*, vol. 12, E. A. Ash and C. R. Hill, eds., New York: Plenum, 1982, pp. 423–433.

14. B. A. Lippman and J. Schwinger. Variational principles for scattering processes, I. *Phys. Rev.* (2d series) 79:469–480 (1950).

15

ULTRASONIC IMAGING

Medical ultrasound has become an important and widely accepted means for the noninvasive imaging of the human body. Studies in a wide range of clinical settings have shown it to be an accurate and versatile technique yielding cross-sectional tomographic images, with little risk or discomfort and with reasonable resolution. Perhaps the most important features of this modality are, first, its ability to produce real-time images of moving structures and, second, its low cost. The first is essential for cardiac and fetal applications; the second imperative for the efficacious practice of medicine.

All diagnostic ultrasound units now in routine clinical service are based on a simple pulse-echo technique in which the backscattered signal from an interrogating ultrasound pulse is detected as a function of time by the same transducer that served as a source. By moving the transducer over a body region or by using an array of such transducers, a cross-sectional image (actually a mapping of echo intensities) can be formed. All current ultrasound imaging systems are based on envelope detection methods and therefore are only capable of displaying echo amplitude (i.e., intensity) information. Although present ultrasound systems have been clinically quite successful, they actually utilize only a small portion of the information available in the echo waveform. For example, phase information is recorded by the transducer, which is a phase-sensitive device but is not utilized in present display or measurement schemes. Other parameters such as the spectral characteristics of the echo wave form are also easily obtained but are not utilized.

In many ways ultrasound has been the poor stepchild of medical imaging: despite technological enhancement and image improvement, today's ultrasound systems have essentially the same block diagram as those from the beginnings of the modality over 40 years ago. There are at least three reasons why ultrasound has remained in its "classical" imaging stage (as defined in Chapter 1) and has yet to utilize, at least on a clinical basis, the reconstruction formalism so much a part of contemporary imaging and the unifying thread for this volume. First, and perhaps the most surprising, is the fact that data rates in ultrasound are higher than even present computer technology can handle. Since ultrasound propagates through tissue fairly slowly (1.5 mm/μsec) each image contains a large number of interactions. Retaining both the phase and amplitude information associated with the echo waveform, the data base associated with a single ultrasonogram can contain several megabytes of information. To record in real time and to process in near real time, a sequence of such data sets poses significant computational demands.

A second reason ultrasound has remained at the classical imaging stage has to do with the fact that the interaction between sound and tissue is an exceedingly complex process. Major factors that describe the propagation of ultrasound in tissue include, as detailed in Chapter 14, the density, elasticity, sound velocity, specific acoustical impedance, absorption, scattering, and the parameter of nonlinearity. In general, these parameters are frequency and temperature dependent and, fortunately, are also a function of tissue type and pathological state. In many cases rather subtle changes in pathology can significantly alter the propagation process. By contrast, the propagation of X rays in tissue is quite simple, determined largely by the density of the material. Thus, in principle, an immense amount of information could be extracted from an analysis of the interaction of sound with tissue. The problem is sorting out what is in effect an overload of complex information in a realistic manner.

Finally, a third reason ultrasonic imaging has not developed further is related to our lack of knowledge of fundamental interactive processes. Although our knowledge of ultrasound physics and of the interaction of ultrasound with tissue has certainly increased recently, our knowledge is still far from complete. Clearly it is difficult to engineer a medical imaging system without all of the basic physics first in place.

In this chapter, after a brief review of conventional or "classical" ultrasound imaging, we examine in some detail the type of information one might extract from the interactions of ultrasound with tissue. We will find that the content of the information so extracted falls naturally into three categories: qualitative imaging (which includes conventional ultrasound), tissue characterization (or the display of appropriate ultrasonic tissue signatures), and quantitative imaging. Our main emphasis here will be on the latter and the various techniques that have been proposed to obtain such displays. It will be useful as a part of our discussions if we reexamine certain aspects of ultrasonic scattering and introduce the propagator/reflector concept as a unifying principle.

It should be emphasized that the various imaging techniques we will discuss largely represent potential possibilities rather than demonstrated methods. Predictions of the ultimate utility of these present techniques or of some future methods have ranged from the ludicrously optimistic to the crushingly pessimistic. We believe that a realistic assessment of their viability must be based on the physics of the ultrasound/tissue interactions. In this manner a better appreciation of the range of information available may be obtained. What cannot be answered here, however, is the medical utility of the extracted information: This is a problem that only protracted clinical trials can resolve.

15-1   INFORMATION CONTENT IN CONVENTIONAL ULTRASONIC IMAGING

All conventional medical ultrasonic imaging systems are based on a simple pulse-echo technique utilizing the backscattered echo waveform. In a simple, yet realistic example, imagine a single-element piezoelectric plane-piston source placed on the abdomen of a human subject. Good acoustical contact between the transducer and the tissue is maintained through the use of mineral oil or some appropriate acoustical gel. Suppose a sharp voltage spike is applied to the mechanically damped transducer. The piezoelectric element attempts to ring at its resonance frequency but because of damping stops after several cycles. Thus the transducer generates a short and relatively broad-band pulse that travels into the tissue. For general abdominal applications, transducers with center frequencies of 3.5 to 5.0 MHz are used. Bandwidths of 60% to 100% are typical. The spectrums are sometimes Gaussian in shape, but other forms are also prevalent.

Perhaps the fundamental design consideration for all ultrasonic imaging devices is the trade off between resolution and attenuation. We would like to operate at the highest frequency possible to obtain the greatest possible resolution. We are restricted, however, because of frequency-dependent attenuation. For soft tissue such attenuation is on the order of 1 dB/cm/MHz.

The short pulse, perhaps a microsecond or so in duration, now travels into tissue with a velocity of about 1.5 mm/μsec. Some form of focusing via a lens or a shaped piezoelectric element is used to ensure a reasonably well collimated beam over an appropriate depth of field. Here, once again, a system design compromise must be made: Any improvements in lateral resolution significantly reduces the depth of field, and vice versa. For abdominal scanning we might expect depths of field between 10 and 15 cm, axial resolutions on the order of a wavelength, and lateral resolutions on the order of 10 wavelengths.

As the pulse propagates in tissue, it will be attenuated, as indicated above, due to absorption and scattering. The backscattered waveform, which will be considerably reduced in amplitude from the incident pulse, is then recorded by the same transducer that produced the original pulse. Since the transducer is a phase-sensitive device, the output voltage of the transducer (produced by the pressure of the backscattered signal on the face of the transducer) will be an rf trace (representational of the backscattered signal) recorded as a function of depth (or more correctly, acoustical travel time) within the tissue. Since the backscattered signals (because of attenuation) span a wide dynamic range (100 to 130 dB), some compression techniques are required if the signals are to be viewed. At least some of the compression is done under front panel control known as TGC (or time gain compensation). This control increases the gain as some function of depth so that signals from a greater depth (which are more attenuated) will be amplified more than signals near the transducer. At some point in this process the received signal is envelope detected, which is important if, as we will soon see, the information is to be incorporated into an image.

The waveform recorded by the transducer, whether rf or envelope detected, can be displayed on an oscilloscope or an appropriate monitor. This trace, which is the amplitude-modulated display of the backscattered signal, is known as an *A-mode display* or *A-scan*.

To make an image, we first take the A-scan and convert the amplitude mode display into a brightness mode display along a vertical axis. This converts a horizontal axis with waveform spikes into a vertical axis with a series of bright dots. Now let us slowly move the transducer over a section of the body and key such motion to the display on the monitor. This motion literally paints an image on the screen. Because the image is formed from a display of bright dots, it is known as a *B-mode display*. Although few scanners today actually move the transducer along the body to produce an image, the principle of scanning is still very much the same. In fact all of the commercial scanners available today produce B-mode images. Constructing an ultrasound B-scan image is still very much an art form. The TGC curve and other controls are changed so as to produce an aesthetically pleasing image. If the structures under view are known to be uniform, then the TGC is set to ensure a constant texture.

A variety of different transducers are utilized in today's ultrasound equipment. Perhaps the most popular is a single crystal mounted in a fluid offset. The crystal rotates sweeping out a sector in real time. This simple sector scanner is perhaps the best known of the ultrasound scanners available today. A variety of transducer arrays are used in present systems. They range from a simple linear array to the more complex ring arrays which focus the beam in depth. Although present array technology does provide a means for beam steering and offers enhanced resolution with depth, true phased arrays with high resolution are beyond today's achievements.

It is instructive at this point to analyze the information content in the signals displayed by conventional ultrasound imaging. The backscattered wave p_s reaching the transducer is given by Eq. (14-153), or

$$p_s(R, t) = \frac{1}{4\pi R} \int A(2R + 2z - c_0 t) H(z)\, dz \qquad (15\text{-}1)$$

where we recall that A is the axial profile of the incident pulse and H is the effective tissue impulse response. The voltage V produced at the transducer by the scattered pressure wave p_s is simply the integral of p_s over the face of the transducer:

$$V(R, t) = d \int_{S(\xi)} p_s(R + \xi, t) \, dS(\xi) \tag{15-2}$$

where d is a constant and represents the response characteristics of the transducer.

To evaluate Eq. (15-2), let us first consider what would happen if a point scatterer were positioned at b:

$$H(z) = \delta(z - b)$$

and Eq. (15-1) becomes

$$p_s(R, t) = \frac{1}{4 \pi R} A(2R + 2b - c_0 t) \tag{15-3}$$

If $h(b)$ is the pulse-echo signal from the point scatterer at b, then, following Eq. (15-2), we can write

$$h(R, t) = \frac{d}{4 \pi R} \int_{S(\xi)} A(2R + 2b + \xi - c_0 t) \, dS(\xi) \tag{15-4}$$

Combining this result with Eqs. (15-1) and (15-2), we have

$$V(R, t) = \int h(2R + 2z - c_0 t) H(z) \, dz \tag{15-5}$$

which is the voltage recorded by the transducer. To form an A-mode ultrasonogram, it is convenient to map this equation into the coordinate set (x, y, z). Note that the A-scan is made in a fixed (x, y) plane, say $x = X_0$ and $y = Y_0$. Then Eq. (15-5) becomes

$$D_A(X_0, Y_0, z) = \int h(x' - X_0, y' - Y_0, 2z' - 2z) H(x', y', z') \, dx' \, dy' \, dz' \tag{15-6}$$

where D_A is the A-mode display. Thus the rf waveform recorded in a conventional A-scan is a convolution between the tissue impulse response and the pulse-echo point spread function. Note that the one-dimensional A-mode display is represented by a three dimensional convolution integral. It should be clear that although one-dimensional analyses may be useful for many simple model studies, the complexities of tissue require a three-dimensional treatment to describe something even as simple as a one-dimensional A-scan.

To form a B-mode ultrasonogram, we take the envelope of Eq. (15-6) for a fixed x and y and form an image by incrementing, say, the y-coordinate. Mathematically this envelope process can be represented as

$$\left| \tilde{D}_A(X_0, Y_0, z) \right| = |\widetilde{h * H}| \tag{15-7}$$

where $\tilde{D}_A$ is the analytic representation of D_A. The reader will recall [1, 2] that the analytic representation of a function f is defined by

$$\tilde{f} \equiv f - i\mathscr{H}(f)$$

where $\mathscr{H}$ is the Hilbert transform operator. If

$$f \equiv p * w$$

then in general

$$|\tilde{f}| \neq |f| \neq |\tilde{p}| * |\tilde{w}| \tag{15-8}$$

Thus the envelope of an A-line (and in turn the complete B-mode display) is a nontrivial function of the tissue impulse response. Moreover the envelope operation so corrupts the backscattered ultrasonic waveform that most information relating to the tissue impulse response is irretrievably lost.

Many workers over the years have tried to obtain additional information about the tissue from an analysis of the B-mode images (or even the envelope detected A-line signals). Attempts have been made at artifact reduction, gray-scale reallocation, resolution enhancement, utilization of multiple images, and a variety of image-processing techniques. From the analysis given above, it should be clear why these attempts have not been successful. The very nature of the data available in a conventional B-mode image has foredoomed most of these techniques to failure. Moreover most of these methods fail to consider the fact that any tissue information in the image is further corrupted by the various instrumentation parameters.

Although conventional ultrasonic imaging has become an important modality for diagnostic medicine, it should be clear that the information content in such images is very limited and that any quantitative information relating to the tissue/sound interactions is irretrievably lost merely as a result of the imaging process. Clearly, as we will see later in our discussion of tissue characterization and quantitative imaging, further advances will largely depend on our ability to capture and utilize the ultrasound data before the data have been altered by instrumentation parameters or the imaging process.

15-2 INFORMATION EXTRACTION FROM ULTRASOUND SCATTERING

Suppose that a pulse of ultrasonic energy is allowed to interrogate a given tissue structure and that we are able to record the signals (assumed to be the result of scattering) produced by such an interaction. Let us now ask two very general questions: What type of information can be obtained from an analysis of such interactions, and how can the information so obtained be usefully presented? Thus we wish to consider the general problem of information extraction from ultrasound scattering.

The known parameters of tissue and ultrasound further define and restrict the information extraction process. For example, the input field can be assumed to be a longitudinal pressure wave, since there is good experimental evidence showing that shear waves do not propagate over significant distances in soft tissues. Frequencies are in the low MHz range. For many applications (but not all) a pulsed field will be employed. There pulses will be broad-band but with a central frequency within the previously indicated range. We can assume that the incident wave is accurately known. There is of course somewhat less certainty in specifying the acoustical properties of the tissue. After all these are the properties we expect to measure via the information extraction process. We can certainly place some general requirements on tissue: It is clearly an inhomogeneous medium varying, in reality, in both space and time. Tissue is also richly structured with spatial correlation lengths spanning a wide spectrum, certainly well beyond the wavelengths ordinarily associated with diagnostic ultrasound. Tissue quickly attenuates ultrasound in the low MHz range at a rate that is near linear with frequency. Since experimental techniques are not sufficiently sophisticated to unambiguously detect nonlinear effects within tissues at the moderate power levels used for imaging, there is no reason to resort to the added complexity of nonlinear acoustics. Soft tissues scatter ultrasound waves via structural inhomogeneities consisting of fluctuations in density and compressibility. The relative strength of scattering is certainly not known, but it can be assumed, based on reasonable experimental evidence, to be in some sense weak. Soft tissues exhibit a complicated composition and thermodynamics and, in some cases, are clearly nonisotropic. The significance of these latter factors has yet to be assessed, is not included in most applications, and will be disregarded for simplicity.

The above discussion suggests that there are only three general approaches to the extraction of information from ultrasound scattering. The first we term *qualitative imaging*. Here some part of the tissue/sound information base is utilized to produce a nonquantitative display such as conventional B-mode imaging. However, parameters other than the echo intensity can, as we will see in Section 15-3, also serve as a basis for qualitative imaging. The second approach to information extraction we term *ultrasonic tissue characterization*. Here we seek to extract the medically significant features from the interaction process and display appropriate tissue signatures or estimates of tissue acoustical properties (see Section 15-4). Finally, the third approach to information extraction we term *quantitative imaging*. Here we seek to map one or more interaction parameters in a truly quantitative way. This approach represents what we, in the context of this book, really mean by "imaging." This topic is discussed in more detail in Sections 15-5 and 15-6.

15-3 QUALITATIVE IMAGING

Conventional pulse-echo imaging maps at least to some degree the location of the scattering structures and the reflecting interfaces but provides little or no information concerning the nature of these reflectors. In all commercial medical ultrasound imaging systems the backscattered echo waveform is envelope detected and, with amplitudes that range well over a 100 dB in dynamic range, compressed for viewing on conventional display devices. As noted in Section 15-1, the typical pulse-echo image is an intensity map, devoid of phase or spectral information, with brightness related only very crudely to scatter strength. Clearly attempts to extract additional information from such images are not likely to be successful.

Although all conventional ultrasound systems are qualitative in nature many nonconventional techniques also fall in this category by virtue of the fact that they also produce a nonquantitative image, in this case, based on an information content other than the echo intensity. Such qualitative imaging schemes include

- various methods to incorporate spectral information into a B-mode format, such as spectracolor ultrasonography [3, 4] and the so-called dual-frequency scanning [5, 6];
- methods to incorporate phase information into a B-mode format [7];
- various novel techniques for interrogating tissue and receiving the echo waveform [8, 9, 10, 11].

All of these methods, regardless of information content or display technique, produce qualitative images, that is, images in which no single parameter is recorded or measured in a quantitative and/or absolute fashion. Even though many of these techniques are interesting and perhaps even clinically useful, it should be clear that further advances in ultrasonic imaging will probably depend upon quantitative rather than qualitative methods.

15-4   ULTRASONIC TISSUE CHARACTERIZATION

We define ultrasonic tissue characterization as the collection of all techniques and methods that seek to extract and separate from an interrogating ultrasonic wave the medically significant features of the ultrasound interactions and to display ultrasonic tissue signatures appropriate for a differential diagnosis or some other medical purpose. Clearly, to be useful or significant, such signatures or measures must be related to tissue pathology or physiology. The reader will recall that as a part of our discussions tissue characterization represents the second general approach to the extraction of information from ultrasound scattering.

Tissue characterization is broad in scope and, in certain cases, can include aspects of both qualitative imaging and quantitative imaging. At its simplest, tissue characterization involves merely a redisplay or recombination of pulse-echo image information in a way that is more pathology specific. Such simple approaches are likely to be of limited value, since they also tend to be machine and operator specific.

In its most useful form, tissue characterization extracts a quantitative and intrinsic measure describing the spatial and/or temporal variations of any mixture (known or unknown) of tissue properties. The interactiveness between, but distinct separateness of, quantitative imaging and tissue characterization should be evident. Thus observations in tissue characterization may lead to new imaging schemes which in turn may lead to additional tissue characterization. In a sense quantitative imaging may well be the precursor to truly successful tissue characterization.

In the several paragraphs that follow we will briefly review a number of tissue characterization methods that have been proposed. Our aim is to foster an understanding and appreciation for the experiences and potentials of the field but not to provide a complete review. For a more extensive coverage the reader is referred to the literature and several reviews [12, 13, 14]. For our discussion of tissue characterization, it will prove useful to separate the various methods and techniques into three very general approaches that can be taken: parameter estimation, structure characterization, and dynamic characterization. We now can consider each of these in turn.

15-4-1   Parameter Estimation

Parameter estimation seeks to measure (or estimate) the value of a particular acoustical property such as impedance, attenuation, or sound velocity. The estimation, of necessity, provides an averaged or mean value of the parameter over some region, which can vary in size from the dimensions of the interrogating pulse to a complete B-mode image. In many cases the parameter is measured with respect to one or more variables (e.g., attenuation is measured as a function of frequency). We now examine in somewhat more detail several parameters that may prove useful for tissue characterization.

Attenuation

Although Wild and Reid [15] made the first crude estimates of attenuation *in vivo* over 40 years ago and demonstrated quantitative differences between normal breast tissue and both malignant and benign lesions, it is only in the last decade that attenuation measurements have become an important area for research. A number of workers used simple spectral analysis to investigate the resulting effects of attenuation [16, 17, 18]. Kuc [19] obtained a statistical estimate of the attenuation from the power spectra of appropriately segmented A-line wave forms. Fink [20] estimated the attenuation from a short-time Fourier analysis of the A-line wave forms. Ferrari and Jones [21] have proposed a zero-crossing technique to estimate the attenuation. A comparison of the various methods is given in [22] and [23].

Impedance

Since the backscattered signal is the result of fluctuations in impedance, it seems reasonable to assume that a profile of impedance can be obtained from the backscattered signal. One such method, known as *impediography* [24], extracts the tissue impulse response function from the backscattered signal. Further processing leads to a profile or map of impedance. Although successful at quantitating several lesions in the eye *in vivo* [25], it has not been as successful in other applications largely because of signal processing difficulties [26, 27]. Impediography represents the first attempt, of which these are now several, to derive basic tissue parameters from pulse-echo information. It may yet have an important role to play in both tissue characterization and quantitative imaging [28].

Velocity

Measurements of velocity or sound speed in tissue are surprisingly difficult, unless recourse is made to transmission methods. If an easily recognizable scattering structure exists in a particular tissue, mean velocities may be estimated by a pulse-echo triangulation technique, involving scanning the structure from a number of different directions [29, 30]. However, this method is prone to refraction errors and the effects of overlying tissue [31].

Other Parameters

A number of other parameters have been used as tissue characterizing features. These include the backscattering coefficient, in terms of Bragg angle scattering [32, 33] as well as integrated backscatter [34]; the parameter of nonlinearity, B/A [35, 36, 37]; and the elasticity [38].

15-4-2   Structure Characterization

This second general approach to tissue characterization seeks to extract from the echo waveform a characterizing signature of the spatial arrangement of tissue. This approach is suggested by the observation that the general pattern of echoes in a conventional B-mode image of a given region may vary dramatically with disease state. Whereas with parameter estimation the goal was to measure or estimate some specific physical property, here we merely seek some signature or characterizing feature.

In some initial attempts intensity data from the image were transformed using rather heuristic methods. More promising results have been obtained using the rf signals (or undermodulated A-lines). Such computations have included the cepstra of echo sequences [39, 40], the histogram of the first peaks in the autocorrelation of the power spectrum [41, 42] the envelope correlation spectrum [43, 44], and a one-dimensional max-min texture algorithm [45, 46]. Some success has also been realized using feature-based methodologies and/or pattern recognition techniques [47, 48, 49, 50, 51].

15-4-3 Dynamic Characterization

The third and final approach to tissue characterization we have termed *dynamic characterization*. The basic underlying idea is that the quantitation of changes within a tissue, rather than the characterization of tissue itself, will be diagnostically significant as well as less sensitive to the problems inherent in other methods. That is, the monitoring of the change of some readily computed feature may be relatively unaffected by overlying tissue layers and system design factors.

There are many changes within the body potentially amenable to investigation. Cyclic changes caused by cardiac action include the study of myocardial contractility and disease, as well as blood perfusion monitoring in tumors and organs. Changes mediated by age, development, or maturity, such as in the placenta, may be amenable to study, although the time scales are much longer. Changes in A-line signatures as a muscle is tensed and then relaxed may well indicate the severity of certain muscle diseases [52, 53]. Charting tissue changes in response to treatment or external stimuli, such as drugs, may also prove useful [54, 55].

Simple correlation analysis [56, 57] and Doppler signatures [58, 59] have been proposed as suitable for dynamic tissue characterization. These approaches rely on their, as yet only hoped for, ability to extract clinically valuable information from either consistently distorted or otherwise poor data, and to achieve that with easily computed echo signatures or indices.

15-5 SCATTERING REVISITED

In Chapter 14 we developed the appropriate formalism for describing the propagation of sound in tissue and for modeling tissue from an acoustical viewpoint. Here we reexamine the scattering process in a much more general way, developing a framework within which we can discuss the various approaches to quantitative imaging.

Let Ψ represent an ultrasound pulse which is propagating in tissue, and let L represent a linear operator that describes the process of propagation and scattering. Then

$$L\Psi = 0 \qquad (15\text{-}9)$$

In general, L will contain both spatial and temporal derivatives. Clearly L will depend on the parameters that define and characterize tissue. A common approach is to decompose the linear operator L as

$$L \equiv P - R \qquad (15\text{-}10)$$

Although this decomposition is not unique, it is usual to ensure that the operator P is independent of tissue parameter fluctuations, these being contained within R. Departing somewhat from the usual conventions, let P also contain large-scale variations in the mean values of the acoustical parameters; R then contains only fluctuations about the mean value. Thus effects such as refraction, and reflection from large-scale smooth tissue interfaces, are considered to be incorporated in P. These are in principle relatively well understood, and solvable problems, so we can still maintain that with the specification of appropriate initial and boundary conditions (and probably with the invocation of realistic approximations) a solution Ψ_0 can be found to the equation

$$P\Psi_0 = 0 \qquad (15\text{-}11)$$

The correct interpretation of Eq. (15-11) cannot be overemphasized. It describes the propagation of the same incident pulse as appropriate to Eq. (15-9) but in an idealized, small-scale, fluctuation free, possibly piecewise continuous medium. In practice we will regard the choice of P to have been such that the solution of Eq. (15-11) represents a possibly distorting, but still bounded, pulse traveling through the medium. Thus the pulse Ψ_0 may depart from its initial path as a result of refraction effects, and "echoes" may be generated at major interfaces: however, no scattered "halo" of ultrasound will follow the pulse as it propagates.

The primary idea underlying the introduction of the operator P is that Ψ_0 presents in some sense an approximate solution to Eq. (15-9). Such an expectation cannot be adequately fulfilled unless the values of the mean tissue parameters appearing in P are known. We assume that this is the case or, at least, that quite reliable estimates may be made. Let us further assume, based on reasonable physical principles, that the solution to Eq. (15-11) can be written as

$$\Psi_0 = P'\Psi_B \qquad (15\text{-}12)$$

Here the pulse within the idealized medium described above is expressed as some kernel P' acting on the known input (i.e., the initial boundary values of the pulse) denoted here as Ψ_B. Given the linearity of the problem, P' is determined in principle by P. For reasons that will soon become clear we term P' the "propagator."

The full solution to Eq. (15-9) is now written in terms of the approximate solution as

$$\Psi = \Psi_0 \otimes \Psi_S \tag{15-13}$$

where Ψ_S remains to be determined and $\otimes$ denotes some, as yet to be defined, operator. The so-called Rytov scheme [60, 61] has as its starting point the choice that $\otimes$ be scalar multiplication. We choose what we believe to be a more transparent and an intuitively more meaningful pathway: We assume that $\otimes$ denotes simple addition. Thus

$$\Psi = \Psi_0 + \Psi_S \tag{15-14}$$

Combining Eqs. (15-9), (15-10), (15-11), and (15-14), we have

$$P\Psi_S = R(\Psi_0 + \Psi_S)$$

Assuming that

$$|R\Psi_S| \ll |R\Psi_0| \tag{15-15}$$

it follows that, to good approximation,

$$P\Psi_S = R\Psi_0 \tag{15-16}$$

This is a linear, inhomogeneous differential equation for Ψ_S and represents a generalized version of the scattering equation developed in Section 14.6. Equation (15-16) can be solved via standard Green function methods:

$$\Psi = \Psi_0 + GR\Psi_0 \tag{15-17}$$

where G is the Green function which is evaluated from P in association with a rather specific boundary condition ultimately derived from the so-called *Sommerfeld radiation condition*. This condition insists that in accordance with our physical intuition, the field scattered from a very small (compared to a wavelength) inhomogeneity should behave as an outgoing (possibly angle modulated) spherical wave at very large distances. Moreover the Ψ_S component of the field will tend to have a similar behavior at large distances from the small-scale inhomogeneous region ($R \neq 0$) because of its dependence on G, as indicated in Eq. (15-17). Clearly the Ψ_S component vanishes if the small-scale tissue fluctuations vanish and arises only from regions where Ψ_0 is nonzero. These properties lead us to associate Ψ_S with our intuitive notions of a scattered field: Equation (15-17) then implies that the actual field within the tissue may be regarded as a sum of an "incident" (Ψ_0) and "scattered" (Ψ_S) field. Note that our treatment has forced us to the conclusion that small-scale fluctuations in any acoustical parameter will give rise to scattering. The essential distinction between what is a scattered and an incident field originated in our ability to call on special methods to solve, with a high degree of accuracy, a wave equation such as Eq. (15-11), which depends on slowly varying, and/or piecewise, continuity of the medium, and our inability to attack the problem in general when small-scale fluctuations are present. This point is clarified when we consider that pulse transmission across a large, smooth impedance discontinuity (say) is a relatively straightforward problem compared to the case when the interface contains significant structure on a wavelength scale. Or compare the problem of a pulse propagating in a medium with slowly varying velocity (where ray "optics" may well be applicable) compared to the case of propagation through a medium showing random, small fluctuations in velocity. Equation (15-15) is a statement that the first Born approximation applies. Given the observed weakness of signals scattered from soft tissues, it is likely that this approximation is valid in most cases. There are certain situations that seem in conflict with this approximation, such as where reverberations are clearly seen in a B-scan image. However, it is often reasonable to interpret these as arising from multiple reflections of the Ψ_0 component of Eq. (15-14), so Eq. (15-15) may hold under rather more general conditions than is at first apparent. It is certainly possible to relax the first Born approximation but at the expense of a rather more cumbersome description.

The Green function G appearing in Eq. (15-17), describes how the wave from a point source propagates within the fictitious medium described in Eq. (15-12). It is thus easy to appreciate that there is an intimate connection between G and the propagator P', as previously introduced. Indeed, a more careful analysis shows that the Green function, when acting as a kernel inside an integral expression as in Eq. (15-17), is equivalent to the propagator P' in Eq. (15-12). We are thus led to a very intuitively appealing conceptual framework for the underlying structure of the scattered field, schematically shown in Fig. 15-1. Consider a known input pulse F incident on some tissue-like medium. We are interested in the scattered field from the small region S depicted in the figure. The pulse actually arriving at S has the form PF, where P is the "propagator" (integral operator) introduced earlier. The region S modifies the pulse in accordance with its scattering properties. We will investigate this in more detail below, but here we describe the modifying effect by the action of an operator R, which may appropriately be referred to as the "reflector." Thus the region S acts as a source of (scattered) sound, described as RPF, and this gives rise to sound waves propagating through the medium. Since this propagation process is described by the propagator P, the field arriving at a detector may be symbolically written as $PRPF$. If the detection process is embodied in the operator D, then it clearly follows that

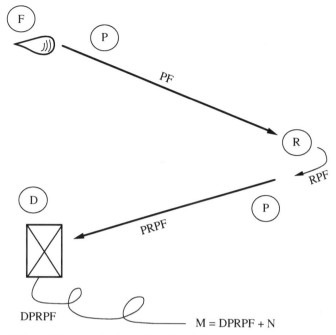

Figure 15-1 Outline of the operator formalism describing scatter imaging. F is the incident pulse, P is the propagator, R is the reflector, D is the detection process, and N is the noise. The scatter image map M is given by the fundamental imaging equation M = DPRPF + N.

the measured signal M is given by

$$M = DPRPF + N \qquad (15\text{-}18)$$

where N denotes possible (additive) noise. The structure of Eq. (15-18), which we refer to as the *fundamental imaging equation*, is intuitively appealing even without recourse to scattering theory. However, the more formal considerations leading to Eq. (15-17) clearly show the close relationship between the two approaches. We emphasize that Eq. (15-18) is written in very symbolic notation and actually involves integrations over many variables, not explicitly shown. In particular, it should be noted that despite the suggestive compactness of S in Fig. 15-1, Eq. (15-18) actually embodies scattering from throughout the medium of interest.

The propagator-reflector approach for the description of ultrasound scattering from human tissues appears to have been first used by Leeman [62] in a derivation of the impediographic equations. Rather similar ideas were used by Berklout et al. [63, 64] in their development of wave extrapolation imaging. The technique has also been used directly by Lefebvre [65]. We feel that the method is rather more general than the implied dependence on the first Born approximation, since it allows phenomenological and heuristic modifications to both the propagator and reflector operators. Some of these will be equivalent to including, at least partially, higher-order corrections. There is also the possibility of incorporating experimental data, such as by modeling the propagator to fit findings in pulse transmission experiments. This last, somewhat surprising, contention may be illustrated in a particularly telling example. Given the absence of small-scale fluctuations (i.e., scattering) in the description of Eq. (15-11), it seems apparent that in a lossy medium the propagator should depend on the absorption characteristics of the medium. However, it does not seem at all unreasonable (in fact it seems rather more appropriate) to model P, in Eq. (15-18), on the measured attenuation properties of the medium, thus including some aspects of higher Born approximations in the treatment.

It may be observed that the propagator, as introduced in Eq. (15-18) is closely associated with the propagation of the coherent wave [60], with the reflector being associated with the incoherent wave. We will not develop this idea further here but will rely on the relatively simple connection with formal scattering theory outlined before.

15-6 QUANTITATIVE IMAGING

We use the term quantitative imaging to refer to those techniques that map the distribution and strength of a single ultrasound/tissue interaction parameter (or at least a well-defined, invirient combination of such parameters) in a truly quantitative way. These methods are largely experimental at present, especially those relying on scattered signals for input.

Conventional pulse-echo B-mode images, despite their medical usefulness, are not quantitative images for two reasons. First, their image densities depend rather strongly on system settings and the choice of transducer. Second, even if such system artifacts could be allowed for, the resultant image would essentially be a reflectivity map of tissue. Unfortunately, reflectivity is a complicated function of both tissue interaction parameters and tissue morphology. The quantitative image in principle will not suffer from these defects: It would be independent of system settings and scanning procedure, and the image density would relate directly to an intrinsic tissue property uncomplicated by geometrical considerations. In this sense the quantitative ultrasound image presents a new dimension of tissue information. However, quantitative imaging also demands elaborate data acquisition arrangements and extensive computer-based manipulation of the acquired data.

Two major approaches to quantitative imaging are being developed: transmission imaging and scatter imaging. Ultrasound computerized tomography, based on X-ray CT and utilizing the transmitted ultrasound wave form, has generated both attenuation and velocity maps of tissue [66, 67, 68, 69]. The velocity images are produced by inputting time-of-flight measurements into the reconstruction process; attenuation images are produced by utilizing measurements of the amplitude of the transmitted signal. Due to the presence of bone and air, these techniques are limited (perhaps fundamentally) to a few body sites such as the female breast or the neonatal head. Ultrasound computerized tomography is more subtle to implement than the X-ray case, since a number of simplifying approximations, such as straight-line propagation, isotropy, and even scalarity of interaction, do not hold in all ultrasound situations. Measurement of the transmitted ultrasound field is complicated by the coherent nature of the generating and detecting devices commonly used. Despite these difficulties reasonable quantitative attenuation and velocity breast images have been obtained *in vivo* [70, 71, 72, 73, 74], but it is yet too early to assess their true diagnostic impact [75, 76, 77].

The second approach to quantitative imaging, which we term scatter imaging, utilizes the scattered signal to produce quantitative maps of tissue interaction parameters. All scatter-imaging methods are related to classical inverse scattering techniques. Here the problems are formidable, and the methods have rarely been applied *in vivo*. The proliferation of scatter-imaging techniques may be conveniently classified by their data acquisition methods. Diffraction tomography [78, 79, 80] and its may variants (including filtered backpropagation) [81, 82] is characterized by the measurement of the scattering into all angles. Impediography [24, 62], including its variant, reflectivity tomography [83], is characterized by the measurement of the backscattered signal only. Wave extrapolation imaging [63, 64, 84] utilizes what may be termed *retro-scattering* (i.e. scattering into a relatively small cone about the strictly backscattered direction). This classification by data acquisition method is in fact dictated by the physics of the ultrasound/tissue interaction. Thus each class of techniques will be expected to measure different parameters (or combinations of parameters) of the interaction, while variants of a given technique are merely different approaches toward mapping the same parameter. It will be useful to discuss each of these techniques in terms of the propagator/reflector formalism of Section 15-5 and Fig. 15-1.

15-6-1 Conventional B-Mode Imaging

In conventional pulse-echo or B-scan imaging systems, P is simple (frequency-independent attenuation) and assumes a homogeneous medium with a constant sound velocity. In most clinical imaging systems time-gain compensation (TGC) hardware corrects for an assumed value of tissue attenuation, and in some cases adjustment is allowed for different values of the attenuation coefficient over different tissue segments. There are at present no hardware corrections for the frequency dependence of attenuation. Thus simple attenuation is only qualitatively allowed for. The nature of the reflector or scatterer R is not considered as such, although simple impedance mismatch ideas are often invoked. D and F are again hardware modified and in some cases adjust for noise, which is otherwise not considered. The resulting image is a nonquantitative artifact-full image of $DPRPF + N$ and not an R image as is usually supposed.

15-6-2 Diffraction Tomography

In this technique the inhomogeneous Helmholtz equation

$$(\nabla^2 + k^2)\tilde{p}(\mathbf{r}, k) = f(\mathbf{r})\tilde{p}(\mathbf{r}, k)$$

where

$$f(\mathbf{r}) = k^2\left[1 - \frac{c_0^2}{c^2(\mathbf{r})}\right]$$

is assumed to govern the propagation of ultrasound through a loss-less or uniformly absorbing (complex k) tissue medium. The solution is obtained via the first Born and Rytov approximations, and knowledge of the attenuation is presupposed. This solution is then used to develop a reconstruction computer-based algorithm to map tissue parameters from observed two-dimensional complex amplitude distributions of the ultrasonic field for the medium of interest. Thus R has a single tissue parameter specification (weak velocity variations) and utilizes a specialized F (plane or spherical wave) and D (4π measurement at all frequencies or at all incident directions). P is relatively simple, and N is disregarded. The result is a quantitative map of the velocity distribution that is as exact as the approximations and measurement allow. Although improvements can be obtained through the use of inverse scattering methods, the image will remain distorted due to the assumption of a uniform input velocity in P and, in the case of a loss-less model, the neglect of absorption. However, in principle good resolution can be obtained. Within the context of Fig. 15-1 diffraction tomography attempts to rewrite the image process as

$$M = \hat{L}R$$

The approximations are then essential in order to obtain a tractable form for $\hat{L}$ and $\hat{L}^{-1}$.

15-6-3 Wave Extrapolation

Wave field extrapolation also uses the inhomogeneous Helmholtz equation in order to describe P. N is not considered, and the fundamental imaging equation is written in discrete form as

$$M(z_0) = D(z_0)\left\{\sum_{i=0}^{N} P(z_i, z_{i+1})R(z_{i+1})P(z_{i+1}, z_i)\right\}F(z_0)$$

R is not clearly specified. However, in principle a highly sophisticated P is possible, although in practice there are insufficient data available, and a uniform velocity with simple attenuation is assumed. R is found by matrix inversion. Hence, if we write the fundamental imaging equation in discrete matrix form, R is given by

$$R = (DP)^{-1}M(PF)^{-1}$$

The evaluation of the inverse matrices $(DP)^{-1}$ and $(PF)^{-1}$ is very time-consuming, and a real-time imaging system based on this technique would at present be inconceivable. The result is a quantitative exact R image with distortion.

15-6-4 Statistical Image Estimation

Statistical image estimation is unique among other scatter-imaging systems in so far as it models and specifically includes N. The theory invisages various D and F arrangements and utilizes a P approximated to that of a uniform medium with frequency-dependent attenuation. R is modeled by a weak random ensemble of isotropic point scatterers. The method requires that $M = DPRPF + N$ be written as $M = HR + N$, where $H = DP \, \delta PF$. The operators are reduced to a matrix form, and linear estimation theory together with signal processing is used to estimate R in the presence of noise. This technique gives a "best estimate" but distorted R image. The method is time-consuming, and it is not at all clear whether it can be applied *in vivo*.

15-6-5 Reflectivity Tomography

Reflectivity tomography maps a tissue scattering parameter by measurement of the backscattered wave field only. Exact inverse methods based on analytical solutions have been reported by Norton and Linzer [83] for variations in both compressibility and density but with absorption neglected and by Blackledge et al. [85] for variations in compressibility with uniform and dispersive absorption. The inverse scattering procedures are based on an exact inversion of a Fredholm integral equation of the first kind to obtain an expression for the scatter function. The technique neglects N, and D involves a 4π measurement aperture; in other words, the field is measured over a complete closed surface as a function of time for CW broad-band insonification. F must be of a specialized form (plane or spherical wave), but the method can accommodate frequency-dependent attenuation and velocity dispersion. The reconstruction is three-dimensional and yields an exact quantitative but distorted map of R (i.e., a scatter function mapping). An important aspect of reflectivity tomography is that, because only the backscattered field is measured, physical considerations indicate that the reflector is a single parameter, namely the impedance which is sometimes called the *reflectivity function*. This suggests that reflectivity tomography is an extension of the next imaging technique we discuss.

15-6-6 Impediography

Impediography is the original quantitative scatter imaging method and utilizes backscattered echos only. Thus the reflector R is specified for weak scattering, as the characteristic tissue impedance Z. P can be extended to include both frequency-dependent attenuation and velocity dispersion, even for pulse insonification from realistic transducers. D and F are both specialized, but N is not specifically taken into account. The method requires that we form the impulse response I given by

$$I = D^{-1}MF^{-1} = PZP$$

A mapping of Z is then obtained by calculating P^{-1} which at present can be obtained analytically for simple media but complicated cases. This technique yields a quantitative but distorted Z image.

15-7 SCATTER IMAGING AND THE INVERSE PROBLEM

Quantitative scatter-imaging methods are nothing but realizations of special solutions to the inverse scattering problem. The first step in solving such a problem is the specification of a wave equation (i.e., a physical model) and the solution of the direct problem, only then is the uncovered relationship between scattering parameters and measured quantities inverted. The specification of the physical model is a crucial step in the procedure, since only those interaction parameters that are incorporated into the original wave equation can be imaged. However, tissue may not conform to the postulated model in all respects, and the measured data may well not be totally compatible with the original wave equation. Under these circumstances the inversion scheme, which would be near exact only under the hypothesis that the postulated physical model applies, produces an image that in some sense is incorrect and thus hardly quantitive.

Much emphasis has been placed on constructing inversion schemes to underpin the quantitative scatter image, but little thought has been given to the limitations of the approach. We may identify three such problem areas:

1. *Resolution.* The attained resolution of the final image is the problem that has received the most attention. This is ultimately a data acquisition and computing problem. In this sense we may relate resolution primarily to the "data model."

2. *Distortion.* The final image may show geometrical distortions of the tissue structures. We include in this category also amplitude distortions, whereby the displayed value of the interaction parameter is distorted from its true value (in an *unknown* way). We have merely to consider the effects of refraction and simple attenuation to appreciate that distortion effects ultimately depend on the correctness of the propagator model.

3. *Fuzziness.* An image displaying the desired interaction parameters (combination) may be corrupted in an unpredictable way by some other interaction parameter(s) not included in the original physical model. Since we are dealing here primarily with quantitative scatter imaging (although our general considerations apply also to transmission imaging), it is clear that fuzziness stems from an incorrect reflector model. Note that a fuzzy image may appear quite sharp (i.e., be apparently highly resolved).

Much attention has focused on the resolution problem: The distortion problem has been addressed mainly within the context of transmission imaging, while fuzziness has been virtually unappreciated as a problem. We emphasize that the three problems in fact are interrelated. Consider a conventional impediography inversion procedure. The three steps involved here are measurement of backscattered signals, deconvolution to obtain the impulse response, and inversion via an "impediography equation" that relates the impedance profile to the impulse response. The actual form of the impediography equation depends on the physical model assumed. Consider a constant velocity model in which frequency-independent attenuation (propagator) and impedance fluctuations only (reflector) are assumed. The final impedogram will be fuzzy if it turns out that backscattering from absorption fluctuations (not included in the inversion scheme) are significant. If the attenuation is frequency dependent, then the ensuing pulse distortions will ensure an incorrect impulse response, which will in turn ensure a resolution loss in the displayed impedogram. However, we will indicate the following scheme bearing in mind that there may be some cross-links between the columns:

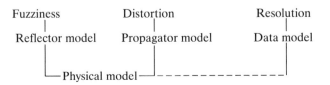

It should be clear that physical modeling underpins the entire framework of quantitative imaging.

An interesting example is afforded by diffraction tomography. Initially the technique was based on the loss-less Helmholtz equation (velocity fluctuations only). Given the measurement of angle scattering on which the technique is based, it is clear that the original technique would give rise to a distorted and fuzzy image. However, a much more detailed analysis by Mueller [86] based on quite a general viscoelastic tissue model has revealed that diffraction tomography, while not being fuzzy, displays an image of a rather unexpected combination of interaction parameters. An appreciation of the fuzziness concept runs deep in Mueller's work, even though the idea is not formulated as above, or analyzed as a general problem of quantitative imaging.

Another interesting, and poorly addressed, problem associated with quantitative imaging is one that we dub "freedom counting." The idea is easily explained by a simple example. Consider a two-dimensional velocity distribution $c(x, y)$. The velocity field shows two degrees of (spatial) freedom, x and y. It is clear that in order to reconstruct the velocity map, measurements with two degrees of freedom will also be needed. For example, in (two-dimensional) transmission tomography a time-of-flight projection (one degree of freedom) must be measured at all angles (second degree of freedom) in order to achieve a reconstruction; in (two-dimensional) diffraction tomography, the field scattered at all angles (one degree of freedom) must be measured for all angles of incidence (second degree of freedom). To measure both the attenuation $\alpha(x, y)$ and velocity distribution $c(x, y)$ of a given (two-dimensional) structure, it is clear that two sets of independent data, each with two degrees of freedom, will be required. The simple expedient of freedom counting often allows a preliminary judgment as to whether an elaborate, and usually highly mathematical, scheme can reconstruct all the postulated interaction parameters, within the context of the suggested data set.

In this section we have considered a number of scatter-imaging techniques in relation to the propagator-reflector concept and the fundamental imaging equation. We have analyzed each technique in the light of this equation, showing the merits and disadvantages of each imaging method. We have shown that quantitative scatter imaging demands exact tissue models, even if computations are approximate. The concept of image fuzziness has been introduced, and its relation to the physical model has been discussed. Thus an inexact model will lead to a fuzzy image, whereas an approximate computation will give poor resolution. Distortion is a common artifact in many of the techniques, and poor physical modeling manifests fuzziness in all the imaging methods. We conclude with a general criticism, common to all these techniques and applicable to all of medical imaging: Too large an emphasis is placed on computation in order to obtain high resolution, but not enough is placed on the accurate modeling of tissue. As a result the images are highly resolved but also badly distorted and often very fuzzy.

REFERENCES

1. R. Bracewell. *The Fourier Transform and Its Applications*. New York: McGraw-Hill, 1965.

2. A. Papoulis. *Probability, Random Variables, and Stochastic Processes*, 2nd ed. New York: McGraw-Hill, 1984.

3. E. Holasek, J. P. Jones, E. W. Purnell, and A. Sokollu. Spectra-color ultrasonography. I: Principles of a technique for incorporating spectral information into a B-scan display. In *Ultrasound in Medicine, 3B*, D. White and R. E. Brown, eds. New York: Plenum, 1977, pp. 1739–1745.

4. J. P. Jones, E. Holasek, E. W. Purnell, and A. Sokollu. Spectra-color ultrasonography. II: Report of a laboratory and clinical evaluation. In *Ultrasound in Medicine, 3B*, D. White and R. E. Brown, eds. New York: Plenum, 1977, pp. 1747–1752.

5. J. P. Jones and R. Kovack. A method for incorporating spectral information into a B-mode display format. *Proc. 1980, Am. Inst. Ultrasound in Medicine*, AIUM Pub., 1982.

6. Y. Hayakawa, J. Egawa, K. Yosioka, and T. Wagai. Multifrequency echoscopy for quantitative acoustical characterization of living tissue. *J. Acoust. Soc. Am.* 69:1838–1840 (1981).

7. L. Ferrari, J. P. Jones, V. Gonzalez, and M. Behrens. Acoustical imaging using the phase of echo waveforms. In *Acoustical Imaging*, vol. 12, E. A. Ash and C. R. Hill, eds. New York: Plenum, 1982, pp. 635–641.

8. T. Yokota and T. Sato. 3-D active incoherent ultrasonic imaging. In *Acoustical Imaging*, vol. 12, E. A. Ash and C. R. Hill, eds. New York: Plenum, 1982, pp. 621–634.

9. F. S. Foster, M. Arditi, M. S. Patterson, D. Lee-Chahal, and J. M. Hunt. Breast imaging with a conical transducer annular array hybrid scanner. *Ultrasound Med. Biol.* 9:151–164 (1983).

10. J. Y. Lu and J. F. Greenleaf. Pulse-echo imaging using a nondiffracting beam transducer. *Ultrasound Med. Biol.* 17:265–281 (1991).

11. P. S. Green, J. S. Ostrem, and T. K. Whitehurst. Combined reflection and transmission ultrasound imaging. *Ultrasound Med. Biol.* 17:283–289 (1991).

12. R. C. Chivers. Tissue characterization. *Ultrasound Med. Biol.* 7:1–20 (1981).

13. M. Linzer and S. J. Norton. Ultrasonic tissue characterization. *Ann. Rev. Biophys. Bioeng.* 11:303–329 (1982).

14. J. P. Jones and S. Leeman. Ultrasonic tissue characterization: A review. *Acta Electronica* 26:3–31 (1984).

15. J. J. Wild and J. M. Reid. Further pilot echographic studies on the histologic structures of tumors of the live intact human breast. *Amer. J. Path.* 28:839–861 (1952).

16. R. C. Waag, R. M. Lerner, and R. Gramiak. Swept frequency ultrasonic determination of tissue macrostructure. In *Ultrasonic Tissue Characterization*, M. Linzer, ed. NBS Special Publ. No. 453, 1976, pp. 213–228.

17. P. P. Lele and H. Senepeti. The frequency spectra of energy backscattered and attenuated by normal and abnormal tissue. In *Recent Advances*, D. H. White, ed. Forest Grove, Oregon: Research Press, 1977, pp. 55–85.

18. F. L. Lizzi and M. A. Laviola. Power spectra measurements of ultrasound backscatter from ocular tissue. *Proc. 1975 IEEE Ultrasonics Symp.* IEEE Pub. 75CH0994-45U, 1975, pp. 29–32.

19. R. Kuc and M. Schwartz. Estimating the acoustic attenuation coefficient slope for liver from reflected ultrasound signals. *IEEE Trans. Sonics Ultrason.* SU-26:353–362 (1979).

20. M. Fink, F. Hottier, and J. F. Cardoso. Ultrasonic signal processing for in vivo attenuation measurements: Short time Fourier analysis. *Ultrasonic Imag.* 5:117–135 (1983).

21. L. Ferrari, J. P. Jones, and V. M. Gonzalez. In vivo measurement of attenuation. *Ultrasonics* 66–72 (1986).

22. S. Leeman, L. Ferrari, J. P. Jones, and M. Fink. Perspectives on attenuation estimation from pulse-echo signals. *IEEE Trans. Sonics Ultrasonics*, SU-31:352–361 (1984).

23. J. Ophir, T. H. Shawker, N. F. Maklad, J. G. Miller, S. W. Flax, P. A. Narayana, and J. P. Jones. Attenuation estimation in reflection: Progress and prospects. *Ultrasonic Imag.* 6:349–395 (1984).

24. J. P. Jones. Ultrasonic impediography and its applications to tissue characterization. In *Recent Advances in Ultrasound in Biomedicine*, D. N. White, ed. Forest Grove, Oregon: Research Press, 1977, pp. 131–156.

25. J. P. Jones and C. Cole-Beuglet. In vivo characterization of several lesions in the eye using ultrasonic impediography. In *Acoustical Imaging*, vol. 8, A. Metherell, ed. New York: Plenum, 1980, pp. 539–546.

26. J. P. Jones. Current problems in ultrasonic impediography. In *Ultrasonic Tissue Characterization*, M. Linzer, ed. NBS Spec. Publ. No. 453, 1976, pp. 253–258.

27. S. Leeman, J. P. Jones, J. M. Blackledge, and D. Seggie. Impedance profiling of human tissues. In *Ultrasonics International*, vol. 83, Z. Novak, ed. London: IPC Science and Tech. Press, 1983.

28. S. Leeman. Impediography revisited. In *Acoustical Imaging*, vol. 9, K. Y. Wang, ed. New York: Plenum, 1980, pp. 513–520.

29. D. E. Robinson, F. Chen, and L. S. Wilson, Measurement of velocity of propagation from ultrasonic pulse-echo data. *Ultrasound Med. Biol.* 8:413–420 (1982).

30. D. E. Robinson, J. Ophir, L. S. Wilson, and C. F. Chen. Pulse-echo ultrasound speed measurements: Progress and prospects. *Ultrasound Med. Biol.* 17:633–646 (1991).

31. I. Cespedes, J. Ophir, and Y. Huang. On the feasibility of pulse-echo speed of sound estimation in small regions: simulation studies. *Ultrasound Med. Biol.* 18:283–291 (1992).

32. R. W. Huggins and J. V. Phelps. Bragg diffraction scanner for ultrasonic tissue characterization in vivo. *Ultrasound Med. Biol.* 2:271–277 (1976).

33. D. Nicholas and A. M. Nicholas. Two-dimensional diffraction scanning of normal and cancerous human hepatic tissue in vitro. *Ultrasound Med. Biol.* 9:283–296 (1983).

34. A. D. Wagoner, J. E. Perez, J. G. Miller, and B. E. Sobel. Differentiation of normal and ischemic right ventricular myocardium with quantitative two-dimensional integrated backscatter imaging. *Ultrasound Med. Biol.* 18:249–253 (1992).

35. T. G. Muir and E. L. Carstensen. Prediction of nonlinear acoustic effects at biomedical frequencies and intensities. *Ultrasound Med. Biol.* 6:345–357 (1980).

36. W. K. Law, L. A. Frizzell, and F. Dunn. Ultrasonic determination of the nonlinearity parameter B/A for biological media. *J. Acoust. Soc. Am.* 69:1210–1212 (1981).

37. K. Yamashita, T. Sato, and K. Y. Jhang. Simultaneous Imaging of movability nonlinearity, and reflectivity of soft tissue. *Ultrasonic Imag.* 14:206 (1992).

38. I. Cespedes, H. Ponnekanti, and J. Ophir. Elastography, experimental results from phantom and biological studies. *Ultrasonic Imag.* 14:189 (1992).

39. J. Fraser, G. S. Kino, and J. Bernholz. Cepstral signal processing for tissue signature analysis. In *Ultrasonic Tissue Characterization II*, M. Linzer, ed. Washington, DC: NBS Special Publ. No. 525, 1979, pp. 287–295.

40. F. L. Lizzi, M. A. Laviola, and D. J. Coleman. Examination of soft tissue histology by frequency domain analysis. In *Ultrasound in Medicine, 3B*, D. White and R. E. Brown, eds. New York: Plenum, 1977, pp. 2079–2080.

41. L. Joynt, R. Martin, and A. Macovski. Techniques for in vivo tissue characterization. In *Acoustical Imaging*, vol. 8, A. Metherell, ed. New York: Plenum, 1980, pp. 527–538.

42. F. G. Sommer, L. Joynt, B. Carroll, and A. Macovski. Ultrasonic characterization of abdominal tissues via digital analysis of backscattered waveforms. *Radiology* 141:811–817 (1981).

43. J. P. Jones, V. Gonzalez, and R. Kovack. Differentiation of abdominal organs and pathologies by the analysis of A-mode ultrasound waveforms. *Proc. 1980 IEEE Ultrasonics Symp.*, IEEE Publ. 80CH1602-2, 1980.

44. J. Gallet and J. P. Jones. The envelope correlation spectrum as a means for characterizing tissue structure. *Ultrasound Med. Biol.* (forthcoming).

45. R. A. Lerski, E. Barnett, P. Morley, P. R. Mills, G. Watkinson, and R. N. M. MacSween. Computer analysis of ultrasound signals in diffuse liver disease. *Ultrasound Med. Biol.* 5:341–350 (1979).

46. V. Gonzalez, J. P. Jones, L. Ferrari, and M. Behrens. The analysis of A-mode waveforms with a one-dimensional texture algorithm. *Proc. 1981, IEEE Ultrasonics Symp.*, IEEE Pub. 81CH1689-9, 1981, pp. 952–955.

47. M. S. Good, J. L. Rose, and B. B. Goldberg. Applications of pattern recognition techniques to breast cancer detection: ultrasonic analysis of 100 pathologically confirmed tissue areas. *Ultrasonic Imag.* 4:378 (1982).

48. D. M. Benson, L. D. Waldroup, A. B. Kurtz, J. L. Rose, M. D. J. Rifkin, and B. B. Goldberg. Ultrasonic tissue characterization of fetal lung, liver, and placenta for the purposes of assessing fetal maturity, *J. Ultrasound Med.* 2:489–494 (1983).

49. S. Finette, A. Bleier, and W. Swindell. Breast tissue classification using diagnostic ultrasound and pattern recognition techniques. I: Methods of pattern recognition. *Ultrasonic Imag.* 5:55–70 (1983).

50. S. Finette, A. Bleier, W. Swindell, and K. Harber. Breast tissue characterization using diagnostic ultrasound and pattern recognition techniques. II: Experimental results. *Ultrasonic Imag.* 5:71–86 (1983).

51. R. F. Wagner, D. G. Brown, K. J. Meyers, and K. A. Wear. Multivariate tissue characterization. *Ultrasonic Imag.* 14:200 (1992).

52. S. Leeman, J. Gehrke, L. Hutchins, and P. Sutton. Cardiac tissue characterization. In *Ultrasonic Tissue Characterization*, J. M. Thijssen, ed. Brussels: Stapen, 1980, pp. 117–123.

53. S. Leeman, J. F. Heckmatt, and V. Dubowitz. Ultrasound imaging in the diagnosis of muscle disease. *J. Pediatrics* 101:656 (1982).

54. D. N. Bateman, S. Leeman, C. Metreweli, and K. Willson. A non-invasive technique for gastric motility measurement. *Br. J. Radiology* 50:526–527 (1977).

55. S. Leeman, P. C. Badcock, J. C. Gore, J. Plessner, and K. Willson. Ultrasonic backscattering assessment of tumor response to treatment. *Tumor Ultrasound* (London) 77 (1977).

56. J. L. Gore, S. Leeman, C. Metreweli, and N. J. Plessner. Dynamic autocorrelation analysis of A-scans, in vivo. In *Ultrasonic Tissue Characterization II*, M. Linzer, ed. NBS. Spec. Pub. No. 525, 1979, pp. 275–280.

57. R. J. Dickinson and C. R. Hill. Measurement of soft tissue motion using correlation between A-scans. *Ultrasound Med. Biol.* 8:263–271 (1982).

58. P. N. T. Wells, M. Halliwell, B. Skidmore, A. J. Webb, and J. P. Woodcock. Tumor detection by ultrasonic Doppler blood flow signals. *Ultrasonics* 15:213–232 (1977).

59. H. Minasian and J. C. Bamber. A preliminary assessment of an ultrasonic Doppler method for the study of blood flow in human breast cancer. *Ultrasound Med. Biol.* 8:357–364 (1982).

60. A. Ishimaru. *Wave Propagation and Scattering in Random Media*, vol. 1. San Diego: Academic Press, 1978.

61. A. C. Kak and M. Slaney. *Principles of Computerized Tomographic Imaging*. New York: IEEE Press, 1988.

62. S. Leeman. The impediography equations. In *Acoustical Imaging*, vol. 8, A. F. Metherell, ed. New York: Plenum, 1980, pp. 517–525.

63. A. J. Berkhout, J. Ridder, and L. F. v.d. Wal. Acoustic imaging by wave field extrapolation. Part I: Theoretical consideration. In *Acoustical Imaging*, vol. 10, P. Alais and A. F. Metherell, eds. New York: Plenum, 1982, pp. 513–540.

64. J. Ridder, A. J. Berkhout, and L. F. v.d. Wal. Acoustic imaging by wave field extrapolation. Part II: Practical aspects. In *Acoustical Imaging*, vol. 10, P. Alais and A. F. Metherell, eds. New York: Plenum, 1982, pp. 541–565.

65. J. P. Lefebvre. Theoretical basis of an ultrasonic investigation method of stratified absorbing media. In *Acoustical Imaging*, vol. 10, P. Alais and A. F. Metherell, eds. New York: Plenum, 1982, pp. 287–293.

66. J. F. Greenleaf, S. A. Johnson, W. F. Samayoa, and F. A. Duck. Algebraic reconstruction of spatial distribution of acoustic velocities in tissue from their time-of-flight profiles. In *Acoustical Holography*, vol. 6, N. Booth, ed. New York: Plenum, 1974, pp. 71–90.

67. J. F. Greenleaf, S. A. Johnson, and A. H. Lent. Measurement of spatial distribution of refractive index in tissues by ultrasonic computer assisted tomography. *Ultrasound Med. Biol.* 3:327–339 (1978).

68. G. H. Glover and J. C. Sharp. Reconstruction of ultrasound propagation speed distributions in soft tissue. Time of flight tomography. *IEEE Trans. Sonics Ultrason.* SU-24:229–234 (1977).

69. G. H. Glover. Computerized time-of-flight ultrasonic tomography for breast examination. *Ultrasound Med. Biol.* 3:117–128 (1977).

70. J. F. Greenleaf, J. J. Gisvold, and R. C. Bahn. A clinical prototype ultrasonic transmission tomographic scanner. In *Acoustical Imaging*, vol. 12, E. A. Ash and C. R. Hill, eds. New York: Plenum, 1982, pp. 579–587.

71. P. L. Carson, C. R. Meyer, A. L. Scherzinger, and T. V. Oughton. Breast imaging in the coronal planes with simultaneous pulse echo and transmission ultrasound. *Science* 214:1141 (1981).

72. P. Harper and E. Kelly-Fry. Ultrasound visualization of the breast in symptomatic patients. *Radiology* 137:465–469 (1980).

73. J. Jellins, G. Kossoff, T. S. Reeve, and B. H. Barraclough. Ultrasonic grey scale visualization of breast disease. *Ultrasound Med. Biol.* 1:393–404 (1975).

74. C. Cole-Beuglet and B. B. Goldberg. Ultrasound in the diagnosis of breast cancer. In *Ultrasound in Cancer, Clinics in Diagnostic Medicine*, B. B. Goldberg, ed. Edinburgh: Churchill Livingstone Press, 1981, pp. 157–166.

75. A. P. Harper, V. P. Jackson, J. Bies, R. Ransburg, E. Kelly-Fry, and J. S. Noe. A preliminary analysis of the ultrasound imaging characteristics of malignant breast masses as compared with X-ray mammographic appearance and the gross and microscopic pathology. *Ultrasound Med. Biol.* 8:365–368 (1982).

76. C. Cole-Beuglet, B. B. Goldberg, A. B. Kurtz, C. S. Rubin, A. S. Patchefsky, and G. S. Shaber. Ultrasound mammography: A comparison with radiographic mammography. *Radiology* 139:639–698 (1981).

77. H. S. Teixidor and E. Kazam. Combined mammographic-sonographic evaluation of breast masses. *Am. J. Cardiology* 128:409–417 (1977).

78. T. R. Coulter, M. Kaveh, R. K. Mueller, and R. L. Rylander. Experimental results with diffraction tomography. *Proc. 1979 Ultrasonics Symp.*, IEEE Publ. 79CHI 482-9, 1979, pp. 405–406.

79. R. K. Mueller, M. Kaveh, and G. Wade. Reconstructive tomography and applications to ultrasonics. *Proc. IEEE* 67:567–587 (1979).

80. J. Ball, S. A. Johnson, and F. Stenger. Explicit inversion of the Helmholtz equation for ultrasound insonification and spherical detection. In *Acoustical Imaging*, vol. 9, E. Y. Wang, ed. New York: Plenum, 1980, pp. 451–461.

81. A. J. Devaney. A filtered backpropagation algorithm for diffraction tomography. *Ultrasonic Imag.* 4:336–350 (1982).

82. A. J. Devaney. A computer simulation study of diffraction tomography. *IEEE Trans. Biomed. Eng.* BME-30:377–386 (1983).

83. S. J. Norton and M. Linzer. Ultrasonic reflectivity imaging in three dimensions. *IEEE Trans. Biomed. Eng.* BME-28:202–220 (1981).

84. A. J. Berkhout, J. Ridder, and M. P. DeGraaff. New possibilities in data measurement, signal processing and information extraction: Philosophy and results. In *Acoustical Imaging*, vol. 12, E. A. Ash and C. R. Hill, eds. New York: Plenum, 1982, pp. 269–279.

85. J. M. Blackledge, M. A. Fiddy, S. Leeman, and L. Zapalowski. Three dimensional imaging of soft tissue with dispersive attenuation. In *Acoustical Imaging*, vol. 12, E. A. Ash and C. R. Hill, eds. New York: Plenum, 1982, pp. 423–433.

86. R. K. Mueller, M. Kaveh, and R. D. Iverson. A new approach to acoustic tomography using diffraction techniques. In *Acoustical Imaging*, vol. 18, A. F. Metherell, ed. New York: Plenum, 1980, pp. 615–628.

V

BIOMAGNETIC IMAGING

16

NEUROMAGNETIC IMAGING

From the preceding chapters it is clear that the introduction of X-ray computed tomography in the 1970s, followed by the emergence of magnetic resonance imaging in the 1980s has made it possible to visualize three-dimensional anatomical details of the human brain with exquisite resolution (less than 1 mm) and clarity never attainable before. Complementing MRI and X-ray CT, nuclear medical imaging techniques, notably positron emission tomography (PET) and single photon emission computed tomography (SPECT), have now evolved to the stage where local biochemical function in the human brain can be mapped to a resolution of about 5 mm. Rapid progress is underway in localized magnetic resonance spectroscopy (MRS) in the 1990s, resulting in a new modality to obtain unique biochemical information pertinent to brain function at a resolution approaching that of PET.

In contrast to the above-mentioned imaging modalities, which provide an excellent depiction of brain anatomy and its function related to metabolism, techniques to visualize or image neural activity directly are relatively undeveloped at the present time. A technique to image the 3-D spatiotemporal distribution of neural activity, either spontaneous activity or activity evoked by specific stimuli, would be of enormous significance to many areas of clinical and basic sciences. For example, it would lead to a better understanding of the neural substrate of complex human behavior, such as speech and language, which is of fundamental importance in many areas of cognitive neuroscience and neural engineering. In addition a technique to identify areas of the brain involved in performing specific functions would be extremely useful in neurosurgery for maneuvering the surgical probes and/or optimizing surgery to avoid damage to any functionally critical regions.

551

Neuromagnetic imaging (NMI) [1] is a relatively new imaging technique based on measuring the magnetic field emitted by neurons during functional activation. The magnetic field emitted from the brain, called the *neuromagnetic field*, is measurable by a superconducting quantum interference device (SQUID) based neuromagnetometer. NMI has great potential in generating 3-D maps of the spatiotemporal distribution of neural activity involved in specific functional tasks. As described below, other noninvasive imaging procedures that detect changes in brain function are based on metabolic differences caused by increased or decreased activity of specific neural areas. For the most part these are single integrated "snapshots" of activity changes over prolonged periods of time. However, most neural functions are associated with activity changes occurring over very short time periods. In humans it has been possible to record changes in neural activity using surface electrodes, such as cortical encephalography (EEG), or in some research animals it has been possible to record the activity changes associated with most "deeper" brain and spinal cord areas using depth electrodes. Thus, some basic information concerning the involvement of certain brain areas in different functions has been obtained. Yet very little is known about the spatiotemporal interactions of brain structures during many sensory/motor functions. Although such information is possible to obtain using recording electrodes, these studies are technically difficult, and they have severe inherent limitations. One serious limitation is that they require invasive procedures that may in fact influence the activity that is being recorded. For example, the use of anesthetics can markedly affect the interactions between different neural areas. The introduction of recording electrodes may also influence activity through damage or irritation. Such recording techniques are also limited in that they do not provide a visual image of the brain. Once developed, SQUID-based NMI in conjunction with existing imaging modalities could overcome these difficulties, and thus provide an excellent opportunity to examine the spatiotemporal interactions of different neural structures during a variety of sensory, motor, and higher-order processing. The basic principles underlying SQUID neuromagnetometry and results of a few key experiments to demonstrate the potential of NMI are described in this chapter.

16-1 BACKGROUND

Neural activation is accompanied by changes in membrane potential, leading to a flow of ions within the dendrites of activated neurons. This ionic flow or current produces two measurable neurophysiologic parameters: electrical potential differences on the surface of the head, and a magnetic field in the space surrounding the head. In principle measurements of either parameter —namely measurements of the electrical potentials on the scalp or measurements of the neuromagnetic field around the head—should enable reconstruction of the underlying neural activity. In practice, however, the task of estimating neural sources from electrical potential measurements becomes very difficult because the electrical current is widely distributed due to volume conduction within the relatively homogeneous brain. Since the higher electrical resistance of the skull disperses currents laterally, neural generators of electrical potential are poorly localizable by scalp electrodes. Furthermore the potential difference between two surface electrode positions is not a direct measure of current because it is impossible to find a truly neutral site for an indifferent reference electrode.

A localization or imaging technique based on the detection of the neuromagnetic field, instead of that based on measuring cortical potentials, could overcome these limitations. In contrast to the electrical potential, which depends on a more diffuse extracellular volume current, the magnetic field is relatively unattenuated by the overlying skull and scalp. The normal component of the neuromagnetic field arises solely from the denser intracellular current flow [2]. Magnetic fields detected beyond the scalp thus provide two major advantages over electrical potential measures: Magnetic fields are measured directly without need for a reference electrode, and spatial resolution is expected to be superior for localizing sources of the underlying neural activity. The quantitative advantages of magnetoencephalography (MEG) over EEG in practical situations, however, are a matter of national debate at the present time, with a reported value of 8 mm for the average error of localization in MEG compared to a 10-mm error in EEG using implanted sources in the human brain [3–6].

The neuromagnetic field, which is on the order of 0.1 to 0.01 pico tesla, can be measured by a SQUID-based neuromagnetometer. A brief description of a SQUID neuromagnetometer is provided in a later section. The neuromagnetometer can be configured to be sensitive only to a gradient of the magnetic field, thereby rejecting the earth's field and other steady fields. Thus, neuromagnetic measurements can be performed in a magnetically unshielded room in a normal hospital environment. SQUID-based single-channel as well as multichannel neuromagnetometers with as many as 37 channels are currently available commercially [7, 8]. Given the recent advances in high-temperature superconductivity, it is very likely that a much larger array of SQUID sensors could be designed in the not too distant future to sample simultaneously the neuromagnetic field surrounding the entire head.

In human studies SQUIDs have been used mainly to record the normal and abnormal magnetoencephalograms [9, 10], visual evoked fields [11, 12], auditory evoked fields [13, 14], somatosensory evoked fields [15], and fields preceding voluntary movement [16]. A review of these measurements is given in Williamson and Kaufman [17]. In most cases the neuromagnetic fields have been localized to a single "equivalent dipolar source" within the brain [17]. For fields evoked by simple iterative stimuli, the computed location of the single dipole agrees closely with neural generators predicted on the basis of known functional anatomy. For example, the somatosensory field evoked in response to repetitive electrical shocks to the little finger was localized to the appropriate region of the contralateral primary sensory cortex. When the thumb was stimulated instead of the little finger, the localized source shifted downward by 2 cm within this sensory representation [18], in agreement with the known functional organization of the primary somatosensory area in the human brain.

In addition to sensory processing referred to above, NMI has the potential of providing unique information on brain processing related to cognitive or higher-order processing. As indicated earlier, PET, SPECT, and MRS are the primary modalities to study brain function at the present time. However, the radiation dose in nuclear medicine and the relatively low sensitivity of MRS represent significant limitations to these modalities. The temporal resolution in PET, SPECT, and MRS is on the order of one to several minutes, which is insufficient to resolve most temporal processing in the brain. For example, a common method of studying brain function in PET is to use F-18 fluorodeoxyglucose (FDG) to map regional brain metabolism [19]. Several minutes of counting after an initial delay of about 30 min are required to produce images. Thus information from transient brain processes occurring with several hundred milliseconds after stimulation is lost. Although gated cerebral blood flow imaging in PET or SPECT, or blood flow/volume related functional MRI, could provide better temporal resolution, there is evidence that regional blood flow does not always accurately reflect either metabolism or ephemeral changes in regional neural activity [20]. Moreover, because of count statistics and the relatively slow kinetics of blood flow, it is highly unlikely that gated blood flow will yield an effective temporal resolution better than 1 sec, which is still more than an order of magnitude worse than that needed to resolve temporal processes in the brain.

NMI provides unique information related to the spatiotemporal distribution of neural activity. It is entirely functional information with very little clue to the corresponding brain anatomy. Thus, to visualize and understand the distribution of neural activity in relation to brain structure, it is necessary to superimpose NMI on an anatomical imaging technique such as MRI. Accurate superposition in turn requires a method to register neuromagnetic and MRI measurements. A registration procedure for this purpose is discussed in Section 16-5-2.

The basic concepts of NMI showing how images of the neural sources responsible for generating the neuromagnetic field could be reconstructed under certain modeling constraints from a sampling of the neuromagnetic field have been described in [1, 21–24]. Although, as indicated above, SQUIDs have been used to record the spontaneous magnetoencephalogram (MEG) and magnetic fields evoked by simple sensory stimuli for over two decades [17], the concept of NMI to produce 3-D images was conceived by Singh et al. [1] recently, and the general imaging problem remains unsolved at the present time. A brief overview of the imaging problem and some model constrained solutions is given in the next section.

16-2   MODELS AND IMAGE RECONSTRUCTION

In general, the inverse problem, where the 3-D distribution of neural sources is determined from a measurement of the neuromagnetic field, has no unique solution. However, the image reconstruction can be constrained from known anatomical and physiological considerations. Under these conditions it becomes possible to find a meaningful solution to the imaging problem.

The neuromagnetic field is produced by the aggregate activity of a large number of neurons. Discretizing the volume of the brain in cubic elements or voxels, the aggregate activity within each voxel could be modeled as a single-current dipole, that is, as a small current source with a certain direction and amplitude. The model may be simplified by the observation that pyramidal-cell-type neurons within the cortex that generate currents through depolarization or hyperpolarization are organized into columns normal to the cortical surface [17]. Thus the orientation of the current dipolar sources could be constrained and determined from MRIs. Also the region within which these dipolar sources lie could be constrained from PET or functional MRI and known physiology, providing enough a priori information to enable reconstruction of the spatiotemporal distribution of neural activity. Similarly models for noncortical sources, such as sources in the hippocampus, could be developed based on anatomical and physiological considerations.

Assuming neural activity to be represented by a distribution of current dipolar sources, the neuromagnetic field at any point above the head is a weighted sum of the field produced by each dipole. The magnetic field produced by a current dipole can be calculated from a straightforward application of the Biot-Savart equation, which in discrete form leads to the following approximation:

$$\underline{B}(\underline{r}_m, t_0) = \frac{\mu}{4\pi} \sum_{n=1}^{N} \frac{\underline{Q}(\underline{r}_n) \times (\underline{r}_m - \underline{r}_n)}{|\underline{r}_m - \underline{r}_n|^3}, \qquad m = 1, M \qquad (16\text{-}1)$$

where $\underline{B}(\underline{r}_m, t_0)$ is the magnetic field at position $\underline{r}_m$, at a single point in time t_0, μ is the permeability of the brain (assumed to be homogeneous), $\underline{Q}(\underline{r}_n)$ denotes the vector current source at location $\underline{r}_n$ at time t_0, N denotes the total number of voxels in the brain, and M denotes the total number of measurement points. The inverse problem posed by Eq. (16-1) is to estimate $\underline{Q}(\underline{r}_n)$ as a function of time, that is, to determine the spatiotemporal distribution of neural activity from measurements of $\underline{B}(\underline{r}_m)$ as a function of time. The conceptual basis of this problem is depicted in Fig. 16-1 where we show

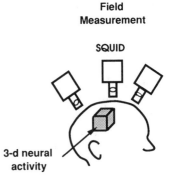

Figure 16-1 A conceptual depiction of how the component of the neuromagnetic field perpendicular to the scalp is measured at several locations around the head by a SQUID neuromagnetometer. A single-channel SQUID is moved from one position to the next to record samples from different locations. Samples are obtained following the curvilinear surface of the head. Multiple-channel SQUIDs perform measurements simultaneously over a large region. The sought-after neural activity is shown distributed within a cubical region inside the head. (Reproduced with permission from ref. [39].)

how measurements of the neuromagnetic field are made in the space surrounding the head. The purpose of NMI is to reconstruct the neural activity inside the head (shown as a cubical region in Fig. 16-1) responsible for producing the measured neuromagnetic field pattern.

In an initial approach designed to reduce the dimensionality of the reconstruction problem, we consider the magnetostatic problem only, ignoring the time dependence of Eq. (16-1), and constrain the dipoles to lie on a single plane modeled as a semi-infinite volume conductor [1, 2, 17]. Since the magnetic field due to a dipole oriented normal to the surface of a semi-infinitive volume conductor is zero everywhere in the nonconducting region [2, 17], only dipoles oriented tangential to the surface (the x, y components of the dipole vector) need to be considered.

Consider the case of dipoles located on a plane $z = 0$ (see Fig. 16-2) and oriented parallel to that plane. Ignoring volume currents the magnetic field measurements on a plane $z = d$ (Fig. 16-2) can be computed using the Biot-Savart Eq. (16-1) after dropping the dependence on time as follows:

$$B_x(k,l) = \kappa \sum_{i=1}^{I} \sum_{j=1}^{J} \frac{Q_y(i,j)\,d}{\text{DEN}} \tag{16-2}$$

$$B_y(k,l) = -\kappa \sum_{i=1}^{I} \sum_{j=1}^{J} \frac{Q_x(i,j)\,d}{\text{DEN}} \tag{16-3}$$

$$B_z(k,l) = \kappa \sum_{i=1}^{I} \sum_{j=1}^{J} \frac{Q_x(i,j)(l-j) - Q_y(i,j)(k-i)}{\text{DEN}}, \tag{}$$

$$k = 1,\ldots,K; l = 1,\ldots,L \tag{16-4}$$

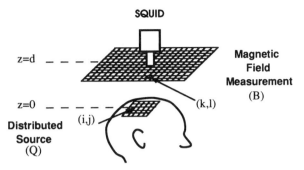

Figure 16-2 The measurement plane and the source plane. Measurements of the normal component of the neuromagnetic field are made by moving the SQUID from one pixel (k, l) to another on the measurement plane. The indices (i, j) denote a pixel within the source plane. The measurement plane is located at a distance d from the source plane.

where

$$\text{DEN} = \left[(k - i)^2 + (l - j)^2 + d^2 \right]^{3/2}$$

$$\kappa = \frac{\mu}{4\pi}$$

k and l are the pixel locations along the x and y direction, respectively, for the B image of dimension $K \times L$, and i and j are the corresponding pixel locations for the Q image of dimension $I \times J$. B_x, B_y, and B_z represent the x, y, and z components of the magnetic field, and Q_x and Q_y the x and y components of the dipoles (lying on the x-y plane).

After neglecting the constant κ, Eqs. (16-2)–(16-4) can be represented as the convolution of the Q images with their corresponding point spread functions (PSFs) as follows:

$$B_x = Q_y * \text{PSF}_{yx} \tag{16-5}$$

$$B_y = Q_x * \text{PSF}_{xy} \tag{16-6}$$

$$B_z = Q_x * \text{PSF}_{xz} + Q_y * \text{PSF}_{yz} \tag{16-7}$$

where

$$\text{PSF}_{yx} = d/\text{DEN}\,2, \quad \text{PSF}_{xy} = -d/\text{DEN}\,2, \quad \text{PSF}_{xz} = j/\text{DEN}\,2$$

$$\text{PSF}_{yz} = -i/\text{DEN}\,2$$

$$\text{DEN}\,2 = \left(i^2 + j^2 + d^2 \right)^{3/2}$$

Taking the discrete Fourier transforms (DFTs) of Eqs. (16-5)–(16-7) leads to

$$\text{DFT}(B_x) = \text{DFT}(Q_y)\text{DFT}(\text{PSF}_{yx}) \qquad (16\text{-}8)$$

$$\text{DFT}(B_y) = \text{DFT}(Q_x)\text{DFT}(\text{PSF}_{xy}) \qquad (16\text{-}9)$$

$$\text{DFT}(B_z) = \text{DFT}(Q_x)\text{DFT}(\text{PSF}_{xz}) + \text{DFT}(Q_y)\text{DFT}(\text{PSF}_{yz}) \quad (16\text{-}10)$$

Then the inverse problem posed under these planar constraints can be solved in Fourier domain from Eqs. (16-8)–(16-10) by a simple division of the DFTs of the magnetic field component images by the corresponding DFTs of the PSF images for the nonzero values of the PSF DFTs. For zero values the corresponding $\text{DFT}(Q)$ is assigned a value of zero.

16-2-1   Simulation Studies

Restricted Orientation
In the case of restricted orientation, we assume that the dipoles are oriented toward either θ or $-\theta$; that is, the directions of all dipoles are either parallel or antiparallel to each other. This constraint is based on the columnar organization of pyramidal cells within a cortical layer, as mentioned earlier [17]. From Eq. (16-10) this constraint implies that either Q_x or Q_y is zero. Thus there is only one Q component to be reconstructed, and the inverse problem can be solved in a straightforward manner from Eq. (16-10) by dividing the DFT of the measured B_z (normal component of the neuromagnetic field) by the DFT of the appropriate PSF (either PSF_{yz} or PSF_{xz}) at a given depth d.

A typical study is presented in Fig. 16-3. The phantom, shown at the top left in Fig. 16-3(a) represents a planar distribution of dipolar sources lying within a disk-shaped region. All dipoles are oriented along the same direction. The normal component of the neuromagnetic field generated by the phantom in accordance with Eq. (16-1) and sampled on 64×64 pixels is shown at the top right in Fig. 16-3(a). An eight-bit gray scale was used to display the field strength, with the upper seven bits assigned to represent positive field values and the lower seven bits assigned to negative fields. The reconstructed images on planes as a function of their depth d are presented in the second and third rows of Fig. 16-3(a). The values of d from left to right are 0.5, 1.0, and 2.0 cm, respectively, for the second row and 3.0, 4.0, and 4.5 cm, respectively, for the third row.

The correct depth of the phantom was 2.0 cm. A plot to determine the depth of the plane, based on a best-focus condition described below [23], is presented in Fig. 16-3(b), correctly locating the depth in this study.

Alternatively, the reconstruction in this case can be carried out by an iterative algorithm. An iterative approach is described in [1], based on measuring the neuromagnetic field on a 17×17 planar grid, whereby a

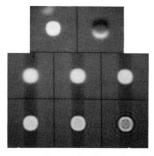

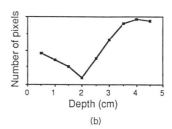

(b)

Figure 16-3   Reconstruction of a planar distribution of dipolar sources. (a) The phantom and the simulated field are shown in the top row (left to right) and the reconstructed images as a function of depth are shown in the middle and bottom rows. (b) A plot to determine the depth of the plane.

17×17 planar source distribution was reconstructed using an algebraic reconstruction technique (ART) incorporating Eq. (16-4). An example of the iterative reconstruction study is presented in Fig. 16-4. The normal component of the neuromagnetic field, generated by a distributed source in accordance with Eq. (16-1) and sampled on 1×1 cm pixels, is shown at the left in Fig. 16-4. As before, an eight-bit gray scale was used to display the field strength, with the upper seven bits assigned to represent positive field values and the lower seven bits assigned to negative fields. A Gaussian noise was added to the sampled field values to produce an SNR of 10 in the measurement. Assuming that the depth of this plane is known (or can be determined as described later), the reconstructed image on a single plane is as shown in Fig. 16-4 at the right. Good convergence was obtained in this case with only two iterations of ART.

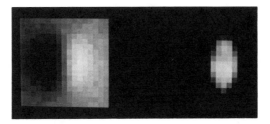

Figure 16-4   At the left computer-simulated samples of the magnetic field on a 17×17 grid, and at the right the planar image reconstructed using ART. A Guassian noise was added to the measurements to yield a SNR of 10.

16-2-2 Unrestricted Orientation in *x-y* Plane

The results of a simulation study corresponding to a planar distribution of dipoles at a known depth, where the dipoles could have any orientation within the *x-y* plane, are presented in Fig. 16-5. From Eqs. (16-8)–(16-10) it is clear that we now need to measure at least two components of the neuromagnetic field to obtain a direct solution. Results of a study assuming that the normal and one of the tangential components of the field would be measured are shown in Fig. 16-5. The phantom is depicted in the top row. Various disk sources with an arrow showing the orientation of the dipoles within each disk are shown at the left, and the horizontal and vertical components of these dipoles are shown at the center and right in the top row, respectively. The reconstructed images from noiseless data are presented in the bottom row following the same sequence as the top row, and they clearly show good reconstructions of both intensity and orientation of dipoles within each disk.

As indicated before, Dallas [25] has outlined a Fourier-space-based general approach to reconstructing current distributions. The technique, however, has been implemented to image planar distributed sources only [26],

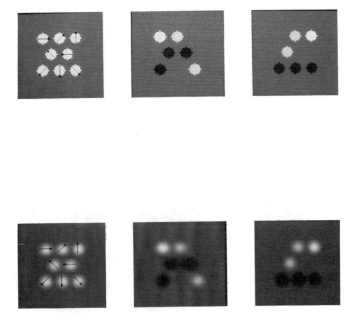

Figure 16-5 A simulation study to reconstruct the intensity and orientation of dipolar sources distributed on a plane. The phantom with its *x* and *y* components separated is depicted in the top row, and reconstructions with noiseless data are presented in the bottom row.

and it is uncertain if it can be extrapolated to three dimensions. Roth et al. [27] have presented a Fourier filtering approach to reconstruct planar distributed current sources with the additional constraint that all return or volume current is confined to the same plane. Under these conditions the continuity equation div $\mathbf{J} = 0$, where $\mathbf{J}$ is the total current density, is valid in two dimensions leading to an analytical solution to the inverse problem [27]. A similar constrained solution has also been derived by Alvarez [28]. Although the approaches in [27] and [28] are appropriate to image currents in electronic circuit boards, they are not readily adaptable to neuromagnetic imaging, since volume currents in the head flow in three dimensions even if the neuromagnetic sources (impressed current) were confined to a single plane. Consequently the continuity equation has to be solved in three dimensions, implying the lack of a unique solution to the 3-D neuromagnetic imaging problem [27].

16-3 INSTRUMENTATION

The SQUID neuromagnetometer is an extremely sensitive instrument to measure the very weak magnetic field emanating from the brain. The instrument comprises a detection coil (called the *pickup coil*), within which a small current is induced by an external magnetic field and an amplification circuitry whose essential component is the SQUID sensor. The SQUID sensor and the pickup coils are immersed in liquid helium contained within a special cryogenic vessel called a *dewar* to form a superconducting circuit to detect weak magnetic fields in the dc to 20 kHz range. The dewar is then mounted on a wooden or plastic gantry and usually suspended from the ceiling such that the neuromagnetometer can be positioned accurately above the head with provisions for x, y, z, and rotational movements. A typical single channel dc-SQUID neuromagnetometer with its associated computer circuitry to generate stimuli and acquire data time-locked to the stimuli, is shown in Fig. 16-6. The pickup coils are typically 2 cm in diameter, and they are designed to measure a specified gradient of the magnetic field (rather than the true magnetic field) to cancel contributions from the earth's magnetic field and from other relatively large but uniform fields in the environment. Measurements are made by placing the tail of the dewar containing the detection coil assemblies in proximity to the head and mechanically moving the probe from one position to the next above the head to sample the neuromagnetic field (Fig. 16-6, bottom). The neuromagnetic samples are digitized, filtered, and stored by a microcomputer (comp1, Fig. 16-6, top), which can also simultaneously acquire cortical electrical potentials from electrodes placed on the head. Stimuli to evoke a neuromagnetic field are generated by a separate microcomputer (comp2) driven synchronously with comp1.

The process of sampling the neuromagnetic field with the single-channel instrument is a very tedious and time-consuming process. The probe has to be adjusted at each position to be normal to the surface of the head so that

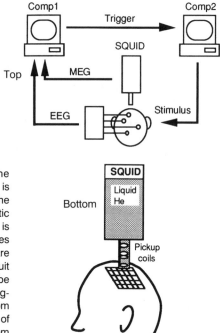

Figure 16-6 A block diagram of the single-channel SQUID neuromagnetometer is shown at the top, and the configuration of the SQUID detector to sample the neuromagnetic field from several locations above the head is conceptually depicted at the bottom. The series of detection coils (pickup coils), which are linked to a superconducting amplification circuit based on a SQUID sensor, are designed to be sensitive to the second-derivative of the magnetic field, thereby to cancel contributions from the relatively homogeneous magnetic field of the earth. (Reproduced with permission from ref. [39].)

the normal component of the neuromagnetic field can be measured with the highest sensitivity and minimum contamination from volume currents flowing within the brain [2]. This problem is greatly reduced by a 37-channel neuromagnetometer, which is commercially available at the present time from two vendors [7, 8]. A few typical experimental studies performed with the 37-channel instrument located at facilities of Biomagnetic Technologies Inc. (BTi) in San Diego are described below.

The 37-channel neuromagnetometer is configured similar to Fig. 16-2 except that it is located in a magnetically shielded room to reduce noise, and special purpose hardware is used to acquire data from the 37 channels simultaneously.

16-4 EXPERIMENTAL MEASUREMENTS WITH TEST OBJECTS

A few typical test-object studies performed to illustrate the planar image reconstruction capabilities of NMI are described in this section. To simulate extended sources lying on a cortical surface, the test-object studies were performed by pulsing a small current (~ 1 μA) through one or two long wires lying on a plane and measuring the resulting magnetic field above the

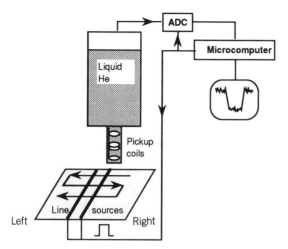

Figure 16-7 The experimental setup for acquiring data from line sources with the SQUID neuromagnetometer.

wires with a single-channel SQUID neuromagnetometer. The direction of current in the two-wire experiment was reversed from that in the single wire. The plane containing the single wire was located at a depth of 2.5 cm, and the plane containing the two wires at a depth of 2.0 cm from the bottom-most pickup coil. The experimental setup is depicted in Fig. 16-7.

Digital samples of the magnetic field were acquired on a 17×17 grid, composed of 1×1 cm pixels. Only the normal component of the magnetic field was measured in these preliminary studies; thus the reconstructions were constrained to only two possible orientations of the dipolar sources. Representative samples of the pulsed magnetic field acquired from the single wire at several locations on the 17×17 grid are shown in Fig. 16-8.

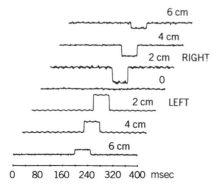

Figure 16-8 Representative magnetic field samples acquired with the neuromagnetometer from a wire carrying a current located 2.5 cm under the pickup coil. Data are shown for the central position of the neuromagnetometer (where the wire-carrying current is directly under the coil) and for positions displaced 2 to 6 cm to the left and right of the central position.

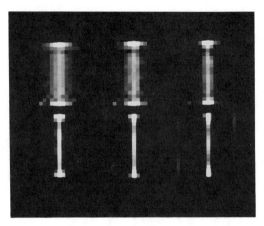

Figure 16-9 Tomographic images reconstructed from the single-wire data on planes at depths of 1.0 to 3.5 cm (left to right) in steps of 0.5 cm.

Tomographic images were reconstructed from the samples of magnetic field acquired with the magnetometer. Images corresponding to the single wire are shown in Fig. 16-9, whereas the images corresponding to the two-wire experiment are shown in Fig. 16-10. These images were reconstructed using the iterative algorithm ART described earlier on 1×1 cm pixels to conform to the 1-cm sampling interval. With the intention of locating the depth of the plane containing the current sources, images were reconstructed on planes lying at depths ranging from 1.0 to 4.0 cm in steps of 0.5 cm. Qualitatively the sharpest images are produced at a depth of 2 to 2.5 cm, which is very close to the correct depth. Note that the images correctly depict the reversal in current flow direction from the single- to the two-wire experiment.

A quantitative method to locate the depth of the plane containing the dipolar sources, based on minimizing the rms error between the forward computed field from each plane and the measured values, has been described in [1]. The method works well for scattered point sources and small distributed sources. However, further studies have shown that the rms criterion breaks down for large extended sources, the main reason being that ART produces a minimum norm solution that favors the plane closest to the detector. Another approach attempted in [23] searches for the "best-focused" plane by identifying the plane containing the minimum number of pixels above an intensity threshold, where the threshold is determined by the noise in the reconstruction. A threshold set at 5% of the maximum intensity value in the reconstructed planes appears to successfully identify the correct plane depth in both experiments as well as simulation studies. Plots of the total number of pixels above the 5% threshold in the experimentally reconstructed images are shown in Fig. 16-11, correctly indicating the depth in each case.

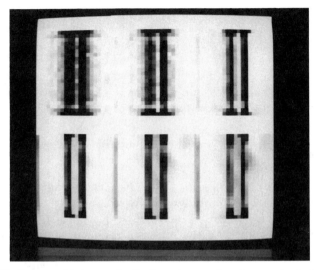

Figure 16-10   Tomographic images for the two-wire experiment, reconstructed on planes as in Fig. 16-9. Note the reversal of intensity in these images, correctly identifying the direction of current flow as opposite to that in Fig. 16-9.

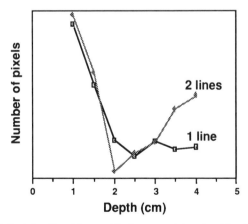

Figure 16-11   A plot of the "best-focused" plane as determined by the least number of pixels above a 5% intensity threshold.

These studies suggest that if cortical sources are modeled to lie on a single layer, it would be possible to (1) reconstruct the distribution of these sources and (2) determine the depth of the cortical layer. The above conclusion is based on measurements of the normal component of the magnetic field and only two possible orientations for the dipolar sources. Measurements of the tangential component of the magnetic field in addition to the normal component could in principle provide a general solution for reconstructing planar sources with no restrictions on their orientation. Extension of these techniques to reconstruct large distributions of sources in three dimensions is a complex problem, and no general solutions to the 3-D reconstruction problem are available at the present time.

16-5   HUMAN STUDIES

A variety of human neuromagnetic studies have been conducted over the last three decades. Most of these studies involve measurements of the neuromagnetic field evoked by a sensory stimulus such as visual, auditory, or somatosensory stimulation [17]. Also various measurements of the spontaneous neuromagnetic field or MEG have been conducted to (1) understand the generation of alpha waves or other spontaneous brain activity under normal conditions and (2) to search for epileptogenic regions involved in epilepsy [10]. As an example of a typical human experiment to measure the evoked

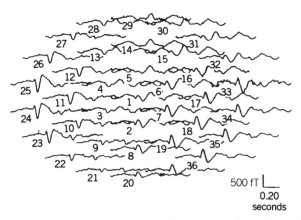

Figure 16-12   An example of the neuromagnetic field data acquired with the BTi 37-channel SQUID system. The neuromagnetic field measured by each channel above the right hemisphere of a subject in response to a 1 kHz tone burst presented to the left ear is shown in a format corresponding to the relative locations of the channels above the head. Each measurement represents an average of 64 time-locked presentations. Prominent peaks are visible at latencies of approximately 90 and 180 msec, with polarity reversed with respect to each other. Reproduced from ref. [34]

neuromagnetic field, details of a study to measure and localize neuronal activity in the brain involved in processing a simple auditory stimulus are presented below. If activities evoked by other types of stimuli—for example, photic stimulation, somatosensory stimulation, or stimuli requiring higher-order processing in the brain—can be investigated in a similar manner, ultimately we will have a detailed map of the spatial and temporal distribution of functional activity.

The measurements were conducted in a magnetically shielded room with a BTi 37-channel neuromagnetometer. The neuromagnetic field emitted in response to a 1-kHz, 200-msec tone burst presented to the left ear was measured above the scalp overlying the contralateral (right) cerebral hemisphere. An example of the evoked magnetic field, simultaneously recorded by each of the 37 channels and averaged over 64 presentations of the stimulus, is presented in Fig. 16-12. The main peaks occur at latencies of approximately 100 and 200 msec after onset of the stimulus. These are the so-called M100 and M200 components, which are presumed to correspond to components contained within the N100 and P200 waves of the evoked electrical potentials [29]. As can be seen in the figure, polarity reversals occur both as a function of latency and as a function of location above the head.

16-5-1   Coordinate Systems

All neuromagnetic measurements were related to a right-handed 3-D cartesian coordinate system based on the subject's head (heretofore referred to as the *head coordinate* system). Using the stylus of a tip digitizer, the subject's nasion and preauricular points were digitized and used to define the head coordinate system in the following manner [30]: The origin was defined as the midpoint between the preauricular points. The x-axis was defined as the line connecting the origin to the nasion. The z-axis was orthogonal to the x-axis, and the plane containing the nasion and the preauricular points and pointed toward the subject's vertex. The y-axis was orthogonal to the x- and z-axes and passed out of the left side of the head from the origin. In addition several other points on the surface of the head were digitized to serve as reference points for registering the neuromagnetic data and MR images of the same subject.

To register the neuromagnetometer in the head coordinate system, the locations of the 37 channels were first specified in a right-handed 3-D cartesian coordinate system (referred to as the *neuromagnetometer coordinate* system) from the known geometry of the pickup coils for each channel and were then transformed to the head coordinate system. Each detection coil has the geometry of a first-order gradiometer (two coaxial coils connected in series and wound in the opposite sense), and the coordinates of both coils in each channel were specified to determine the orientation of each channel. The transformation between the head (x, y, z) and the neuromagnetometer

(x^*, y^*, z^*) coordinate systems is of the form

$$\begin{bmatrix} x^* \\ y^* \\ z^* \end{bmatrix} = \begin{bmatrix} b_1 \\ b_2 \\ b_3 \end{bmatrix} + \begin{bmatrix} c_{11} & c_{12} & c_{13} \\ c_{21} & c_{22} & c_{23} \\ c_{31} & c_{32} & c_{33} \end{bmatrix} \begin{bmatrix} x \\ y \\ z \end{bmatrix} \qquad (16\text{-}11)$$

where the coefficients b_1, b_2, b_3, define the translation between the two systems, and the coefficients c_{kl} (which define a rotation around two orthogonal axes) satisfy the condition [31]:

$$\sum_{l=1}^{3} c_{kl} c_{ml} = \delta_{km}, \qquad k, m = 1, 2, 3 \qquad (16\text{-}12)$$

where δ_{km} is the Kronecker delta. Equations (16-11) and (16-12) imply that the coordinate transformation can be accomplished uniquely if the coordinates of the same three points (not collinear with the origin of either system) are known in each system to serve as reference points or landmarks. A probe position indicator (PPI) comprising a transmitter attached to the neuromagnetometer dewar and a set of three receivers attached to the subject's head by a Velcro band was used for this purpose. The position of the three receivers was determined in the head coordinate system by the tip digitizer and in the neuromagnetometer system by the transmitter, thereby providing the data to specify the location and orientation of each neuromagnetometer channel in the head coordinate system.

Spin-echo magnetic resonance images of the subject were subsequently acquired with a 1.5-tesla system using a spin-echo time $TE = 20$ msec and repetition time $TR = 500$ msec. Multiple plane 2-D images (5 mm thick, 2.5-mm gap between slices) were reconstructed after positioning the subject and selecting the orientation of the planes to be imaged so that the MR images and the neuromagnetic data would be represented, as close as possible, by the same 3-D coordinate system. However, due to difficulties in aligning a subject precisely within the scanner, subject and slice positioning cannot always provide exact registration. This is seen in the data shown in Fig. 16-13 representing a superposition of the MR images and the neuromagnetic reference points (the two preauricular points, nasion, and several points on the surface of the head) in which matching of the two modalities was attempted by positioning alone. Even if one were able to position the subject and set the alignment of the MRI scans to match a specified plane within the subject's head to a specified plane in the MR images, there is no assurance that there will be a perfect match in 3-D space due to inherent distortions in spatial coordinates within a stack of MR images.

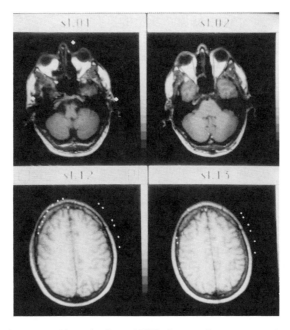

Figure 16-13 A superposition of selected MRI slices and neuromagnetic reference points. The reference points correspond to the nasion (arrow), preauricular points, and several points on the surface of the head (bright dots). Note the misregistration. (Reproduced from ref. [3]).

16-5-2 Registration

A first-order registration algorithm incorporating a shift, scaling, and rotation in three dimensions was developed to register the two modalities. The general approach represents an extension to three dimensions of a 2-D registration procedure described in [32]. The algorithm involves an estimation of the coordinate transformations needed to register the two modalities. We formulate the coordinate transformation as follows:

$$x = f_x(u_k, v_k, w_k)$$

$$y = f_y(u_k, v_k, w_k)$$

$$z = f_z(u_k, v_k, w_k)$$

where (x, y, z) is the final coordinate system and (u_k, v_k, w_k) the coordinate system of modality k. Using a polynomial expansion, we can express the transformation by the following equations:

$$x = a_0 + a_1 u_k + a_2 v_k + a_3 w_k + a_4 u_k v_k + a_5 v_k w_k + a_6 u_k w_k + a_7 u_k^2 + \cdots$$

$$y = b_0 + b_1 u_k + b_2 v_k + b_3 w_k + b_4 u_k v_k + b_5 v_k w_k + b_6 u_k w_k + b_7 u_k^2 + \cdots$$

$$z = c_0 + c_1 u_k + c_2 v_k + c_2 w_k + c_4 u_k v_k + c_5 v_k w_k + c_6 u_k w_k + c_7 u_k^2 + \cdots$$

The coefficients $a_0 \cdots a_n, b_0 \cdots b_n, c_0 \cdots c_n$, are estimated by least square regression using a set of landmarks previously measured. The order of the transformation and the number of landmarks required for an accurate estimate depends on the degree of distortion between the different modalities. As mentioned earlier, the nasion, preauricular points, and several additional points on the surface of the head were digitized during the neuromagnetic measurements. Corresponding points were detected manually in the MRIs from the displayed anatomy. Using these landmarks, a first-order correction procedure was implemented (i.e., only the first four coefficients in the above equations were estimated) in registering the neuromagnetic measurements and the MRIs. Higher-order corrections may be implemented if necessary.

16-5-3   Neuromagnetic Localization

The objective of NMI is to reconstruct the 3-D spatiotemporal distribution of multiple sources as a function of latency to image the neural activity involved in specific cerebral processing. The study described below, however, was restricted to reconstructing only one source per time window and following its location and orientation as a function of latency. It is expected that these studies will lay the foundation for future attempts at reconstructing the full 3-D distribution.

The reconstruction or localization of a single-point source was accomplished through a parameter optimization approach. From the Biot-Savart Eq. (16-1), the weighted least squares objective function to be minimized was

$$\sum_{m=1}^{M} w_m \left[\underline{B}(\underline{r}_m, t) - \underline{\hat{B}}\left(\underline{r}_m, t; \underline{\hat{Q}}(\underline{r}_n, t)\right) \right]^2$$

where $\underline{\hat{Q}}$ and $\underline{\hat{B}}$ represent the estimated dipolar sources and the magnetic field values, respectively, and w_m the weight assigned to each neuromagnetometer channel based on its signal-to-noise performance. The objective function was then minimized using the Nelder-Mead simplex algorithm [33] to estimate six parameters of each source (the three position coordinates x, y, z, and the three components of the dipole strength vector) as a function of latency. An estimate was obtained for sources within the latency range of 70 to 230 msec in steps of 11 msec.

16-5-4   Results and Discussion

The results of the registration algorithm are shown in Fig. 16-14. Compared with Fig. 16-13, a much better match between the neuromagnetic reference points and their anatomical locations in the MR images is now obtained [34]. The spatiotemporal distribution of the neuromagnetic sources in a format showing a superposition of the neuromagnetic sources on magnetic resonance images are presented in Fig. 16-15. Results are shown for four representative time windows lying within the 70 to 230 msec latency range investigated in this work. The orientation of the dipoles, which are not shown in Fig. 16-15 due to lack of a suitable display method, vary as a function of latency and show a complete reversal between the M100 and M200 peaks, as expected from the data shown in Fig. 16-12. Also the MR images reveal that the estimated sources shift as a function of latency but remain within the superior temporal gyrus of the right temporal lobe, which is consistent with the location of the primary auditory cortex. These results suggest the viability of superposing neuromagnetically localized sources on MRIs to depict accurately the spatiotemporal distribution of neural activity.

The main sources of errors in these spatiotemporal images are expected to be due to spatial localization factors and not temporal factors, since the

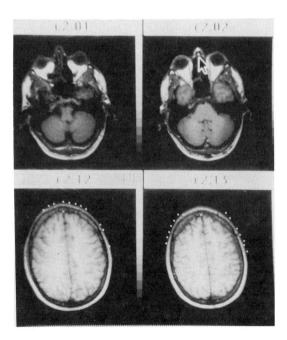

Figure 16-14 A superposition of selected MRI slices and neuromagnetic reference points after applying a first-order coordinate transformation to achieve registration. Compared with Fig. 16-14; the two modalities now show better registration. (Reproduced from ref. [34]).

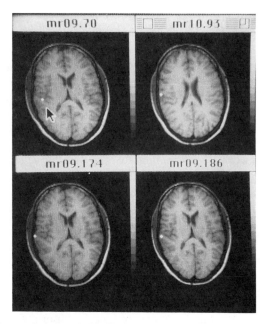

Figure 16-15 The spatiotemporal distribution of neuromagnetically localized neural activity (bright dots) in response to simple auditory stimulation. Results are shown for four representative time windows corresponding to latencies of 70 and 93 msec (top row) and 174 and 186 msec (bottom row).

temporal resolution in the neuromagnetic field measurements is about 1 msec, and the time jitter between the 37 channels is also on the order of 1 msec, both of which are an order of magnitude smaller than the 11-msec temporal window used in the localizations. Also, the fluctuations in the response latency among the time-averaged 64 presentations are expected to have minimal, if any, significant effect within the 11-msec temporal window.

Spatial localization errors can arise from the neuromagnetic localization algorithm as well as from errors in registering the neuromagnetic measurements to the MR images. Since each neuromagnetic channel is treated as an independent sensor in 3-D space without being constrained to any specific head shape, the errors are expected to be comparable to the "multisphere" iterative least squares method of Weinberg et al. [35] based on the simplex algorithm. Using a gel-filled human skull, they report a mean 3-D location error of 3.5 mm for three dipoles. However, as mentioned earlier, recent preliminary studies of humans with implanted electrodes show a location error of 8 mm [3]. Thus the absolute accuracy of the results described here is subject to further studies.

The accuracy of the localization in relation to brain anatomy is dependent on the accuracy of (1) locating the neuromagnetometer channels in relation to the head, (2) locating the landmarks in each modality, and (3) the registration algorithm to superpose neuromagnetic measurements on MRIs. Each of the three procedures to define landmarks—by the PPI system, manual recording by the tip digitizer, and locating the landmarks in the MRI —are estimated to have an uncertainty of ± 1 mm.

Some investigators, such as Pantev et al. [36] and Yamamoto et al. [30], register the two modalities by aligning the subject so that three landmarks appear in a specified plane of the MR image. Registration based on subject alignment alone, however, can be prone to errors, not only because it is difficult to align a subject (or align the slices in an MRI scanner) so that three points lie exactly within a single plane but, more important, because there are inherent 3-D geometrical distortions in MR images, implying that matching a single plane is insufficient to prevent superposition errors in 3-D space. MRI distortions are instrument, pulse sequence, and image dependent and difficult to predict. For example, Cutler et al. [37] report axial skewing of as much as 8 to 10 mm in their MRI scans, and additional misalignment when multiple acquisitions are stacked or interleaved (which is a common method of acquiring 3-D data in MRI). The first-order registration approach would allow for correction of skew (besides rotation and translation) and is therefore expected to be more accurate than approaches based on matching three points alone. The registration procedure can further be extended to compensate for higher-order distortions as better accuracy is sought in determining the site of neuromagnetic sources.

16-6 CONCLUSIONS AND FUTURE PROSPECTS

In this chapter we have presented an overview of a relatively new functional imaging technique termed *neuromagnetic imaging*, or NMI, based on measuring the magnetic field emanating from the brain during specific stimulation. From a theoretical standpoint we have shown how under certain conditions the underlying sources of evoked neural activity in response to specific stimuli are localizable from measurements of the evoked magnetic field. In humans, we have demonstrated that the neuromagnetic field during auditory stimulation is measurable and localizable. Although the localizations in the human study reported here have been restricted to an equivalent single current dipole whose location and orientation vary as a function of latency, more general localizations in two or three dimensions are expected as additional information from PET and MRI scans are incorporated into the NMI measurements. The neuromagnetic data have been superposed on corresponding MRIs to depict both function and anatomy. Registration problems inherent to such multimodality representation have been addressed and an approach to achieve accurate superposition has been investigated using experimental data acquired from a 37-channel SQUID neuromagnetometer system and a 1.5-tesla clinical magnetic resonance imager.

In addition to evoked responses the spontaneous magnetoencephalogram, or MEG, which is the counterpart of the EEG, carries unique information on brain function and is detectable with SQUID neuromagnetometry. For example, several investigators have demonstrated the potential of localizing interictal spike activity using MEG [10, 38], information which is vital to neurosurgeons to locate epileptogenic regions of the brain. Existing imaging modalities often yield inadequate information for accurately pinpointing the location or locations of epileptogenic foci. Surgically implanted depth electrodes, which represent a risky, invasive procedure, are often used prior to surgery. Reconstruction of images from the MEG may be able to provide, noninvasively, a depiction of the 3-D location of these foci and the resulting discharges during seizure. This information, when fused with MRI or X-ray CT anatomical images, should greatly facilitate surgery to remove the epileptogenic regions.

In addition to applications of direct benefit to neurosurgery [39], the knowledge gained by NMI is expected to be of vast importance to neuroscientists and clinicians dealing with illness affecting brain function. Examples of potential clinical examples include:

Alzheimer's disease

Head trauma and stroke

Parkinson's disease

Psychiatric disorders such as schizophrenia

Vision defects of neurologic origin

AIDS dementia

Memory functions

Neuro- and psychopharmacology

Learning disorders

Finally, no single imaging technique can provide all the information required to generate precise spatiotemporal images of the brain depicting both anatomy and various types of brain function. Each modality yields different, yet complementary, information. A synergistic fusion of information derived from multiple anatomical and functional imaging techniques including NMI holds great promise in advancing the area of brain visualization.

REFERENCES

1. M. Singh, D. Doria, V. Henderson, et al. Reconstruction of images from neuromagnetic fields. *IEEE Trans. Nucl. Sci.* NS-31:585–589 (1984).
2. B. N. Cuffin and D. Cohen. Magnetic fields of a dipole in special volume conductor shapes. *IEEE Trans. Biomed. Eng.* BME-24:372–381 (1977).

3. D. Cohen, B. N. Cuffin, K. Yunokuchi, et al. *Ann. Neurol.* 28:811–817 (1990).

4. S. J. Williamsom. *Ann. Neurol.* 30:222 (1991).

5. R. Hari, M. Hamalainen, R. Ilmoniemi, and O. V. Lounasmaa. *Ann. Neurol.* 30:222 (1991).

6. R. P. Crease. News and comment. *Science* 25:374–375 (1991).

7. Biomagnetic Technologies Inc., San Diego, CA.

8. Siemens Medical Systems, Inc., Iselin, NJ.

9. D. Cohn. *Science* 175:664–666 (1972).

10. D. S. Barth, W. Sutherling, J. Engel, Jr., and J. Beatty. *Science* 218:891–894 (1982).

11. D. Brenner, S. J. Williamson, and L. Kaufman. *Science* 190:480–482 (1975).

12. T. J. Teyler, B. N. Cuffin, and D. Cohen. *Life Sci.* 17:683–692 (1975).

13. M. Reite, J. T. Zimmerman, and J. E. Zimmerman. *Elec. Clin. Neurophysiol.* 53:643–651 (1982).

14. G. L. Romani, S. J. Williamson, and L. Kaufman. *Science* 216:1339–1340 (1982).

15. D. Brenner, J. Lipton, L. Kaufman, and S. J. Williamson. *Science* 199:81–83 (1978).

16. H. Weinberg, L. Deecke, P. Brickett, and J. Boschert. *4th Int. Workshop on Biomagnetism*, Rome, 1982, p. 103.

17. S. J. Williamson and L. Kaufman. Biomagnetism. *J. Magnetism and Magnetic Matter* 22:129–201 (1981).

18. Y. C. Okada, R. Tanenbaum, S. J. Williamson, and L. Kaufman. *Clin. Brain Research* 56:197–205 (1984).

19. M. E. Phelps, J. C. Mazziotta, and S. C. Huang. Study of cerebral function with positron computed tomography. *J. Cerebral Blood Flow Metab.* 2:113–152 (1982).

20. W. Powers et al. The effect of carotid artery disease on the cerebrovascular response to physiological stimulation, *Neurology* 38:1475–1478 (1988).

21. B. Jeffs, R. Leahy, and M. Singh. An evaluation of methods for neuromagnetic image reconstruction. *IEEE Trans. Biomed. Eng.* BME-34:713–723 (1987).

22. M. Singh, B. Wong, R. Brechner, and C. Horne. Basics of neuromagnetic imaging: A potential new modality for functional brain imaging. *SPIE* 671 (Physics and Engineering of Computerized Multidimensional Imaging and Processing): 108–113 (1986).

23. M. Singh and R. R. Brechner. SQUID tomographic neuromagnetic imaging. *Int. J. Imag. Sys. Tech.* 1:218–222 (1989).

24. M. Singh, R. Brechner, K. Oshio, R. Leahy, and V. Henderson. SQUID neuro-magnetometric reconstruction of brain activity. *SPIE* 1351 (Digital Image Synthesis and Inverse Optics): 417–426 (1990).

25. W. J. Dallas. Fourier space solution to the magnetostatic imaging problem. *Appl. Opt.* 24:4543–4546 (1985).

26. W. Kullmann and W. J. Dallas. Fourier imaging of electrical currents in the human brain from their magnetic fields. *IEEE Trans. Biomed. Eng.* BME-34:837–842 (1987).

27. B. J. Roth, N. G. Sepulveda, and J. P. Wikswo, Jr. Using a magnetometer to image a two-dimensional current distribution. *J. Appl. Phys.* 65:361–372 (1989).

28. R. E. Alvarez. Biomagnetic Fourier imaging. *IEEE Trans. Med. Imag.* 9:299–304 (1990).

29. R. Naatanen and T. Picton. The N1 wave of the human electric and magnetic response to sound: A review and an analysis of the component structure. *Psychophysiology* 24:375–425 (1987).

30. T. Yamamoto, S. J. Williamson, L. Kaufman, et al. Magnetic localization of neuronal activity in the human brain. *Proc. Natl. Acad. Sci.* 85:8732–8736 (1988).

31. E. Kreyszig. *Advanced Engineering Mathematics*. New York: Wiley, 1979, pp. 397–401.

32. M. Singh, W. Frei, T. Shibata, G. Huth, and N. Telfer. A digital technique for accurate change detection in nuclear medical images—With application to myocardial perfusion studies using thallium-201. *IEEE Trans. Nucl. Sci.* NS-26:565–575 (1979).

33. J. Nelder and R. Mead. *A simplex method for function minimization*. Comput. J. 4:308–313 (1965).

34. M. Singh, R. R. Brechner, and V. W. Henderson. Neuromagnetic localization using magnetic resonance imaging. *IEEE Trans. Med. Imag.* 11:129–136, 1992.

35. H. Weinberg, P. Brickett, F. Coolsma, and M. Baff. Magnetic localisation of intracranial dipoles: Simulation with a physical model. *Electroencep. Clin. Neurophys.* 64:159–170 (1986).

36. C. Pantev, M. Hoke, K. Lehnertz, et al. Identification of sources of brain neuronal activity with high spatiotemporal resolution through combination of neuromagnetic source localization (NMSL) and magnetic resonance imaging (MRI). *Electroencep. Clin. Neurophys.* 75:173–184 (1990).

37. P. D. Culter, S. Sinha, M. Dahlbom, and E. J. Hoffman. Correction of spatial distortions in MR and PET images for structure-function registration. *Soc. of Nuclear Medicine, 36th Meeting*. WIP#1132, 1989, p. 37.

38. J. Tiihonen, R. Hari, M. Kajola, et al. Localization of epileptic foci using a large area magnetometer and functional brain anatomy. *Ann. Neurol.* 27:283–290 (1990).

39. M. Singh. Neuromagnetic Imaging: A new window on brain function. In *Neurosurgery for the Third Millennium*, Michael J. Apuzzo, ed., Park Ridge, IL: American Association of Neurological Surgeons, 1992.

INDEX

577